Virology II

Advanced Issues

Virology II – Advanced Issues

Publisher: iConcept Press Ltd.
Cover design: Pineapple Design Ltd.
Interior design: iConcept Press Ltd.
Typesetting and copy editing: iConcept Press Ltd. and Pineapple Design Ltd.

ISBN:9781922227454

Printed in the United States of America

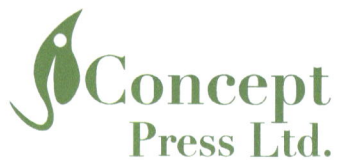

iConcept
Press Ltd.

www.iconceptpress.com

Contents

Preface

A virus is a small infectious agent that replicates within living cells of organisms. Viruses infect all types of organisms, from animals and plants to bacteria and archaea. Today, around 5,000 viruses have been reported in detail, although there are potentially millions. Viruses are found in almost every ecosystem on Earth and are the most abundant type of biological entity. The study of viruses is known as virology, a sub-speciality of microbiology. *Virology* has two volumes. Volume 1 mainly discusses the latest research related to Human Immunodeficiency Virus (HIV). Volume 2 (this volume) discusses other important issues and trends within the research community.

There are totally 17 chapters in this book. Chapter 1 highlights seminal findings from the basic sciences and describes the benefits and risks of current medications based on the recent advances in genetics, immunology, diagnostic imaging, medicinal chemistry, clinical therapeutics and health-care systems. Chapter 2 presents a brief description of foot-and-mouth disease virus (FMDV) and the different functions of various viral proteins, with the main focus on our current knowledge of the strategies that FMDV utilizes to circumvent the host protective response and the results of stimulating host innate immunity to control disease. Chapter 3 proposes a model, in which humoral immunity against monomer capsid protein (CP) is immunopathogenic; whereas antibodies generated in response to the intact virion results in protective immunity. Chapter 4 discusses current understandings of human innate immune responses to respiratory viral infections in the airways, viral evasion strategies, and abnormalities in the immune responses in people with chronic airways diseases, leading to increased susceptibility and worsened outcome.

Chapter 5 presents three replication modes: normal, rolling circle, and double rolling circle replication (DRCR). Herpes simplex virus, chloroplast and yeast 2-micron plasmid DNA replicate through DRCR, which is highly recombinogenic. Amplification of drug-resistance genes in higher eukaryotes is also caused by DRCR, during which hyper recombination between large numbers of transposable elements results in elimination of genes disadvantageous to the cell and amplification of resistance genes. Chapter 6 considers the evidence for transmission of the flavivirus West Nile Virus (WNV) by ticks in addition to the major transmission vector, mosquitoes. Although experimental (and field) evidence points to ticks being competent vectors of the virus we consider their likely role within the enzootic cyle of this virus. Chapter 7 describes two tick-borne viruses that may be circulating in the Iberian Peninsula: the Crimean-Congo Hemorrhagic Fever Virus (CCHFV) and the European Tick-Borne Encephalitis Virus (TBEV). It is possible that some of the encephalitic syndromes diagnosed in the Iberian Peninsula are caused by TBEV, and an outbreak of CCHF may occur at any time. Chapter 8 reviews the evidences supporting the contribution of miRNA regulation to Retinoic Acid (RA)-induced differentiation of neuroblastoma cells. The authors put forward the idea that miRNA regulation is part of the RA signaling pathway, and that miRNAs are essential mediators of the actions of RA in neuroblastoma cells.

Chapter 9 summarizes recent findings shedding light on how multiple geminiviral proteins interact with post-translational modification pathways, and how these interactions impact pathogenicity. The results highlight the important role of post-translational modifications in the outcome of plant-virus interactions, and illustrate how viruses evolve elaborate strategies to ultimately achieve infection. Chapter 10 summarizes the structure and function of immunoregulatory molecule CD150 (SLAM), known also as a receptor of an important human pathogen, measles virus. Understanding the signaling events upon CD150 ligation with measles virus hemagglutinin may answer the multiple questions concerning the molecular mechanism of measles virus mediated immunosuppression. Chapter 11 attempts to develop an *E.coli* expression and purification system that utilises the insoluble nature of inclusion bodies to produce soluble and endotoxin-free Bovine Viral Diarrhoea Virus (BVDV) E2 protein suitable for *in vivo* applications. Chapter 12 reviews how adenovirus alternative splicing is regulated during a lytic virus infection. Special emphasis is devoted to the significance of cellular protein kinases, phosphatases and SR proteins on the function of the adenovirus L4-33K alternative splicing factor.

Chapter 13 provides an overview of the potential of resistance development to influenza antivirals in the enivironment due to the discharge of pharmaceutical residues. Furthermore, the possibility of antiviral resistance re-entering the human population is discussed, and gaps in the knowledge and potential future research areas are identified. Chapter 14 describes the chronic phase of a disease called Chikungunya in a cohort of affected patients. Chikungunya, a mosquito-borne disease, recently emerged as a significant public health problem in South Asian islands. Chapter 15 reviews the incidence of Mokola virus, an unusual member of the Lyssavirus genus in southern Africa and the subsequent antigenic and genetic studies thereof. Although several isolations of this Lyssavirus have been made throughout the African continent, the reservoir host(s) has not yet been identified. Such information can only be obtained through improved and integrated surveillance of Lyssaviruses. Chapter 16 presents a review on the advances made so far in search of novel drug targets against the HCV (Hepatitis C virus)-encoded non-structural protein, NS3, which has recently emerged as a promising drug target for anti-viral therapy.

Chapter 17 reviews, the potential role of eltrombopag in the context of hepatitis C virus (HCV)-related thrombocytopenia. Eltrombopag may have a role in priming up platelet levels to help initiate antiviral therapy, although it is deemed very expensive and probably not cost-effective. Also, there are some legitimate concerns about the safety profile of this novel agent (most importantly, portal vein thrombosis, bone marrow fibrosis and hepatotoxicity).

Editing and publishing a book is never an easy task. Each chapter in this book has gone through a peer review, a selection and an editing process so as to guarantee its quality. Without the supports and contributions of the authors and reviewers, this book can never be able to complete. We would like to thank all of the authors in this book and all of the reviewers who participated in the reviewing process: Samad Amini-Bavil-Olyaee, Prasert Auewarakul, Domingo Barettino, Wibke Bayer, Lesley Bell-Sakyi, Gioia Capelli, Neil D. Christensen, Alexander T. Ciota, Marco Ciotti, Rik L. de Swart, José G. B. Derraik, Sabine Druillennec, Koray Ergünay, Camille Escadafal, Assane G Fall, Anthony R. Fooks, Mario Giacobini, Laurent Gillet, roger grand, Efrain Guzman, Toshiyuki Hikita, Fred L. Homa, Chienjin Huang, Masaharu Iwasaki, Wim Jennes, S.M. Kadri, Benedikt B. Kaufer, Alhossain Khalafallah, C. Kiffner, Marion C. Lanteri, Y L Lau, Miguel A. Martín-Acebes, Charles E. McGee, Thomas E. Morrison, Daniel O. Ochiel, Motoyuki Otsuka, Deborah S. Parris, Leonidas A. Phylactou, Lesya M Pinchuk, William K. Reisen, Mohammad Rostami Nejad, Daniel Ružek, Farhad Safarpoor Dehkordi, Heiner Schaal, Oliver Schildgen,

Sibylle Schneider-Schaulies, Harald Schulze, Soroush Sharbati, Marcelo A. Soares, Julio Sotelo, Ashley L. St. John, Luminita A. Stanciu, Frank Tacke, Frank L.W. Takken, Joshua M. Tebbs, Ikuo Tsunoda, John W Upham, David H. Walker, Jinbao Wang, Matthew D. Weitzman, Jeffrey Wilusz, Donglai Wu, Xianfu Wu and Katsuyuki Yui. We hope that you, the reader, will find this book interesting and useful. Any advices please feel free and are always welcome to tell us.

iConcept Press Ltd
March 2014

Multiple Sclerosis: Fundamental Concepts & Clinical Perspectives

Douglas R. Allington
University of Montana, USA

Andrew Davis
University of Montana, USA

Jesse Sutton
Meriter Hospital, USA

Michael P. Rivey
University of Montana, USA

1   Introduction

The first modern-era description of multiple sclerosis (MS) pairing clinical presentation with central nervous system lesions (CNS) is attributed to Dr. Charcot in 1865 (Butler & Bennett, 2003). Physicians and scientists have unsuccessfully searched for the definitive cause(s) of MS since that time. However, advances in genetics, immunology, diagnostic imaging, medicinal chemistry, clinical therapeutics and health-care systems have created a wealth of knowledge that has led to new, novel medications and significant improvements in care of MS patients. This chapter will highlight seminal findings from the basic sciences and describe the benefits and risks of current medications.

2   Epidemiology

Studies of epidemiology have been instrumental in providing clues to important factors associated with the acquisition of MS. Early, seminal MS population-based epidemiology studies implicated two broad categories of influence; genetics and environmental factors. Differing rates of MS have been linked to gender, race, geographic location and shared genetic content. Women of all races develop MS at relative rates approximately 2-3 times more frequent than men (Wallin *et al.*, 2004). After adjusting for gender, study results indicate a racial predominance among whites slightly greater than rates found in blacks and markedly greater than rates observed in other races (Wallin *et al.*, 2004). Individuals living farther from the equator in the northern and southern hemispheres appear to have a higher likelihood of acquiring MS. However, the influence of latitude on the development of MS appears to be declining in present day (Wallin *et al.* 2012). Incidence rates reflect the number of new cases developing in a population over a fixed time period, typically one year. MS incidence rates range from 7-8 per 100,000 people yearly. Prevalence rates quantify the number of cases in a given population at any point in time, also referred to as point prevalence. MS prevalence rates of 20-30 per 100,000 people are commonly reported for populations living near the equator whereas rates of 80-120 per 100,000 people have been documented in the United Kingdom, Scandinavia, United States and Australia (Kurtzke, 1980). However, variation in prevalence rates are common even within regions lending some investigators to speculate on the influence of vitamin D levels, fish consumption or other environmental factors associated with MS acquisition (Kampman & Brustad, 2008).

   Early epidemiologic studies suggested a genetic predisposition because of family clusters of MS (Schapira *et al.*, 1963) but more robust population-based studies were not available until the 1980s (Sadovnick, 2002). If MS risk is linked to genetic content, the disease should occur with a greater frequency among closest family members and less frequently as the genetic pool diversifies. The highest rate of MS concordance occurs among monozygotic twins who have identical genetic makeup. In comparison to the general population the age-adjusted lifetime risk of MS in identical twins is approximately 30%, 3% for siblings and 2% for parents or children (Compston & Coles, 2002). Several recent, excellent articles on epidemiology and MS exist (Ramagopalan & Sadovnick, 2011; Kock-Henriksen & Sorensen, 2010).

3   Genetics

The genetic inheritance pattern for MS is both complex and polygenic. Serology studies in the 1970s first identified an association between MS and the human leukocyte antigen (HLA) gene cluster, major histocompatibility complex (MHC) class I and II regions, on chromosome 6 (Jersild *et al.*, 1973; Thorsby *et al.*, 1977). The HLA MHC region consists of almost four million base pairs and this region exhibits a high degree of polymorphism. This number of base pairs and high degree of polymorphism creates immense potential for genotype and haplotype diversity (Oksenberg *et al.*, 2001).

Single nucleotide polymorphism (SNP) is the substitution of a single nucleotide (A, T, C, or G) in a genome sequence. Variation of two alternative base pairs at a single nucleotide occurs at a frequency greater than 1% in the human population. Genetic diversity also exists among combinations of alleles (haplotypes) observed at closely linked sites. Microsatellites consist of multiple repeats of base pairs in a short sequence, usually 2-8 base pairs. Microsatellites differ considerably between individuals and most people exhibit heterogeneity at any single locus (Burton *et al.*, 2005). Identifying, mapping, and genotyping of SNPs in the human genome give researchers a powerful tool for studying genetic influence on disease.

During meiosis, the probability is low that two genes sharing close proximity on a single chromosome will separate during recombination. Relative distances between two genes on the chromosome can be determined by studying the number of recombinants. The genes are linked if the two loci are transmitted together from parent to child more frequently than calculated by independent inheritance that is less than 50%. Linkage disequilibrium occurs when two loci occur on the same haplotype more frequently than expected across the population (Teare & Barrett, 2005). Linkage is calculated by using a logarithm of odds (LOD) score that is a function of the loci recombination fraction (θ) or the chromosomal position measured in centimorgan (cM). Positive scores define linkage or cosegregation with higher scores reflecting greater evidence for linkage (Teare & Barrett, 2005). LOD scores greater than 3 are considered proof of linkage. (Baranzini, 2011) In 2005, there were over 10 million known SNPs in the human genome with half of these independently validated (Burton *et al.*, 2005).

3.1 Linkage analysis studies

Linkage analysis or MS pedigree studies identify potential chromosomal sites or candidate genes by comparing inheritance patterns among MS affected and non-affected family members. Diseases with complex inheritance patterns that include minor to moderate influence from multiple genes, such as MS, lead to numerous potential candidate genes. Data generated from individual linkage studies requires extensive replication to separate true linkage from simple random variation or co-segregation (Oksenberg *et al.*, 2008). Sifting through the long list of potential candidate genes is complicated by inconclusive and often contradictory results during replication testing (Risch & Merikangas, 1996).

Numerous MS linkage analysis studies were conducted from the 1970s to early 1990s. The studies were limited by small study sizes, crude DNA markers, slow throughput times and a lack of statistical power to detect small influences. Once linkage screening studies identify candidate gene regions, higher density markers covering distances of 5-10cM are used to further refine candidate genes status. In 2005, a MS linkage screen study in over 2600 individuals from 730 multi-case families using more than 4500 SNPs produced a LOD of 11.7 for the HLA MHC 6p21 candidate gene site (Sawcer *et al.*, 2005). Overall, candidate linkage studies have generated numerous potential candidate genes but only the MHC HLA-class II site on chromosome 6p21.3 has been statistically associated with MS (Oksenberg *et al.*, 2008).

First generation whole genome-wide linkage scans were conducted in MS patients from the US, UK, Canada, and Finland beginning in the 1990s. These whole-genome screens identified many gene regions of interest but replication of sites of interest between the different studies was minimal (Fernald *et al.*, 2005). At least 11 major genome wide linkage studies of MS patients were completed between 1995 and 2005 but none identified linkage with genome wide significance other than the previously recognized HLA MHC site.

3.2   Genome-Wide Association Studies

Advances in laboratory and analytical techniques have made genome-wide association studies (GWAS) possible since 2007. GWAS seek to identify the differences in alleles from unrelated individuals with MS to closely matched controls from the same population. (Kellar-Wood *et al.*, 1995) Association studies allow for detailed mapping of genetic loci and it is the better testing method for detecting genes that produce smaller effect sizes (Cordell & Clayton, 2005). Efficient simultaneous genotyping of several hundred thousand SNPs throughout the genome is now possible through chip-based technology (Hoffjan & Akkad, 2010).

GWAS commonly use data from international consortiums to boost enrollments in the MS and control populations. Since numerous tests are run in parallel during GWAS only p-values of 10^{-7} or 10^{-8} are deemed statistically significant (Gourraud *et al.*, 2012). A review of seven GWAS of MS patients demonstrated that the HLA-DRB1 risk locus demonstrated the strongest association with a $p < 1 \times 10^{-32}$ but evidence also supported 12 other non-HLA loci. By studying the HLA allele sharing by descent in siblings it is estimated that, at most, HLA locus only accounts for approximately 20-60% of the genetic propensity in MS (Baranzini 2011). Notable non-HLA loci that have shown strong associations with MS during GWAS include cell adhesion molecule CD58, interleukin 2 receptor (IL2RA), IL7, ribosomal protein L5 (EV15/RPL5) and C-type lectin domain (CLEC16A). Despite the strong associations of these allele variants with MS, individually these alleles produce weak effects on MS susceptibility (D'Netto, *et al.*, 2009).

The largest GWAS was conducted in 2011 with collaboration between the International Multiple Sclerosis Genetics Consortium (IMSGC) and the Wellcome Trust Case Control Consortium (WTCCC). Results from this study identified 29 novel loci in addition to the 23 previously identified sites associated with MS. However, many of the non-HLA allele variants also share disease susceptibility inheritance with, or protection from other autoimmune disorders including type-1 diabetes, Graves' disease and rheumatoid arthritis (Baranzini 2011). Results from these studies are being used to map autoimmune disease-gene networks that quantify the allele relationships between several autoimmune diseases. Several excellent, in-depth reviews detailing the history and promise of genetic testing in MS are available (Baranzini, 2011; McElroy & Oksenberg, 2011).

4   Environmental Factors

Several key myelin peptide regions have been associated with MS. Myelin basic protein (MBP $_{84-102}$) peptide region is essential for MHC class II binding and for T cell receptor (TCR) recognition (Wucherpfenning & Strominger, 1995). A number of viral and some bacterial peptides are capable of activating human MBP$_{85-99}$ specific T cell clones developed from MS patients (Wucherpfenning & Strominger, 1995). Greer *et al.* identified two overlapping myelin proteolipid-protein peptides (PLP$_{184-199}$ and PLP$_{190-209}$) that demonstrated increased proliferative responses during peptide screenings using mononuclear cells from MS patients and healthy controls (Greer *et al.*, 1997).

Traditional epidemiologic studies have also been used to examine the influence of environment on MS risk. Infection as the environmental cause of MS was first purposed in the late 1890s (Kakalacheva *et al.*, 2011). Population migration studies suggest viral infections acquired during childhood or adolescences are a risk factor for MS. Migrants moving from regions with high MS rates to areas with low rates have an intermediate risk of acquiring MS while those moving from low to high risk areas retain a low risk profile (Visscher *et al.*, 1977). Individuals migrating after age 15 retain MS rates reflective of their originating regions although no specific age differential for risk is proven (Detels *et al.*, 1978). So called outbreaks or epidemics of MS such as one that occurred in the Faroe Islands after posting of British troops during World War II (Kurtzke & Hyllested *et al.*, 1979) supports a post infection hypothesis but evidence of an epidemic has been questioned (Poser & Hibberd., 1988).

Infections caused by spirochetes (Steiner, 1952), chlamydia pneumoniae (Munger *et al.*, 2003; Morre *et al.*, 2000), and a plethora of viruses have been investigated as possible MS triggers. Human herpesvirus-6 (HHV-6) and Epstein-Barr virus (EBV), and varicella zoster virus VZV are herpes family viruses that continue to generate considerable interest in the research community. (Table 1) Other evidence exist suggesting human endogenous retroviruses HERV-H and HERV-W could be linked to MS (Petersen *et al.* 2012). Infections including varicella, mumps, measles, and rubella have been thoroughly investigated in case control trials but overwhelming and conclusive evidence for an association of MS with any of these viruses is lacking (Marrie 2004).

Viruses	Evidence of association	Reference
Herpesviruses		
A. Epstein-Barr (EBV)	A-1.Prior mononucleosis and increased MS risk.	A-1. Thacker *et al.*, 2006; Hernan *et al.*, 2001
	A-2.EBV seroprevalence virtually universal in MS patients	A-2. Serafini *et al.*, 2007; Alotaibi *et al.*, 2004
	A-3.EBNA1-specific T cell reactivity with myelin proteins	A-3. Lünemann *et al.*, 2008
	A-4. Strong EBV-specific CD8+ T cell response	A-4. Jilek *et al.*, 2008
B. Human Herpes Virus-6 (HHV-6)	B-1. Viral DNA at MS plaques	B-1. Challoner *et al.*, 1995
	B-2. Elevated HHV-6 antibodies in CSF.	B-2. Ablashi *et al.*, 1998
	B-3. DNA from serum/peripheral mononuclear cells (Mixed findings).	B-3. Akhyani *et al.*, 2000; Mayne *et al.*, 1998
	B-4. Higher HHV-6 gene expression in oligodendrocytes of MS patients.	B-4. Opsahl & Kennedy, 2005
C. Varicella-Zoster Virus (VZV)/Herpes Simplex Virus (HSV)	C-1. Increased VZV/HSV infection in MS patients	C-1. Perez-Cesari *et al.*, 2005
	C-2. Elevated HSV-1 during acute MS exacerbations	C-2. Ferrante *et al.*, 2000

Table 1: Common viruses and Multiple Sclerosis

5   Experimental Autoimmune Encephalomyelitis

Experimental autoimmune encephalomyelitis (EAE) is an animal model used to study MS (Kasper & Shoemaker, 2010; Batoulis *et al.*, 2011; Chen *et al.*, 2012, Croxford *et al.*, 2011). EAE is generally accepted as the best model to study the pathogenesis of demyelinating diseases and to investigate new drug therapies. The EAE model was first developed in the 1930s by immunizing monkeys with rabbit brain emulsion (Batoulis *et al.*, 2011). Inoculated animals develop a flaccid paralysis, perivascular infiltrates, and central nervous system demyelination (Baxter, 2007; Mix *et al.*, 2010). The basic brain emulsion is now bolstered with adjuvants including Freund's and others, to more efficiently produce rapid EAE signs with fewer injections (Baxter, 2007).

The EAE model has been adapted to other species, most notably rats and mice. Smaller animals are easier to care for and less expensive, allowing for studies with a greater number of subjects. The EAE model was traditionally used to study T lymphocyte functions. Discovery and use of 'knockout' and transgenic mice have advanced the EAE model even further. These more diverse EAE models produce a broader array of more specific immune cell actions, central nervous system lesions (CNS), immunologic responses, and relapsing-remitting or progressive clinical patterns with close similarities to MS in humans (Baxter, 2007; Batoulis *et al.*, 2011; Croxford *et al.*, 2011).

6   Overview of Autoimmune Pathogenesis Seen in EAE & MS

6.1   Direct Immunization of EAE

EAE is induced by two methods which are direct immunization with antigen or passive, sometimes referred to as adoptive, transfer of autoreactive T-cells (Desai & Barton, 1989; Batoulis *et al.*, 2011; Croxford *et al.*, 2011). EAE is directly induced by immunizing animals with myelin-derived proteins or peptides which act as antigens. MBP, myelin-oligodendrocyte glycoprotein (MOG), PLP, CNS homogenate and other myelin constituents all act as antigens to directly induce EAE. After injection, the myelin derived proteins react with autoimmune effector cells (T cells, B cells) already present in the animal to induce EAE.

6.2   Passive Induction of EAE

Alternatively, EAE is passively induced by transferring autoreactive $CD4^+$ T cells specific for myelin-derived peptides (i.e. adoptive transfer of MBP-sensitized T cells) to naïve animals [Desai & Barton, 1989; Batoulis *et al.*, 2011; Croxford *et al.*, 2011). Passive induction does not occur in MS.

Once the EAE inflammatory cascade is induced, T cells originating in the periphery cross through the blood-brain barrier (BBB) with the assistance of endothelial adhesion molecules and matrix metalloproteinases (MMPs). On entering the CNS, antigen presenting cells (APCs), (i.e. dendritic cells, macrophages, and B cells) reactivate lymphocytes and the inflammatory cascade is perpetuated.

Damage to the CNS is caused through multiple pathways. Macrophages release inflammatory cytokines such as interleukins (IL-1, IL-6), tumor necrosis factor alpha (TNFα) and nitric oxide (NO) which causes demyelination through the production of reactive oxygen species. $CD8^+$ cytotoxic T lymphocytes directly attack oligodendrocytes and neurons (Chen *et al.*, 2012; Kasper & Shoemaker, 2010). Recent comprehensive reviews of the contributions and limitations of the EAE model are available (Batoulis *et al.*, 2011; Croxford *et al.*, 2011).

7   Role of Individual Cell Types in Autoimmunity / Historical Overview

Early EAE research focused primarily on the role of T lymphocytes. This focus influenced beliefs regarding MS pathogenesis for many years. Two distinct CD4$^+$ T helper (Th) cells subsets, Th1 and Th2 cells, were considered responsible for the inflammatory immune reaction underlying the development of MS. The Th1 cell pathway was believed to be inflammatory and Th2 cell pathway was believed to be regulatory. An early theory held that autoimmunity in MS was caused by a shift in the Th1/Th2 balance towards Th1 mediated inflammation. Although Th1 cells are clearly involved, more recent evidence suggests EAE and MS pathogenesis includes significant contributions from additional T lymphocytes (Th17), B lymphocytes, cytokines, chemokines, and adhesion molecules. The link between MS and autoimmunity is clearly complex and poorly understood, involving a wide variety of immune cells (See Figure 1).

7.1   CD4$^+$ T Helper: Th1 cells

CD4$^+$ Th1 cells were historically believed to be the primary pathogenic T cell in EAE and MS (Batoulis et al., 2011; Kasper & Shoemaker, 2010). Th1 cells differentiate from naïve CD4$^+$ T cells when exposed to IL-12 (Kasper & Shoemaker, 2010). Differentiated Th1 cells produce large amounts of inflammatory cytokines such as interferon gamma (IFN-γ), TNF-α, and IL-15. In the healthy immune system, Th1 cells respond to intracellular pathogens (i.e. bacteria). However, evidence also supports a role for Th1 cells in autoimmunity. Th1 cells and their associated cytokines (IL-12, IFN-γ) are prevalent in the CSF, blood, and inflammatory lesions of MS patients (Olsson et al., 1990; Soderstrom et al., 1993). Th1-related cytokine levels increase during MS and EAE relapse and decrease during remission (Iman et al., 2007; Killestein et al., 2001). IFN-γ causes macrophages to release nitric oxide and induces apoptosis of oligodendrocytes, which protect and support axons (Misko et al., 1995; Molina-Holgado et al., 2001; Vartanian et al., 1995).

7.2   CD4$^+$ T Helper: Th17 cells

While Th1 cells are a likely major contributor to the inflammation and demyelination in MS, Th17 cell discovery in the late 1990s changed the traditional Th1 cell driven view of MS (Bettelli et al., 2007; Hofstetter et al., 2005). Th17 cells differentiate from naïve CD4$^+$ T helper cells on exposure to IL-6, tumor growth factor (TGF-β), and IL-21 and subsequent expression of the transcription factor: retinoic-acid-related orphan receptor γt (RORγt) (Kimura et al., 2007; Bettelli et al., 2007; Torchinsky & Blander, 2010). Differentiated Th17 cells require IL-23 for homeostasis (Kimura et al., 2007) and Th 17 cells secrete the potent proinflammatory cytokine IL-17 and granulocyte-macrophage colony-stimulating factor (GM-CSF) (Hofstetter et al., 2005; Kasper & Shoemaker, 2010). In the healthy immune system, Th17 cells defend against extracellular pathogens by recruiting neutrophils and macrophages to sites of infection (Torchinsky & Blander, 2010). Like Th1, amplified Th17 cell response is also implicated in autoimmunity.

The existence of Th17 cells was discovered during EAE model research (Bettelli et al., 2007). Researchers blocked IFN-γ secretion (from Th1 cells) expecting to find symptomatic improvement in EAE; however, paralysis symptoms worsened. These findings led to identification of the IL-17 producing CD4$^+$ Th17 cells (Bettelli et al., 2007). In many EAE models, IL-17 producing Th17 cells cause inflammation, demyelination, and subsequent paralysis (Hofstetter et al., 2005; Langrish et al., 2005). IL -17 production positively correlates with EAE disease activity and produces CNS ectopic lymphoid follicles,

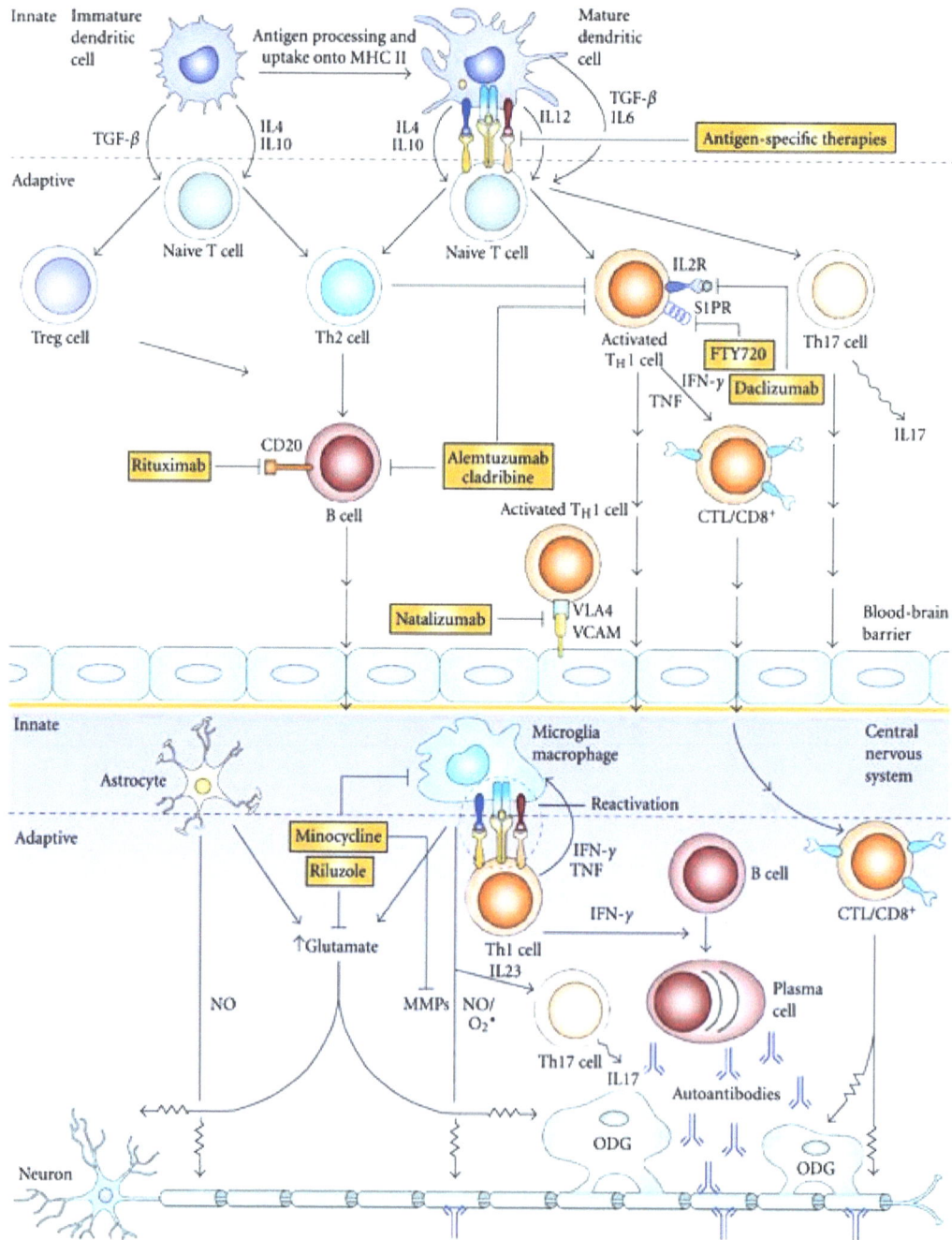

Figure 1: Chen *et al*. 2012, open access article. Hindawi Publishing Corporation.

a rare characteristic of MS (Berghams *et al*., 2011; Peters *et al*., 2011). Pretreatment of mice with anti-IL-17 antibodies protects against passive EAE induction (Berghams *et al*., 2011). Th17 cells readily disrupt the BBB and infiltrate the CNS prior to EAE onset (Kebir *et al*., 2007; Murphy *et al*., 2010). Temporal relationships between Th17, Th1, and EAE signs suggest Th17 has a predominant role in *initiating* the inflammatory process (Kebir *et al*., 2007; Murphy *et al*., 2010).

In humans, IL-17 expression and IL-17 receptors are increased in active acute and chronic MS lesions (Tzartos *et al.*, 2008; Durelli *et al.*, 2009). Important cytokines in the IL-17/Th17 pathway, IL-23 and IL-6, are also identified on MS lesions as well as activated macrophages and microglia (Li *et al.*, 2007). Moreover, IL-17 levels correlate with MS lesion activity on MRI (Hedegaard *et al.*, 2008). These findings suggest IL-17 expressing Th17 cells have a critical role in initiating inflammation, demyelination, and damage within the CNS.

7.3 B Cells

In addition to T cells, B cells are essential for coordinating the autoimmune response in MS (Dalakas, 2008). B cells originate from hematopoietic stem cells and differentiate into naïve B cells (Dalakas, 2008). Naïve B cells are activated on antigen exposure and differentiate through multiple steps to plasma cells (Dalakas, 2008). CD19 and CD20 are two important surface antigens expressed on maturing B cells but are absent on fully differentiated plasma cells (Dalakas, 2008). Pharmacotherapies directed against CD20 are currently available such as rituximab or undergoing Phase II, ofatumumab, (GlaxoSmithKline, 2012) or Phase III, ocrelizumab, (Hoffman-LaRoche, 2012) trials. In addition to the CD19 and CD20 antigens on B cells, there are also several important cytokines and chemokines in B cell homeostasis and MS pathogenesis. B cell activating factor (BAFF) and a proliferation-inducing ligand (APRIL) are cytokines that promote B cell differentiation and population expansion. BAFF and APRIL also prevent apoptosis, and maintain germinal centers and IgG production (Hase *et al.*, 2004; Kalled , 2005; Kalled, 2006; Mackay *et al.*, 2003, Mackay & Browning, 2002; Schiemann *et al.*, 2001).Chemokine (C-X-C motif) ligand 13 (CXCL 13) is responsible for attracting B cells to the CNS (Khademi *et al.*, 2011).

Ample evidence exists linking B cell contributions to the complex autoimmune pathogenesis seen in MS patients (Dalakas, 2008; Ragheb *et al.*, 2011). In post mortem brains of MS patients, B cells are numerous in active MS lesions while absent in those that are quiescent (Traugott *et al.*, 1983; Hauser *et al.*, 1986; Nyland *et al.*, 1982). B cells, plasma cells, and antibodies are found in the cerebral spinal fluid (CSF), CNS plaques, and CNS lesions of MS patients (Breij *et al.*, 2008; Obermeier *et al.*, 2008; Obermeier *et al.*, 2011). Oligoclonal bands (OCBs) that are autoantibodies secreted by B cells, are present in greater than 95% of MS patients and represent a hallmark laboratory finding in the disease (Obermeier *et al.*, 2008). The expression of BAFF, APRIL, and CXCL 13 significantly increases during active MS and correlate with acute disease relapses (Alter *et al.*, 2003; Kowarik *et al.*, 2012; Ragheb *et al.*, 2011). The most compelling evidence to support B-cells role in MS pathogenesis is the success of B-cell depleting therapies in MS trials (Disanto *et al.*, 2012).

Traditionally, B cells were implicated in MS pathogenesis as precursor plasma cells that simply produced autoantibodies (Dalakas, 2008; Ragheb *et al.*, 2011). B cells are now known to contribute to the disease process through four mechanisms: antigen presentation, cytokine and chemokine production, autoantibody secretion (after maturing to a plasma cell), and formation of ectopic germinal centers (Dalakas, 2008; Dalakas, 2008; Browning, 2006). First, B cells serve as potent APCs leading to activation of the immune response. Second, B cells produce several cytokines and chemokines that shift the immune response towards inflammation. Third, B cells mature to plasma cells and secrete antibodies that activate complement when exposed to antigen. Fourth, the cytokine lymphotoxin β that is expressed on B cells, leads to B cell follicle formation with ectopic infiltrates. The follicles produce intrathecal IgG and are the source for the persistent OCBs seen in MS (Dalakas, 2008; Dalakas, 2008; Browning, 2006).

7.4   CD8$^+$ Cytotoxic T cells

Most MS autoimmune studies focus on the role of CD4$^+$ T cells or B cells as effector cells, but evidence also supports a similar role for CD8$^+$ cytotoxic T cells. Cytotoxic T cells target and kill cells expressing the MHC class I molecules (Zozulya & Wiendi, 2008). MHC class I molecules are prevalent in CNS oligodendrocytes and neurons (Zozulya & Wiendi, 2008). CD8+ T cells are plentiful in MS plaques and, in fact, outnumber CD4$^+$ T cells (Hauser *et al.*, 1986).

7.5   Regulatory T cells (T reg)

Dysfunction of regulatory immune cells is another hypothesized component of MS autoimmune pathogenesis. Dysregulation of CD4$^+$ Th2 cells, CD4$^+$CD25$^+$FoxP3$^+$ Tregs, and CD8$^+$ Tregs are implicated in MS. Th2 cells differentiate from naïve CD4$^+$ T cells when exposed to IL-4 (Kasper & Shoemaker, 2010). In the healthy immune system, Th2 cells respond to extracellular pathogens (i.e. parasites) and mediate humoral immunity (Kasper & Shoemaker, 2010). Th2 cells produce anti-inflammatory cytokines IL-4, IL-6, and IL-13 (Kasper & Shoemaker, 2010). A decrease in Th2 cells has been found to correlate with MS relapse (Kieseier, 2011).

CD4$^+$CD25$^+$FoxP3$^+$ Tregs also differentiate from naïve CD4$^+$ T cells when exposed to TGF-β and retinoic acid (Kasper & Shoemaker, 2010). CD4$^+$CD25$^+$FoxP3$^+$ Treg expression has been shown to be low in patients with relapsing-remitting multiple sclerosis (RRMS) (Venken *et al.*, 2010). CD4$^+$CD25$^+$FoxP3$^+$ Tregs promote self-tolerance by inhibiting myelin-specific Th1 cell line expansion (Venken *et al.*, 2010). Decreased CD8$^+$ T reg expression is observed during MS exacerbations. Additionally, MS patients have a high expression of CD94/NKG2A, a natural killer (NK) receptor that inhibits CD8$^+$ Treg activity (Correale & Villa, 2008). CD8$^+$ Tregs modulate immune pathogenesis by lysing myelin-reactive CD4$^+$ T cells and secreting IL-10 which down regulates the inflammatory cytokine IFNγ (Endharti *et al.*, 2005; Niederkom, 2008). Although the role of regulatory cells in MS autoimmune pathogenesis is not well understood, available evidence suggests dysfunction of regulatory immune cells has a role in MS autoimmune pathology.

7.6   Cell Trafficking

An important step in the disease progression is migration of immune cells across the blood-brain barrier (BBB) endothelium and into the CNS. Immune cell trafficking across the BBB is a complex process involving chemokine and chemokine receptor interactions, adhesion molecules, and proteinases. In the periphery, T and B cell lymphocytes primed by antigen exposure circulate through the blood stream and lymphatic system. Selectins, a cell adhesion molecule subtype, interact with the circulating lymphocytes causing them to tether and roll along BBB endothelial cells. The interaction between selectins and lymphocytes leads to the activation of additional cell adhesion molecules called integrins (Holman *et al.*, 2011; Englehardt, 2006.).

Integrins cause the lymphocytes to stop moving and adhere to the BBB endothelial cells. Additional cell adhesion molecules, lymphocyte function-associated antigen-1 (LFA-1), very late antigen-4 (VLA-4), vascular cell adhesion molecule-1 (VCAM-1), and intercellular adhesion molecule 1 (ICAM-1) then facilitate lymphocyte migration across the BBB (Holman *et al.*, 2011). The chemokine and receptor interactions between monocyte chemotactic protein-1 (MCP-1) and its chemokine (C-C motif) receptor CCR2, IL-8 and receptors CCR1 and CCR2, and CXCL13 and receptor CCR5 are integral to the recruitment and facilitation processes during lymphocyte migration into the CNS (Alter *et al.*, 2003; Dalakas, 2008; Meinl *et al.*, 2006). Matrix metalloproteinases (MMPs) are proteolytic enzymes that break down the BBB endothelium, thereby enhancing lymphocyte migration across the BBB endothelium (Leppert *et al.*, 2001).

Additional lymphocytes and other immune cells (macrophages and natural killer cells) migrate to the CNS, cross the BBB endothelium, and cause inflammation and demyelination. An in depth discussion of these individual interactions is beyond the scope of this chapter. Several reviews cover these topics (Holman *et al.*, 2011; Englehardt, 2006).

8   Pathology

MS is characterized by focal areas of inflammation that lead to demyelinating lesions in the brain and spinal cord. Lesions primarily occur in the white matter and a classification scheme that consists of four lesion subtypes has been proposed. Newly formed lesions reflect acute inflammatory changes dominated by T-cell and B-cell infiltration (Patterns I & II) while older, chronic lesions demonstrate primary glial damage and sparse remyelination (Patterns III & IV). Lesion patterns appeared heterogenous between patients but were homogenous within the same patient (Lucchinetti *et al.*, 2000). Another classification scheme is based upon lesion staining characteristics using hematoxylin-eosin and luxol fast blue and immunohistochemistry analysis with anti-CD 68 that yields lesion sample types of acute, chronic active, or chronic inactive based upon the degree of demyelinating activity. Acute lesions exhibit pronounced inflammatory cell infiltration with fragments of myelin in the lesion. Axonal damage can occur in normal appearing white matter even before demyelination is evident (Sabada *et al.* 2012).

Cortical or gray matter lesions are not easily identified with traditional MRI T-2 weighted imaging and are not readily detectable at autopsy due to unique histological staining requirements. (Trapp & Nave, 2008) Nevertheless, a separate classification scheme consisting of three types (I-III) has been proposed to describe different cortical demyelination patterns (Peterson *et al.*, 2001).

Conceptually, classification schemes serve to simplify complex immunological responses, identify potential therapeutic targets, and help explain phenotypic clinical course evolution from relapsing-remitting multiple sclerosis (RRMS) to secondary progressive multiple sclerosis (SPMS). However, the classification systems are static and fail to account for patients who present with multiple lesion types (Frohman *et al.*, 2006).

9   Diagnosis

Diagnostic criteria for MS have undergone significant changes over the past 40 years, primarily as a result of advances in neuroimaging. The Schumacher (1961) and Poser (1983) criteria were replaced by the McDonald Criteria in 2001. The original McDonald Criteria were revised in 2005 and 2010 (Poser & Briner, 2001; Polman *et al.*, 2011). The presence of symptoms or signs caused by demyelination that are disseminated in time (DIT) or space (DIS) were included in original criteria and remain crucial elements for diagnosis. Diagnosis is aided by MRI results and paraclinical laboratory evidence, mostly from cerebrospinal fluid (CSF) analysis and visual-evoked potentials (VEP) (Freedman *et al.*, 2005). (See Table 2)

9.1   Clinically Isolated Syndrome

Clinically isolated syndrome (CIS) is the first episode of dysfunction resulting in a neurological sign or symptom consistent with but not fully matching criteria of MS (Miller *et al.*, 2008). Limb sensory dys

Clinical Features	Additional Requirement(s) for Diagnosis
2 or more attacks[a]; objective evidence of 2 or more lesions or objective evidence of 1 lesion with reliable history of previous attack[b]	None needed[c]
2 or more attacks; objective evidence of 1 lesion	Proof of Dissemination in Space (DIS): 1 or more T2 lesions in a minimum of 2 of 4 MS-typical lesions of the CNS (juxtacorticol, infratentorial, periventricular or spinal cord)[d]; or wait until second confirmed attack from a different CNS site
1 attack; objective evidence of 2 or more lesions	Proof of Dissemination in Time (DIT): At any time, concurrent presence of gadolinium-enhancing and non-enhancing lesions; or A new T2 and/or gadolinium-enhancing lesion(s) on follow-up MRI, irrespective of timing as it pertains to the baseline scan; or wait until a second clinical attack occurs
1 attack; objective evidence of 1 lesion (Clinically isolated syndrome)	For DIS: 1 or more T2 lesions in a minimum of 2 of 4 MS-typical lesions of the CNS (juxtacorticol, infratentorial, periventricular or spinal cord); or wait until second confirmed attack from a different CNS site. For DIT:): At any time, concurrent presence of gadolinium-enhancing and non-enhancing lesions:or A new T2 and/or gadolinium-enhancing lesion(s) on follow-up MRI, irrespective of timing as it pertains to the baseline scan; or wait until a second clinical attack occurs
Insidious neurological progression suggestive of primary progressive MS (PPMS)	Disease progression of 1 year, determined retrospectively or prospectively, plus 2 of 3 remaining criteria:[d] 1.) Evidence for DIS in brain: 1 or more T2 lesions in MS-typical regions of CNS (juxtacorticol, infratentorial, periventricular). 2.) Evidence for DIS in spinal cord: 2 or more T2 lesions in spinal cord. 3.) Positive CSF findings of oligoclonal bands and/or elevated IgG index

[a] Attacks (exacerbations or relapses) can be patient-reported or objectively diagnosed must be consistent with acute demyelinating inflammatory event with a minimum duration of 24 hours.

[b] Objective clinical evidence of 2 or more attacks is the most secure clinical diagnosis for MS.

[c] No additional testing is required if patient has clinical evidence of 2 or more clinical attacks. However, imaging results can be useful especially in patients with negative imaging & CSF findings.

[d] Gadolinum-enhancing lesions are not required. Polman *et al* 2011.

Table 2: Key Features of 2010 McDonald Criteria of multiple sclerosis

function, pyramidal tract abnormalities, optic nerve dysfunction, bladder and bowel dysregulation, diplopia, and ataxia are hallmark CIS signs and symptoms (Frohman *et al.*, 2003). Individuals with CIS and concurrent MRI abnormalities who do not meet MS diagnostic criteria are more likely to progress to clinically definite multiple sclerosis (CDMS), often within 2-5 years (Goodin & Bates, 2009). Compared to placebo, using beta interferons 1a or 1b or glatiramer acetate in individuals with CIS has reduced conversion rates from CIS to CDMS. Products, dosages, efficacy rates and MRI data for medications used in treating CIS are presented in Table 3.

9.2   Radiologically Isolated Syndrome

Radiologically isolated syndrome (RIS) is a term used to describe an individual with MRI evidence suggestive of demyelination but without any clinical sign or neurological symptom associated with MS. Specific diagnostic criteria intended to standardize RIS nomenclature has been proposed (Okuda *et al.*,

Product\Study\Year	Therapy Groups	Conversion to Clinically Definite Multiple Sclerosis CDMS
Interferon β-1a Avonex®\CHAMPS[a] 2000	IFNβ-1a 30 ug i.m. once weekly Placebo	Cumulative probability at 3 years: IFNβ-1a: 35% Placebo: 50% MRI: significant reductions in T2 lesion volume, fewer new or enlarging lesions
Interferon β-1a Rebif®\ETOMS[b]	IFNβ-1a 22 ug s.c. once weekly Placebo	Cumulative probability at 2 years: IFNβ-1a: 34% Placebo: 45% MRI: significantly fewer new T2 weighted lesions; IFNβ-1a delayed time to CDMS
Interferon β-1b Betaseron®\BENEFIT[c]	IFNβ-1b 250 ug (8mIU) s.c. every other day Placebo	Cumulative probability at 2 years. IFNβ-1b: 28% Placebo: 45% Significant reductions in newly active T2 lesions, lesion volume. Delayed progression to CDMS.
Glatiramer acetate Copaxone®\PreCISe[d]	Glatiramer 20mg sc daily Placebo	Cumulative probability at 2 years. Glatiramer: 25% Placebo: 43% Delayed time to CDMS
Teriflunimide (TOPIC)[e]	Teriflunomide 7mg/day Teriflunomide 14mg/day Placebo	Ongoing: Estimated Primary Completion Date: June 2013 Primary endpoint: conversion from CIS to CDMS

[a] CHAMPS: Jacobs *et al.* 2000
[b] ETOMS: Comi *et al.* 2001
[c] BENEFIT:Kappos *et al.* 2006
[d] PRECISE:Marinelli *et al.* 2009
[e] TOPIC: data obtained from ClinicalTrials.gov, accessed November 1, 2012

Table 3: Clinically Isolated Syndrome Studies

2009). Results of small studies of individuals followed for mean or median timeframes between 5 – 6 years indicate that progression from RIS to CIS or CDMS occurs in approximately 25-33% patients (Okuda *et al.*, 2009; Lebrun *et al.*, 2009). Larger studies are needed to define the natural history of RIS and to identify which individuals are at highest risk for progression to CDMS. Studies using medications to prevent or alter the conversion of RIS to CDMS have not been conducted.

10   Clinical Course

Approximately 85% of MS patients experience a relapsing-remitting disease course (RRMS) character-ized by periods of neurological deterioration called exacerbations followed by periods of symptom reso-lution and improved function (Compston & Coles, 2002). Accumulating lesion burden over time and sus-tained damage leads to secondary progressive MS (SPMS) in approximately 50% of RRMS patients, of-ten within 10 years (Hauser & Oksenburg, 2006). Approximately 10 – 15% of MS patients experience a primary progressive disease course (PPMS). Attempts have been made to standardize clinical course terminology to aid researchers and clinical investigators (Lublin & Reingold, 1996). PPMS patients experience persistent ongoing neurological and functional deterioration with no clear periods of remission. Patients with PPMS usually have significant disability within 10 years of initial diagnosis (Noseworthy *et al.*, 2000).

The prognosis once MS is diagnosed varies considerably among patients and no method has been developed to accurately predict an individual's disease course or timeframe for progression. Epidemiology studies indicate that a benign course with little sustained disability for over 20 years is experienced by approximately 10% of patients with MS (Noseworthy *et al.*, 2000) whereas death within months occurs in rare circumstances for some patients with PPMS (Compston & Coles, 2002). Patients with brain-stem dysfunction, optic neuritis and gait or coordination disturbances typically have a poorer prognosis whereas individuals with predominately sensory or visual symptoms have a more positive prognosis (McDonald *et al.*, 2001).

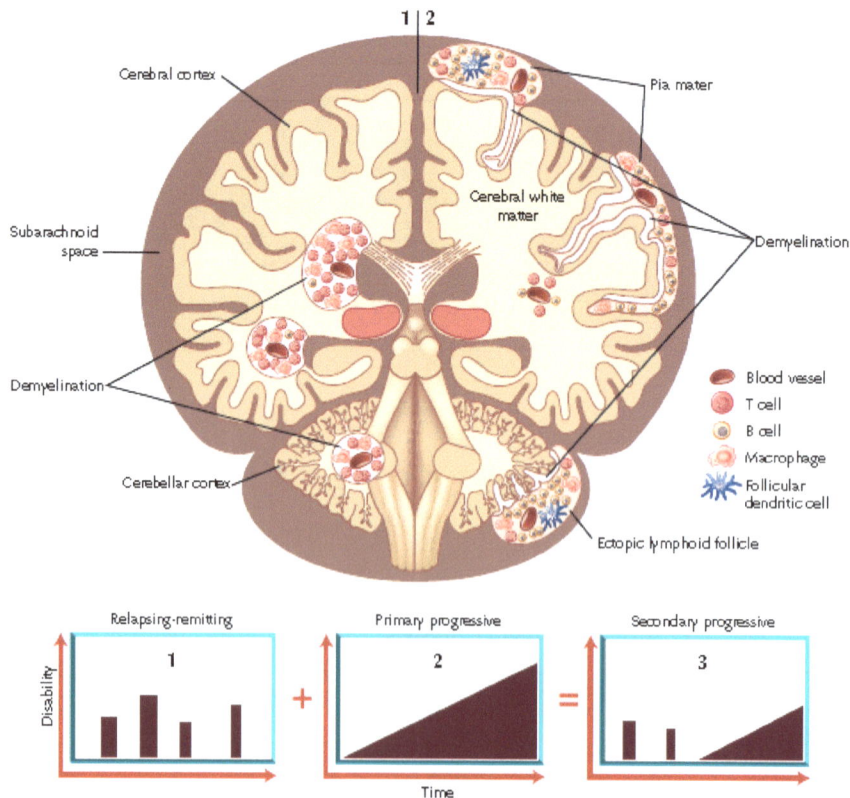

Figure 2: Different clinical courses of MS. (From Pender & Greer, 2007).

11   Medications

11.1   Traditional Therapy for MS

Acute exacerbations of MS are commonly treated with short courses of intravenous methylprednisolone, typically 3-7 days duration, this therapy may or may not be followed by tapering doses of oral prednisone. Corticosteroid administration decreases inflammation and shortens the duration of a MS exacerbation but does not affect the overall course of disease. Adverse effects from short courses of corticosteroids are generally mild and transient but repeated or prolonged steroid courses increase the risk of osteoporosis and bone fracture (Pithaldia *et al.*, 2009).

11.2   Interferon-Beta

The use of disease-modifying agents was introduced in the 1990s for the treatment of RRMS. Beta interferons (INFβ) are family members of cytokines involved during inflammatory cascade signaling and gene regulation. There are three different beta interferon products, each differ in their manufacturing process, dose, biological activity or routes of administration. The full spectrum of INFβ 1a and 1b effects are unknown but they have been shown to alter the number and activation of T-cells, MHC Class I and II expression, and adhesion molecule expression (Karp *et al.*, 2001). INFβ 1a and 1b reduce annual MS relapse rates by 29-37% and development of new, gadolinium-enhancing (GdE+) lesions on MRI (IFNB, 1993; Jacobs *et al.*, 1996; PRISMS., 1998; Johnson *et al.*, 1995). Moreoever, a reduction in the progression of disability as measured by EDSS has been observed in trials. As noted, most individuals with RRMS progress to SPMS. INFβ products have been shown to continue to reduce relapse rates but their effects at slowing disease progression in patients with SPMS is modest, at best (Bermel & Rudick, 2007).

Individuals receiving INFβ often develop neutralizing antibodies (NAbs) that can block interferon-receptor binding or receptor mediated functions. The presence of NAbs, especially in high titers, has been associated with reduced efficacy. However, some experts question the overall clinical impact of NAbs (Bermel & Rudick, 2007). Injection of beta interferon is most commonly associated with pain, erythema, and other minor injection site reactions but serious injection site infections and necrosis can occur. Biosimilar products for several INFβ products exist in different countries. Biosimilar products are sometime also referred to a biogenerics and are meant to mirror the biological activity of the original, innovator drug. However, limited, small numbers of product analysis studies indicate these biosimilar products contain lower levels of non-aggregated (i.e. active) INFβ (Rudick & Goelz, 2011).

INFβ products do not reverse pre-existing CNS damage (Schwid & Bever, 2001) or significantly alter the eventual course of MS (Compston & Coles 2002; Bermel & Rudick 2007). Several large clinical trials have assessed the benefits of INFβ on slowing the progression of disability in patients with SPMS. The European Interferon-β 1b study demonstrated reductions in disease progression for individuals receiving INFβ 8mIU administered subcutaneously every other day but other studies were either halted early (Panitch *et al.*, 2004) or failed to demonstrate reductions in EDSS progression (Kappos *et al.*, 2001; SPECTRIMS, 2001; Andersen *et al.*, 2004). A more recent study compared RRMS individuals receiving INFβ products with untreated contemporary and historical control groups. Each group had similar disease progression rates even after adjusting for baseline confounders such as sex, baseline EDSS score, age or disease duration (Shirani *et al.*, 2012).

11.3   Glatiramer Acetate

Glatiramer acetate (Copaxone® or Copolymer 1) is a synthetic analog of myelin basic protein (MBP) composed of a defined ratio of four L-amino acids (Blanchette & Neuhaus, 2008). Glatiramer increases serum interleukin (IL)-10, decreases TNF-α mRNA, and enhances secretion of anti-inflammatory cytokines (Racke *et al.*, 2010). Early successful use of glatiramer acetate in RRMS patients in a pilot study (Bornstein *et al.* 1987) led to a large trial that demonstrated significant reductions in annual relapse rates of 29% and more favorable EDSS and ambulation index scores (Johnson *et al.*, 1995). Glatiramer acetate has also been shown to reduce emergence of new enhancing lesions, new T2-weighted images, and the volume of enhancing lesions during a multicenter study (Comi *et al.*, 2001). Unfortunately, glatiramer acetate has not been effective in reducing disease progression in patients with chronic progressive MS (Bornstein *et al.*, 1991) or in patients with PPMS (Wolinsky *et al.*, 2007). At one point it was believed that *oral* administration of glatiramer acetate might be effective but it was proven unsuccessful in treating patients with RRMS (Fillipi *et al.*, 2006).

Interferon products and glatiramer acetate remain first line recommendations in major US and European MS treatment guidelines regardless of the discovery and approval of new medications for MS. These guidelines offer excellent reviews of the advantages, adverse effects, and limitations of these historic agents (Goodin *et al.*, 2002; Sorensen *et al.*, 2005).

11.4   Natalizumab

Natalizumab received United States Food and Drug Administration (USFDA) approval for treatment of RRMS in 2004. Natalizumab is a monoclonal antibody that binds to the alpha-4 chain (α-4β-1) receptor that blocks leukocyte trafficking from the peripheral circulation across the BBB. Natalizumab is administered in doses of 300mg intravenously over approximately 1 hour given every 4 weeks. Patients allocated to the natalizumab compared to placebo arm in the AFFIRM trial had a 68% annual clinical relapse rate reduction at 1 year, a 42% reduction in sustained disability over two years, and decreased MRI lesion activity (Polman *et al.*, 2006).

Reports of progressive multifocal leukoencephalopathy (PML), a rare demyelinating disorder produced after reactivation of the JC virus, were linked to natalizumab use following approval of the drug. Three known risk factors including the presence of anti-JCV antibodies, prior treatment with immunosuppressant medications and longer duration of natalizumab use (especially periods longer than 24 months) increases the likelihood of acquiring PML. As of October 2, 2012 there have been approximately 96,582 patients treated with natalizumab and 201 reported cases of PML (USFDA, 2012). Patients, prescribers, infusion centers and pharmacies must be registered with the manufacturer and the TOUCH™ Prescribing Program to receive, prescribe, or infuse natalizumab. This restricted access program is to ensure close patient monitoring by qualified healthcare professionals. Natalizumab concentrations persist for months following repeated maintenance doses and some patients have chosen to receive immunoadsorption or plasma exchange to lower levels of natalizumab after being diagnosed with PML (Tan *et al.* 2011). Immune reconstitution inflammatory syndrome (IRIS) has occurred in some patients following immunoadsorption or plasma exchange (National Multiple Sclerosis Society. Accessed October 2, 2012).

11.5   Fingolimod

Fingolimod is the first approved *oral* disease-modifying agent for chronic treatment of RRMS. Fingolimod is a sphingosine-1 phosphate-1 (S1P1) receptor modulator that prevents lymphocyte egress from lymph tissue. The TRANSFORMS and FREEDOMS trials were comparisons of fingolimod versus INFβ and placebo, respectively. Fingolimod treatment was associated with greater reductions in annualized relapse rates in each trial, fewer multiple relapses and more days to first relapse in TRANSFORMS and slower disease progression based on EDSS progression in FREEDOMS. Nearly 90% of all patients enrolled in both trials completed the studies. (Cohen *et al.*, 2010; Kappos *et al.*, 2010) (See Table 4).

During clinical trials of fingolimod, the majority of adverse effects were judged to be of mild or moderate severity but higher rates of first and second degree heart block and bradycardia were reported in the fingolimod treatment arms. Several patients died while receiving fingolimod following the drug's

Study	Subjects	Regimen	Duration	Study Outcomes
TRANS-FORMS	RRMS with a relapse in the past year	Fingolimod 1.25 mg PO daily (n= 420) Fingolimod 0.5 mg PO daily (n=429) INFβ-1a 30μg IM weekly (n=431)	12 months	Clinical: Annualized relapse rate (ARR): Fingolimod 1.25 mg : 0.2 (p <0.001) Fingolimod 0.5 mg: 0.16 (p<0.001) INFβ-1a: 0.33 MRI: Mean gadolinium-enhancing (Gd+) lesions per patient: Fingolimod 1.25 mg : 0.14 (p <0.001) Fingolimod 0.5 mg: 0.23 (p<0.001) INFβ-1a: 0.51 Patients with no Gd+ lesions: Fingolimod 1.25 mg : 321 (p <0.001) Fingolimod 0.5 mg: 337 (p<0.001) INFβ-1a: 286 Mean new or enlarging T2 weighted lesions per patient: Fingolimod 1.25 mg : 1.5 +/- 2.7 (p <0.001) Fingolimod 0.5 mg: 1.7 +/- 3.9 (p<0.01) INFβ-1a: 2.5 +/- 5.8
FREE-DOMS	RRMS with a relapse in the past year	Fingolimod 1.25 mg PO daily (n= 429) Fingolimod 0.5 mg PO daily (n=425) Placebo (n=418)	24 Months	Clinical: Annualized relapse rate (ARR): Fingolimod 1.25 mg : 0.16 (p <0.001) Fingolimod 0.5 mg: 0.18 (p<0.001) Placebo: 0.40 MRI data: Subset of patients Mean gadolinium-enhancing (Gd+) lesions per patient: Fingolimod 1.25 mg : 0.2 (p <0.001) Fingolimod 0.5 mg: 0.2 (p<0.001) Placebo: 1.1 Patients with no Gd+ lesions: Fingolimod 1.25 mg : 308 (p <0.001) Fingolimod 0.5 mg: 331(p<0.001) Placebo: 216 Mean new or enlarging T2 weighted lesions per patient: Fingolimod 1.25 mg : 2.5 +/- 5.5 (p <0.001) Fingolimod 0.5 mg: 2.5 +/- 7.2 (p<0.001) Placebo: 9.8 +/- 13.2

Abbreviations: RRMS – relapse remitting multiple sclerosis, SPMS – secondary progressive multiple sclerosis, T1-Gd – gadolinium enhancing, EDSS – expanded disability status scale

Table 4: Hallmark Phase III Trials of fingolimod

approval, prompting the FDA and EMA (European Medicine Agency) to review the drug's safety. Revised prescribing information was issued after the FDA and EMA reviews. MS patients being considered for fingolimod treatment must be carefully screened for certain common cardiac conditions or conduction defects and therapy with Class Ia or IIIa anti-arrhythmic drugs which preclude its use. Patients receiving their first dose of fingolimod must be observed for a minimum of 6 hours.

11.6   Teriflunomide

Teriflunomide is a recently appproved oral medication used for RRMS. Teriflunomide inhibits proliferating T and B lymphocytes in the periphery by selectively inhibiting mitochondrial enzyme dihydroorate (DHODH). Since DHODH is the rate limiting enzyme in the de novo synthesis of pyrimidines, inhibition of DHODH causes cell cycle arrest in the G1 phase of rapidly dividing cells, B- and T-cells (Dalakas, 2008; Bruneau et al., 1998). Teriflunomide in the 2 year TEMSO trial reduced annualized MS relapse rates by 54% versus placebo 37% and confirmed disability progression was 21.7% in the active treatment group versus 27.3% in the placebo group. In the TENERE trial, teriflunomide demonstrated statistically significant superiority over INFβ (Rebif®) for the primary composite endpoint which was the risk of treatment failure.

Teriflunomide is well tolerated and no life threatening adverse effects have emerged during the Phase II and Phase III trials. Discontinuation rates due to ADRs were approximately 11% in the teriflunomide arm compared to 8.1% in the placebo group in TEMSO trial. Several large Phase III trials are ongoing. (See Table 5).

11.7   Combination Therapy

Despite considerable improvements in reducing relapse rates and the development of new CNS lesions achieved by first line therapies for RRMS, they have not produced complete suppression of symptoms or arrested progression of cumulative disability. The complexity of immunologic pathways and variable clinical states of MS suggest that combination therapy might be a more logical approach to therapy. Selecting medications with differing mechanisms of actions could provide additive or synergistic effects. As proof of the theory, combination therapy is a standard of care for other complex, autoimmune diseases such as rheumatoid arthritis. Data from combination therapy trials in MS are limited but the area is becoming the focus of intensive research. Three small investigations that explored the use of mitoxantrone with INFβ (Correale et al., 2005) or glatiramer acetate as sequential therapy following mitoxantrone (Ramatahal et al., 2006) or cyclophosphamide with INFβ (Patti et al., 2004) have demonstrated limited benefits.

11.8   Natalizumab Combination Trials

Trials combining natalizumab with intramuscular INFβ-1a (SENTINEL) or glatiramer acetate (GLANCE) have shown relapse rate reductions and significantly fewer new or expanding lesions detected by MRI compared to their respective monotherapy active treatment arms of INFβ-1a or glatiramer actetate. Patients who received the combination therapy in the SENTINEL and GLANCE trials developed antibodies to natalizumab at a higher rate. The higher rate of antibodies appeared to be related to more frequent relapses, adverse effects and cumulative probability of disease progression. A single case of PML was detected in the SENTINEL trial that caused early trial termination whereas no evidence of PML was discovered during the GLANCE trial or its extension phase (Rudick et al., 2006, Goodman et al., 2009).

Study	Subjects	Regimen	Duration	Study Outcomes
TEMSO phase III N=1088	RRMS SPMS	Teriflunomide 7 mg/day Teriflunomide 14mg/day Placebo	108 wks	Clinical: Annualized relapse rate (ARR): Relative Rate Reduction (RRR)-versus placebo Teriflunomide 7mg: RRR 31.2% (p=0.0002) Teriflunomide 14mg: RRR 31.7% (p=0.0005) Sustained Disease Progression (EDSS): Teriflunomide 7mg: NS- not significant Teriflunomide 14mg: RRR 29.8% (p=0.0279) MRI: RRR versus placebo: Total lesion volume: Teriflunomide 7mg: 39.4% (p= 0.03) Teriflunomide 14mg: 67.4% (p=0.001) Volume of T1-weighted images: Teriflunomide 7mg: 16.7 (p= 0.19) Teriflunomide 14mg: 31.3 (p=0.02) Volume of T2-weighted images: Teriflunomide 7mg: 44.0 (p=0.04) Teriflunomide 14mg: 76.7 (p<0.001)
TEMSO open-label extension N=556	RRMS SPMS	Active treatment groups	≥108 wks	Ongoing extension study Primary endpoint: safety/tolerability Secondary endpoints: EDSS ARR, MRI
TOWER[a] phase III N=1110*	Relapsing MS	Teriflunomide 7 mg/day Teriflunomide 14mg/day Placebo	≥ 48 wks	Ongoing : Estimated Primary Completion Date: August 2015 Primary endpoint: ARR Secondary endpoint: disability progression
TENERE[a] phase III N=300*	Relapsing MS	Teriflunomide 7 mg/day Teriflunomide 14mg/day IFN-β 1a 44µg three times weekly	≥ 48 weeks	Ongoing: Estimated Primary Completion Date: June 2015 Primary endpoint: time to failure (1st occurrence or relapse or permanent study treatment discontinued for any cause – whichever outcome occurs first) Secondary endpoint: ARR
TERACLES[a] phase III N=1455*	Relapsing MS	Teriflunomide7mg/day + IFN-β1a (stable dose) Teriflunomide 14mg/day + IFN-β1a (stable dose) PBO + IFN-β1a (stable dose)	48 – 152 weeks	Ongoing: Estimated Primary Completion Date: April 2014 Primary endpoint: ARR Secondary endpoint: MRI, EDSS, change in abnormal brain volume

Notes: [a] data obtained from ClinicalTrials.gov, accessed November 1, 2012; * planned recruitment total
Abbreviations: RRMS – relapse remitting multiple sclerosis, SPMS – secondary progressive multiple sclerosis, T1-Gd – gadolinium enhancing, EDSS – expanded disability status scale

Table 5: Hallmark Phase III and Ongoing Teriflunomide Trials

11.9   Steroid Combination Trials

The combination of steroid plus INFβ-1a in two trials, NORMIMS (Sorensen *et al.*, 2009) and MECOMBIN (Ravnborg *et al.*, 2010), led to reductions in relapse rates compared to monotherapy with INFβ-1a but the time to sustained progression of disease was unaffected (MECOMBIN). Moreover, individuals assigned to the steroid and INFβ-1a combination arms in each trial, NORMIMS and MECOMBIN, experienced more frequent adverse effects. These trials were also limited by low enrollments and high dropout rates. Two other trials combined INFβ-1a 30μg intramuscular injections once weekly plus steroids: one using high dose methylprednisolone with/without methotrexate (Cohen *et al*, 2009) and another combining low dose oral prednisone with oral azathioprine (Havrdova *et al.* 2009), neither trial produced significant reductions in the primary outcome of reduced relapse rates.

12   General Therapy Algorithm

The use of INFβ products or glatiramer acetate as initial therapies have been shown to reduce the progression rate of CIS patients and reduce relapse rates and short term progression of disease for RRMS patients. Patients who fail to respond to the initially selected first line agent most frequently are switched to the alternative first-line drug. INFβ-1b (Betaseron®) and INFβ-1a subcutaneously (Rebif®) have been shown to offer some benefit in patients with SPMS. Natalizumab and fingolimod often the promise of more significant reductions in relapse rates but also carry the risk of more serious adverse effects. None of the current therapies have been shown to be effective in PPMS.

13   Management of Secondary Complications

Symptomatic management is as important as disease-modifying therapies (DMT) in MS patients since effective therapy improves overall function and quality of life. Individuals with MS experience a wide variety of symptoms throughout the course of their disease progression. The various symptoms should be carefully and thoroughly assessed on a routine basis, and treatment should be individualized for each patient. Optimal symptomatic management includes a multidisciplinary approach with all types of healthcare professionals, and specialists when required. Unfortunately, there are very few well designed trials that address the treatment of symptoms in MS. Rather, the therapy recommended to treat a given symptom of MS is commonly based on evidence provided by investigations in other disease states. In the following sections, tables are provided to briefly summarize the various trials that have specifically been carried out in MS patients. Other medications or therapies that have been proposed as beneficial, but not specifically studied in the MS population, will be discussed in the narrative portions.

14   Neurogenic Bladder

Neurogenic bladder dysfunction is a common affliction in MS patients and the prevalence increases with duration of the disease. It is estimated that more than 70% of patients experience urinary dysfunction (Samkoff & Goodman, 2011; Thompson *et al.*, 2010). Symptoms are thought to arise from interruption of communication between the pontine and sacral micturition center (Thompson *et al.*, 2010). Three types of neurogenic bladder occur in MS patients including detrusor hyperreflexia, hyporeflexive bladder, and detrusor-sphincter dyssynergia. Diagnosis of the correct type of bladder dysfunction is important for proper treatment, but cannot be based solely on symptoms as they can be similar between different types. Post-micturition volumes are helpful for distinguishing between different forms and should always be assessed by ultrasonography or catheterization to aid in proper diagnosis (DasGupta & Fowler, 2003; Samkoff & Goodman, 2011). It is also important to rule out urinary tract infection prior to initiation of any therapy (Fowler *et al.*, 2009; Samkoff & Goodman, 2011; Thompson *et al.*, 2010). Table 6 lists medications that have been studied in MS patients with neurogenic bladder.

Medication	Study design	Comments
Detrusor Overactivity		
Solifenacin	Prospective, open-label study (van Rey & Heesakkers, 2011)	Solifenacin significantly decreased number of pads used and micturitions per day. Incontinence was not improved although many patients were not incontinent at baseline. Only 2 patients discontinued therapy due to side effects (van Rey & Heesakkers, 2011).
Dual therapy (oxybutynin, tolterodine, trospium)	Randomized unblinded comparative study (Amend *et al.*, 2008)	There were impressive improvements in incontinence events in 85% of patients who had unsatisfactory response to monotherapy. Dual-therapy was well tolerated. All patients had incontinence originating from spinal abnormalities, but only 2 patients included had MS (Amend *et al.*, 2008).
Oxybutynin vs. intravesicular atropine	Randomized, double-blind, comparative, crossover study (Fader *et al.*, 2007).	Atropine increased bladder capacity 24mL more than oral oxybutynin. Voiding frequency and incontinence events and were similar in both groups. Atropine had significantly fewer adverse events compared to oxybutynin (Fader *et al.*, 2007).
Oxybutynin vs. propantheline	Prospective, randomized study (Gajewski & Awad, 1986)	67% and 36% of oxybutynin and propantheline patients had good responses respectively. Four patients in each group dropped out due to adverse events (Gajewski & Awad, 1986).
Botulinum toxin A	Randomized, double-blind, placebo-controlled study (Cruz *et al.*, 2011). Retrospective unblinded study (Deffontaines-Rufin *et al.*, 2011). Prospective, open-label study (Khan *et al.*, 2011). Systematic review (Habek *et al.*, 2010)	In all studies, patients achieved full continence, or incontinence was improved (Cruz *et al.*, 2011; Deffontaines-Rufin *et al.*, 2011; Habek *et al.*, 2010; Khan *et al.*, 2011) Two studies reported increased QOL (Cruz *et al.*, 2011; Habek *et al.*, 2010). Botulinum toxin may be useful even in patients refractory to oral anticholinergics (Deffontaines-Rufin *et al.*, 2011). Duration of disease seems to correlate with unresponsiveness to treatment (Deffontaines-Rufin *et al.*, 2011). Typically, all patients will require CISC after treatment, but this has not been shown to adversely affect QOL (Khan *et al.*, 2011).
Hyporeflexive Bladder		
Indoramin	Randomized, single-blind, placebo-controlled study (O'Riordan *et al.*, 1995)	Mean peak flow improved 41% with the alpha-1 antagonist compared to a 7.4% deterioration in placebo group. However, the effects were mild and only approximately half of patients continued treatment after the study (O'Riordan *et al.*, 1995).
Nocturia		
Desmopressin	Meta-analysis (Bosma *et al.*, 2005)	Voiding frequency, incontinence, and nighttime awakenings were all improved with desmopressin. Effects typically lasted only 6 to 8 hours (Bosma *et al.*, 2005).

Table 6: Medications studied in MS for neurogenic bladder

14.1 Neurogenic Detrusor Overactivity

Neurogenic detrusor overactivity (also referred to as detrusor hyperreflexia) is the most common type of neurogenic bladder (DasGupta & Fowler, 2003). Overactivity of the detrusor muscle results in frequent feelings of urgency even with small residual volumes, and can progress to urge incontinence with urinary leakage (DasGupta & Fowler, 2003; Samkoff & Goodman, 2011). Based on results from small trials, an anticholinergic agent is the mainstay of therapy (Samkoff & Goodman, 2011; Thompson *et al.*, 2010). However, anticholinergic side effects may precipitate new, or exacerbate preexisting symptoms in MS patients including constipation and cognitive impairment. As such, selective anticholinergics such as darifenacin and solifenacin that are less likely to cross the blood-brain-barrier may be more appropriate in patients with cognitive impairment (Samkoff & Goodman, 2011). Intravesical injection of botulinum toxin has also been shown to be effective in treating symptoms of neurogenic detrusor overactivity and represents an option for patients unresponsive to oral anticholinergic medications. The effects of botulinum toxin typically last around 10 to 12 months and treatments may be repeated if desired (Khan *et al.*, 2011).

14.2 Hyporeflexive Bladder

Hyporeflexive bladder generally presents with symptoms of frequency with incomplete emptying. Hyporeflexive bladder has been shown to occur in up to 20% of MS patients with neurogenic bladder (Litwiller *et al.*, 1999). Treatment depends on the post-micturition residual volume. If the volume is less than 100mL, an alpha-1 antagonist can improve incomplete emptying and reduce residual volume in some patients (O'Riordan *et al.*, 1995). Conversely, if the post-micturition volume is greater than 100mL, an alpha-1 antagonist will not be sufficiently effective and clean intermittent self-catheterization (CISC) is indicated (Fowler *et al.*, 2009). CISC should be performed at least once daily (Samkoff & Goodman, 2011). If CISC is not feasible or becomes impractical due to increasing disability, a suprapubic indwelling catheter should be established (Fowler *et al.*, 2009).

14.3 Detrusor-Sphincter Dyssynergia

Of MS patients with neurogenic bladder, it has been estimated that 25% of MS patients will experience this form (Litweller *et al.*, 1999). With detrusor-sphincter dyssynergia, urinary retention results from constriction of the detrusor muscle and external urinary sphincter at the same time (Samkoff & Goodman, 2011). Feelings of hesitancy, frequency, and incomplete emptying typically result. CISC is usually necessary and the preferred treatment in most instances. Anticholinergic therapy may be effective by inhibiting detrusor contraction, but in most cases should be used concurrently with CISC management (Mahfouz & Corcos, 2011).

14.4 Miscellaneous Bladder Symptoms

Nocturia can be an issue with MS patients and intranasal desmopressin has been demonstrated to increase the periods of uninterrupted sleep and decrease the number of nighttime voiding episodes (Bosma *et al.*, 2005). Hyponatremia can occur in up to 5% of patients receiving desmopressin, and should be monitored (Thompson *et al.*, 2010). Diuretics given in the afternoon may also be considered in patients that urinate frequently during the night (Fowler *et al.*, 2009).

It is clear from the studies summarized in Table 6 that treatment with medication for neurogenic bladder symptoms may not be effective or produce optimal effects in individuals with MS. In this instance, it may be necessary to employ general strategies aimed at improving urinary dysfunction. Patients with nocturia or detrusor hyperreflexia should attempt to reduce their fluid intake 25% to improve symptoms of urgency and frequency. Some patients may avoid fluid intake due to the increasing symptoms it causes. One to two liters a day of fluid is generally recommended to maintain adequate hydration, and should be encouraged. Alcohol intake should be limited and caffeine intake should be restricted to less than 100 mg a day to improve symptoms of urgency and frequency (Ben-Zacharia, 2011; Fowler *et al.*, 2009). Proper and routine bowel emptying is also recommended to improve bladder function (Fowler *et al.*, 2009). Lastly, pelvic floor exercises can improve symptoms in some patients with mild disability who have hyperreflexia (Fowler *et al.*, 2009). In cases where there are irreversible complications or intractable symptoms from long term catheters, procedures such as bladder augmentation or urinary diversion may be beneficial (Thompson *et al.*, 2010).

15   Neurogenic Bowel

Neurogenic bowel is a common problem in MS patients with 50% of patients experiencing constipation, and 30-40% experiencing incontinence (Ben-Zacharia, 2011). Despite the frequent occurrence, little data is available to support different treatment options, resulting in a treatment approach based on trial and error. Establishing a routine for bowel evacuation at a convenient time of the day is arguably the most important factor in either constipation or incontinence bowel dysfunction. An established routine will help prevent impaction due to constipation, and decrease the risk of incontinence episodes throughout the day (Coggrave *et al.*, 2006). Evacuation can be accomplished using enemas, rectal stimulants (such as glycerin or bisacodyl suppositories), or by manual means (Ben-Zacharia, 2011; Fowler *et al.*, 2009; Samkoff & Goodman, 2011; Thompson *et al.*, 2010). All individuals should be encouraged to maintain adequate fluid intake, consume a well balanced diet, and participate in regular exercise (Fowler *et al.*, 2009).

The treatment of constipation in MS employs a similar approach to the general population and, therefore, a wide range of medications are utilized. Bulking drugs (e.g. psyllium or methylcellulose) soften and increase the bulk of stool, and promote peristalsis. Stool softeners (e.g. docusate) are surfactants and increase water uptake into the stool. Stimulant laxatives (e.g. senna or bisacodyl) cause localized mucosal irritation and successive stimulation of bowel movement, but chronic use may cause impaired colonic function. Osmotic laxatives like polyethylene glycol 3350 or lactulose result in distention in the bowel, promoting peristalsis (Howard-Thompson, 2012). Any one of these classes of medications can generally be recommended because they increase motility without subsequent incontinence (Thompson *et al.*, 2010). Laxative medications may be used in conjunction with other medications or methods for routine evacuation.

Fecal incontinence is a much more challenging symptom to treat pharmacologically. Rarely, the anti-motility agent, loperamide is used (Ben-Zacharia, 2011; Samkoff & Goodman, 2011; Thompson *et al.*, 2010). However, the mainstay of treatment is routine evacuation as aforementioned (Fowler *et al.*, 2009; Thompson *et al.*, 2010). Surgical interventions such as sphincter repair, artificial bowel sphincter placement, or sacral nerve stimulation may be considered in patients without improvement, although these procedures have not been assessed in MS patients (Thompson *et al.*, 2010).

Biofeedback has been shown to be effective for mildly or moderately disabled patients with either constipation or incontinence and may be an appropriate alternative or adjunct to try (Wiesel *et al.*, 2000). If treatment failure occurs with either incontinence or constipation, end stoma (such as a colostomy or ileostomy) may be an appropriate option (Thompson *et al.*, 2010). A review of a patient's current medication therapy should always be performed to assess for possible medication causes of incontinence or constipation.

16   Sexual Dysfunction

Sexual dysfunction in MS patients is typical in both genders. 84% of men will have either reduced libido, erectile dysfunction (ED), or premature ejaculation and 85% of females will experience reduced libido, difficulty in achieving orgasm, or decreased vaginal lubrication (Tepavcevic *et al*., 2008). Symptoms of sexual dysfunction may not be readily disclosed by the patient and therefore should be assessed on a routine basis. The only sexual dysfunction that has been studied in men with MS is ED (see Table 7). Phosphodiesterase-5 (PDE5) inhibitors are considered first-line therapy for ED in MS males (Ben-Zacharia, 2011; Samkoff & Goodman, 2011; Thompson *et al*., 2010). However, it is important to note that the studies were performed in younger, ambulatory men and it is therefore uncertain if medication benefits extend to patients with more significant disability. The adverse effects associated with PDE5 inhibitors are generally well tolerated. An option for men with ED who are unresponsive or intolerant to PDE5 inhibitors include intracavernous or intraurethral alprostadil (Ben-Zacharia, 2011; Samkoff & Goodman, 2011; Thompson *et al*., 2010). Pharmacotherapy for women with MS and sexual dysfunction is limited. Sildenafil was evaluated in women with MS and sexual dysfunction in a study that yielded disappointing results (Dasgupta *et al*., 2004). Therefore, sildenafil is not recommended for women. Topical estrogens have been shown to increase vaginal moisture and increase clitoral sensitivity in non-MS women and represent a treatment option (Ben-Zacharia, 2011). Nonpharmacologic lubricants may be a better choice for women who wish to avoid side effects of topical estrogen therapy (Ben-Zacharia, 2011; Samkoff & Goodman, 2011; Thompson *et al*., 2010). Vibratory stimulation may be helpful in women achieving orgasm (Samkoff & Goodman, 2011; Thompson *et al*., 2010). The clitoral vacuum pump is the only FDA approved treatment for women with sexual dysfunction, and is intended to improve arousal (Ben-Zacharia, 2011).

Medication	Study design	Comments
Sildenafil	Two randomized, double-blind, placebo-controlled studies (Fowler, 2005; Safarinejad, 2009)	Sildenafil significantly improves the number of erections (Fowler, 2005; Safarinejad, 2009). Also, successful penetrations increased significantly compared to placebo (Safarinejad, 2009). QOL was reported to improve with sildenafil therapy (Fowler, 2005). Adverse events with treatment are fairly common, but are usually mild in nature (Safarinejad, 2009).
Tadalafil	Prospective, open-label study (Lombardi *et al*., 2010)	Overall, erections and sexual satisfaction scores were improved in almost 80% of the patients. Two patients discontinued therapy due to moderate adverse events (Lombardi *et al*., 2010).

Table 7: Medications studied in MS for sexual dysfunction

17   Cognitive Dysfunction

Cognitive dysfunction is estimated to occur in 40-60% of MS patients (Lovera & Kovner, 2012). The most common domains affected are speed of information processing, working memory, verbal fluency, verbal memory, executive function, and visual memory (Lovera & Kovner, 2012). Cognitive impairment can significantly affect a patient's social life and has been shown to be correlated with social isolation, unemployment, and family role changes (Ben-Zacharia, 2011; Samkoff & Goodman, 2011; Thompson *et al.*, 2010). Concurrent depression or fatigue may exacerbate cognitive dysfunction and therefore proper assessment and treatment, if these symptoms are present, is important.

Disease modifying therapies (DMT) can improve or lessen the progression of cognitive function. Interferon beta-1a and beta-1b both have been shown to have beneficial effects on cognition in MS patients in several trials (Barak & Achiron, 2002; Fischer *et al.*, 2000; Melanson *et al.*, 2010; Patti *et al.*, 2010; Pliskin *et al.*, 1996). In addition, natalizumab has been shown to significantly reduce the development or worsening cognitive function in patients with MS (Iaffaldano *et al.*, 2012; Lang *et al.*, 2012; Mattioli, Stampatori, & Capra, 2011; Mattioli *et al.*, 2011). Despite the positive effect on cognition that seems to occur with DMT, patients with cognitive impairment still require specific treatment for cognitive function in most instances.

Clinical trials of acetylcholinesterase inhibitors donepezil and rivastigmine have produced mixed results (see Table 8). The findings suggest that cognitive impairment in MS and Alzheimer's patients have different pathologies (Ben-Zacharia, 2011). It seems likely that certain subsets of MS patients benefit from an acetylcholinesterase inhibitor but methods to identify these patients are not available. Although memantine is commonly used for cognitive impairment in Alzheimer's patients, it should never be used in MS patients as it has been found to worsen cognitive function (Lovera *et al.*, 2010; Villoslada *et al.*, 2009).

Physical exercise should be encouraged as it may improve or prevent worsening of cognitive function, and it has no adverse effects associated with it. However, data is inconclusive at this time whether or not exercise truly is effective (Lovera & Kovner, 2012).

Other therapies may prove useful in the future. Small studies have revealed that cognitive rehabilitation (or exercises) may offer significant benefits (Lovera & Kovner, 2012). Also, the stimulants L-amphetamine, methylphenidate, and modafinil have shown promising results in small MS patient studies (see Table 8).

18   Pain

There are several types of pain that can occur in MS patients. Pain is a fairly frequent finding in MS and it is estimated that some form of pain occurs in over 40% of patients (Solaro & Messmer, 2010). Trials for pain in MS patients are limited, and there is a wide range of recommendations by experts. Guidelines for other disease states are commonly followed when treating MS patients with pain. This section will focus on analgesic medications that have been specifically studied in MS patients (see Table 9) and others that are commonly used.

18.1   Central Neuropathic Pain

Central neuropathic pain has been reported to be the most common type of pain in MS (Solaro & Messmer, 2010). It usually presents as a chronic burning sensation that affects the lower extremities, although it can also affect the upper extremities (Samkoff & Goodman, 2011). Tricyclic antidepressants are arguably the most commonly used medications to treat central neuropathic pain in MS (Samkoff & Goodman, 2011; Solaro & Messmer, 2010; Thompson *et al.*, 2010), despite the fact that there are no randomized controlled trials to document their efficacy for pain in MS patients. Moreover, the adverse events from these medications include drowsiness, constipation, and urinary retention, which may exacerbate concurrent MS symptoms. Consequently, some experts recommend the use of serotonin and norepinephrine reuptake inhibitors such as venlafaxine or duloxetine which have less adverse events compared to tricy

Medication	Study design	Comments
Donepezil	Two randomized, double-blind, placebo-controlled studies (Krupp *et al.*, 2011; Krupp *et al.*, 2004)	The most recent study showed no significant differences in any primary or secondary outcomes relating to cognitive function between placebo and donepezil (Krupp *et al.*, 2011). Another study showed significant improvements in memory, and clinician and patient reports (Krupp *et al.*, 2004).
Rivastigmine	Two randomized, double-blind, placebo-controlled studies (Huolman *et al.*, 2011; Mäurer *et al.*, 2012)	A single dose of rivastigmine improved processing speed in MS patients compared to placebo and an MRI scan revealed changes in brain activation patterns of MS patients to resemble those of the healthy control group (Huolman *et al.*, 2011). However, a second, 16-week trial showed numerical, but not significant improvements in total recall scores compared to placebo (Mäurer *et al.*, 2012). Adverse events cause a fair amount of discontinuation of treatment (Mäurer *et al.*, 2012).
Memantine	Two randomized, double-blind, placebo-controlled studies (Lovera *et al.*, 2010; Villoslada *et al.*, 2009)	One trial did not show any improvements in any primary or secondary cognitive impairment outcomes (Lovera *et al.*, 2010). The other trial was stopped early due to approximately half of the patients reporting worsening of their neurologic symptoms, which was reversible upon discontinuation of memantine (Villoslada *et al.*, 2009). Adverse events are more common than placebo and include fatigue and neurological symptoms (Lovera *et al.*, 2010).
Methylphenidate	Randomized, double-blind, single-dose, placebo-controlled study (Harel *et al.*, 2009).	MS patients with impaired attention received a single dose of methylphenidate or placebo. Significant improvements in attention were seen with methylphenidate while none were seen with placebo (Harel *et al.*, 2009).
L-Amphetamine	Randomized, double-blind, placebo-controlled, single-dose crossover study (Benedict *et al.*, 2008). Randomized, double-blind, placebo-controlled, dose-titration study (Morrow *et al.*, 2009).	In the single-dose study, the highest dose resulted in significant improvements in processing speed and working memory, but episodic memory was not significantly different between the groups (Benedict *et al.*, 2008). In the second study, cognition and processing speed were not different between placebo and L-amphetamine, but auditory and visual memory was improved in the active drug group (Morrow *et al.*, 2009).
Modafinil	Randomized, single-blind, parallel-group study (Wilken *et al.*, 2008). Randomized, double-blind, placebo-controlled study (Möller *et al.*, 2011).	Modafinil plus interferon beta-1a compared to interferon beta-1a alone had significantly better improvements in attention span, working memory, and phonemic verbal fluency (Wilken *et al.*, 2008). However, the other study reported modafinil being more effective in one neuropsychological test and placebo being more effective in a different neuropsychological test (Möller *et al.*, 2011).

Table 8: Medications studied in MS for cognitive impairment

clic antidepressants (Ben-Zacharia, 2011; Samkoff & Goodman, 2011).

Antiepileptic medications have been investigated in small studies for use in central neuropathic pain in MS. Carbamazepine is commonly utilized (Ben-Zacharia, 2011) but has no studies to support its use, leading some experts to question its efficacy in the context of a drug with a substantial side effect profile (Solaro & Messmer, 2010).

Morphine has been studied for central neuropathic pain in MS patients but with poor results in that a minority of patients responded to morphine and only at high dosages (Kalman *et al.*, 2002). The results support the notion that opioids are usually not adequate for treating pain of neuropathic origin.

Cannabinoids have been tested in well-designed trials for the treatment of pain in MS. In virtually all of the studies, cannabinoids have provided significant reductions in pain (see Table 9). However, the utility of the results are limited because of the lack of standardized pharmaceutical products. Currently, only an oral mucosal spray of cannabinoids is awaiting FDA approval.

Medication	Study design	Comments
Central Neuropathic Pain		
Lamotrigine	Prospective, open-label study (Cianchetti *et al.*, 1999). Randomized, double-blind, placebo-controlled, crossover study (Breuer *et al.*, 2007).	In one study, lamotrigine was added onto existing therapy in unresponsive patients. About half of the patients had some extent of improvement in their pain scores (Cianchetti *et al.*, 1999). In a more recent controlled study, lamotrigine did not significantly improve mean pain intensity or QOL compared to placebo (Breuer *et al.*, 2007).
Gabapentin	Prospective, open-label study (Houtchens *et al.*, 1997)	Excellent to moderate pain relief was reported in two thirds of patients. Half of patients experienced adverse events (primarily somnolence and GI upset), but only 5 discontinued treatment (Houtchens *et al.*, 1997).
Levetiracetam	Randomized, prospective, single-blind, placebo-controlled study (Rossi *et al.*, 2009). Randomized, double-blind, placebo-controlled, crossover study (Falah *et al.*, 2012).	In one study, all outcomes related to pain were improved with levetiracetam compared to placebo (Rossi *et al.*, 2009). In a more recent study, there were no differences between placebo and levetiracetam in any pain outcome; however, patients with lancinating pain experienced significant reductions in pain (Falah *et al.*, 2012). Somnolence appears to be fairly common with levetiracetam treatment (Rossi *et al.*, 2009).
Pregabalin	Prospective, open-label study (Solaro *et al.*, 2009)	9 of 16 patients refractory to other medical therapy achieved complete and sustained recovery. Study also included patients with TN, and painful tonic spasms (Solaro *et al.*, 2009).
Oral cannabinoids	Randomized, double-blind, placebo-controlled study (Rog *et al.*, 2005) with an uncontrolled, open-label, two-year extension (Rog *et al.*, 2007)	Mean intensity pain score and sleep disturbance were improved with treatment (Rog *et al.*, 2005). A 2-year extension showed that pain reduction was maintained and tolerance was not seen (Rog *et al.*, 2007). 92% of patients experienced an adverse event with nausea and dizziness being the most common. 25% of patients withdrew due to adverse events in the 2 year follow-up (Rog *et al.*, 2007).
Trigeminal Neuralgia (TN)		
Carbamazepine	Retrospective, observational study (Hooge & Redekop, 1995)	Carbamazepine treatment in 27 patients resulted in complete or partial pain relief in 20 patients. Four discontinued treatment due to adverse events (Hooge & Redekop, 1995).
Gabapentin	Three prospective, open-label studies (Khan, 1998; Solaro *et al.*, 2000; Solaro *et al.*, 1998)	The majority of patients in every trial received full or at least partial pain control (Khan, 1998; Solaro *et al.*, 2000; Solaro *et al.*, 1998). Studies show that when used as an add on to patients not receiving adequate relief from other treatments, most patients may be able to completely discontinue, or lower the dose, of the previous medication (Khan, 1998; Solaro *et al.*, 2000). In all studies, gabapentin was well tolerated, with very few adverse events (Khan, 1998; Solaro *et al.*, 2000; Solaro *et al.*, 1998).

Lamotrigine	Prospective, open-label study (Lunardi *et al.*, 1997). Prospective, physician-blinded study (Leandri *et al.*, 2000).	Majority of patients received complete or near complete remission of pain. Skin rash was a fairly common adverse event, but with proper dosing and management, patients can still receive lamotrigine treatment (Lunardi *et al.*, 1997; Leandri *et al.*, 2000).
Topiramate	Prospective, open-label study (Zvartau-Hind *et al.*, 2000)	Five of six patients were able to discontinue their current therapy and receive complete relief with topiramate only. Treatment with topiramate was well tolerated (Zvartau-Hind *et al.*, 2000).
Misoprostol	Two prospective, open-label studies (DMKG, 2003; Reder & Arnason, 1995)	Misoprostol achieved resolution or partial resolution of pain in most patients that were refractory to other therapies (DMKG, 2003; Reder & Arnason, 1995) GI effects and menorrhagia can occur with a fairly high frequency (DMKG, 2003).
Painful Tonic Spasms		
Gabapentin	Prospective, open-label study (Solaro & Uccelli, *et al.*, 2000)	Almost all patients in this study had resolution or amelioration of discomfort with treatment. Four patients experienced adverse events (Solaro & Uccelli, *et al.*, 2000).
Botulinum toxin A	Prospective, open-label study (Restivo *et al.*, 2003)	Four or five patients had improvements in their pain intensity score and number of episodes per day. Effects lasted at least 90 days after the injection (Restivo *et al.*, 2003).

Table 9: Medications studied in MS for pain

18.2   Trigeminal Neuralgia

Trigeminal neuralgia (TN) is characterized as paroxysmal facial pain and has been estimated to occur at prevalence twenty times greater in MS patients compared to the general population (Samkoff & Goodman, 2011). TN is thought to be caused by demyelinated lesions forming where the trigeminal nerve enters the pons. These lesions are thought to cause abnormal firing of electrical impulses thereby causing episodes of pain (Solaro *et al.*, 2013). Despite its significantly higher incidence in MS patients, TN is still is a relatively infrequent symptom and is reported to occur only in around 5% of patients with MS (Solaro & Messmer, 2010). Since the pain can be excruciating and debilitating to patients, management is essential.

Because placebo-controlled trials in patients with TN are considered unethical, available studies have been open-label. Traditionally, carbamazepine and lamotrigine have been recommended as first line therapy (Samkoff & Goodman, 2011; Solaro & Messmer, 2010; Thompson *et al.*, 2010) but a number of other options may be more suitable (see Table 9). Misoprostol has been shown to be fairly effective but should be relegated to last-line therapy for patients refractory or intolerant to other medications, due to its greater incidence of adverse events.

Some patients present with an atypical face pain that should not be classified as TN. These patients usually describe a dull and almost continuous facial pain originating from different sites (Solaro & Messmer, 2010). Treatment with amitriptyline as a single bedtime dose for several months has been recommended (Solaro & Messmer, 2010).

18.3   Lhermitte's Sign

It has been estimated that 40% of MS patients will experience Lhermitte's sign at some point in their disease course (Al-Araji & Oger, 2005). Lhermitte's sign is a transient, usually self-limiting, paroxysmal sensation related to neck flexion that radiates down the spine and limbs. While symptoms after an episode will typically resolve in weeks to months it has persisted in rare instances for the rest of a patients disease course (Al-Araji & Oger, 2005). In a study of 122 MS patients who experienced Lhermitte's sign, no patient asked for treatment at any time during their episode (Al-Araji & Oger, 2005). In patients who require therapy, low dose carbamazepine has been recommended to help reduce the severity and frequency (Solaro & Messmer, 2010).

18.4   Painful Tonic Spasms

Painful tonic spasms (PTS) are distinct from the type of pain experienced with spasticity and occur in approximately 10% of MS patients. PTS usually occur at night and are triggered by movement. It typically involves only the extremities and is described as a cramping, pulling type pain. There have been few MS patient studies to assess the efficacy of treatments for PTS (see Table 9) and empiric treatment is common with anti-spasticity medications including baclofen, benzodiazepines, and carbamazepine (Restivo et al., 2003; Solaro & Messmer, 2010).

19   Mood Disorders

19.1   Depression

Depression occurs in approximately 40 to 50% of MS patients (Ben-Zacharia, 2011). The rate is higher than that observed in other chronic systemic neurologic illnesses, suggesting MS may have a unique pathophysiologic process causing depression (Samkoff & Goodman, 2011). The impact of depression on patients with MS is immense, potentially leading to impaired quality of life and relationships, deteriorating cognitive function, suicidal ideation and attempt, and reduced adherence with DMT (Feinstein, 2011). There has been a long-standing debate about whether DMT causes depression but data proving such a connection are unavailable and patients receiving DMT who develop depression should be treated appropriately without alteration or discontinuation of DMT (Feinstein, 2011).

Despite its prevalence, there have only been three studies that assess antidepressant use for depression in MS patients (see Table 10). Since data specific to the treatment of depression in MS patients are lacking, guidelines for treating depression in the general population are typically followed. SSRIs are considered first-line agents for the treatment of depression associated with MS. TCAs and serotonin plus norepinephrine reuptake inhibitors may be considered for the patient with concomitant neuropathic pain (Samkoff & Goodman, 2011).

Cognitive behavioral therapy (CBT) has been shown to be more effective than group-based therapy for MS-based depression (Mohr et al., 2001). Cognitive behavioral therapy may also be utilized as an adjunct to antidepressant medications (Samkoff & Goodman, 2011; Thompson et al., 2010).

19.2   Pseudobulbar Affect

Pseudobulbar affect is defined as episodes of involuntary and uncontrollable crying or laughing without an apparent trigger. This disorder has been estimated to affect approximately 10% of patients with MS (Ben-Zacharia, 2011). Only two medications have been studied for the treatment of this disorder in MS patients (see Table 10). One of these medications, a combination of dextromethorphan and quinidine (DMq), is the only FDA approved treatment for pseudobulbar affect.

Medication	Study design	Comments
Depression		
Sertraline	Prospective, open-label study (Mohr *et al.*, 2001)	Sertraline was compared to CBT and group psychotherapy. Sertraline was equally effective as CBT and more effective than group psychotherapy at improving depression scores. Drop-out rates were not significantly different between treatment groups (Mohr *et al.*, 2001).
Paroxetine	Randomized, double-blind, placebo-controlled study (Ehde *et al.*, 2008)	There were no significant differences in depression scores between placebo and paroxetine treatment arms. However, in those that completed the study, there was a better response with paroxetine compared to placebo suggesting paroxetine may be of benefit to a specific patient subgroup (Ehde *et al.*, 2008).
Desipramine	Randomized, double-blind, placebo-controlled study (Schiffer & Wineman, 1990)	All patients in this study received concurrent psychotherapy. Desipramine decreased depression scores significantly compared to placebo in one but not both depression rating scales used. Adverse events occurred in 12 of the patients receiving desipramine, but did not cause discontinuation of treatment (Schiffer & Wineman, 1990).
Pseudobulbar Affect		
DMq	Two randomized, double-blind, placebo-controlled studies (Panitch *et al.*, 2006; Pioro *et al.*, 2010)	DMq reduced the number of daily episodes compared to placebo. It also improved QOL, quality of relationships, and scores for a validated questionnaire for pseudobulbar affect (Panitch *et al.*, 2006; Pioro *et al.*, 2010). Overall, adverse events did not occur significantly more, with the exception of dizziness (Panitch *et al.*, 2006).
Amitriptyline	Double-blind, placebo-controlled, crossover study (Schiffer *et al.*, 1985)	8 of 12 patients experienced significant improvement with treatment (Schiffer *et al.*, 1985).

Table 10: Medications studied in MS for mood disorders

20   Fatigue

Fatigue is a common symptom occurring in an estimated 70 to 90% of MS patients and usually is worse during the afternoon (Ben-Zacharia, 2011; Zifko, 2004). Between 50 to 60% of patients with fatigue describe it is as their most debilitating symptom (Zifko, 2004). Fatigue is unrelated to the duration or disability of MS and may be transient or chronic in nature (Zifko, 2004). There are two types of fatigue in MS: primary and secondary. Primary fatigue occurs due to an unknown cause and typically requires treatment. Secondary fatigue can be due to a variety of different causes that should be assessed before treatment is initiated. Medications (particularly antispasticity agents, anticonvulsants, muscle relaxants, etc.), infections, depression, and sleep disorders are common secondary causes of fatigue (Zifko, 2004). Medications for the treatment of fatigue should be taken in the morning when possible, so as to not interrupt a patients sleep schedule (Ben-Zacharia, 2011).

Several medications have been studied in MS-related fatigue (see Table 11). Modafinil has been the most studied treatment of fatigue in MS patients, with predominantly favorable results. Amantadine has shown benefit in trials, but mild adverse events can occur in up to 40% of patients (Pucci *et al.*, 2007). Levocarnitine has recently shown improvements in fatigue scores with good tolerability, mainly in patients treated with DMT. Experts have also recommended using CNS stimulants such as methylphenidate or dextroamphetamine and amphetamine products (Ben-Zacharia, 2011; Samkoff & Goodman, 2011). Stimulating antidepressants, mainly the SSRIs, are recommended in patients suffering from depression-related fatigue (Ben-Zacharia, 2011; Zifko, 2004).

Medication	Study design	Comments
Modafinil	Two randomized, double-blind, placebo-controlled studies (Lange et al., 2009; Stankoff et al., 2005). Prospective, single-blind study (Rammohan et al., 2002). Prospective, open-label study (Zifko et al., 2002).	All four studies showed improvements in fatigue with modafinil treatment (Lange et al., 2009; Rammohan et al., 2002; Stankoff et al., 2005; Zifko et al., 2002). However, in one study, modafinil was no better than placebo (Stankoff et al., 2005). Effects were sustained up to 8 weeks (Lange et al., 2009), but another study had no improvement two weeks after a dose increase (Rammohan et al., 2002). Modafinil seems to be well tolerated (Zifko et al., 2002).
Amantadine	Two double-blind, placebo-controlled, crossover studies (Cohen et al., 1989; Rosenberg & Appenzeller, 1988). Two randomized, double-blind, placebo-controlled studies (Krupp et al., 1995; Murray, 1985).	Three studies showed significantly better subjective fatigue scores with amantadine compared to placebo (Krupp et al., 1995; Murray, 1985; Rosenberg & Appenzeller, 1988). In one study, with rating scales for fatigue, scores were improved in one rating scale compared to placebo but not another (Krupp et al., 1995). In another study, there was a nonsignificant trend toward overall reduction in fatigue for patients treated with amantadine versus placebo, and only overall energy level, concentration, problem solving, and sense of well-being were significantly improved (Cohen et al., 1989).
Levocarnitine	Prospective, open-label study (Lebrun et al., 2006). Randomized, double-blind, comparative, crossover study (Tomassini et al., 2004).	MS patients who have been administered DMT appear to have lower levels of carnitine. Despite this, both patients treated with DMT and those who were not had improved fatigue symptoms with levocarnitine treatment (Lebrun et al., 2006). Levocarnitine administration seems to improve fatigue scores significantly more than amantadine, and also looks to be better tolerated (Tomassini et al., 2004).

Table 11: Medications studied in MS for fatigue.

Although drug therapy for MS-related fatigue is an attractive treatment option, nonpharmacologic therapy should always be initiated first. Ensuring that a patient has a proper amount of sleep at night and a regular sleep schedule is important (Samkoff & Goodman, 2011; Thompson et al., 2010). Conducting strenuous activities in the morning, taking daytime naps or rest periods, and rearranging activities for the day are other interventions that can benefit patients (Ben-Zacharia, 2011; Thompson et al., 2010).

There is some evidence that an exercise program in MS patients with moderate disability results in an improvement in fatigue and overall quality of life (Nicholas & Rashid, 2012; Zifko, 2004). Exercise programs studied include mostly aerobic workouts, but resistance training has been studied as well. Since exercise has no known safety issues, it should be recommended and evaluated in all candidate patients before pharmacologic therapy is considered (Nicholas & Rashid, 2012; Zifko, 2004).

21   Spasticity

Spasticity is one of the most common symptoms in MS, reported to occur in up to 90% of patients at some point in their disease course (de Sa *et al.*, 2011). Spasms that are not controlled can lead to pain, reduced mobility, limited range of movement, and involuntary contractures (Thompson *et al.*, 2010). In contrast, spasticity may in some cases be beneficial to a MS patient by strengthening the stability of lower limbs that may be too weak to support weight in the absence of spasticity (de Sa *et al.*, 2011; Thompson *et al.*, 2010). Therefore, proper assessment must be performed before and routinely after spasticity treatment is initiated.

Physiotherapy is considered the foundation for the treatment of spasticity (de Sa *et al.*, 2011). Stretching, exercise, and repetitive movements are all techniques that can be beneficial (de Sa *et al.*, 2011; Samkoff & Goodman, 2011). Repeated functional electric stimulation to the thigh muscles also appears to help reduce spasticity (de Sa *et al.*, 2011).

Several agents have been evaluated for the treatment for spasticity in MS patients (see Table 12). While baclofen is typically the first pharmacologic agent prescribed for MS patients with spasticity, other agents including tizanidine and diazepam have been shown to be as effective as baclofen in comparative trials. However, diazepam is rarely used because of the profound sedation that accompanies treatment (Ben-Zacharia, 2011; Nicholas & Rashid, 2012; Samkoff & Goodman, 2011; Thompson *et al.*, 2010).

Limited data indicate gabapentin is especially well tolerated when used for spasticity in MS patients. Therefore, it may be a valid option in patients intolerant of other therapies. It may also be considered as an adjunct to other therapies. Dantrolene has been shown to be effective in a limited number of studies. However, it's poor safety profile has resulted in it being rarely used for treatment of MS related spasticity (Thompson *et al.*, 2010).

Botulinum toxin has demonstrated significant reduction in spasticity when injected locally into symptomatic muscles. Advantages of this therapy are minimum systemic side effects and long-lasting effects, however treatment is expensive (Nicholas & Rashid, 2012; Thompson *et al.*, 2010). It generally takes one to two weeks to reach full effect, but the benefit lasts 3 to 6 months in most cases depending on the injected dose and target muscle (Ben-Zacharia, 2011; Thompson *et al.*, 2010). Side effects that were more frequent than placebo in trials included diarrhea, back pain, and weakness of non-injected muscles.

Intrathecal baclofen was approved by the FDA in 1992 for treatment of spasticities that are spinal in nature and is administered by continuous infusion through an implantable pump. Intrathecal baclofen is an effective strategy that is employed when spasticity is intractable to other medications, when a patient is intolerable to other treatments, or in patients with severe disability (Ben-Zacharia, 2011; Samkoff & Goodman, 2011; Thompson *et al.*, 2010).

By administering baclofen intrathecally, adverse events associated with large dosages of oral baclofen are significantly reduced. Drowsiness occurs in only 21% of patients receiving intrathecal baclofen compared to over 60% of patients taking oral baclofen. The sole adverse effect more common with intrathecal compared to oral baclofen is hypotonia resulting in muscle weakness that occurs in 21% and 15% of patients, respectively (Lioresal tablet [package insert], 1998; Lioresal intrathecal [package insert], 2011). Intrathecal baclofen also appears to be safer in pregnancy than oral baclofen (Dalton et al., 2008).

A new oral mucosal spray (Sativex®; GW Pharmaceuticals, UK) that is a mixture of two different cannabinoids (Δ(9)-tetrahydrocannabinol and cannabidiol) has been approved in eight countries for the treatment of MS-related spasticity and is currently undergoing USFDA review for the same indication. It is generally used as add-on therapy for spasticity that is not well controlled. Adverse events associated with this therapy have included dizziness, disturbance in attention, impaired balance, and blurred vision (Nicholas & Rashid, 2012).

Medication	Studies	Results & Comments
Baclofen	Randomized, double-blind, placebo-controlled study (Sachais et al.,1977). Four randomized, double-blind, placebo-controlled, crossover studies (Brar et al., 1991; Feldman et al., 1978; Orsnes et al., 2000; Sawa & Paty, 1979)	Treatment with baclofen has been shown to improve spasticity with effects lasting up to three years in studies (Brar et al., 1991; Feldman et al., 1978; Orsnes et al., 2000; Sachais et al., 1977; Sawa & Paty, 1979). Implementing stretching exercises concurrently with baclofen may help improve spasticity more than treatment with baclofen alone (Brar et al., 1991). Baclofen may also be used in non-ambulatory patients with advanced disease, as reducing spasms has been shown to make immobility more bearable (Feldman et al., 1978). Adverse events are common, but well tolerated in the studies (Orsnes et al., 2000; Sachais et al., 1977; Sawa & Paty, 1979). A common and problematic adverse event is increased muscle weakness. Therefore, baclofen should be avoided in some patients who require spasticity for support and daily function (Sawa & Paty, 1979). In contrast, it may actually help other patients who have gait disorders (Orsnes et al., 2000). Therefore, it is important to properly stratify which patients will receive benefit from baclofen treatment.
Tizanidine	Four randomized, double-blind, placebo-controlled studies (Lapierre et al., 1987; Nance et al., 1997; Smith et al., 1994; United Kingdom Tizanidine Trial Group, 1994). Randomized, double-blind, placebo-controlled, crossover study (Vakhapova et al., 2010).	Only one study did not show significant improvements in spasticity with tizanidine treatment (Smith et al., 1994). All other studies have shown improvements in spasticity and hyperreflexia (Lapierre et al., 1987; Nance et al., 1997; United Kingdom Tizanidine Trial Group, 1994; Vakhapova et al., 2010). However, studies that assessed changes in functional status or activities of daily living showed no differences compared to placebo (Lapierre et al., 1987; United Kingdom Tizanidine Trial Group, 1994). Adverse events are dose-dependent and the most common are dry mouth and sedation (Lapierre et al., 1987; Nance et al., 1997). One study has shown that nighttime administration of tizanidine improves spasticity without the adverse effect of daytime somnolence (Vakhapova et al., 2010).
Baclofen vs. Tizanidine	Three randomized, controlled studies (Eyssette et al., 1988; Smolenski et al., 1981; Stien et al., 1987). Two randomized, double-blind, crossover studies (Bass et al., 1988; Hoogstraten et al., 1988).	Baclofen and tizanidine appear to be equally effective in reducing muscle spasms (Bass et al., 1988; Eyssette et al., 1988; Hoogstraten et al., 1988; Smolenski et al., 1981; Stien et al., 1987). The most common, serious adverse effect of baclofen is muscle weakness (Bass et al., 1988; Hoogstraten et al., 1988; Smolenski et al., 1981). In contrast, muscle strength seems to improve with tizanidine; however, dry mouth and sedation are frequent, problematic adverse events (Bass et al., 1988; Hoogstraten et al., 1988; Smolenski et al., 1981).
Baclofen vs. Diazepam	Two randomized, controlled studies (Cartlidge et al., 1974; From & Heltberg, 1975)	Both diazepam and baclofen appear to be equally effective in treating spasticity (Cartlidge et al., 1974; From & Heltberg, 1975). The rates of adverse events between the two drugs are about equal. However, diazepam appears to cause more sedation, while baclofen has a broader range of adverse events (From & Heltberg, 1975).
Intrathecal baclofen	Systematic Review (Beard et al., 2003). Two long-term follow-up	15 studies were included in a 2003 systematic review. Patients included all had severe spasticity unresponsive to oral therapy. All 15 studies showed impressive outcomes in terms of reducing spasticity for

	studies (Rekand & Grønning, 2011; Sadiq & Wang, 2006).	patients treated with intrathecal baclofen. However, complications were frequent and occurred primarily with the pump and catheter. Adverse events due to baclofen were uncommon (Beard *et al.*, 2003). In two long-term follow-up studies, intrathecal baclofen had maintained it's benefit on spasticity for up to 12 to 13 years in some cases (Rekand & Grønning, 2011; Sadiq & Wang, 2006). Intrathecal baclofen therapy does not seem to be associated with loss of ambulatory function (Sadiq & Wang, 2006).
Gabapentin	Two randomized, double-blind, placebo-controlled, crossover studies (Cutter *et al.*, 2000; Mueller *et al.*, 1997)	Significant improvements in spasticity were seen in both studies for all outcomes measured (Cutter *et al.*, 2000; Mueller *et al.*, 1997). In one study, gabapentin was used as an add-on therapy if the patient was already on current oral therapies for spasticity (Mueller *et al.*, 1997). Gabapentin has these favorable effects without causing worsening concentration or fatigue (Cutter *et al.*, 2000).
Botulinum Toxin	Two randomized, double-blind, placebo-controlled, crossover studies (Grazko *et al.*, 1995; Snow *et al.*, 1990). Randomized, double-blind, placebo-controlled study (Hyman *et al.*, 2000). Randomized, single-blind, placebo-controlled study (Giovannelli *et al.*, 2007).	In all studies, botulinum toxin improved spasticity outcomes in MS patients and was well tolerated (Giovannelli *et al.*, 2007; Grazko *et al.*, 1995; Hyman *et al.*, 2000; Snow *et al.*, 1990). Improvement in nursing care was also noted (Snow *et al.*, 1990). In one study, botulinum toxin when added to oral treatments did not decrease spasticity more than placebo but did significantly decrease muscle tone (Hyman *et al.*, 2000). Efficacy and adverse events appear to be dose-dependent (Hyman *et al.*, 2000; Sobolewski, 2007). When exercise and stretching regimens are added to botulinum toxin treatment, there is greater improvement in spasticity than treatment with botulinum toxin alone (Giovannelli *et al.*, 2007).
Oral Cannabinoids	Meta-analysis (Wade *et al.*, 2010). Randomized, double-blind, placebo-controlled study (Novotna *et al.*, 2011). Open-label follow-up safety trial (Serpell *et al.*, 2012).	Three randomized, placebo-controlled trials were evaluated in the meta-analysis (Wade *et al.*, 2010). A more recent trial only included patients who had initially responded to treatment with nabiximols (Novotna *et al.*, 2011). Results of all four studies revealed a greater reduction in spasticity symptoms when treated with nabiximols compared to placebo as an add-on to current therapies (Novotna *et al.*, 2011; Wade *et al.*, 2010). Up to 79% of patients can experience some type of adverse event (Wade *et al.*, 2010). These are usually mild, but up to 14% of patients discontinue therapy because of them (Serpell *et al.*, 2012). Dizziness (24.7 %) and fatigue (12.3 %) are the most common events (Serpell *et al.*, 2012). Serious adverse events are rare and have resolved upon discontinuation of treatment. In patients responding to treatment, the reduction in spasticity was shown to persist up to a year (Serpell *et al.*, 2012).

Table 12: Medications studied in MS for spasticity.

22   Impaired Gait

Impairment of ambulation may have a sudden onset or gradually worsen over time in MS (Ben-Zacharia, 2011). It has been reported that 64% of MS patients have trouble walking at least twice weekly (Samkoff

& Goodman, 2011). The mainstay of therapy has traditionally been physiotherapy and this treatment modality should always be considered for patients with ambulation difficulties (Ben-Zacharia, 2011; Thompson *et al.*, 2010).

Dalfampridine was approved by the FDA in 2010 for improving ambulation in MS patients. Approval was based on two phase III clinical trials. In one study, 229 patients were treated with dalfampridine and 72 with placebo (Goodman *et al.*, 2008). Efficacy was evaluated by the time it took to walk 25 feet. Significant benefit was observed with dalfampridine, with 35% of patients responding. The responders improved walking speed by 25%. In the second study, efficacy was assessed by the same 25-foot walking test (Goodman *et al.*, 2010). In this study, 43% of individuals receiving dalfampridine improved their ambulation with a 25% increase in their walking speed. Although this increase in walking speed is statistically significant, its clinical significance is debatable and identifying which individuals would be responders remains difficult. Nevertheless, this is the first pharmacologic therapy that has shown promising results for impaired gait in MS. Due to the medication's potential to cause seizures at high doses, it is contraindicated in patients with impaired renal function or a history of seizures. Experts recommend a trial of 2 to 4 weeks to determine if the drug is effective (Samkoff & Goodman, 2011).

References

Ablashi, D.V., Lapps, W., Kaplan, M., Whitman, J.E., Richert, J.R., & Pearson, G.R. (1998). Human Herpesvirus-6 (HHV-6) infection in multiple sclerosis: a preliminary report. Multiple Sclerosis, 4, 490-496.

Akhyani, N., Berti, R., Brennan, M.B., Soldan, S.S., Eaton, J.M., McFarland, H.F., & Jacobson, S. (2000). Tissue distribution and variant characterization of human herpesvirus (HHV)-6: Increased prevalence of HHV-6A in patients with multiple sclerosis. Journal of Infectious Disease, 182, 1321-1325.

Al-Araji, A.H. & Oger, J. (2005). Reappraisal of Lhermitte's sign in multiple sclerosis. Multiple Sclerosis,11(4), 398-402.

Alotaibi, S., Kennedy, J., Tellier, R., Stephens, D., & Banwell, B. (2004). Epstein-Barr virus in pediatric multiple sclerosis. Journal of the American Medical Association, 291, 1875-1879.

Alter, A., Duddy, M., & Hebert, S. et al. (2003). Determinants of human B cell migration across brain endothelial cells. Journal of Immunology, 170, 4497-4505.

Amend, B., Hennenlotter, J., Schäfer, T., Horstmann, M., Stenzl, A., & Sievert, K.D. (2008). Effective treatment of neurogenic detrusor dysfunction by combined high-dosed antimuscarinics without increased side-effects. European Urology, 53(5), 1021-1028.

Anderson, O., Elovaara, I., & Färkkilä, M., et al. (2004). Multicentre, randomised, double blind, placebo-controlled, phase III study of weekly, low dose, subcutaneous interferon beta-1a in secondary progressive multiple sclerosis. Journal of Neurology, Neurosurgery, and Psychiatry,75, 706-710.

Barak, Y. & Achiron, A. (2002). Effect of interferon-beta-1b on cognitive functions in multiple sclerosis. European Neurology, 47(1), 11-14.

Baranzini, S.E. (2011). Revealing the genetic basis of multiple sclerosis: are we there yet? Current Opinion   Genetics   & Development, 21, 317-324.

Bass, B., Weinshenker, B., Rice, G.P., Noseworthy, J.H., Cameron, M.G., Hader, W., et al. (1988). Tizanidine versus baclofen in the treatment of spasticity in patients with multiple sclerosis. The Canadian Journal of Neurological Sciences, 15(1), 15-19.

Batoulis, H., Recks, M.S., Addicks, K., & Kuerten, S. (2011). Experimental autoimmune encephalomyelitis – achievements and prospective advances. APMIS,119, 819-830.

Baxter, A.G. (2007). The origin and application of experimental autoimmune encephalomyelitis. Nature, 7, 904-912.

Beard, S., Hunn, A., & Wight, J. (2003). Treatments for spasticity and pain in multiple sclerosis: a systematic review. Health Technology Assessment, 7(40), 1-111.

Benedict, R.H., Munschauer, F., Zarevics, P., Erlanger, D., Rowe, V., Feaster, T., et al. (2008). Effects of l-amphetamine sulfate on cognitive function in multiple sclerosis patients. Journal of Neurology, 255(6), 848-852.

Berghams, N., Nuyts, A., Uyttenhove, C., Van Snick, J., Opdenakker, G., & Heremans, H. (2011). Interferon-γ orchestrates the number and function of Th17 cells in experimental autoimmune encephalomyelitis. Journal of Interferon & Cytokine Research, 31(7):575-587.

Bermel, R.A. & Rudick, R.A. (2007). Interferon-β treatment for multiple sclerosis. Neurotherapeutics,4:633-646.

Bettelli, E., Oukka, M., & Kuchroo, V.K. (2007). T_H-17 cells in the circle of immunity and autoimmunity. Nature Immunology, 8(4):345-350.

Ben-Zacharia, A.B. (2011). Therapeutics for multiple sclerosis symptoms. The Mount Sinai Journal of Medicine, New York, 78(2), 176-191.

Blanchette, F. & Neuhaus, O. (2008) Glatiramer Acetate. Evidence for a dual mechanism of action. Journal of Neurology, 255:26-36.

Bornstein, M.B., Miller, A., Slagle, S., Weitzman, M., Crystal, H., Drexler, E., Keilson, M., Merriam, A., Wassertheil-Smoller, S., & Spada, V. et al. (1987). A pilot trial of Cop 1 in exacerbating-remitting multiple sclerosis. New England Journal of Medicine, 317:408-414.

Bosma, R., Wynia, K., Havlíková, E., De Keyser, J., & Middel, B. (2005). Efficacy of desmopressin in patients with multiple sclerosis suffering from bladder dysfunction: a meta-analysis. Acta Neurologica Scandinavica, 112(1), 1-5.

Brar, S.P., Smith, M.B., Nelson, L.M., Franklin, G.M., & Cobble, N.D. (1991). Evaluation of treatment protocols on minimal to moderate spasticity in multiple sclerosis. Archives of Physical Medicine and Rehabilitation, 72(3), 186-189.

Breij, M.H., Brink, B.P., & Veerhuis, R. et al. (2008). Homogeneity of active demyelinating lesions in established multiple sclerosis. Annals of Neurology, 63,16-25.

Breuer, B., Pappagallo, M., Knotkova, H., Guleyupoglu, N., Wallenstein, S., & Portenoy, R.K. (2007). A randomized, double blind, placebo-controlled, two-period, crossover, pilot trial of lamotrigine in patients with central pain due to multiple sclerosis. Clinical Therapeutics, 29(9), 2022-2030.

Browning, J.L. (2006). B cells move to center stage: novel opportunities for autoimmune disease treatment. Nature Reviews. Drug Discovery, 5(7):564-576.

Bruneau, J.M., Yea, C.M., Spinella-Jaegle, S., Fudali, C., Woodward, K., & Robson, P.A., et al. (1998). Purification of human dihydro-orotate dehydrogenase and its inhibition by A77 1726, the active metabolite of leflunomide. The Biochemical Journal, 336(2):299-303.

Burton, P.R., Tobin, M.D., & Hopper, J.L. (2005). Key concepts in genetic epidemiology. Lancet, 366, 941-951.

Butler, M.A. & Bennett, T.L. (2003). In Search of a Conceptualization of Multiple Sclerosis: A Historical Perspective. Neuropsychology Review. 13, 93-112.

Cartlidge, N.E., Hudgson, P., & Weightman, D. (1974). A comparison of baclofen and diazepam in the treatment of spasticity. Journal of the Neurological Sciences, 23(1), 17-24.

Challoner, P.B., Smith, K.T, Parker, J.D., MacLeod, D.L., Coulter, S.N., & Rose, T.M., et al. (1995). Plaque- associated expression of human herpesvirus 6 in multiple sclerosis. Proceedings of the National Academy of Sciences of the United States of America, 92, 7440-7444.

Chen, S.J., Wang, Y.L., Fan, H.C., Lo, W.T., Wang, C.C., & Sytwu, H.K. (2012). Current status of the immunomodulation and immunomediated therapeutic strategies for multiple sclerosis. Clinical and Developmental Immunology, Volume 2012 (2012), Article ID 970789, 16 pages doi:10.1155/2012/970789

Cianchetti, C., Zuddas, A., Randazzo, A.P., Perra, L., & Marrosu, M.G. (1999). Lamotrigine adjunctive therapy in painful phenomena in MS: preliminary observations. Neurology, 53(2), 433.

Coggrave, M., Wiesel, P.H., & Norton, C. (2006). Management of faecal incontinence and constipation in adults with central neurological diseases. Cochrane Database of Systematic Reviews (Online), (2), CD002115.

Cohen, R.A. & Fisher, M. (1989). Amantadine treatment of fatigue associated with multiple sclerosis. Archives of Neurology, 46(6), 676-680.

Cohen, J.A., Barkhof, F., & Comi, G., et al for the TRANSFORMS Study Group. (2010). Oral fingolimod or intramuscular interferon for relapsing multiple sclerosis. New England Journal of Medicine, 362: 402-415.

Cohen, J.A., Imrey, P.B., & Calabresi, P.A., et al for the ACT Investigators. (2009). Results of Avonex Combination Trial(ACT) in relapsing-remitting MS. Neurology, 72:535-541.

Comi, G., Filippi, M., & Wolinsky, J. (2001). European/Canadian multicenter, double-blind, randomized, placebo-controlled study of the effectds of glatiramer acetate on magnetic resonance imaging-Measured disease activity and burden in patients with relapsing multiple sclerosis. European/Canadian Glatiramer Acetate Study Group. Annals of Neurology,49:290-297.

Comi, G., Filippi, M., Barkof, F., Durelli, L., Edan, G., Fernandez, O., et al. (2001) Effect of early interferon treatment on conversion to definite multiple sclerosis: a randomised study. Lancet 357:1576-1582.

Comi, G., Martinelli, V., Rodegher, M., Moiola, L., Bajenaru, O., Carra, A., et al. (2002) Effect of glatiramer acetate on conversion to clinically definite multiple sclerosis in patients with clinically isolated syndrome (PreCISe study); a randomised, double-blind, placebo-controlled trial. Lancet 374, 1503-1511.

Compston, A. & Coles, A. (2002). Multiple sclerosis. Lancet 359, 1221-1231.

Cordell, H.J. & Clayton, D.G. (2005). Genetic epidemiology 3: Genetic association studies. Lancet, 366, 1121-1131.

Correale, J., Rush, C., Amengual, A., & Goicochea, M.T. (2005). Mitoxantrone as rescue therapy in worsening relapsing remitting MS patients receiving IFN-β. Journal of Neuroimmunology,162:173-183.

Correale,J. & Villa, A. (2008). Isolation and characterization of CD8+ regulatory T cells in multiple sclerosis. Journal of Neuroimmunology, 195(1-2):121-134.

Croxford, A.L., Kurschus, F.C., & Waisman, A. (2011). Mouse models for multiple sclerosis: historical facts and future implications. Biochimica et Biophysica Acta 1812(2):177-183.

Cruz, F., Herschorn, S., Aliotta, P., Brin, M., Thompson, C., Lam, W., et al. (2011). Efficacy and safety of onabotulinumtoxin A in patients with urinary incontinence due to neurogenic detrusor overactivity: a randomised, double-blind, placebo-controlled trial. European Urology, 60(4), 742-750.

Cutter, N.C., Scott, D.D., Johnson, J.C., & Whiteneck, G. (2000). Gabapentin effect on spasticity in multiple sclerosis: a placebo controlled, randomized trial. Archives of Physical Medicine and Rehabilitation, 81(2), 164-169.

Dalakas, M.C. (2008). B cells as therapeutic targets in autoimmune neurological disorders. Nature Clinical Practice. Neurology, 10:557-567.

Dalakas, M.C. (2008). Invited article: inhibition of B cell functions implications for neurology. Neurology, 70:2252-2260.

Dalton, C.M., Keenan, E., Jarrett, L., Buckley, L., & Stevenson, V.L. (2008). The safety of baclofen in pregnancy: intrathecal therapy in multiple sclerosis. Multiple Sclerosis, 14(4), 571-572.

DasGupta, R. & Fowler, C.J.(2003). Bladder, bowel and sexual dysfunction in multiple sclerosis: management strategies. Drugs, 63(2), 153-166.

DasGupta, R., Wiseman, O.J., Kanabar, G., Fowler, C.J., & Mikol, D.D. (2004). Efficacy of sildenafil in the treatment of female sexual dysfunction due to multiple sclerosis. The Journal of Urology, 171(3), 1189-1193.

de Sa, J.C., Airas, L., Bartholome, E., Grigoriadis, N., Mattle, H., Oreja-Guevara, C., et al. (2011). Symptomatic therapy in multiple sclerosis: a review for a multimodal approach in clinical practice. Therapeutic Advances in Neurological Disorders,4(3), 139-168

Deffontaines-Rufin, S., Weil, M., Verollet, D., Peyrat, L., & Amarenco, G. (2011). Botulinum toxin A for the treatment of neurogenic detrusor overactivity in multiple sclerosis patients. International Brazilian Journal of Urology, 37(5), 642-648.

Desai, S. & Barton, R. (1989). Pharmacological comparison of active and passive experimental allergic encephalomyelitis in the rat. Agent and Actions, 27, 351-355.

Detels, R., Visscher, B.R., Hile, R., Malmgren, R.M., Dudley, J.P., & Coulson, A.H. (1978). Multiple sclerosis and age at migration. American Journal of Epidemiology,108:386-393.

Disanto, G., Morahan, J.M., Barnett, M.H., Giovannoni, G., & Ramagopalan, S.V. (2012). The evidence for a role of B cells in multiple sclerosis. Neurology, 78(11):823-832.

DMKG study group. (2003). Misoprostol in the treatment of trigeminal neuralgia associated with multiple sclerosis. Journal of Neurology, 250(5), 542-545.

D'Netto, M.J., Ward, H., & Morrison, K.M., et al. (2009). Risk alleles for multiple sclerosis in multiplex families. Neurology, 72, 1984-1988.

Durelli, L., Conti, L., & Clerico, M. et al. (2009). T-helper 17 cells expand in multiple sclerosis and are inhibited by interferon beta. Annals of Neurology, 65(5), 499-509.

Ehde, D.M., Kraft, G.H., Chwastiak, L., Sullivan, M.D., Gibbons, L.E., & Bombardier, C.H. (2008). Efficacy of paroxetine in treating major depressive disorder in persons with multiple sclerosis. General Hospital Psychiatry, 30(1), 40-48.

Endharti, A.T., Shi, R.Z., & Fukuoka, Y. et al. (2005) Cutting edge: $CD8^+ CD122^+$ regulatory cells produce IL-10 to suppress IFN-gamma production and proliferation of $CD8^+$ T cells. Journal of Immunology, 175, 7093-7097.

Englehardt, B. (2006). Molecular mechanisms involved in T cell migration across the blood-brain barrier. Journal of Neural Transmission, 113:477-485.

Eyssette, M., Rohmer, F., Serratrice, G., Warter, J.M., & Boisson, D. (1988). Multi-centre, double-blind trial of a novel antispastic agent, tizanidine, in spasticity associated with multiple sclerosis. Current Medical Research and Opinion, 10(10), 699-708.

Fader, M., Glickman, S., Haggar, V., Barton, R., Brooks, R., Malone-Lee, J. (2007). Intravesical atropine compared to oral oxybutynin for neurogenic detrusor overactivity: a double-blind, randomized crossover trial. The Journal of Urology, 177(1), 208-213.

Falah, M., Madsen, C., Holbech, J.V., & Sindrup, S.H. (2012). A randomized, placebo-controlled trial of levetiracetam in central pain in multiple sclerosis. European Journal of Pain, 16(6), 860-869.

Feinstein, A. (2011). Multiple sclerosis and depression. Multiple Sclerosis, 17(11), 1276-1281.

Feldman, R.G., Kelly-Hayes, M., Conomy, J.P., & Foley, J.M. (1978). Baclofen for spasticity in multiple sclerosis. Double-blind crossover and three-year study. Neurology, 28(11), 1094-1098.

Fernald, G.H., Yeh, R.F., Hauser, S.L. , Oksenberg, J.R., & Baranzini, S.E. (2005). Mapping gene activity in complex disorders: Integration of expression and genomic scans for multiple sclerosis. Journal of Neuroimmunology, 167, 157-169.

Ferrante, P., Mancuso, R., Pagani, E., Guerini, F.R., Calvo, M.G., Saresella, M., Speciale, L ., & Caputo, D. (2000). Molecular evidences for a role of HSV-1 in multiple sclerosis clinical acute attack. Journal of Neurovirology, 6 Suppl 2, S109-S114.

Fillipi M, Wolinsky JS, Gomi G. CORAL study group. (2006). Effects of oral glatiramer acetate on clinical and MRI-monitored disease activity in patients with relapsing multiple sclerosis: a multicentre,double-blind, randomized, placebo-controlled study. Lancet Neurology, 5:213-220.

Fischer, J.S., Priore, R.L., Jacobs, L.D., Cookfair, D.L., Rudick, R.A., Herndon, R.M., et al. (2000). Neuropsychological effects of interferon beta-1a in relapsing multiple sclerosis. Multiple Sclerosis Collaborative Research Group. Annals of Neurology, 48(6), 885-892.

Fowler, C.J., Miller, J.R., Sharief, M.K., Hussain, I.F., Stecher, V.J., & Sweeney, M. (2005). A double blind, randomised study of sildenafil citrate for erectile dysfunction in men with multiple sclerosis. Journal of Neurology, Neurosurgery, and Psychiatry, 76(5), 700-705.

Fowler, C.J., Panicker, J.N., Drake, M., Harris, C., Harrison, S.C., Kirby, M., et al. (2009). A UK consensus on the management of the bladder in multiple sclerosis. Postgraduate Medical Journal, 85(1008), 552-559.

Freedman, M.S., Thompson, E.J., & Deisenhammer, F., et al. (2005). Recommended standard of cerebrospinal fluid analysis in the diagnosis of multiple sclerosis: a consensus statement. Archives of Neurology, 62:865-870.

Frohman, E.M., Racke, M.K., & Raine, C.S. (2006). Multiple Sclerosis- The plaque and its pathogenesis. New England Journal of Medicine, 354:942-955.

Frohman, E.M., Goodin, D.S., & Calabresi, P.A., et al. (2003). The utility of MRI in suspected MS: Report of the Therapeutics and Technology Assessment Subcommittee of the American Academy of Neurology. Neurology, 61:602-611.

From, A. & Heltberg, A. (1975). A double-blind trial with baclofen (Lioresal) and diazepam in spasticity due to multiple sclerosis. Acta Neurologica Scandinavica. 51(2). 158-166.

Gajewski, J.B. & Awad, S.A. (1986). Oxybutynin versus propantheline in patients with multiple sclerosis and detrusor hyperreflexia. The Journal of Urology, 135(5), 966-968.

Giovannelli, M., Borriello, G., Castri, P., Prosperini, L., & Pozzilli, C. (2007). Early physiotherapy after injection of botulinum toxin increases the beneficial effects on spasticity in patients with multiple sclerosis. Clinical Rehabilitation, 21(4), 331-337.

GlaxoSmithKline. Ofatumumab Subcutaneous Administration in Subjects With Relapsing-Remitting Multiple Sclerosis (MIRROR). In: Clinical Trials.gov [Internet]. Bethesda (MD): National Library of Medicine (US). 2000-[Cited 2012 Nov 14]. Available from: http://www.clinicaltrials.gov/ct2/show/NCT01457924 NLM Identifier: NCT01457924.

Goodin, D.S. & Bates, D. (2009). Treatment of early multiple sclerosis: the value of treatment initiation after a first clinical episode. Multiple Sclerosis 15:1175-1182.

Goodin, D.S., Frohman, E.M., & Garmany, G.P. Jr., et al. (2002). Disease modifying therapies in multiple sclerosis: report of the Therapeutics and Technology Assessment Subcommittee of the American Academy of Neurology and the MS Council for Clinical Practice Guidelines. Neurology, 58,169–178.

Goodman, A.D., Brown, T.R., Cohen, J.A., Krupp, L.B., Schapiro, R., Schwid, S.R., et al. (2008). Dose comparison trial of sustained-release fampridine in multiple sclerosis. Neurology, 71(15), 1134-1141.

Goodman, A.D., Rossman,H., & Bar-Or. A., et al for the GLANCE investigators. (2009). GLANCE results of a phase 2, randomized, double-blind, placebo-controlled study. Neurology, 72, 806-812.

Goodman, A.D., Brown, T.R., Edwards, K.R., Krupp, L.B., Schapiro, R.T., Cohen, R., et al. (2010). A phase 3 trial of extended release oral dalfampridine in multiple sclerosis. Annals of Neurology, 68(4), 494-502.

Gourraud, P.A., Harbo, H.F., Hauser, S.L., & Baranzini, S.E. (2012). The genetics of multiple sclerosis: an up-to-date review. Immunological Reviews 248, 87-103.

Grazko, M.A., Polo, K.B., & Jabbari, B. (1995). Botulinum toxin A for spasticity, muscle spasms, and rigidity. Neurology, 45(4), 712-717.

Greer J.M., Csurhes P.A., Cameron, K.D., McCombe, P.A., Good, M.F., & Pender, M.P. (1997). Increased immunoreactivity to two overlapping peptides of myelin proteolipid protein in multiple sclerosis. Brain, 120, 1447-1460.

Habek, M., Karni, A., Balash, Y., & Gurevich, T. (2010). The place of the botulinum toxin in the management of multiple sclerosis. Clinical Neurology and Neurosurgery, 112(7), 592-596.

Harel, Y., Appleboim, N., Lavie, M., & Achiron, A. (2009). Single dose of methylphenidate improves cognitive performance in multiple sclerosis patients with impaired attention process. Journal of the Neurological Sciences, 276(1-2), 38-40.

Hase, H., Kanno, Y., & Kojima, M. et al. (2004). BAFF/BLyS can potentiate B-cell selection with the B-cell coreceptor complex. Blood 103(6), 2257-2265.

Hauser, S.L., Bhan, A.K., Gilles, F., Kemp, M., Kerr, C., & Weiner, H.L. (1986) Immunohistochemical analysis of the cellular infiltrate in multiple sclerosis lesions. Annals of Neurology, 19(6):578-587.

Hauser, S.L. & Oksenberg, J.R. (2006). The neurobiology of multiple sclerosis: genes, inflammation, and neurodegeneration. Neuron 52:61-76.

Havrdova, E., Zivadinov, R., & Krasensky, J., et al. (2009) Randomized study of interferon beta-1a, low-dose azathioprine, and low-dose corticosteroids in multiple sclerosis. Multiple Sclerosis, 15:965-976.

Hedegaard, C.J., Krakauer, M., Bendtzen, K., Lund, H., Sellenbjerg, F., & Nielsen, C.H. (2008). T helper cell type 1 (Th1), Th2, and Th17 responses to myelin basic protein and disease activity in multiple sclerosis. Immunology 125(2):161-169.

Hernan, M.A., Zhang, S.M., & Lipworth, L., et al. (2001). Multiple sclerosis and age at infection with common viruses. Epidemiology, 12, 301–306.

Hoffjan, S. & Akkad, D.A. (2010). The genetics of multiple sclerosis: An update 2010. Molecular and Cellular Probes, 24:237-243.

Hoffman La Roche. A Study of Ocrelizumab in Comparison With Interferon Beta-1a (Rebif) in Patients With Relapsing Multiple Sclerosis. In: Clinical Trials.gov [Internet]. Bethesda (MD): National Library of Medicine (US). 2000- [Cited 2012 Nov 14]. Available from: http://www.clinicaltrials.gov/ct2/show/NCT01247324 NLM Identifier: NCT01247324

Hofstetter, H.H., Ibrahim, S.M., & Koczan, D., et al. (2005). Therapeutic efficacy of IL-17 neutralization in murine experimental autoimmune encephalomyelitis. Cellular Immunology, 237(2), 123-130.

Holman, D.W., Klein, R.S., & Ransohoff, R.M. (2011). The blood-brain barrier, chemokines, and multiple sclerosis. Biochimica et Biophysica Acta, 1812(2), 220-230.

Hooge, J.P. & Redekop, W.K. (1995). Trigeminal neuralgia in multiple sclerosis. Neurology, 45(7), 1294-1296.

Hoogstraten, M.C., van der Ploeg, R.J., vd Burg, W., Vreeling, A., van Marle, S., & Minderhoud, J.M. (1988). Tizanidine versus baclofen in the treatment of spasticity in multiple sclerosis patients. Acta Neurologica Scandinavica, 77(3), 224-230.

Houtchens, M.K., Richert, J.R., Sami, A., & Rose, J.W. (1997). Open label gabapentin treatment for pain in multiple sclerosis. Multiple Sclerosis, 3(4), 250-253.

Howard-Thompson, A. (2012). Nonprescription medications. In APhA: Complete review for pharmacy 9th ed. Washington, DC: American Pharmacists Association. (pp. 631-658).

Huolman, S., Hämäläinen, P., Vorobyev, V., Ruutiainen, J., Parkkola, R., Laine, T., et al. (2011). The effects of rivastigmine on processing speed and brain activation in patients with multiple sclerosis and subjective cognitive fatigue. Multiple Sclerosis, 17(11), 1351-1361.

Hyman, N., Barnes, M., Bhakta, B., Cozens, A., Bakheit, M., Kreczy-Kleedorfer, B., et al. (2000). Botulinum toxin (Dysport) treatment of hip adductor spasticity in multiple sclerosis: a prospective, randomised, double blind, placebo controlled, dose ranging study. Journal of Neurology, Neurosurgery, and Psychiatry, 68(6), 707-712.

Iaffaldano P, Viterbo RG, Paolicelli D, Lucchese G, Portaccio E, Goretti B, et al. (2012). Impact of natalizumab on cognitive performances and fatigue in relapsing multiple sclerosis: a prospective, open-label, two years observational study. PLoS One. 7(4). e35843.

The IFNB Multiple Sclerosis Study Group. (1993). Interferon beta-1b is effective in relapsing-remitting multiple sclerosis: I. clinical results of a multicenter, randomized, double-blind, placebo-controlled trial. Neurology 43, 655-661.

Iman, S.A., Guyton, M.K., & Haque, A., et al. (2007). Increased calpain correlates with Th1 cytokine profile in PBMCs from MS patients. Journal of Neuroimmunology 190, 139-145.

Jacobs, L.D., Cookfair, D.L., & Rudick, R.A., et al, and The Multiple Sclerosis Collaborative Research Group. (1996). Intramuscular interferon beta-1a for disease progression in relapsing multiple sclerosis. Annals of Neurology, 39, 285-294.

Jacobs, L.D., Beck, R.W., Simon, J.H., Kinkel, R.P., Brownscheidle, C.M., Murray, T.J., et al. (2000). Intramuscular interferon beta-1a therapy initiated during a first demyelinating event in multiple sclerosis. CHAMPS Study Group. New England Journal Medicine 343 (13):898-904.

Jersild, C., Hansen, G.S., Svejgaard, A., Fog, T., Thomsen, M., & Dupont, B. (1973). Histocompatibility determinants in multiple sclerosis, with special reference to clinical course. Lancet 2, 1221-1225.

Jilek, S., Schluep, M., Meylan, P., Vingerhoets, F., Guignard, L., & Monney, A., et al. (2008) Strong EBV-specific CD8+ T-cell response in patients with early multiple sclerosis. Brain 131, 1712-1721.

Johnson, K.P., Brook, B.R., Cohen, J.A., Ford, C.C., Goldstein, J., Lisak, R.P., Myers, L.W., Panitch, H.S., Rose, J.W., & Schiffer, R.B., et al. (1995). Copolymer 1 reduces relapse rate and improves disability in relapsing-remitting multiple sclerosis: Results of a phase III multicenter, double-blind, placebo-controlled trial. Neurology, 45,1268-1276.

Kakalacheva, K., Münz, C., & Lünemann, J.D. (2011). Viral triggers of multiple sclerosis. Biochimica et Biophysica Acta, 1812(2),132-140.

Kalled, S.L. (2005). The role of BAFF in immune function and implications for autoimmunity. Annual Review of Immunology, 204, 43-54.

Kalled, S.L. (2006). Impact of the BAFF. BR3 axis on B cell survival, germinal center maintenance and antibody production. Seminars in Immunology, 18(5), 290-296.

Kampman, M.T., & Brustad, M. (2008). Vitamin D: a candidate for the environmental effect in multiple sclerosis-observations from Norway. Neuroepidemiology, 30, 140-146.

Kappos, L., Radue, E.W., & O'Connor ,P., et al for the FREEDOMS Study Group. (2010). A placebo-controlled trial of oral fingolimod in relapsing multiple sclerosis. New England Journal of Medicine, 362:387-401.

Kappos, L., Weinshenker, B., & Pozzilli, C., et al: European (EU-SPMS) Interferon beta-1b in Secondary Progressive Multiple Sclerosis Trial Steering Committee and Independent Advisory Board; North American (NA-SPMS) Interferon beta-1b in Secondary Progressive Multiple Sclerosis Trials Steering Committee and Independent Advisory Board. (2001). Inteferon beta-1b in secondary progressive MS: a combined analysis of the two trials. Neurology, 56:1496-1504.

Kappos, L., Polman, C.H., Freedman, M.S., Edan, G., Hartung, H.P., Miller, D.H., et al. (2006) Treatment with interferion beta-1b delays conversion to clinically definite and McDonald MS in patients with clinically isolated syndromes. Neurology, 67(7):1242-9.

Karp, C.L., van Boxel-Dezaire, A.H., Byrnes, A.A., & Nagelkerken, L. (2001). Interferon-beta in multiple sclerosis: altering the balance of interleukin-12 and interleukin 10? Current Opinion in Neurology, 14:361-368.

Kasper, L.H. & Shoemaker, J. (2010). Multiple sclerosis immunology: the healthy immune system vs the MS immune system. Neurology, 74(suppl 1):S2-S8.

Kebir, H., Kreymborg, K., & Ifergan, I., et al. (2007). Human T_H17 lymphocytes promote blood-brain barrier disruption and central nervous system inflammation. Nature Medicine, 13(10):1173-1175.

Kellar-Wood, H.F., Wood, N.W., Holmans, P., Clayton, D., Robertson, N., & Compston, D.A.S. (1995). Multiple sclerosis and the HLA-D region: linkage and association studies. Journal of Neuroimmunology, 58, 183-190.

Khademi, M., Kockum, I., & Andersson, M.L. et al. (2011). Cerebrospinal fluid CXCL 13 in multiple sclerosis: a suggestive prognostic marker for the disease course. Multiple Sclerosis, 17:335-343.

Khan OA. (1998). Gabapentin relieves trigeminal neuralgia in multiple sclerosis patients. Neurology. 51(2). 611-614.

Khan S, Game X, Kalsi V, Gonzales G, Panicker J, Elneil S, et al. (2011). Long-term effect on quality of life of repeat detrusor injections of botulinum neurotoxin-A for detrusor overactivity in patients with multiple sclerosis. The Journal of Urology. 185(4). 1344-1349.

Kieseier, B.C. (2011). The mechanism of action of interferon-β in relapsing multiple sclerosis. CNS Drugs, 25(6), 491-502.

Killestein, J., Rep, M.H., & Barkhof, F. et al. (2001). Active MRI lesion appearance in MS patients is preceded by fluctuations in circulating T-helper 1 and 2 cells. Journal of Neuroimmunology, 118(2):286-294.

Kimura, A., Naka, T., & Kishimoto,T. (2007). IL-6-dependent and –independent pathways in the development of interleukin 17-producing T helper cells. Proceedings of the National Academy of the Sciences of the United States of America, 104(29), 12099-12104.

Kock-Henriksen, N. & Sorensen, P.S. (2010). The changing demographic pattern of multiple sclerosis epidemiology. Lancet Neurology 9, 520-532.

Kowarik, M.C., Cepok, S., & Sellner, J., et al. (2012). CXCL13 is the major determinant for B cell recruitment to the CSF during neuroinflammation. Journal of Neuroinflammation 9(1):93 [abstract].

Krupp LB, Christodoulou C, Melville P, Scherl WF, MacAllister WS & Elkins LE. (2004). Donepezil improved memory in multiple sclerosis in a randomized clinical trial. Neurology. 63(9). 1579-1585.

Krupp LB, Christodoulou C, Melville P, Scherl WF, Pai LY, Muenz LR, et al. (2011). Multicenter randomized clinical trial of donepezil for memory impairment in multiple sclerosis. Neurology. 76(17). 1500-1507.

Kurtzke, J.F. (1980). Geographic distribution of multiple sclerosis: An update with special reference to Europe and the Mediterranean region. Acta Neurologica Scandinavica, 62, 65-80.

Kurtzke, J.F. & Hyllested, K. (1979). Multiple sclerosis in the Faroe Islands: i. clinical and epidemiological features. Annals of Neurology, 5, 6-21.

Lang, C., Reiss, C., & Mäurer, M. (2012). Natalizumab may improve cognition and mood in multiple sclerosis. European Neurology, 67(3), 162-166.

Lange, R., Volkmer, M., Heesen, C., & Liepert, J. (2009). Modafinil effects in multiple sclerosis patients with fatigue. Journal of Neurology, 256(4), 645-650.

Langrish, C.L., Chen, Y., Blumenschein, W.M., et al. (2005). IL-23 drives a pathogenic T cell population that induces autoimmune inflammation. Journal of Experimental Medicine, 201(2):233-240.

Lapierre, Y., Bouchard, S., Tansey, C., Gendron, D., Barkas, W.J., & Francis, G.S. (1987). Treatment of spasticity with tizanidine in multiple sclerosis. The Canadian Journal of Neurological Sciences, 14(3 Suppl), 513-517.

Leandri, M., Lundardi, G., Inglese, M., Messmer-Uccelli, M., Mancardi, G.L., Gottlieb, A., et al. (2000). Lamotrigine in trigeminal neuralgia secondary to multiple sclerosis. Journal of Neurology, 247(7), 556-558.

Lebrun, C., Alchaar, H., Candito, M., Bourg, V., & Chatel, M. (2006). Levocarnitine administration in multiple sclerosis patients with immunosuppressive therapy-induced fatigue. Multiple Sclerosis, 12(3), 321-324.

Lebrun, C., Bensa, C., & Debouverie, M., et al. (2009). Association between clinical conversion to multiple sclerosis in radiologically isolated syndrome and magnetic resonance imaging, cerebrospinal fluid, and visual evoked potential: follow-up of 70 patients. Archives of Neurology, 66:841-846.

Leppert, D., Lindberg, R.L., Kappos, L., & Leib, S. (2001). Matrix metalloproteinases: multifactorial effectors of inflammation in multiple sclerosis and bacterial meningitis. Brain Research Reviews, 36(2-3):249-257.

Li, Y., Chu, N., Hu, A., Gran, B., Rostami, A., & Zhang, G.X. (2007). Increased IL-23p19 expression in multiple sclerosis lesions and its induction in microglia. Brain 130(2):490-501.

Lindberg, C., Andersen, O., Vahlne, A., Dalton, M., & Runmarker, B. (1991). Epidemiological investigation of the association between infectious mononucleosis and multiple sclerosis. Neuroepidemiology,10, 62-65.

Lioresal (baclofen) tablet [package insert]. (1998). East Hanover, NJ: Novartis Pharmaceuticals.

Lioresal Intrathecal (baclofen injection) [package insert]. (2011). Minneapolis, MN: Medtronic Incorporated.

Litweller., S.E., Frohman, E.M., & Zimmern, P.E. (1999). Multiple sclerosis and the urologist. Journal of Urology, 161(3), 743 757.

Lombardi, G., Macchiarella, A., & Del Popolo, G. (2010). Efficacy and safety of tadalafil for erectile dysfunction in patients with multiple sclerosis. The Journal of Sexual Medicine, 7(6), 2192-2200.

Lovera, J. & Kovner, B. (2012). Cognitive Impairment in Multiple Sclerosis. Current Neurology and Neuroscience Reports, 12(5), 618-627.

Lovera, J.F., Frohman, E., Brown, T.R., Bandari, D., Nguyen, L., Yadav, V., et al. (2010). Memantine for cognitive impairment in multiple sclerosis: a randomized placebo-controlled trial. Multiple Sclerosis, 16(6), 715-723.

Lublin F.D. & Reingold S.C., (1996) Defining the clinical course of multiple sclerosis: Results of an international survey. Neurology 46, 907-911.

Lucchinetti, C., Bruck, W., Parisi, J., Scheithauer, B., Rodriguez, M., & Lassmann, H. (2000). Heterogeneity of multiple sclerosis lesions: implications for the pathogenesis of demyelination. Annals of Neurology, 47:707-717.

Lunardi, G., Leandri, M., Albano, C., Cultrera, S., Fracassi, M., Rubino, V., et al. (1997). Clinical effectiveness of lamotrigine and plasma levels in essential and symptomatic trigeminal neuralgia. Neurology, 48(6), 1714-1717.

Lüneman, J.D., Huppke, P., Roberts, S., Brück, W., Gärtner, J., & Münz, C. (2008). Broadened and elevated humoral immune response to EBNA1 in pediatric multiple sclerosis. Neurology, 71, 1033-1037.

The International HapMap Consortium (2003). The International HapMap Project. Nature, 18, 789–796.

Mackay, F. & Browning, J.L. (2002). BAFF: a fundamental survival factor for B cells. Nature Reviews. Immunology, 2(7), 465-475.

Mackay, F., Schneider, P., Rennert, P., & Browning ,J. (2003). BAFF and APRIL: a tutorial on B cell survival. Annual Review of Immunology, 21:231-264.

Mahfouz, W. & Corcos, J. (2011). Management of detrusor external sphincter dyssynergia in neurogenic bladder. European Journal of Physical and Rehabilitation Medicine, 47(4), 639-650.

Marrie RA. (2004). Environmental risk factors in multiple sclerosis aetiology. Lancet Neurology, 3, 709-718.

Mattioli, F., Stampatori, C., Bellomi, F., & Capra, R. (2011). Natalizumab efficacy on cognitive impairment in MS. Neurological Sciences, 31 Suppl 3, 321-323.

Mattioli, F., Stampatori, C., & Capra, R. (2011). The effect of natalizumab on cognitive function in patients with relapsing-remitting multiple sclerosis: preliminary results of a 1-year follow-up study. Neurological Sciences: official journal of the Italian Neurological Society and of the Italian Society of Clinical Neurophysiology, 32(1), 83-88.

Mäurer, M., Ortler, S., Baier, M., Meergans, M., Scherer, P., & Hofmann, W. (2012). Randomised multicentre trial on safety and efficacy of rivastigmine in cognitively impaired multiple sclerosis patients. Multiple Sclerosis, doi:10.1177/1352458512463481.

Mayne, M., Krishnan, J., Metz, L., Nath, A., Auty, A., Sahai, B.M., & Power, C. (1998). Infrequent detection of human herpesvirus 6 DNA in peripheral blood mononuclear cells from multiple sclerosis patients. Annals of Neurology, 44:391-394.

McDonald, W., Compston, A., & Edan, G. (2001). Recommended diagnostic criteria for multiple sclerosis: guidelines from the international panel on the diagnosis of multiple sclerosis. Annals of Neurology, 50:121-127.

McElroy, J.P. & Oksenberg, J.R. (2011). Multiple Sclerosis: Genetics 2010. Neurologic Clinics, 29, 219-231.

Meinl, E., Krumbholz, M., & Hohlfeld, R. (2006). B lineage cells in the inflammatory central nervous system environment: migration, maintenance, local antibody production, and therapeutic modulation. Annals of Neurology, 59:880-892.

Melanson, M., Grossberndt, A., Klowak, M., Leong, C., Frost, E.E., Prout, M., et al. (2010). Fatigue and cognition in patients with relapsing multiple sclerosis treated with interferon β. The International Journal of Neuroscience, 120(10), 631-640.

Miller, D.H., Weinshenker, B.G., & Filippi, M., et al. (2008). Differential diagnosis of suspected multiple sclerosis:a consensus approach. Multiple Sclerosis, 14:1157-1174.

Misko, T.P., Trotter, J.L., & Cross, A.H. (1995). Mediation of inflammation by encephalitogenic cells: interferon gamma induction of nitric oxide synthase and cyclooxygenase 2. Journal of Neuroimmunology, 61(2):195-204.

Mix, E., Meyer-Rienecker, H., & Hartung, H.P. et al. (2010). Animal models of multiple sclerosis- Potentials and limitations. Progress in Neurobiology, 92:386-404.

Mohr, D.C., Boudewyn, A.C., Goodkin, D.E., Bostrom, A., & Epstein, L. (2001). Comparative outcomes for individual cognitive-behavior therapy, supportive-expressive group psychotherapy, and sertraline for the treatment of depression in multiple sclerosis. Journal of Consulting and Clinical Psychology, 69(6), 942-949.

Molina-Holgado, E., Vela, J.M., Arevalo-Martin, A., & Guaza, C. (2001). LPS/IFN-gamma cytotoxicity in oligodendroglial cells: role of nitric oxide and protection by the anti-inflammatory cytokine IL-10. European Journal of Neuroscience, 13(3),493-502.

Möller, F., Poettgen, J., Broemel, F., Neuhaus, A., Daumer, M., & Heesen, C. (2011). HAGIL (Hamburg Vigil Study): a randomized placebo-controlled double-blind study with modafinil for treatment of fatigue in patients with multiple sclerosis. Multiple Sclerosis, 17(8), 1002-1009.

Morre, S.A., De Groot, C.J.A., & Kellestein, J., et al. (2000). Is Chlamydia pneumoniae present in the central nervous system of multiple sclerosis patients? Annals of Neurology, 48, 399.

Morrow, S.A., Kaushik, T., Zarevics, P., Erlanger, D., Bear, M.F., Munschauer, F.E., et al. (2009). The effects of L-amphetamine sulfate on cognition in MS patients: results of a randomized controlled trial. Journal of Neurology, 256(7), 1095-1102.

Mueller, M.E., Gruenthal, M., Olson, W.L., & Olson, W.H. (1997). Gabapentin for relief of upper motor neuron symptoms in multiple sclerosis. Archives of Physical Medicine and Rehabilitation, 78(5), 521-524.

Munger, K.L., Peeling, R.W., & Hernan, M.A., et al. (2003). Infection with Chlamydia pneumonia and risk of multiple sclerosis. Epidemiology 14, 141-147.

Murphy, A.C., Lalor, S.J., Lynch, M.A., & Mills, K.H.G. (2010). Infiltration of Th1 and Th17cells and activation of microlia in the CNS during the course of experimental autoimmune encephalomyelitis. Brain, Behavoir, and Immunity, 24, 641-651.

Murray, T.J. (1985). Amantadine therapy for fatigue in multiple sclerosis. The Canadian Journal of Neurological Sciences, 12(3), 251-254.

Nance, P.W., Sheremata, W.A., Lynch, S.G., Vollmer, T., Hudson, S., Francis, G.S., et al. (1997). Relationship of the anti-spasticity effect of tizanidine to plasma concentration in patients with multiple sclerosis. Archives of Neurology, 54(6), 731-736.

National Multiple Sclerosis Society: Update on Tysabri and PML: Sponsor and FDA provide information on cases and risks. http://www.nationalmssociety.org/news/news-detail/index.aspx?nid=2308 /Accessed October 2, 2012.

Nicholas, R. & Rashid, W. (2012). Multiple sclerosis. Clinical Evidence (Online), pii:1202.

Niederkom, J.Y.(2008). Emerging concepts in CD8$^+$ T regulatory cells. Current Opinion in Immunology, 20(3):327-331.

Noseworthy, J., Lucchinetti, C., Rodriguez, M., & Weinshenker, B. (2000). Multiple Sclerosis. New England Journal of Medicine, 343:938-952.

Novotna, A., Mares, J., Ratcliffe, S., Novakova, I., Vachova, M., Zapletalova, O., et al. (2011). A randomized, double-blind, placebo-controlled, parallel-group, enriched-design study of nabiximols (Sativex®), as add-on therapy, in subjects with refractory spasticity caused by multiple sclerosis. European Journal of Neurology, 18(9), 1122-1131.

Nyland, H., Mork, S., & Matre, R. (1982). In-situ characterization of mononuclear cell infiltrates in lesions of multiples sclerosis. Neuropathology and Applied Neurobiology, 8(5),403-411.

Obermeier, B., Mentele, R., & Matlotka, J., et al. (2008). Matching of oligoclonal immunoglobulin transcriptomes and proteomes of cerebrospinal fluid in multiple sclerosis. Nature Medicine, 14(6), 688-693.

Obermeier, B., Lovato, L., & Mentele, R., et al. (2011). Related B cell clones that populate the CSF and CNS of patients with multiple sclerosis produce CSF immunoglobulin. Journal of Neuroimmunology, 233(1-2):245-248.

Oksenberg, J.R., Baranzini, S.E., Barcellos, L.F., & Hauser, S.L. (2001). Multiple sclerosis: genomic rewards. Journal of Neuroimmunology, 13, 171-184.

Oksenberg, J.R., Baranzini, S.E., Sawcer, S., & Hauser, S.L. (2008). The genetics of multiple sclerosis: SNPs to pathways to pathogenesis. Nature, 9, 516-526.

Okuda, D.T., Mowry, E.M., & Beheshtian, A., et al. (2009). Incidental MRI anomalies suggestive of multiple sclerosis: The radiologically isolated syndrome. Neurology 72:800-805.

Olsson, T., Zhi, W.W., & Hojeberg, B., et al. (1990). Autoreactive T lymphocytes in multiple sclerosis determined by antigen induced secretion of interferon-gamma. Journal of Clinical Investigation, 86(3), 981-985.

Opsahl, M.L. & Kennedy P.G.E. (2005). Early and late HHV-6 gene transcripts in multiple sclerosis lesions and normal appearing white matter. Brain, 128, 516–527.

O'Riordan, J.I., Doherty, C., Javed, M., Brophy, D., Hutchinson, M., & Quinlan, D. (1995). Do alpha-blockers have a role in lower urinary tract dysfunction in multiple sclerosis? The Journal of Urology, 153(4), 1114-1116.

Orsnes, G.B., Sørensen, P.S., Larsen, T.K., & Ravnborg, M. (2000). Effect of baclofen on gait in spastic MS patients. Acta Neurologica Scandinavica, 101(4), 244-248.

Panitch, H., Miller, A., Paty, D., & Weinshenker, B. (2004) North American Study Group on Interferon beta- 1b in Secondary Progressive MS. Interferon beta-1b in secondary progressive MS: results from a 3-year controlled study. Neurology, 63, 1788-1795.

Panitch, H.S., Thisted, R.A., Smith, R.A., Wynn, D.R., Wymer, J.P., Achiron, A., et al. (2006). Randomized, controlled trial of dextromethorphan/quinidine for pseudobulbar affect in multiple sclerosis. Annals of Neurology, 59(5), 780-787.

Patti, F., Amato, M.P., Filippi, M., Gallo, P., Trojano, M., & Comi, G.C. (2004). A double blind, placebo-controlled, phase II, add-on study of cyclophosamide (CTX) for 24 months in patients affected by multiple sclerosis on a background therapy with interferon-beta study denomination. CYCLIN. Journal of the Neurological Sciences, 223:69-71.

Patti, F., Amato, M.P., Bastianello, S., Caniatti, L., Di Monte, E., Ferrazza, P., et al. (2010). Effects of immunomodulatory treatment with subcutaneous interferon beta-1a on cognitive decline in mildly disabled patients with relapsing-remitting multiple sclerosis. Multiple Sclerosis, 16(1), 68-77.

Pender, M.P., Greer, J.M. (2007). Immunology of multiple sclerosis. Current allergy and asthma reports. 7, 285-292.

Perez-Cesari, C., Saniger, M.M., & Sotelo, J. (2005). Frequent association of multiple sclerosis with varicella and zoster. Acta Neurologica Scandinavica 112, 417–419.

Peters, A., Pitcher, L.A., & Sullivan, J.M,, et al. (2011). Th17 cells induce ectopic lymphoid follicles in central nervous system tissue inflammation. Immunity 35(5):986-996.

Petersen T., Moller-Larsen A., Ellermann-Eriksen S, Thiel S, Christensen T. (2012) Effects of interferon-beta therapy on elements in the antiviral immune response towards the human herpesviruses EBV, HSV, VZV, and to the human endogenous retroviruses HERV-H and HERV-W in multiple sclerosis. Journal of neuroimmunology 249, 105-108.

Peterson, J.W., Bo, L., Mork, S., Chang, A., & Trapp, B.D. (2001). Transected neurites, apoptotic neurons and reduced inflammation in cortical MS lesions. Annals of Neurology, 50, 389-400.

Pioro, E.P., Brooks, B.R., Cummings, J., Schiffer, R., Thisted, R.A., Wynn, D., et al. (2010). Dextromethorphan plus ultra low dose quinidine reduces pseudobulbar affect. Annals of Neurology, 68(5), 693-702.

Pithaldia, A., Jain, S., & Navale, A. (2009). Pathogenesis and treatment of multiple sclerosis (MS). Internet Journal of Neurology, 10(2):1-20.

Pliskin, N.H., Hamer, D.P., Goldstein, D.S., Towle, V.L., Reder, A.T., Noronha, A., et al. (1996). Improved delayed visual reproduction test performance in multiple sclerosis patients receiving interferon beta-1b. Neurology, 47(6), 1463-1468.

Polman, C.H., Reingold, S.C., Banwell, B., Clanet, M., Cohen, J.A., & Filippi, M. et al. (2011). Diagnostic criteria for multiple sclerosis: 2010 revisions to the McDonald Criteria. Annals of Neurology, 69:292-302.

Polman, C.H., O'Connor, P.W., & Havrdova, E., et al, for the AFFIRM Investigators. (2006). A randomized, placebo-controlled trial of natalizumab for relapsing multiple sclerosis. New England Journal of Medicine, 354:899-910.

Poser, C.M. & Hibberd, P.L. (1998). Analysis of the 'epidemic' of multiple sclerosis in the Faroe Islands I. clinical and epidemiological aspects. Neuroepidemiology 7, 168-180.

Poser, C.M., & Brinar, V,V. (2001). Diagnostic criteria for multiple sclerosis. Clinical Neurology and Neurosurgery,103:1-11.

PRISMS Study Group. (1998). Randomised double-blind placebo-controlled study of interferon β-1a in relapsing/remitting multiple sclerosis. Lancet 352:1498-1504.

Pucci, E., Branãs, P., D'Amico, R., Giuliani, G., Solari, A., & Taus, C. (2007). Amantadine for fatigue in multiple sclerosis. Cochrane Database of Systematic Reviews (Online), (1), CD002818.

Racke, M.K., Lovett-Racke, A.E., & Karandikar, N.J. (2010). The mechanism of action of glatiramer acetate treatment in multiple sclerosis. Neurology, 74, S25-S30.

Ragheb, S., Li, Y., Simon, K., et al. (2011). Multiple sclerosis: BAFF and CXCL 13 in cerebrospinal fluid. Multiple Sclerosis, 17(7):819-829.

Ramagopalan, S.V. & Sadovnick, A.D. (2011). Epidemiology of multiple sclerosis. Neurologic Clinics, 29, 207-217.

Rammohan, K.W., Rosenberg, J.H., Lynn, D.J., Blumenfeld, A.M., Pollak, C.P., Nagaraja, H.N. (2002). Efficacy and safety of modafinil (Provigil) for the treatment of fatigue in multiple sclerosis: a two centre phase 2 study. Journal of Neurology, Neurosurgery, and Psychiatry, 72(2), 179-183.

Ramtahal, J., Jacob, A., Das, K., & Boggild, M. (2006). Sequential maintenance treatment with glatiramer acetate after mitoxantrone is safe and can limit exposure to immune-suppression in very active,relapsing remitting multiple sclerosis. Journal of Neurology, 253:1160-64.

Reder, A.T. & Arnason, B.G. (1995). Trigeminal neuralgia in multiple sclerosis relieved by a prostaglandin E analogue. Neurology, 45(6), 1097-1100

Rekand, T. & Grønning, M. (2011). Treatment of spasticity related to multiple sclerosis with intrathecal baclofen: a long-term follow-up. Journal of Rehabilitation Medicine, 43(6), 511-514.

Restivo, D.A., Tinazzi, M., Patti, F., Palmeri, A., & Maimone, D. (2003). Botulinum toxin treatment of painful tonic spasms in multiple sclerosis. Neurology, 61(5), 719-720.

Risch, N. & Merikangas, K. (1996). The future of genetic studies of complex human diseases. Science, 273, 1516-1571.

Rog, D.J., Nurmikko, T.J., Friede, T., & Young, C.A. (2005). Randomized, controlled trial of cannabis-based medicine in central pain in multiple sclerosis. Neurology, 65(6), 812-819.

Rog, D.J., Nurmikko, T.J., & Young, C.A. (2007). Oromucosal delta9-tetrahydrocannabinol/cannabidiol for neuropathic pain associated with multiple sclerosis: an uncontrolled, open-label, 2-year extension trial. Clinical Therapeutics, 29(9), 2068-2079.

Rosenberg, G.A. & Appenzeller, O. (1988). Amantadine, fatigue, and multiple sclerosis. Archives of Neurology, 45(10), 1104-1106.

Rossi, S., Mataluni, G., Codecà, C., Fiore, S., Buttari, F., Musella, A., et al. (2009). Effects of levetiracetam on chronic pain in multiple sclerosis: results of a pilot, randomized, placebo-controlled study. European Journal of Neurology, 16(3), 360-366.

Rudick, R.A., Stuart, W.H., & Calabresi, P.A., et al for the SENTINEL Investigators. (2006). Natalizumab plus interferon beta-1a for relapsing multiple sclerosis. New England Journal of Medicine, 354, 911-923.

Rudick, R.A. & Goelz, S.E. (2011). Beta-interferon for multiples sclerosis. Experimental Cell Research, 317;1301-1311.

Sabada M.C., Tzartos J., Paino C., Garcia-Villanueva M., Alvarez-Cermeno J.C.,Villar L.M. et al. (2012) Axonal and oligodendrocyte-localized IgM and IgG deposits in MS lesions. Journal of Neuroimmunology 247, 86-94.

Sachais, B.A., Logue, J.N., & Carey, M.S. (1977). Baclofen, a new antispastic drug. A controlled, multicenter trial in patients with multiple sclerosis. Archives of Neurology, 34(7), 422-428.

Sadiq, S.A. & Wang, G.C. (2006). Long-term intrathecal baclofen therapy in ambulatory patients with spasticity. Journal of Neurology, 253(5), 563-569.

Sadovnick, A.D. (2002). The genetics of multiple sclerosis. Clinical Neurology and Neurosurgery, 104, 199-202.

Safarinejad, M.R. (2009). Evaluation of the safety and efficacy of sildenafil citrate for erectile dysfunction in men with multiple sclerosis: a double-blind, placebo controlled, randomized study. The Journal of Urology, 181(1), 252-258.

Samkoff, L.M. & Goodman, A.D. (2011). Symptomatic management in multiple sclerosis. Neurologic Clinics, 29(2), 449-463.

Sawa, G.M. & Paty, D.W. (1979). The use of baclofen in treatment of spasticity in multiple sclerosis. The Canadian Journal of Neurological Sciences, 6(3), 351-354.

Sawcer, S. Ban, M., Maranian, M., Yeo, T.W., Compston, A., & Kirby, A., et al. (2005). A high-density screen for linage in multiple sclerosis. American Journal of Human Genetics, 77, 454-467.

Schapira, K., Poskanzer, D.C., & Miller, H. (1963). Familial and conjugal multiple sclerosis. Brain 86, 315-332.

Schiemann, B., Gommerman, J.L., & Vora, K., et al. (2001). An essential role for BAFF in the normal development of B cells through a BCMA-independent pathway. Science, 293 (5537), 2111-2114.

Schiffer, R.B., Herndon, R.M., & Rudick, R.A. (1985). Treatment of pathologic laughing and weeping with amitriptyline. The New England Journal of Medicine, 312(23), 1480-1482.

Schiffer, R.B. & Wineman, N.M. (1990). Antidepressant pharmacotherapy of depression associated with multiple sclerosis. The American Journal of Psychiatry, 147(11), 1493-1497.

Schwib, S.R., & Bever, C.T. Jr. (2001). The cost of delaying treatment in multiple sclerosis: what is lost is not regained. Neurology, 56:1620.

Secondary Progressive Efficacy Clinical Trial of Recombinant Interferon-beta-1a in MS (SPECTRIMS) Study Group. (2001). Randomized controlled trial of interferon beta-1a in secondary progressive AMS: clinical results. Neurology, 56:1496-1504.

Serafini, B., Rosicarelli, B., Franciotta, D., Magliozzi, R., Reynolds, R., & Cinque, P. (2007). Dysregulated Epstein-Barr virus infection in the multiple sclerosis brain. Journal of Experimental Medicine, 204, 2899-2912.

Serpell, M.G., Notcutt, W., & Collin, C. (2012). Sativex long-term use: an open-label trial in patients with spasticity due to multiple sclerosis. Journal of Neurology, doi: 10.1007/s00415-012-6634-z.

Smith, C., Birnbaum, G., Carter, J.L., Greenstein, J., & Lublin, F.D. (1994). Tizanidine treatment of spasticity caused by multiple sclerosis: results of a double-blind, placebo-controlled trial. US Tizanidine Study Group. Neurology, 44(11 Suppl 9) S34-42; discussion S42-3.

Smolenski, C., Muff, S., & Smolenski-Kautz, S. (1981). A double-blind comparative trial of new muscle relaxant, tizanidine (DS 103-282), and baclofen in the treatment of chronic spasticity in multiple sclerosis. Current medical Research and Opinion, 7(6), 374-383.

Snow, B.J., Tsui, J.K., Bhatt, M.H., Varelas, M., Hashimoto, S.A., & Calne, D.B. (1990). Treatment of spasticity with botulinum toxin: a double-blind study. Annals of Neurology, 28(4), 512-515.

Sobolewski, P. (2007). The application of botulinum toxin type A in the treatment of spastic paraparesis [abstract]. Przegląd Lekarski, 64 Suppl 2:3-7.

Soderstrom, M., Link, H., & Sun, J.B., et al. (1993). T cells recognizing multiple peptides of myelin basic protein are found in blood and enriched cerebrospinal fluid in optic neuritis and multiple sclerosis. Scandinavian Journal of Immunology, 37(3):355-368.

Solaro, C., Boehmker, M., & Tanganelli, P. (2009). Pregabalin for treating paroxysmal painful symptoms in multiple sclerosis: a pilot study. Journal of Neurology, 256(10), 1773-1774.

Solaro, C., Lunardi, G.L., Capello, E., Inglese, M., Messmer Uccelli, M., Uccelli, A., et al. (1998). An open-label trial of gabapentin treatment of paroxysmal symptoms in multiple sclerosis patients. Neurology, 51(2), 609-611.

Solaro, C., Messmer Uccelli, M., Uccelli, A., Leandri, M., & Mancardi, G.L. (2000). Low-dose gabapentin combined with either lamotrigine or carbamazepine can be useful therapies for trigeminal neuralgia in multiple sclerosis. European Neurology, 44(1), 45-48.

Solaro, C. & Messmer Uccelli, M. (2010). Pharmacological management of pain in patients with multiple sclerosis. Drugs, 70(10), 1245-1254.

Solaro, C., Trabucco, E., Messmer Uccelli, M. (2013). Pain and multiple sclerosis: pathophysiology and treatment. Current Neurology and Neuroscience Reports, 13(1), 320.

Solaro, C., Uccelli, M.M., Guglieri, P., Uccelli, A., & Mancardi, G.L. (2000). Gabapentin is effective in treating nocturnal painful spasms in multiple sclerosis. Multiple Sclerosis, 6(3), 192-193.

Sorensen, P.S., Deisenhammer, F., & Duda, P., et al. (2005). Guidelines on use of anti-IFN-beta antibody measurements in multiple sclerosis: report of an EFNS Task Force on IFN-beta antibodies in multiple sclerosis. European Journal of Neurology, 12:817-827.

Sorensen, P.S., Mellgren, S.I., & Svenningsson, A., et al. (2009). NORdic trial of oral methylprednisoloine as add-on therapy to Interferon beta-1a for treatment of relapsing-remitting Multiple Sclerosis (NORMIMS study): a randomised, placebo-controlled trial. Lancet Neurology, 8:519-529.

Sospedra, M. & Martin, R. (2006). Molecular mimicry in multiple sclerosis. Autoimmunity, 39, 3-8.

SPECTRIMS Study Group, Hughes RAC. (2001) Randomized controlled trial of interferon-beta-1a in secondary progressive MS: clinical results. Neurology, 56:1496–504.

Spurkland, A., Ronningen, K., Vandvik, B., Thorsby, E., & Vartdal, F. (1991). HLA-DQA1 and HLA-DQB1 genes may jointly determine susceptibility to develop multiple sclerosis. Human Immunology, 30, 69-75.

Stankoff, B., Waubant, E., Confavreux, C., Edan, G., Debouverie, M., Rumbach, L., et al. (2005). Modafinil for fatigue in MS: a randomized placebo-controlled double-blind study. Neurology, 64(7), 1139-1143.

Steiner, G. (1952). Acute plaques in multiple sclerosis, their pathogenetic significance and the role of spirochetes as etiological factor. Journal of Neuropathology and Experimental Neurology. 11, 343-372.

Stien, R., Nordal, H.J., Oftedal, S.I., & Slettebø, M. (1987). The treatment of spasticity in multiple sclerosis: a double-blind clinical trial of a new anti-spastic drug tizanidine compared with baclofen. Acta Neurologica Scandinavica, 75(3), 190-194.

Tan I.L., McArthur J.C., Clifford D.B., Major E.O., Nath A. (2011) Immune reconstitution inflammatory syndrome in natalizumab-associated PML. Neurology 77, 1061-1067.

Teare, M.D. & Barrett, J.H. (2005). Genetic linkage studies. Lancet, 17, 1036-1044.

Tepavcevic, D.K., Kostic, J., Basuroski, I.D., Stojsavljevic, N., Pekmezovic, T., & Drulovic, J. (2008). The impact of sexual dysfunction on the quality of life measured by MSQoL-54 in patients with multiple sclerosis. Multiple Sclerosis, 14(8), 1131-1136.

Thacker, E.L., Mirzaei, F., & Ascherio, A. (2006). Infectious mononucleosis and risk for multiple sclerosis: a meta-analysis. Annals of Neurology, 59, 499-503.

Thompson, A.J., Toosy, A.T., & Ciccarelli, O. (2010). Pharmacological management of symptoms in multiple sclerosis: current approaches and future directions. Lancet Neurology, 9(12), 1182-1199.

Thorsby, E., Helgesen, A., Solheim, B.C., & Vandvik, B. (1977). HLA antigens in multiple sclerosis. Journal of the Neurological Sciences, 32, 187-193.

Tomassini, V., Pozzilli, C., Onesti, E., Pasqualetti, P., Marinelli, F., Pisani, A., et al. (2004). Comparison of the effects of acetyl L-carnitine and amantadine for the treatment of fatigue in multiple sclerosis: results of a pilot, randomised, double-blind, crossover trial. Journal of the Neurological Sciences, 218(1-2), 103-108.

Torchinsky, M.B. & Blander, J.M. (2010). T helper 17 cells: discovery, function, and physiological trigger. Cellular and Molecular Life Sciences, 67:1407-1421.

Trapp, B.D. & Nave, K.A. (2008). Multiple sclerosis: An immune or neurodegenerative disorder? Annual Review of Neuroscience, 31:247-269.

Traugott, U., Reinherz, E.L., & Raine, C.S. (1983) Multiple sclerosis: distribution of T cell subsets within active chronic lesions. Science, 219(4582):308-310.

Tzartos, J.S., Friese,M.A., & Craner, M.J., et al. (2008). Interleukin-17 production in central nervous system-infiltrating T cells and glial cells is associated with active disease in multiple sclerosis. American Journal of Pathology, 172(1):146-155.

United Kingdom Tizanidine Trial Group. (1994). A double-blind, placebo-controlled trial of tizanidine in the treatment of spasticity caused by multiple sclerosis. Neurology, 44(11 Suppl 9), S70-8.

U.S. Food and Drug Administration: FDA Drug Safety Communication: New risk factor for Progressive Multifocal Leukoencephalopathy (PML) associated with Tysabri (natalizumab) http://www.fda.gov/drugs/drugsafety/ucm288186.htm Accessed October 02, 2012.

Vakhapova, V., Auriel, E., & Karni, A. (2010). Nightly sublingual tizanidine HCl in multiple sclerosis: clinical efficacy and safety. Clinical Neuropharmacology, 33(3), 151-154.

van Rey, F. & Heesakkers, J. (2011). Solifenacin in multiple sclerosis patients with overactive bladder: a prospective study. Advances in Urology, 2011:834753, doi: 10.1155/2011/834753.

Vartanian, T., Li,Y., Zhao, M., & Stefansson, K. (1995). Interferon-gamma-induced oligodendrocyte cell death: implications for the pathogenesis of multiples sclerosis. Molecular Medicine (Cambridge, Mass), 1(7):732-743.

Venken, K., Hellings, N., Liblau, R., & Stinissen, P. (2010). Disturbed regulatory T cell   homeostasis in multiple sclerosis. Trends in Molecular Medicine, 16(2):58-68.

Villoslada, P., Arrondo, G., Sepulcre, J., Alegre, M., & Artieda, J. (2009). Memantine induces reversible neurologic impairment in patients with MS. Neurology, 72(19), 1630-1633.

Visscher, B.R., Detels, R., Coulson, A.H., Malmgren, R.M., & Dudley, J.P. (1977). Latitude, migration, and the prevalence of multiple sclerosis. American Journal of Epidemiology, 106, 470-475.

Wade, D.T., Collin, C., Stott, C., & Duncombe, P. (2010). Meta-analysis of the efficacy and safety of Sativex (nabiximols), on spasticity in people with multiple sclerosis. Multiple Sclerosis, 16(6), 707-714.

Wallin, M.T., Page, W.F., & Kurtzke, J.F. (2004). Multiple sclerosis in US veterans of the Vietnam era and later military service: race, sex, and geography. Annals of Neurology, 55, 65-71.

Wallin, M.T., Culpepper, W.J., Coffman, P., Pulaski, S., Maloni, H., Mahan, C.M., Haselkorn, J.K., & Kurtzke, J.F. (2012). The Gulf War era multiple sclerosis cohort: age and incidence rates by race, sex and service. Brain 135, 1778-1785.

Wiesel, P.H., Norton, C., Roy, A.J., Storrie, J.B., Bowers, J., & Kamm, M.A. (2000). Gut focused behavioural treatment (biofeedback) for constipation and faecal incontinence in multiple sclerosis. Journal of Neurology, Neurosurgery, and Psychiatry, 69(2), 240-243.

Wilken, J.A., Sullven, C., Wallin, M., Rogers, C., Kane, R.L., Rossman, H., et al. (2008). Treatment of multiple sclerosis-related cognitive problems with adjunctive modafinil. International Journal of MS Care, 10, 1-10.

Wolinsky, J.S., Narayana, P.A., O'Conner, P., Coyle, P.K., Ford, C., Johnson, K., Miller, A., & Pardo, L., et al. PROMise Trial Study Group. (2007). Glatiramer acetate in primary progressive multiple sclerosis; results of a multinational, multicenter, double-blind, placebo-controlled trial. Annals of Neurology. 61:14-24.

Wucherpfenning, K.W. & Strominger, J.L. (1995). Molecular mimicry in T cell-mediated autoimmunity: Viral peptides activate human T cell clones specific for myelin basic proteins. Cell 80, 695-705.

Zifko, U.A., Rupp, M., Schwarz, S., Zipko, H.T., & Maida, E.M. (2002). Modafinil in treatment of fatigue in multiple sclerosis: results of an open-label study. Journal of Neurology, 249(8), 983-987.

Zifko, U.A. (2004). Management of fatigue in patients with multiple sclerosis. Drugs, 64(12), 1295-1304.

Zozulya, A.L. & Wiendi, H. (2008). The role of CD8 suppressors versus destructors in autoimmune central nervous system inflammation. Human Immunology, 69(11):797-804.

Zvartau-Hind, M., Din, M.U., Gilani, A., Lisak, R.P., & Khan, O.A. (2000). Topiramate relieves refractory trigeminal neuralgia in MS patients. Neurology, 55(10), 1587-1588.

Understanding the Mechanisms of Interferon-Induced Protection against Foot-and-Mouth Disease

Fayna Diaz-San Segundo

Plum Island Animal Disease Center, North Atlantic Area, Agricultural Research Service
U.S. Department of Agriculture, USA

Nestor Montiel

Plum Island Animal Disease Center, North Atlantic Area, Agricultural Research Service
U.S. Department of Agriculture, USA

Teresa de los Santos

Plum Island Animal Disease Center, North Atlantic Area, Agricultural Research Service
U.S. Department of Agriculture, USA

Marvin J. Grubman

Plum Island Animal Disease Center, North Atlantic Area, Agricultural Research Service
U.S. Department of Agriculture, USA

1   Introduction

At the end of the nineteenth century, foot-and-mouth disease (FMD) became the first animal disease shown to be caused by a virus, earning a place in history. Although the earliest recognition of the clinical entity of FMD is generally credited to Fracastorius's observations in the 16th century (Fracastorius, 1546), it was not until 1897 when Loeffler and Frosch demonstrated that this disease was caused by a filterable agent (Loeffler & Frosch, 1897). In its acute form, FMD affects livestock and wild cloven-hoofed animals and is characterized by fever, lameness, and vesicular lesions of the feet, tongue, snout and teats. With high morbidity, low mortality rates, and its notorious debilitating effects, FMD is responsible for severe losses in livestock productivity, including weight loss, decreased milk production, and loss of draught power. The highly contagious nature of this disease and the severity of the associated economic impact caused by an outbreak have led to the recognition of FMD as the most important disease in the livestock industry, limiting trade of animals and animal products throughout the world (Leforban, 1999). In fact, countries that are FMD-free prohibit imports of livestock or animal products from countries where the disease is enzootic. The economic impact of an FMD outbreak can be significant, as observed during recent outbreaks in Europe, Japan, Taiwan, South Korea, and other countries, that resulted in losses of billions of dollars (Grubman & Baxt, 2004). Furthermore, worldwide concerns following the 2001 terrorist attacks in the United States has raised awareness about the possibility of terrorist groups or rogue states attempting to use FMD virus (FMDV) as a bioweapon to target the $100-billion/year U.S. livestock industry.

The virus spreads from animal to animal in a number of ways including direct contact between an infected animal and non-infected animals and indirect spread when an animal eats food that has been contaminated by the virus (from saliva, for example). The virus can also become airborne, particularly when it has been exhaled, thus an infection in one herd can quickly become widespread over the countryside (Alexandersen et al., 2003). However, experimental studies use direct inoculation including subcutaneous, intradermal, intramuscular and intravenous inoculation, intranasal instillation, and exposure to artificially created aerosols.

Current methods of disease control include limiting movement of susceptible animals and animal products, slaughtering of infected and susceptible in-contact animals, except in countries in which the disease is enzootic, disinfection of affected areas, and vaccination with a chemically inactivated whole virus antigen vaccine (Grubman & Baxt, 2004). However, in case of an outbreak occurring in previously FMD-free countries, the use of vaccination is problematic since The World Organization for Animal Health (OIE) favors slaughtering or vaccination followed by slaughtering, rather than vaccination alone in order to rapidly regain FMD free status. Countries that slaughter all infected and susceptible in-contact animals can regain FMD-free status, and thus re-engage in trade, by documenting and demonstrating absence of disease for the next three consecutive months after the last case. On the other hand, countries that do not slaughter vaccinated animals must wait six months to regain FMD-free status. Although the conventional inactivated vaccine and a newly developed recombinant replication-defective human adenovirus 5 (Ad5) FMDV subunit vaccine are effective in controlling disease, they require approximately 7 days to induce full protection in swine and cattle (Golde et al., 2005; Moraes et al., 2002; Pacheco et al., 2005; Grubman et al., 2010). Therefore, in the event of an outbreak, induction of rapid protection, prior to the development of vaccine-induced adaptive immunity, is critical and necessary to limit disease dissemination and potentially reduce the number of animals that need to be eliminated.

A number of studies have demonstrated that FMDV initially infects epithelial cells of the naso-pharynx attaching to these cells via integrin receptors and then the virus spreads to epithelial cells in the lungs (Alexandersen et al., 2003; Arzt et al., 2011; Monaghan et al., 2005; O'Donnell et al., 2008). The viremic phase of FMDV infection generally occurs and peaks during the first 24 to 48 hours, and coincides with appearance of clinical signs. It is during this period that an infected individual can secrete copious amounts of virus into the environment transmitting the disease to susceptible animals. To achieve such a rapid takeover of the host, FMDV manipulates the early immune response ensuring a window of opportunity to replicate and spread before the onset of effective adaptive immunity. Thus, understanding early host-pathogen interactions and the contributions of innate versus adaptive immune responses has become a central topic in FMDV research. The role of the immune response in disease progression and pathology is fundamental to an effective and rational design of early intervention strategies. This review will present a brief description of FMDV and the different functions of various viral proteins, with the main focus on our current knowledge of the strategies that FMDV utilizes to circumvent the host protective response and the results of stimulating host innate immunity to control disease.

2   The Agent

Foot-and-mouth disease virus is the prototype member of the *Aphthovirus* genus of the *Picornaviridae* family and contains a single-stranded, positive-sense RNA genome of approximately 8,500 nucleotides surrounded by an icosahedral capsid composed of 60 copies each of four structural proteins (VP1 [1D], VP2 [1B], VP3 [1C], and VP4 [1A]) (Figure 1a) (Grubman and Baxt, 2004; Rueckert, 1996; Rueckert and Wimmer, 1984). The viral genome consists of a long open reading frame (ORF) flanked by 5' and 3' highly structured untranslated regions (5' and 3'UTRs) (Figure 1a). Upon infection, the viral ORF is translated as a single polyprotein that is cotranslationally processed by three virus-encoded proteinases, leader (L^{pro}), 2A, and $3C^{pro}$, into the four structural proteins and a number of nonstructural (NS) proteins (Mason et al., 2003; Rueckert, 1996). L^{pro} is a papain-like proteinase that cleaves itself from the nascent polypeptide chain (Strebel & Beck, 1986) and as later explained in this chapter, interacts with the host, playing a critical role in virulence. 2A is a peptide of 18 amino acids that, using a unique cleavage mechanism, is responsible for processing P1-2A from the remainder of the polyprotein (Donnelly et al., 2001a and 2001b). Most of the viral polyprotein is enzymatically processed by the cysteine-proteinase $3C^{pro}$ (Klump et al., 1984; Vakharia et al., 1987) which also plays an important role in virulence. $3C^{pro}$ is involved in the cleavage of various host proteins including histone H3, Sam68, NEMO, cytoskeleton proteins, and translation initiation factors eIF-4A and eIF-4G (Armer et al., 2008; Belsham et al., 2000; Falk et al., 1990; Lawrence et al., 2012; Wang et al., 2012). Other NS viral proteins are involved in various aspects of the viral replication cycle: 3D is the viral RNA-dependent RNA polymerase; 3B (also termed VPg) is a protein covalently linked to the 5' end of virion RNA that is involved in the initiation of RNA synthesis; 2C binds single-stranded RNA nonspecifically, has ATPase activity and its interaction with cellular protein Beclin1 modulates autophagy pathways allowing for virus survival (Gladue et al., 2012); 2B, 2C, and 3A are also involved in membrane rearrangements required not only for viral RNA replication, but for capsid assembly (Grubman & Baxt, 2004). Furthermore, recent evidence has demonstrated that some of the NS proteins or their precursors also have additional roles in controlling the host response including inhibition of protein trafficking by 2B and 2C or 2BC (Moffat et al., 2005, 2007). This latter function may be responsible for the decrease in surface expression of major histocompatibility class I

(a)

(b)

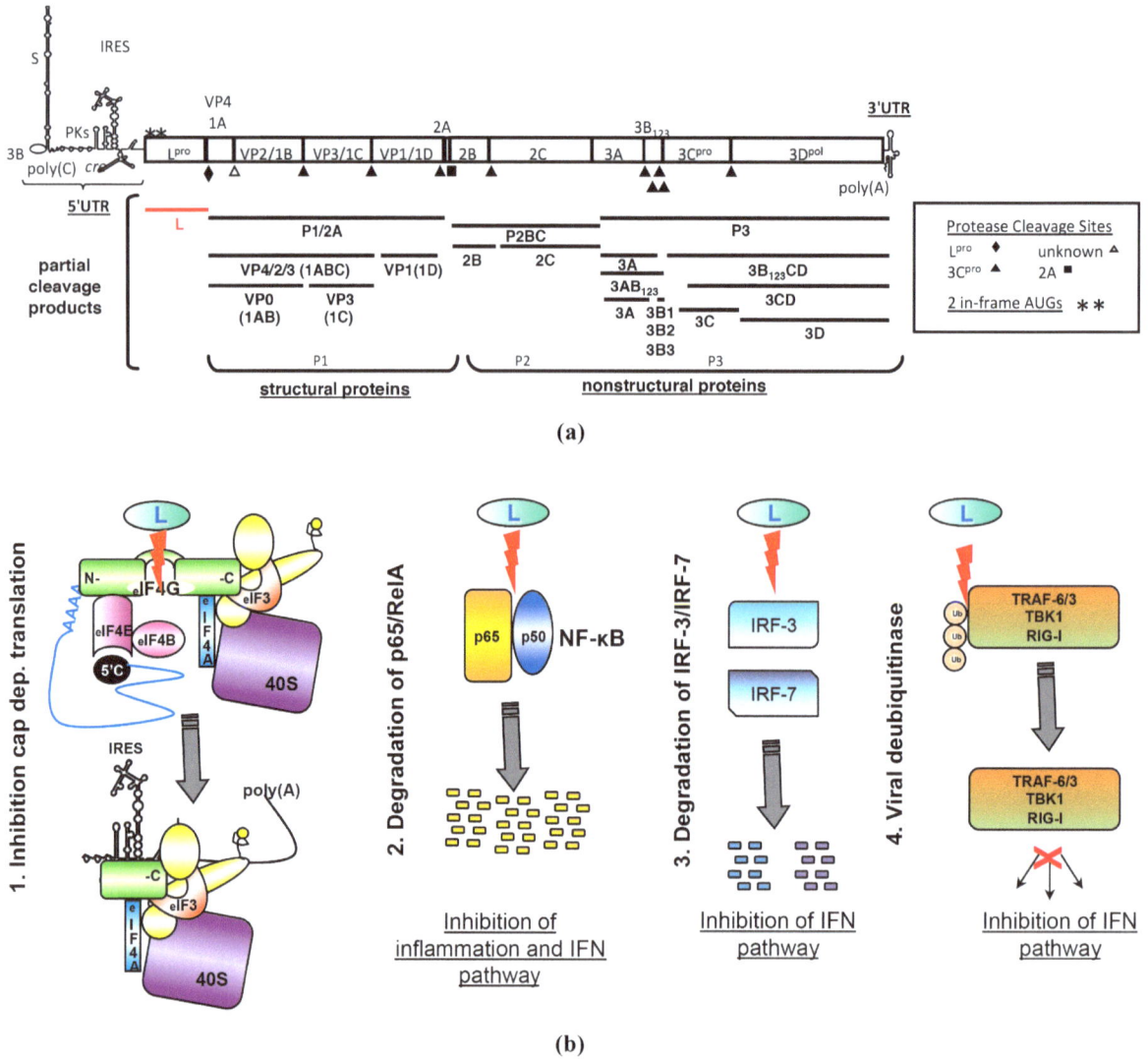

Figure 1: (a) Schematic map of the FMDV genome. The ORF is shown in the boxed area, with the viral proteins named according to the nomenclature of Rueckert and Wimmer (1984), lines indicate RNA structures. Thick lines below the genome diagram indicate prominent partial cleavage products. S fragment, short fragment of the genome, poly(C), poly cytosine tract, PK, pseudoknot, *cre*, *cis*-acting replicative element, IRES, internal ribosome entry site. The sites of the primary cleavages and the proteases responsible are indicated (adapted from Mason *et al.*, 2003). **(b)** Schematic diagram illustrating the known biological activities of FMDV L^{pro} which affect the host response. 1. L^{pro} cleaves the translation initiation factor eIF4G resulting in the shutoff of host cap dependent protein synthesis. eIF4A, eIF4B, eIF4G, eIF4E and eIF3 are translation initiation factors. 40S and 60S are ribosomal subunits. 2. L^{pro} is directly or indirectly involved in the cleavage of the transcription factor NF-kB. p65/p50 represents the NF-kB heterodimer. 3. L^{pro} is involved in the degradation of IFN regulatory factor (IRF)-3 and IRF-7, resulting in the inhibition of the IFN pathway. 4. L^{pro} acts as a viral deubiquitinase removing ubiquitin (Ub) moieties from TNF receptor-associated factor 6 (TRAF-6), and TRAF-3, retinoic acid-inducible gene I (RIG-I) and TANK-binding kinase 1 (TBK1), key signaling molecules in activation of type I IFN response. (adapted from Grubman *et al.*, 2008).

molecules upon FMDV infection resulting in a delay in the host adaptive immune response (Sanz-Parra *et al.*, 1998).

As mentioned above the leader proteinase is the first viral protein translated upon infection. L^{pro} cleaves itself from the polyprotein precursor and early in infection cleaves host translation initiation factor eIF-4G, resulting in the shut off of host cap-dependent mRNA translation (Fig. 1B; Devaney *et al.*, 1988; Medina *et al.*, 1993, Strebel & Beck, 1986). Translation of FMDV mRNA remains unaffected since it proceeds by a cap-independent mechanism, via an internal ribosome entry site (IRES) present within the 5' UTR of the viral genome that does not require intact eIF-4G (Belsham & Brangwyn, 1990; Kuhn *et al.*, 1990). Thus, as a result of FMDV infection, host cell protein synthesis is rapidly suppressed without affecting translation of viral mRNA, thereby diverting the cell protein synthesis machinery towards the production of large amounts of new virus.

L^{pro} is a virulence factor and viruses can be attenuated *in vitro* and *in vivo* by removing the leader coding region (leaderless virus) or by inserting mutations in some domains within the L^{pro} coding sequence (Chinsangaram *et al.*, 1998; de los Santos *et al.*, 2009; Diaz-San Segundo *et al.*, 2012, Mason *et al.*, 1997; Piccone *et al.*, 1995, 2010). It has been shown that the attenuated phenotype of the leaderless virus results from its inability to block the host innate immune response, in particular the production of type I interferon (IFN-α/β) (Chinsangaram *et al.*, 1999). FMDV L^{pro} also blocks the induction of IFN-β transcription (de los Santos *et al*, 2006), which requires the translocation of biologically active L^{pro} to the nucleus of infected cells and subsequent degradation of p65/RelA, a subunit of the transcription factor nuclear factor kappa B (NF-κB) (Fig. 1B; de los Santos *et al*, 2007). Structure-function analysis of L^{pro} has demonstrated that, in addition to the proteinase activity, an intact protein motif, SAP (SAF-A/B, acinus, and PIAS domain), is required for FMDV virulence (de los Santos *et al.*, 2009). Others have demonstrated that L^{pro} is involved in the degradation of IFN regulatory factors (IRF)-3 and -7, affecting specific gene transcription (Fig. 1B; Wang *et al.*, 2010) and causes de-ubiquitination of RIG-I, TBK-1, TRAF-1 and TRAF-6, affecting IFN and IFN stimulated gene (ISG) transcription (Figure 1B; Wang *et al.*, 2011). Thus, FMDV L^{pro} helps subvert the host innate response by inhibiting the induction of antiviral molecules at both transcriptional and translational levels thereby blocking the action of IFNs and other cytokines that would naturally prevent virus replication and dissemination.

3   Evading the Host Immune Response

As a successful pathogen, FMDV has developed several mechanisms to counteract or evade the host innate and adaptive immune response (Grubman *et al.*, 2008; Golde *et al.*, 2008).

Dendritic cells (DCs), a heterogeneous group of potent antigen-presenting cells (APCs), are the master regulators of the immune response and are functionally situated at the interphase between the innate and the adaptive immune system (Banchereau & Steinman, 1998). In order to fulfill their role as sentinels of the immune system, DCs express several families of specialized pattern recognition receptors (PRRs) which recognize virus specific products termed pathogen-associated molecular patterns (PAMPs). PRRs include Toll-like receptors (TLRs), nucleotide-binding oligomerization domain (NOD)-like receptors (NLRs), retinoic acid-inducible gene I (RIG-I)-like receptors (RLRs) and C-type lectin receptors (CLRs) all reacting directly with pathogen components (Kawai & Akira, 2011; Lee & Kim, 2007; Robinson *et al.*, 2006; Trinchieri & Sher, 2007). The most common division of DCs is into two major groups, conventional DCs (cDCs) and plasmacytoid DCs (pDCs). While cDCs have been described to have a unique capacity for naive T cell priming (Banchereau & Steinman, 1998), pDCs have the unique property of secreting IFN-α/β in response to viruses and/or virus-derived nucleic acids (Reizis et al., 2011). The cross-talk between DCs and natural killer (NK) cells leads to the activation of NK cells to modulate the initial barriers of the cellular host defense against pathogens (Vivier et al., 2011). In addition, DCs inter-actions with T and B lymphocytes modulate the cellular and humoral adaptive immune response (Iwasaki & Kelsal, 2000; Wykes et al., 1998). Thus, it is not surprising that FMDV has evolved mechanisms to prevent these cell populations from functioning optimally throughout the course of infection. During the course of FMD, the virus interacts with different DCs populations, either by direct infection or as a con-sequence of DCs phagocytosing the virus in peripheral tissues for antigen presentation (Merad & Manz, 2009).

Several studies have documented the interaction between FMDV and different DC populations (Bautista et al., 2005; Diaz-San Segundo et al., 2009; Nfon et al., 2008; Ostrowski et al., 2005; Robinson et al., 2011). FMDV can infect cDCs ex vivo leading to the synthesis of viral NS proteins. Although in most cases this interaction is abortive and no virions are produced in infected cDCs (Diaz-San Segundo et al., 2009; Ostrowski et al., 2005), it has been demonstrated that the presence of specific anti-FMDV anti-bodies enhances infection through the interaction of virus-antibody complexes with FcγR receptors locat-ed on the surface of DCs. In cattle, uptake of these complexes by DCs results in productive infection and cell death (Robinson et al., 2011). In addition, FMDV can modulate adaptive immune responses by means of its interaction with DCs. During acute infection the virus stimulates DCs to produce interleukin (IL)-10, thus directing adaptive immunity towards the development of a stronger humoral rather than a T-cell mediated response (Diaz-San Segundo et al., 2009; Robinson et al., 2011). It has been shown that interaction of FMDV with bovine cDCs, in vitro, results in productive infection; however attempts to recover virus from DCs derived from FMDV infected swine have been unsuccessful. Nevertheless, FMDV affects monocytes extracted from pigs during acute stages of FMDV blocking their ability to dif-ferentiate into mature cDCs (Diaz-San Segundo et al., 2009) and to respond to stimulation with TLR lig-ands (Nfon et al., 2008).

Langerhan cells (LCs), which are a DC subset found in all layers of the epidermis and express langerin (Valladeau et al., 2000), are also affected by FMDV (Bautista et al., 2005; Nfon et al., 2008). Although these cells constitutively express type I IFN, in vitro studies demonstrated that FMDV is able to attach and become internalized by these cells; however, there is no evidence of viral RNA replication or production of viral proteins (Bautista et al., 2005). Furthermore, LCs from FMDV infected pigs show a reduction in IFN-α production after ex vivo stimulation, although their ability to present antigen remains normal (Nfon et al., 2008). These findings suggest that whereas FMDV enhances pathogenesis in infect-ed animals during the acute phase of infection, DCs antigen presentation is preserved as it is critical to the host for the relatively rapid induction of a strong adaptive immune response and recovery.

pDCs are not susceptible to FMDV in vitro, unless the virus is internalized as part of immune complexes bound to FcγRII surface receptors, and uptake of these complexes results in abortive virus replication (Guzylack-Piriou et al., 2006). However, during acute infection of swine, the pDC population is depleted in blood, and the remaining pDCs are less able to produce IFN-α in response to TLR ligands or FMDV (Nfon et al., 2010). Similarly, FMDV can be internalized by bovine pDCs as immune com-plexes recognized by FcγRII receptors, but the ability of these cells to produce large amounts of type I IFN is not affected (Reid et al., 2011).

Macrophages are part of the innate responses to virus infections and are fundamental for rapid "clean up" of viral pathogens at the sites of infection. Similar to pDCs, FMDV also utilizes an antibody-dependent internalization process via the FcγRII receptor to enter macrophages (Baxt & Mason, 1995; McCullough *et al.*, 1988). Interestingly, it has been reported that, in the absence of productive infection of porcine macrophages, FMDV remains infectious for 10 to 24 hours after internalization by macrophages (Ridgen *et al.*, 2002). Implications of these observations favor the role of macrophages as transporters and disseminators of viable virions to distant sites of the body where the virus can infect and replicate in other cells.

As mentioned before, NK cells occupy a critical position during the initial host responses against pathogens, particularly during virus infections (Vivier *et al.*, 2011). *In vitro*, stimulation of NK cells with proinflammatory cytokines induced lysis of FMDV-infected cells and expression of IFN-γ (Toka, *et al.*, 2009). In addition, Toka *et al.*, (2009) also demonstrated that direct activation of cytokine-secreting accessory cells by TLR7 and TLR8 agonists and at least partial activation of NK cells by these compounds, caused cytotoxitciy against FMDV-infected cells through enhanced secretion of IFN-γ and storage of perforin granules (Toka, *et al.*, 2009). Interestingly, the same group later demonstrated that during FMDV infection of swine there is a reduced capacity of NK cells to lyse target cells and secrete IFN-γ (Toka *et al.*, 2009). The later *in vivo* results contrast with the former (*in vitro*) results, which is not entirely unexpected given the complexity of host-virus interactions and immune responses during FMDV infection. Natural killer cell dysfunction during the viremic phase of acute infection with FMDV suggest that the virus can effectively block NK function and evade the host's immune system allowing the virus to replicate and disseminate within the host. Several mechanisms attempt to explain, synergistically, the inhibition or lack of activation of NK cells during FMDV infection. Upregulation of TLR3 and more transiently of SOCS3 mRNA can lead to a block in IFN-α gene expression, which is necessary for NK activation. Additionally, inhibitory effects on protein synthesis, specifically cytokines of importance in NK activation such as IL-12, IL-15, and IL-18, can render NK cells hyporeactive to FMDV. Although it is know that a number of surface receptors with inhibitory and activating functions modulate responses of NK cells to infected cells, measurement of mRNA expression for some of these molecules such as NKG2D, NKp80, and granzyme B was minimally altered in infected animals. Nevertheless, these cells were dysfunctional. Although productive infection of NK cells could not be demonstrated the authors did not rule out the possibility of low levels of viral replication. While specific mechanisms explaining NK cell dysfunction remain unresolved, it is evident that FMDV infection induces negative effects in NK cell function, including reduced cytotoxicity, impaired expression of NK cell receptors, and reduced capacity to secrete cytokines, ultimately allowing the virus to effectively evade the host antiviral responses to FMDV infection.

FMDV also has an effect on other lymphocytic populations. It has been demonstrated that there is a transient lymphopenia during the peak of viremia in infected swine and cattle (Bautista *et al.*, 2003; Diaz-San Segundo *et al.*, 2006; Perez-Martin *et al.*, 2012). T and B cell subsets are affected and severe lymphoid depletion in lymphoid organs has been reported (Diaz-San Segundo *et al.*, 2006). In addition, the T cell function during early stages of infection is significantly impaired (Bautista *et al.*, 2003; Diaz-San Segundo *et al.*, 2006; Ostrowski *et al.*, 2005). One possible mechanism that can explain such diminished T cell responses could be related to the elevated amounts of IL-10 produced by the cDCs during infection (Diaz-San Segundo *et al.*, 2009; Ostrowski *et al.*, 2005), as IL-10 has been reported to have a role in inducing immunosuppression *in vivo* (Brooks *et al.*, 2006). However, the exact mechanisms involved in FMDV-induced lymphopenia remain poorly understood. While infection of lymphocytes with FMDV has been described in swine and cattle (Diaz-San Segundo *et al.*, 2006; Joshi *et al.*, 2009), infection could not be associated with cell death, suggesting that lymphopenia during infection might not be related to virus-mediated killing.

Effects on the early host innate and subsequent adaptive immune responses, such as modulation of DC and NK cells and transient lymphopenia, may provide favorable conditions for the virus to both spread systemically within the animal and shed infectious particles into the environment. Although there is a rapid B cell depletion after FMDV infection, the host is still able to mount a very fast antibody response that clears virus within 4-5 days postinfection. Ultimately, the infected host will induce production of serum IgM detectable as early as 3-4 days post-infection followed by maximum IgA and then IgG titers 1 to 2 weeks later (Collen *et al.*, 1989; Juleff *et al.*, 2009; Pacheco *et al.*, 2010; Salt *et al.*, 1996). Using a murine experimental model, it was demonstrated that an effective neutralizing antibody response seems to occur despite absence of T-cell help. Spleen cells of mice were adoptively transferred into irradiated recipients and only B cells were able to control viremia in FMDV-infected animals (Borca *et al.*, 1986). Similarly, it was shown that FMDV-infected DCs can stimulate CD9+ B-cells producing neutralizing anti-FMDV immunoglobulin M antibodies without T-lymphocyte collaboration. Therefore, it is suggested that early protective thymus-independent antibody responses to FMDV is mediated, in mice, by splenic B lymphocytes (Otrowski *et al.*, 2007). Similar results have been reported in cattle (Juleff *et al.*, 2009). In this regard, the specific mechanism of B-cell activation in the absence of T-cell activation in swine and cattle requires further investigation.

4   FMDV is Susceptible to IFN

IFNs are the first line of the host innate immune defense against viral infection in mammals (**Ank et al., 2006;** Basler, and Garcia-Sastre, 2002; Frese *et al.*, 2002). Three families of IFNs have been described, type I, II and III, based on their receptor specificity (Fensterl & Sen, 2009). Type I IFNs (IFN-α and IFN-β) signal through a heterodimeric receptor complex formed by IFNAR1/IFNAR2, type II IFN (IFN-γ) signals through the complex IFN-γR1/IFN-γR2, and type III IFNs bind the receptor complex IL-28Rα/IL-10Rβ. IFNs have some overlapping biologic activities but unique functional roles in the innate and adaptive immune response. Type I IFNs, are primarily responsible for inducing direct antiviral responses in virus infected cells and do so with more potency than IFN-γ (Tan *et al.*, 2005), but type I IFNs can also stimulate DC maturation and NK cell activation (Tilg, 1997). IFN-γ is mainly produced by activated T lymphocytes and NK cells (Schoenborn & Wilson, 2007). In addition to having antiviral activity, IFN-γ also activates components of the cell-mediated immune system such as cytotoxic T lymphocytes, macrophages, and NK cells, favoring Th1 responses. Type III IFNs are also induced in response to recognition of PAMPs and activation of transcription factors, such as NF-κB and IRF-3 and -7, and are mainly produced by DCs (Iversen *et al.*, 2010). However, expression of the type III IFN receptor in a tissue-specific manner, particularly in epithelia, has been proposed as one of the mechanisms that some organisms utilize to prevent and protect themselves from viral invasion through the skin and mucosal surfaces (Sommereyns *et al.*, 2008). Despite the receptor differences, the three families of IFN transduce signals through the JAK-STAT pathways and type I and type III IFNs induce redundant responses. After the IFN pathway is stimulated transcriptional up-regulation of hundreds of effector genes occurs to block viral infection and spread (Der at al., 1998; Takaoka & Yanai, 2006).

As explained above and similar to many other viruses, FMDV counteracts the innate immune response at least in part by blocking the expression of IFN (Chinsangaram *et al.*, 1999; de los Santos *et al.*

2006). In fact, L^pro is the major FMDV protein responsible for this blocking effect. This was initially observed in supernatants from leaderless virus-infected primary cells, which contain higher levels of IFN-α/β antiviral activity than supernatants from wild-type (WT) virus-infected cells (Chinsangaram et al., 1999). Furthermore, it has been demonstrated that pretreatment of cell cultures with type I, type II, and type III IFNs can dramatically inhibit replication of all seven FMDV serotypes (Chinsangaram et al., 1999, 2001; Diaz-San Segundo et al., 2011; Moraes et al., 2007). To determine whether IFN could block FMDV replication in vivo in swine and/or cattle, replication defective human Ad5 vectors that express type I, II and III IFNs were constructed (Grubman et al., 2012). These vectors have the advantage of allowing for a sustained production of IFN in treated animals reducing the need for multiple inoculations of relatively high doses of IFN protein that could lead to undesirable adverse effects (Lukaszewski and Brooks, 2000; Qin et al., 1998; Santodonato et al., 2001). In addition, unlike humans, livestock do not have pre-existing antibodies to human Ad5 vectors and thus administration of this vector containing various foreign transgenes can efficiently induce an immune response to the transgenes in swine and cattle (Graham & Previc, 1992; Mayr et al., 1999). Swine pretreated with Ad5 vectors expressing either porcine IFN-α (Ad5-poIFN-α), porcine IFN-γ (Ad5-poIFN-γ) or porcine IFN-λ (Ad5-poIFN-λ) are completely protected when challenged with different FMDV serotypes one day post inoculation (Chinsangaram et al., 2003; Dias et al., 2011; Moraes et al., 2003, 2007; Perez-Martin et al., manuscript in preparation) and protection lasts 3-5 days (Moraes et al., 2003). Interestingly, the synergistic actions of type I in combination with type II IFN can block virus replication in vivo; swine inoculated with a combination of Ad5-poIFN-α and Ad5-poIFN-γ, at doses that alone do not protect against FMDV, are completely protected against clinical disease and do not develop viremia (Moraes et al., 2007). In cattle, the use of type I or type II IFNs has had only limited success (Wu et al., 2003). However, treatment of cattle with an Ad5 vector expressing type III IFN (Ad5-boIFN-λ3) followed by exposure to aerosolized FMDV, resulted in protection for at least 9 days post challenge (Perez-Martin et al., 2012).

5   IFNs Induce Tissue-Specific Innate Immune Cell Infiltration and Stimulate ISGs Expression against FMDV

Although the critical importance of the IFN system in regulating FMDV pathogenesis is now well established, it is still unclear how IFN inhibits FMDV replication and dissemination. The action of IFNs can involve upregulation of hundreds of IFN-stimulated genes (ISGs) and activation of different aspects of the immune system. It has been recently demonstrated that the actions of IFN can not only be virus-specific, but also ISGs- and tissue specific (Fensterl et al., 2012; Schoggins & Rice, 2011).

In vitro studies demonstrated that at least two ISGs, double-stranded-RNA-dependent protein kinase (PKR) and 2', 5' oligoadenylate synthetase (OAS)/RNase L, are involved in inhibition of FMDV replication (Chinsangaram et al., 2001; de los Santos et al., 2006). Subsequently in Ad5-IFN-treated animals, we showed that numerous ISGs were induced and that protection against FMDV correlated with an increase of the 10-kDa IFN-γ-inducible protein (IP-10) mRNA expression in peripheral blood mononuclear cells (PBMCs) as well as in all analyzed FMDV infected tissues (Figure 2; Diaz-San Segundo et al., 2010; Moraes et al., 2007;), including isolated skin DCs and NK cells (Figure 2; Diaz-San Segundo et al., 2010,2011). This chemokine is known to be involved in the recruitment, proliferation, and activation of NK cells (Taub et al., 1995) and has been demonstrated to have a protective effect in mice infected with a number of viruses including mouse hepatitis virus (Trifilo et al., 2004), coxsackievirus B3 (Yu

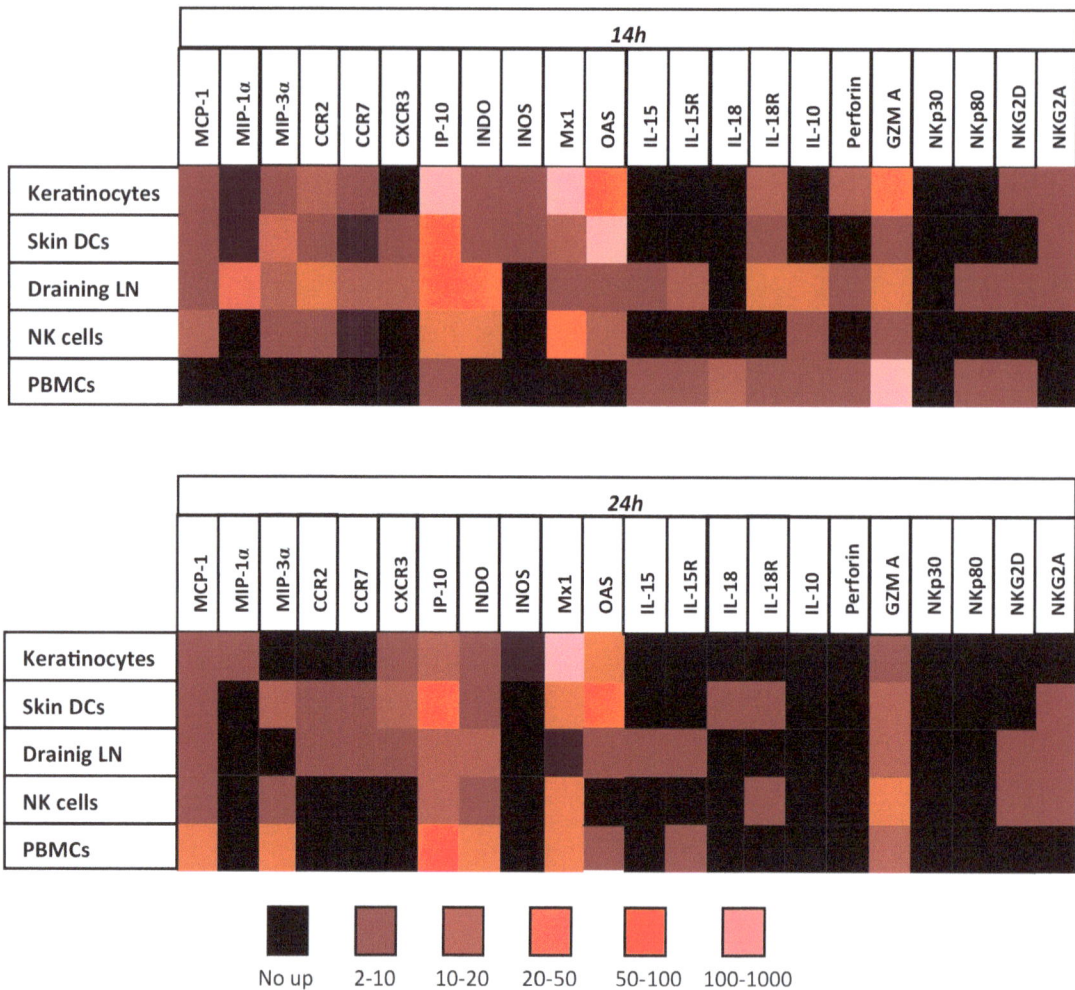

Figure 2: Induction of interferon stimulated genes (ISGs) in PBMCs, keratinocytes, skin DCs, NK cells, and the draining lymph node (LN) of swine. Real time RT-PCR was used to analyze upregulation of ISGs in different organs. Relative mRNA levels were determined by comparative cycle threshold analysis utilizing as a reference the samples at 0 dpi from the control group and upregulation of genes at different time-points are represented in different shades of red as indicated in the figure.

an et al., 2009), dengue virus (Chen et al., 2006), and respiratory syncytial virus (Lindell et al., 2008), but not in Theiler's murine encephalomyelitis virus (TMEV) infected mice (Tsunoda et al., 2004). To determine whether IP-10 has a role in the IFN-induced protection against FMDV, we used a mouse model for FMDV developed by Salguero et al. (2005). IP-10 knockout (ko) or WT C57Bl/6 mice were treated with murine IFN-α (muIFN-α) or PBS 4 h prior to challenge. Although IFN treatment protected 100% of WT C57Bl/6 mice, protection was significantly reduced to only 30% survival when the IP-10 gene was absent, (Diaz-San Segundo et al., submitted). These results indicated that IP-10 is directly involved in protection induced by IFN against FMDV.

The major replication organ for FMDV and the main site of macroscopic lesions in infected animals is the skin (Alexandersen *et al.*, 2003). We have observed that the totality of animals inoculated with an Ad5 vector expressing IFN not only show statistically significant higher numbers of epidermal DCs, but also these cells appear larger and displayed more dendrites 24 h after IFN treatment (Figure 3; Diaz-San Segundo *et al.*, 2010). LCs migrate selectively to areas with higher concentrations of MIP-3α (via CCR6), a chemokine that is secreted by keratinocytes (Charbonnier *et al.*, 1999). In studies in swine inoculated with Ad5-poIFN-α, we found systemic antiviral activity in plasma and high levels of poIFN-α in serum (Figure 4), and there are increased mRNA levels of MIP-3α in keratinocytes and skin DCs 14 h after inoculation (Figure 2). Other IFN-regulated chemokines including monocyte chemotactic protein-1 (MCP-1), macrophage inflammatory protein (MIP)-1α, and IP-10 are not only involved in migration, but also in epidermal DC maturation (Fujita *et al.*, 2005). We showed that upregulation of both, MCP-1 and IP-10, occurs in keratinocytes and LCs of Ad5-poIFN-α treated animals (Figure 2). Furthermore, the IP-10 receptor, chemokine (C-X-C motif) receptor (CXCR) 3, is also upregulated in skin DCs (Figure 2). These results indicate that the migratory capacity of skin DCs is enhanced following IFN treatment. Most importantly, this enhancement correlates with protection against FMDV.

In addition, several studies have shown that IFN-α can induce rapid differentiation of monocytes into activated DCs (Longhi *et al.*, 2009). In order to verify the correlation between these upregulated chemokines and swine skin DCs maturation, we analyzed skin DC status in pigs treated with type I IFN. DC maturation is a multi-step process characterized by phenotypic changes including: redistribution of major histocompatibility complex (MHC) molecules from intracellular endocytic compartments to the cell membrane surface, down-regulation of antigen internalization, increase in antigen processing, increase in the surface expression of co-stimulatory molecules (CD80/86), and morphological changes (*e.g.* formation of dendrites). As previously described, there is an increase in the number of LCs and a significant increase in size and number of dendrites in the skin of Ad5-IFN-α-treated swine. Furthermore, we found that skin DCs extracted from pigs treated with Ad5-poIFN-α showed increased antigen processing capacity (Figure 5a), increased expression of CD80/86 (Figure 5b), and decreased phagocytic activity (Figure 5c). However, no changes were observed in micropinocytosis activity or in the expression of MHC II molecules (Figure 5d). These data indicate that IFN-α induces partial maturation of skin DCs. Moreover, upregulation of mRNA levels of IL-18 and IL-15 at 24 and 48 h respectively after treatment with IFN-α has been observed in the skin (Diaz-San Segundo *et al.*, 2010). These two cytokines are produced by activated DCs (Andoniou *et al.*, 2005, Lucas *et al.*, 2007) and are functionally involved in porcine NK cell proliferation and activation (Toka *et al.*, 2009). In recent *ex vivo* experiments in which skin DCs from pigs were treated with type I IFN, we also found upregulation of IL-18 and IL-18R mRNA expression was also noticed (Figure 2). Furthermore, supernatants obtained from the *ex vivo* assay used to purify skin DCs, showed increased levels of IL-18 with significant amounts by 24 h after treatment (Figure 4b). IL-18 was also detected in the serum of IFN-treated animals at 24 h post-treatment (Figure 4a), indicating that IL-18 secretion by DCs was systemic. Increased expression of IL-18R was also observed in enriched populations of NK cells obtained from PBMCs extracted from IFN-α-treated swine (Figure 2). These results suggest that IFN-α dependent expression of IL-18 and IL-15 by DCs might be responsible for enhanced NK activity. Infiltration of NK cells in the skin of IFN treated swine was not detected by immunophenotype analysis (CD2⁺/CD8⁺/CD3⁻) using an immunofluorescence technique; however an increase in the number of these cells in draining lymph nodes was noticeable (Diaz-San Segundo *et al.*, 2010). We also detected upregulation of perforin and granzyme A in draining lymph nodes, as well as genes associated with NK cell regulation (NKp80, NKG2A and NKG2D) (Figure 2).

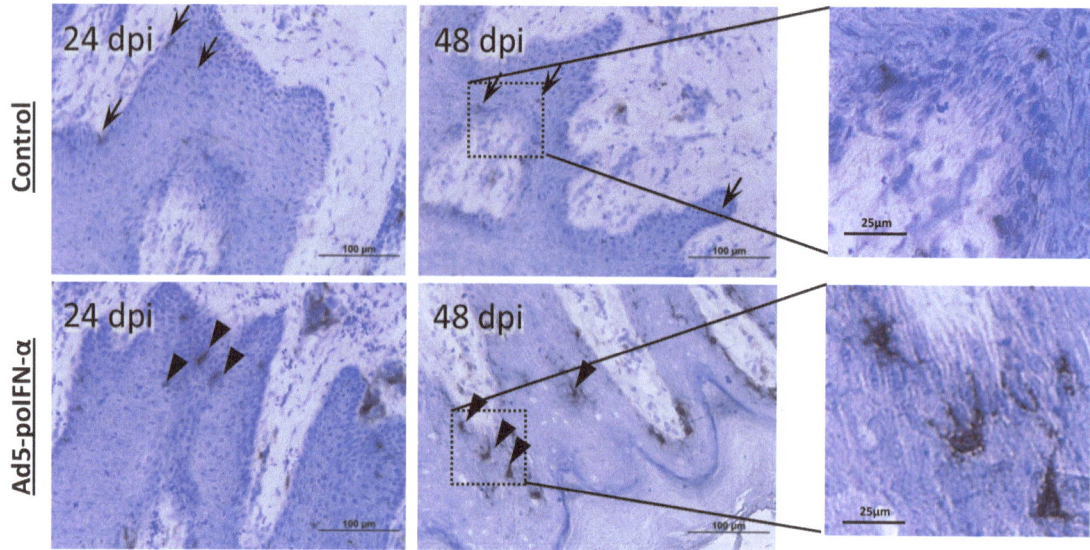

(a)

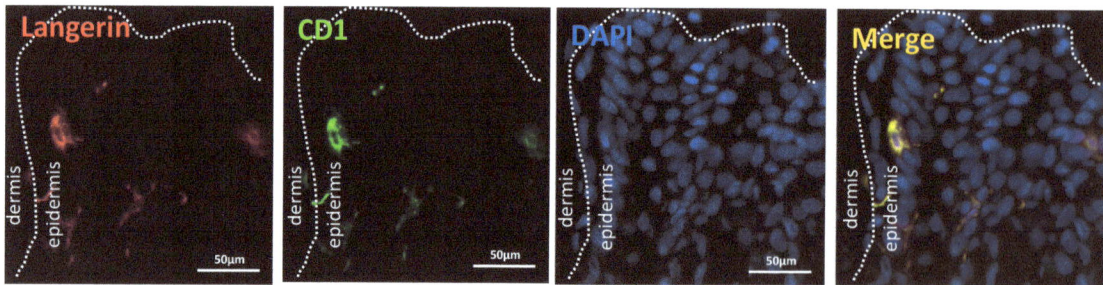

(b)

Figure 3: Immunohistochemical detection of DCs in skin from the heel-bulb of swine. a. Skin from control non-treated animals or Ad5-poIFN-α-inoculated swine was harvested 24 and 48 h after Ad5 treatment. **a.** CD1[+] cells were detected by immunohistochemistry (IHC) using the avidin-biotin-peroxidase complex technique and developed with 3,3′-diaminobenzidine which gives a brown product where primary antibody binds (dark brown); sections were counterstained with Harry's hematoxylin. Arrows indicate positive staining for DCs in control animals; these cells were small and appeared localized in the stratum basale of the epidermis. Arrowheads indicate the positive staining of DCs in treated animals; these cells appeared larger than positive cells in control animals, showed dendrites, and were localized along the stratum spinosum. **b.** Double-Immunofluoresence (IFA) detection of CD207/Langerin (red) and CD1 (green) in the epidermis of the heel-bulb. Nuclei were stained with DAPI (blue) (adapted from Diaz-San Segundo *et al.*, 2010).

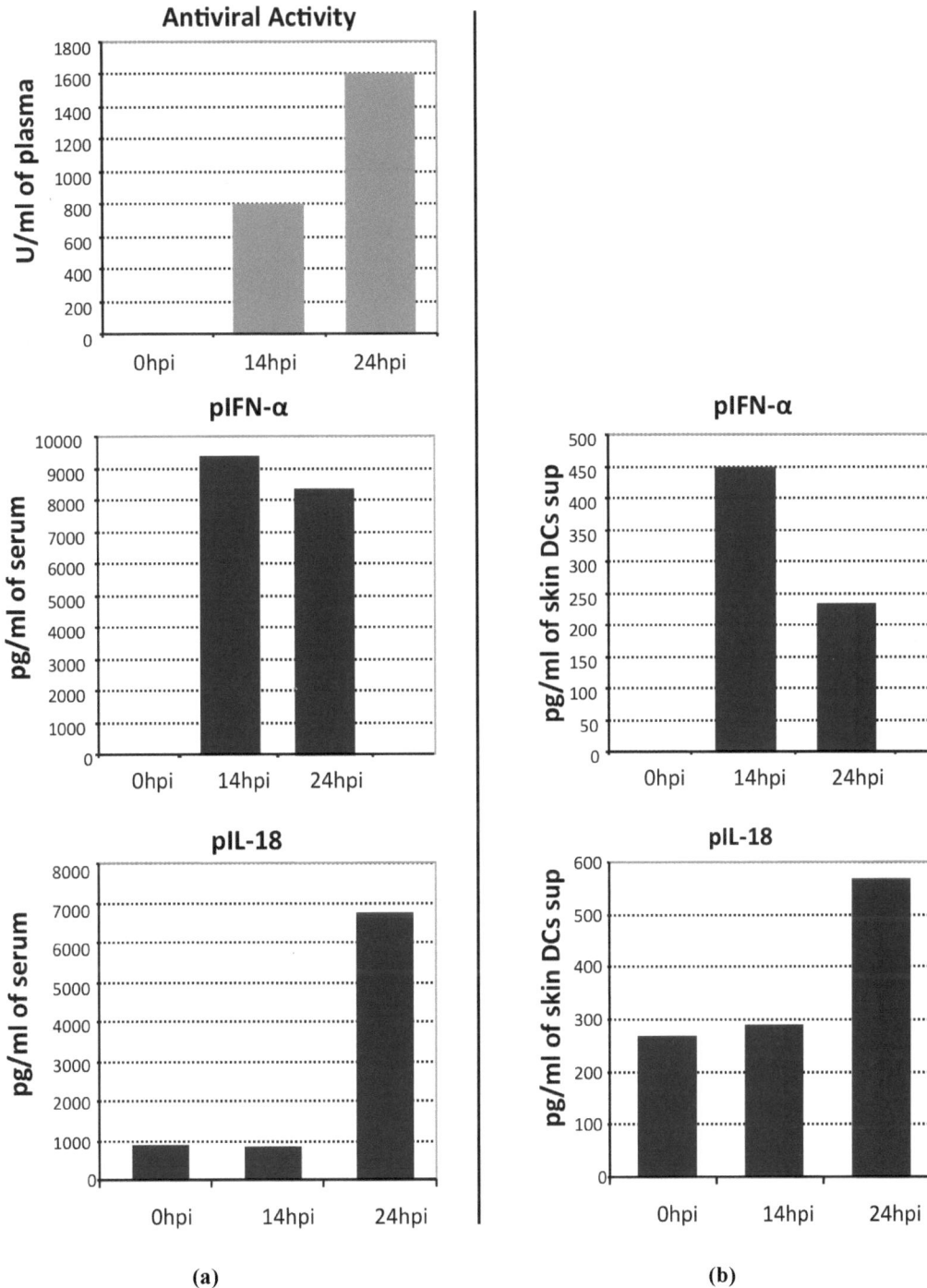

Figure 4: Effect of IFN treatment in swine. Systemic effect (serum and plasma) (a) or effects in skin DCs (b) were evaluated by measuring antiviral activity or levels of poIFN-α and IL-18 in plasma, serum or supernatant of skin DCs, 14 and 24 h after IFN treatment. Antiviral activity was detected in a porcine cell line and is expressed as Units (U) per milliliter of plasma. Amounts of IFN-α and IL-18 were detected by ELISA and are expressed in picograms per milliliter (pg/ml).

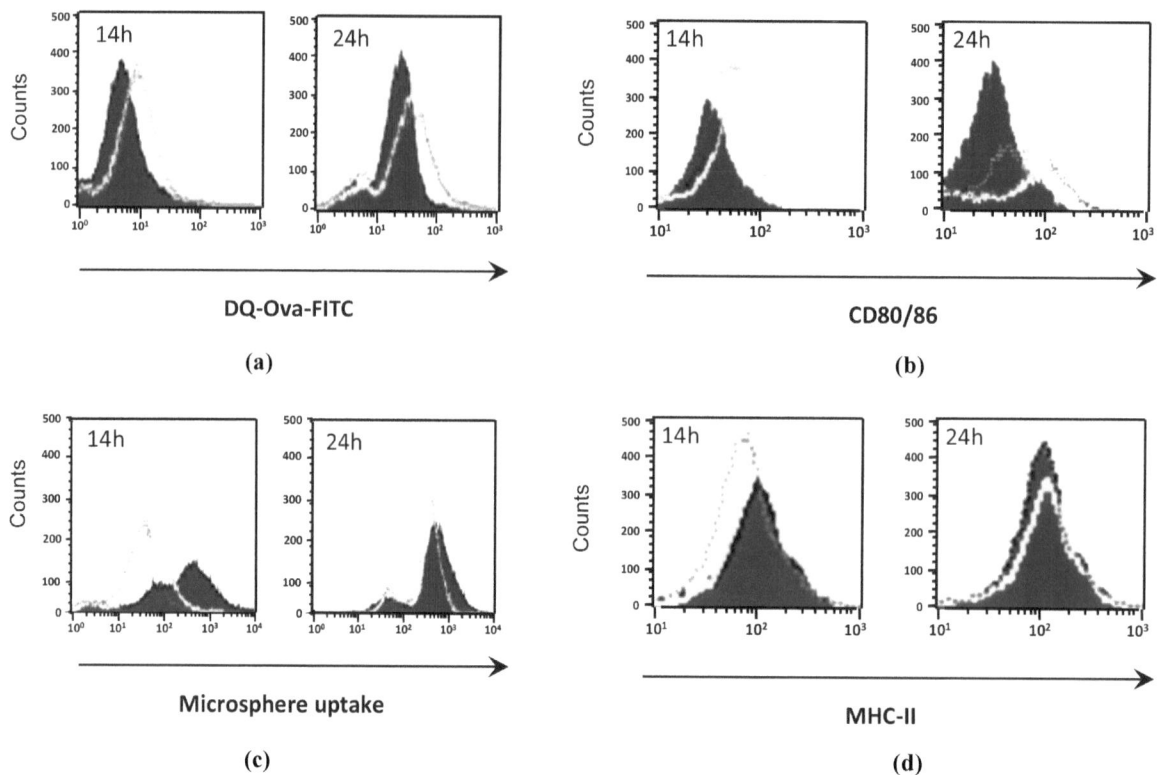

Figure 5: Maturation of skin DCs induced by IFN treatment. Antigen processing (a.), co-stimulatory molecules expression (CD80/86) (b.), phagocytosis (c.), and expression of MHC-II (d.) were evaluated on swine skin DCs extracted at 14 or 24 h after type I IFN treatment. **a.** Isolated skin DCs were incubated with 2 µg/ml DQ-OVA-FITC at 37°C for 2 h. DQ-OVA processing in DCs was assessed by comparing the intensity of FITC signal of cells from treated animals (open histograms) with that obtained from a control untreated pig (filled histogram). **b.** CD80/86 surface staining was analyzed by flow cytometry from freshly isolated skin DCs from treated and control animals at 14 and 24 h after treatment. **c.** Isolated skin DCs were incubated with fluorescent labeled polystyrene microspheres of 2 µm diameter at 37°C for 2 h. Phagocytosis was assessed by comparing the intensity of microspheres signal of cells from treated animals (open histograms) with that obtained from a control untreated pig (filled histogram). **d.** MHC-II surface staining was analyzed by flow cytometry from freshly isolated skin DCs from treated and control animals at 14 and 24 h after treatment. Analysis was performed on a FACSCalibur® flow cytometer using the Cell Quest® software (Becton Dickinson, San Jose, CA).

However, whether NK cells in the draining lymph node display an increased killing activity after IFN treatment requires further research. It has been previously described that NK cells are rapidly recruited to lymph nodes upon DC activation (Longhi *et al.*, 2009). It is possible that IFN-induced DCs maturation is involved in NK cells recruitment to the lymph nodes via IL-18 and IL-15 stimuli. In fact, we also observed upregulation of IL-15 and IL-18 mRNA levels in draining lymph nodes of IFN treated animals (Figure 2 and Diaz-San Segundo *et al.*, 2010).

Cytotoxicity of NK cells can be enhanced by many activating cytokines. Type I IFN is one of the most potent activators of NK cells in both humans and in mice (Biron *et al.*, 1999); however, as mentioned earlier, the underlying mechanism of enhanced NK cytotoxicity remains incompletely understood. It has been proposed that IL-15 produced by accessory DCs in response to type I IFN can activate NK cells (Lucas *et al.*, 2007). Furthermore, type I IFN-induced granzyme B and perforin were found to be required for NK cell activation in response to vaccinia virus infection in mice (Martinez *et al.*, 2008). These results suggest that type I IFN can activate NK cells by direct and indirect mechanisms. To this end, it is evident that intricate pathways involving NK cell cytokine responses that depend on cross-talk with activated/mature DCs exists, and systemic antiviral effects induced by FMDV infection add complexity to the current understanding of virus-host interactions. Further studies are required to understand the role of NK cells in protection against FMDV infection.

6   Concluding Remarks

Similar to most viruses, FMDV is highly sensitive to the action of IFNs. Acting in a concerted manner hundreds of IFN stimulated genes control viral infection through the induction of direct antiviral activity and the modulation of multiple cellular responses. Concurrently, FMDV has evolved numerous strategies to effectively counteract the effects of IFN, thus establishing infection. The studies described herein will contribute to a better understanding of the intricate relationships between FMDV and the host immune response and will hopefully lead to the development of new and improved disease control strategies.

Acknowledgements

This research was supported in part by the Plum Island Animal Disease Research Participation Program administered by the Oak Ridge Institute for Science and Education through an interagency agreement between the U.S. Department of Energy and the U.S. Department of Agriculture (appointment of Nestor Montiel), by CRIS project number 1940-32000-057-00D, ARS, USDA (M. J. Grubman and T. de los Santos) and by grants through an interagency agreement with the Science and Technology Directorate of the U.S. Department of Homeland Security under the Award Numbers HSHQDC-09-X00373 and HSHQDC-11-X-00189 (M. J. Grubman and T. de los Santos). We thank the animal care staff at PIADC for their professional support and assistance

References

Alexandersen, S., Zhang, Z., Donaldson, A. I. & Garland, A. J (2003). The pathogenesis and diagnosis of foot-and-mouth disease. Journal of Comparative Pathology, 129, 1-36.

Andoniou, C. E., van Dommelen, S. L. H., Voigt, V., Andrews, D. M., Brizard, G., Asselin-Paturel, C., Delale, T., Stacey, K. J., Trinchieri, G., & Degli-Esposti., M. A. (2005). Interaction between conventional dendritic cells and natural killer cells is integral to the activation of effective antiviral immunity. Nature Immunology, 214, 331-341.

Ank N., West, H., & Paludan, S. R. (2006). IFN-lambda: novel antiviral cytokines. Journal of Interferon Cytokine Research, 26, 373-379.

Armer, H., Moffat, K., Wileman, T., Belsham, G. J., Jackson, T., Duprex, W. P., Ryan, M., & Monaghan, P. (2008). Foot-and-mouth disease virus, but not bovine enterovirus, targets the host cell cytoskeleton via the nonstructural protein 3Cpro. Journal of Virology, 82, 10556-10566.

Arzt, J., Juleff, N., Zhang, Z., & Rodriguez, L. L. (2011). The pathogenesis of foot-and-mouth disease I: viral pathways in cattle. Transboundary and Emerging Diseases, 58, 291-304.

Banchereau, J., & Steinman, R. M. (1998). Dendritic cells and the control of immunity. Nature. 392, 245-252.

Basler, C. F., & Garcia-Sastre, A. (2002). Viruses and the type I interferon antiviral system: induction and evasion. Internal Reviews of Immunology, 21, 305-337.

Bautista, E. M., Gregg, D., & Golde, W. T. (2002). Characterization and functional analysis of skin-derived dendritic cells from swine without a requirement for in vitro propagation. Veterinary Immunology and Immunopathology, 88, 131-148.

Bautista, E. M., Ferman, G. S., & Golde, W. T. (2003). Induction of lymphopenia and inhibition of T cell function during acute infection of swine with foot and mouth disease virus (FMDV). Veterinary Immunology and Immunopathology 92, 61-73.

Bautista, E. M., Ferman, G. S., Gregg, D., Brum, M. C., Grubman, M. J., & Golde, W. T. (2005). Constitutive expression of alpha interferon by skin dendritic cells confers resistance to infection by foot-and-mouth disease virus. Journal of Virology, 79, 4838-4847.

Baxt, B., & Mason. P. W. (1995). Foot-and-mouth disease virus undergoes restricted replication in macrophage cell cultures following Fc receptor-mediated adsorption. Virology 207, 503-509.

Belsham, G. J., & Brangwyn, J. K. (1990). A region of the 5' noncoding region of foot-and-mouth disease virus RNA directs efficient internal initiation of protein synthesis within cells: involvement with the role of L protease in translational control. Journal of Virology, 64, 5389-5395.

Belsham, G. J., McInerney, G. M., & Ross-Smith, N. (2000). Foot-and-mouth disease virus 3C protease induces cleavage of translation initiation factors eIF4A and eIF4G within infected cells. Journal of Virology, 74, 272-280.

Biron, C. A., Nguyen, K. B., Pien, G. C., Cousens, L. P., & Salazar-Mather, T. P. (1999). Natural killer cells in antiviral defense: function and regulation by innate cytokines. Annual Reviews of Immunology, 17, 189-220.

Borca, M.V., Fernandez, F.M., Sadir, A.M., Braun, M., & Schudel, A. A. (1986). Immune response to foot-and-mouth disease virus in a murine experimental model: effective thymus-independent primary and secondary reaction. Immunology, 59, 261–267.

Brooks D. G., Trifilo, M. J., Edelmann, K. H., Teyton, L., McGavern, D. B., & Oldstone. M. B. A. (2006). Interleukin-10 determines viral clearance or persistence in vivo. Nature Medicine, 12, 1301-1309.

Charbonnier, A. S., Kohrgruber, N., Kriehuber, E., Stingl, G., Rot, A., & Maurer, D. (1999). Macrophage inflammatory protein 3alpha is involved in the constitutive trafficking of epidermal langerhans cells. Journal of Experimental Medicine, 190, 1755-1768.

Chen, J. P., Lu, H. L., Lai, S. L., Campanella, G. S., Sung, J. M., Lu, M. Y., Wu-Hsieh, B. A., Lin, Y. L., Lane, T. E., Luster, A. D., & Liao, F. (2006). Dengue virus induces expression of CXC chemokine ligand 10/IFN-γ-inducible protein 10, which competitively inhibits viral binding to cell surface heparin sulfate. Journal of Immunology, 177, 3185-3192.

Chinsangaram, J., Beard, C., Mason, P. W., Zellner, M. K., Ward, G., & Grubman, M. J. (1998). Antibody response in mice inoculated with DNA expressing foot-and-mouth disease virus capsid proteins. Journal of Virology, 72, 4454-4457.

Chinsangaram, J., Piccone, M. E. & Grubman, M. J. (1999). Ability of foot-and-mouth disease virus to form plaques in cell culture is associated with suppression of alpha/beta interferon. Journal of Virology, 73, 9891-9898.

Chinsangaram, J., Koster, M., & Grubman, M. J. (2001). Inhibition of L-deleted foot-and-mouth disease virus replication by alpha/beta interferon involves double-stranded RNA-dependent protein kinase. Journal of Virology, 75, 5498-5503.

Chinsangaram, J., Moraes, M. P., Koster, M., & Grubman, M. J. (2003). Novel viral disease control strategy: adenovirus expressing alpha interferon rapidly protects swine from foot-and-mouth disease. Journal of Virology, 77, 1621-1625.

Collen, T., Pullen, L. & Doel, T. R. (1989). T-cell-dependent induction of antibody against foot-and-mouth- disease virus in a mouse model. Journal of General Virology, 70, 395–403.

de los Santos, T., de Avila Botton, S., Weiblen, R. & Grubman, M. J. (2006). The leader proteinase of foot-and-mouth disease virus inhibits the induction of beta interferon mRNA and blocks the host innate immune response. Journal of Virology, 80, 1906-1914.

de los Santos T., Diaz-San Segundo, F., & Grubman, M. J. (2007). Degradation of nuclear factor kappa B during foot-and-mouth disease virus infection. Journal of Virology, 81, 12803-12815.

de los Santos T., Diaz-San Segundo, F., Zhu, J., Koster, M., Dias, C. C., & Grubman, M. J. (2009). A conserved domain in the leader proteinase of foot-and-mouth disease virus is required for proper subcellular localization and function. Journal of Virology, 83, 1800-1810.

Der, S. D., Zhou, A., Williams, B. R. G., & Silverman, R. H. (1998). Identification of genes differentially regulated by interferon α, β, or γ using oligonucleotide arrays. Proceedings of the Natural Academy of Science, 95, 15623-15628.

Devaney, M. A., Vakharia, V. N., Lloyd, R. E., Ehrenfeld, E., & Grubman, M. J. (1988). Leader protein of foot-and-mouth disease virus is required for cleavage of the p220 component of the cap-binding protein complex. Journal of Virology, 62, 4407-4409.

Dias, C. C., Moraes, M. P., Diaz-San Segundo, F., de los Santos, T., & Grubman, M. J. (2011). Porcine type I interferon rapidly protects swine against challenge with multiple serotypes of foot-and-mouth disease virus. Journal Interferon Cytokine Research, 31, 227-236.

Diaz-San Segundo, F., Dias, C. C., Moraes, M. P., Weiss, M., Pérez-Martín, E., Owens, G, Custer, M., Kamrud, K., de los Santos, T., & Grubman, M. J. (2012). Venezuelan equine encephalitis replicon particles can induce rapid protection against foot-and-mouth disease virus. Submitted.

Diaz-San Segundo, F., Weiss, M., Pérez-Martín, E., Dias, C. C., Grubman, M. J., & de los Santos, T. (2012). Inoculation of swine with foot-and-mouth disease SAP-mutant virus induces early protection against disease. Journal of Virology, 86, 1316-27.

Diaz-San Segundo, F., Weiss, M., Pérez-Martín, E., Koster, M. J., Zhu, J., Grubman, M. J., & de los Santos, T. (2011). Antiviral activity of bovine type III interferon against foot-and-mouth disease virus. Virology. 413, 283-292.

Diaz-San Segundo, F., Moraes, M. P., de Los Santos, T., Dias, C. C., & Grubman, M. J. (2010). Interferon-induced protection against foot-and-mouth disease virus infection correlates with enhanced tissue-specific innate immune cell infiltration and interferon-stimulated gene expression. Journal of Virology, 84, 2063-2077.

Diaz-San Segundo, F., Rodriguez-Calvo, T., de Avila, A., & Sevilla, N. (2009). Immunosprression during acute infection with foot-and-mouth disease virus in swine is mediated by IL-10. PLoS One 4, 1-11.

Díaz-San Segundo, F., Salguero, F. J., de Avila, A., de Marco, M. M., Sanchez-Martín, M. A., & Sevilla, N. (2006). Selective lymphocyte depletion during the early stage of the immune response to foot-and-mouth disease virus infection in swine. Journal of Virology, 80, 2369-2379.

Donnelly, M. L., Hughes, L. E., Luke, G., Mendoza, H., ten Dam, E., Gani, D., & Ryan, M. D. (2001a). The 'cleavage' activities of foot-and-mouth disease virus 2A site- directed mutants and naturally occurring '2A-like' sequences. Journal of General Virology, 82, 1027-1041.

Donnelly, M. L., Hughes, L. E., Luke, G., Mendoza, H., ten Dam, E., Gani, D., & Ryan, M. D. (2001b). Analysis of the aphthovirus 2A/2B polyprotein 'cleavage' mechanism indicates not a proteolytic reaction, but a novel translational effect: a putative ribosomal 'skip'. Journal of General Virology, 82, 1013-1025.

Falk, M. M., Grigera, P. R., Bergmann, I. E., Zibert, A., Multhaup, G., & Beck, E. (1990). Foot-and-mouth disease virus protease 3C induces specific proteolytic cleavage of host cell histone H3. Journal of Virology, 64, 748-56.

Fracastorius, H. (1546). De alijs differentijs contagionis. De sympathia et antipathia rerum Liber unus. De Contagione et Contagiosis Morbis et Curatione (libri iii), pp. 36–38. Heirs of L.A. Junta Book 1.

Fenster,l V., & Sen, G. C. (2009). Interferons and viral infections. Biofactors, 35, 14–20.

Fensterl, V., Wetzel, J. L., Ramachandran, S., Ogino, T., Stohlman, S. A., Bergmann, C. C., Diamond, M. S., Virgin, H. V. & Sen, G. C. (2012). Interferon-induced Ifit2/ISG54 protects mce from lethal VSV neuropathogenesis. PLoS Pathogens, 8, e1002712.

Frese, M., Schwärzle, V., Barth, K., Krieger, N., Lohmann, V., Mihm, S., Haller, O., & Bartenschlager, R. (2002). Interferon-gamma inhibits replication of subgenomic and genomic hepatitis C virus RNAs. Hepatology, 35, 694-703.

Gladue D. P., O'Donnell, V., Baker-Branstetter, R., Holinka, L. G., Pacheco, J. M., Fernandez Sainz, I., Lu, Z., Brocchi, E., Baxt, B., Piccone, M. E., Rodriguez, L., & Borca, M. V. (2012). Foot and mouth disease virus non structural protein 2C interacts with Beclin1 modulating virus replication. Journal of Virology, 86, 12080-12090.

Golde, W. T., Pacheco, J. M., Duque, H., Doel, T., Penfold, B., Ferman, G. S., Gregg, D. R. & Rodriguez, L. L. (2005). Vaccination against foot-and-mouth disease virus confers complete clinical protection in 7 days and partial protection in 4 days: Use in emergency outbreak response. Vaccine, 23, 5775-5782.

Golde, W. T., Nfon, C. K. & Toka, F. N. (2008). Immune evasion during foot-and-mouth disease virus infection of swine. Immunological Reviews, 225, 85-95.

Graham, F. L. & Prevec, L. (1992). Adenovirus-based expression vectors and recombinant vaccines. Biotechnology, 20, 363-390.

Grubman, M. J., & Baxt, B. (2004). Foot-and-mouth disease. Clinical Microbiology Reviews, 17, 465-493.

Grubman, M. J., Moraes, M. P., Díaz-San Segundo, F., Pena, L., & de los Santos, T. (2008). Evading the host immune response: how foot-and- mouth disease virus has become an effective pathogen. FEMS Immunology and Medical Microbiology, 53, 8-17.

Grubman, M. J., Moraes, M. P., Shutta, C., Barrera, J., Neilan, J., Ettyreddy, D., Butman, B. T., Brough, D. E., & Brake, D. A. (2010). Adenovirus serotype 5-vectored foot-and-mouth disease subunit vaccines: the first decade. Future Virology, 5, 51-64.

Grubman, M. J., Diaz-San Segundo, F., Dias, C. C., Moraes, M. P., Perez-Martin, E. & de los Santos, T. (2012). Use of replication-defective adenoviruses to develop vaccines and biotherapeutics against foot-and-mouth disease. Future Virology, 7, 767-778.

Guzylack-Piriou L., Bergamin, F., Gerber, M., McCullough, K. C., & Summerfield, A. (2006). Plasmacytoid dendritic cell activation by foot-and-mouth disease virus requires immune complexes European Journal of Immunology, 36, 1674-1683.

Haller, O., Staeheli, P., & Kochs, G. (2007). Interferon-induced Mx proteins in antiviral host defense. Biochimie. 89, 812-818.

Iversen, M. B., Ank, N., Melchjorsen, J. & Paludan, S. R. (2010). Expression of type III interferon (IFN) in the vaginal mucosa is mediated primarily by dendritic cells and displays stronger dependence on NF-kappaB than type I IFNs. Journal of Virology, 84, 4579-4586.

Iwasaki, A., & Kelsall, B. L. (2000). Localization of distinct Peyer's patch dendritic cell subsets and their recruitment by chemokines macrophage inflammatory protein (MIP)-3alpha, MIP-3beta, and secondary lymphoid organ chemokine. Journal of Experimental Medicine, 191, 1381–1394.

Joshi, G., Sharma, R. & Kakker, N. K. (2009). Phenotypic and functional characterization of T-cells and in vitro replication of FMDV serotypes in bovine lymphocytes. Vaccine, 27, 6656-6661.

Juleff, N., Windsor, M., Lefevre, E. A., Gubbins, S., Hamblin, P., Reid, E., McLaughlin, K., Beverley, P. C., Morrison, I. W. & Charleston, B. (2009). Foot-and-mouth disease virus can induce a specific and rapid CD4+ T-cell-independent neutralizing and isotype class-switched antibody response in naïve cattle. Journal of Virology, 83, 3626-3636.

Kawai, T., & Akira, S. (2011). Regulation of innate immune signalling pathways by the tripartite motif (TRIM) family proteins. EMBO Molecular Medicine, 3, 513-327.

Kleina, L. G., & Grubman, M. J. (1992). Antiviral effects of a thiol protease inhibitor on foot-and-mouth disease virus. Journal of Virology, 66, 7168-7175.

Kochs, G., & Haller, O. (1999). Interferon-induced human MxA GTPase blocks nuclear import of Thogoto virus nucleocapsids. Proceedings of the Natural Academy of Science, 96, 2082-2086.

Kuhn, R., Luz, N. & Beck, E. (1990). Functional analysis of the internal translation initiation site of foot- and-mouth disease virus. Journal of Virology, 64, 4625-4631.

Klump, W., Marquardt, O. & Hofschneider, P. H. (1984). Biologically active protease of foot-and-mouth disease virus is expressed from cloned viral cDNA in Escherichia coli. Proceedings of the Natural Academy of Science, 81, 3351-3355.

Lawrence P., Schafer, E. A., & Rieder, E. (2012). The nuclear protein Sam68 is cleaved by the FMDV 3C protease redistributing Sam68 to the cytoplasm during FMDV infection of host cells.Virology. 425, 40-52.

Lee M. S., & Kim, Y. J. (2007). Signaling pathways downstream of pattern-recognition receptors and their cross talk. Annual Reviews of Biochemistry, 76, 447–480.

Leforban, Y. (1999). Prevention measures against foot-and-mouth disease in Europe in recent years. Vaccine, 17, 1755-1759.

Lindell, D. M., Lane, T. E., & Lukacs, N. W. (2008). CXCL10/CXCR3-mediated responses promote immunity to respiratory syncytial virus infection by augmenting dendritic cell and CD8+ T cell efficiency. European Journal of Immunology, 38:2168-2179.

Loeffler, F., & Frosch, P. (1897). Summarischer Bericht ueber der Ergebnisse der Untersuchungen zur Erforschung der Maul- und Klauenseuche. ZentBl. Bakt. Parasitkde 22, 257–259.

Longhi, M. P., Trumpfheller, C., Idoyaga, J., Caskey, M., Matos, I., Kluger, C., Salazar, A. M., Colonna, M., & Steinman, R. M. (2009). Dendritic cells require a systemic type I interferon response to mature and induce CD4+ Th1 immunity with poly IC as adjuvant. Journal of Experimental Medicine, 206, 1589-1602.

Lucas, M., Schachterle, W., Oberle, K., Aichele, P., & Diefenbach, A. (2007). Natural killer cell-mediated control of infections requires production of interleukin 15 by type I IFN-triggered dendritic cells. Immunity, 26, 503–517.

Lukaszewski, R. A., & Brooks, T. J. (2000). Pegylated alpha interferon is an effective treatment for virulent Venezuelan equine encephalitis virus and has profound effects on the host immune response to infection. Journal of Virology, 74, 5006–5015.

Martinez, J., Huang, X. & Yang, Y. (2008). Direct action of type I IFN on NK cells is required for their activation in response to vaccinia viral infection in vivo. Journal of Immunology, 180, 1592–1597.

Mason, P. W., Piccone, M. E., McKenna, T. S., Chinsangaram, J., & Grubman, M. J. (1997). Evaluation of a live-attenuated foot-and-mouth disease virus as a vaccine candidate. Virology, 227, 96-102.

Mason, P. W., Chinsangaram, J., Moraes, M.P., Mayr, G.A., & Grubman, M. J. (2003). Engineering better vaccines for foot-and-mouth disease. Developments in Biologicals (Basel), 114, 79-88.

Mayr, G. A., Chinsangaram, J., & Grubman, M. J. (1999). Development of replication-defective adenovirus serotype 5 containing the capsid and 3C protease coding regions of foot-and-mouth disease virus as a vaccine candidate. Virology, 263, 496-506.

McCullough, K.C., Parkinson, D. & Crowther, J. R. (1988). Opsonization-enhanced phagocytosis of foot-and-mouth disease virus. Immunology, 65, 187-191.

Medina, M., Domingo, E., Brangwyn, J. K. & Belsham, G. J. (1993). The two species of the foot-and-mouth disease virus leader protein, expressed individually, exhibit the same activities. Virology, 194, 55-359.

Merad, M., & Manz, M. G. (2009). Dendritic dells homeostasis. Blood, 113, 3418-3427.

Moffat, K., Howell, G,. Knox, C,. Belsham, G. J., Monaghan, P., Ryan, M. D. & Wileman, T. (2005). Effects of foot-and-mouth disease virus nonstructural proteins on the structure and function of the early secretory pathway: 2BC but not 3A blocks endoplasmic reticulum-to-Golgi transport. Journal of Virology, 79, 4382-4395.

Moffat, K., Knox, C., Howell, G., Clark, S. J., Yang, H., Belsham, G. J., Ryan, M., & Wileman, T. (2007). Inhibition of the secretory pathway by foot-and-mouth disease virus 2BC protein is reproduced by coexpression of 2B with 2C, and the site of inhibition is determined by the subcellular location of 2C. Journal of Virology, 81, 1129-1139.

Monaghan, P, Gold, S, Simpson, J, Zhang, Z, Weinreb, P. H., Violette, S. M., Alexandersen, S., & Jackson, T. (2005). The avb6 integrin receptor for foot-and-mouth disease virus is expressed constitutively on the epithelial cells targeted in cattle. Journal of General Virology, 86, 2769-2780.

Moraes, M. P., Chinsangaram, J., Brum, M. C. S., & Grubman, M. J. (2003). Immediate protection of swine from foot-and-mouth disease: a combination of adenoviruses expressing interferon alpha and a foot-and-mouth disease virus subunit vaccine. Vaccine, 22, 268-279.

Moraes, M. P., de los Santos, T., Koster, M., Turecek, T., Wang, H., Andreyev, V. G., & Grubman, M. J. (2007). Enhanced antiviral activity against foot-and-mouth disease virus by a combination of type I and II porcine interferons. Journal of Virology, 81, 7124-7135.

Moraes, M. P., Mayr, G. A., Mason, P. W. & Grubman, M. J. (2002). Early protection against homologous challenge after a single dose of replication-defective human adenovirus type 5 expressing capsid proteins of foot-and-mouth disease virus (FMDV) strain A24. Vaccine, 20, 1631-1639.

Nfon, C. K., Dawson, H., Toka, F. N. & Golde, W. T. (2008). Langerhans cells in porcine skin. Veterinary Immunology and Immunopathology, 126, 236-247.

Nfon, C. K., Ferman, G. S., Toka, F. N., Gregg, D. A., & Golde, W. T. (2008). Interferon-alpha production by swine dendritic cells is inhibited during acute infection with foot-and-mouth disease virus. Viral Immunology, 21, 68-77.

Nfon, C. K., Toka, F. N., Kenney, M., Pacheco, J. M., & Golde, W. T. (2010). Loss of plasmacytoid dendritic cell function coincides with lymphopenia and viremia during foot-and-mouth disease virus infection. Viral Immunology, 23, 29-41. Erratum in: Viral Immunology, 23, 339.

O'Donnell, V., Pacheco, J. M., Gregg, D., & Baxt, B. (2008). Analysis of foot-and-mouth disease virus integrin receptor expression in tissues from naive and infected cattle. Journal of Comparative Pathology, 141, 98-112.

Okuse, C., Rinaudo, K J., Farrar, A., Wells, F., & Korba, B. E. (2005). Enhancement of antiviral activity against hepatitis C virus in vitro by interferon combination therapy. Antiviral Research, 65, 23-34.

Ostrowski, M., Vermeulen, M., Zabal, O., Geffner, J. R., Sadir, A. M. & Lopez, O. J. (2005). Impairment of thymus-dependent responses by murine dendritic cells infected with foot-and-mouth disease virus. Journal of Immunology, 175, 3971-3979.

Ostrowski, M., Vermeulen, M., Zabal, O., Zamorano, P. I., Sadir, A. M., Geffner, J. R. & Lopez. O. J. (2007). The early protective thymus-independent antibody response to foot-and-mouth disease virus is mediated by splenic CD9+ B lymphocytes. Journal of Virology, 81, 9357-9367.

Pacheco, J. M., Brum, M. C. S., Moraes, M. P., Golde, W. T., & Grubman, M. J. (2005). Rapid protection of cattle from direct challenge with foot-and-mouth disease virus (FMDV) by a single inoculation with an adenovirus vectored FMDV subunit vaccine. Virology, 337, 205-209.

Pacheco, J.M., Butler, J.E., Jew, J., Ferman, G.S., Zhu, J., & Golde, W.T. (2010). IgA antibody response of swine to foot-and-mouth disease virus infection and vaccination. Clinical and Vaccine Immunology, 17, 550–558.

Perez-Martin E., Weiss, M., Diaz-San Segundo, F., Pacheco, J. M., Arzt, J., Grubman, M. J., & de los Santos, T. (2012). Bovine type III interferon significantly delays and reduces the severity of foot-and-mouth disease in cattle. Journal of Virology, 86, 4477-4487.

Piccone, M. E., Rieder, E., Mason, P. W., & Grubman, M. J. (1995). The foot and- mouth disease virus leader proteinase gene is not required for viral replication. Journal of Virology, 69, 5376-5382.

Piccone, M. E., Pacheco, J. M., Pauszek, S. J., Kramer, E., Rieder, E., Borca, M. V., & Rodriguez, L. L. (2010). The region between the two polyprotein initiation codons of foot-and-mouth disease virus is critical for virulence in cattle. Virology, 396, 152-159.

Qin, X.Q., Tao, N., Dergay, A., Moy, P., Fawell, S., Davis, A., Wilson, J.M., & Barsoum, J. (1998). Interferon-beta gene therapy inhibits tumor formation and causes regression of established tumors in immune-deficient mice. Proceedings of the Natural Academy of Science, 95, 14411–14416.

Reid, E., Juleff, N., Gubbins, .S, Prentice, H., Seago, J., & Charleston B. (2011). Bovine plasmacytoid dendritic cells are the major source of type I interferon in response to foot-and-mouth disease virus in vitro and in vivo. Journal of Virology, 85, 4297-4308.

Reizis, B., Bunin, A., Ghosh, H, S., Lewis, K. L., & Sisirak V. (2011). Plasmacytoid dendritic cells: recent progress and open questions. Annual Review in Immunology, 29, 163-183.

Rigden, R. C., Carrasco, C. P., Summerfield, A., & McCullough, K. C. (2002). Macrophage phagocytosis of foot-and-mouth disease virus may create infectious carriers. Immunology, 106, 537-548.

Roberts, P. J., & Belsham, G. J. (1995). Identification of critical amino acids within the foot-and-mouth disease virus leader protein, a cysteine protease. Virology, 213, 140-146.

Robinson, M. J., Sancho, D., Slack, E. C., LeibundGut-Landmann, S., & Reis e Sousa. C. (2006). Myeloid C-type lectins in innate immunity. Nature Immunology, 7, 1258-1265.

Robinson, L., Windsor, M., McLaughlin, K., Hope, J., Jackson, T., & Charleston, B. (2011) Foot-and-mouth disease virus exhibits an altered tropism in the presence of specific immunoglobulins, enabling productive infection and killing of dendritic cells. Journal of Virology, 85, 2212-2223.

Rueckert, R. R. (1996). Picornaviridae: the viruses and their replication. In "Field's Virology" (B. N. Fields, D.M. Knipe, and P.H. Howley, Ed.), pp. 609-654. Lippincott-Raven, Philadelphia and New York.

Rueckert R. R., & Wimmer, E. (1984). Systematic nomenclature of picornavirus proteins. Journal of Virology, 50, 957-959.

Salguero, F. J., Sánchez-Martín, M. A., Díaz-San Segundo, F., de Avila, A., & Sevilla, N.. (2005). Foot-and-mouth disease virus (FMDV) causes an acute disease that can be lethal for adult laboratory mice. Virology. 332:384-396.

Salt, J. S., Mulcahy, G., & Kitching, R. P. (1996). Isotype-specific antibody responses to foot-and-mouth disease virus in sera and secretion of 'carrier' and 'non-carrier' cattle. Epidemiology and Infection, 117, 349-360.

Santodonato, L., Ferrantini, M. Palombo, F., Aurisicchio, L., Delmastro, P., La Monica, N., Di Marco, S., Ciliberto, G., Du, M. X., Taylor, M. W., & Belardelli, F. (2001). Antitumor activity of recombinant adenoviral vectors expressing murine IFN-alpha in mice injected with metastatic IFN-resistant tumor cells. Cancer Gene Therapy, 8, 63–72.

Sanz-Parra, A., Sobrino, F., & Ley, V. (1998). Infection with foot-and-mouth disease virus results in a rapid reduction of MHC class I surface expression. Journal of General Virology, 79, 433-436.

Schoenborn, J. R., & Wilson,, C. B. (2007). Regulation of interferon-gamma during innate and adaptive immune responses. Advances in Immunology, 96, 41–101.

Schoggins, J. W., & Rice, C. M. (2011). Interferon stimulated genes and their antiviral effector functions. Current Opinion on Virology, 6, 519-525.

Skern, T., Fita, I. & Guarne, A. (1998). A structural model of picornavirus leader proteinases based on papain and bleomycin hydrolase. Journal of General Virology, 79, 301-307.

Sommereyns, C., Paul, S., Staeheli, P., & Michiels, T. (2008). IFN-lambda (IFN-lambda) is expressed in a tissue-dependent fashion and primarily acts on epithelial cells in vivo. PLoS Pathogens, 4, e1000017.

Strebel, K., & Beck, E. (1986). A second protease of foot-and-mouth disease virus. Journal of Virology, 58, 893-899.

Summerfield, A., & McCullough, K. C. (2009). The porcine dendritic cell family. Developmental and Comparative Immunology, 33, 299-309.

Takaoka, A., & Yanai, H. (2006). Interferon signalling network in innate defence. Cell Microbiology, 8, 907-922.

Tan, H., Derrick, J., Hong, J., Sanda, C., Grosse, W., M., Edenberg, H. J., Taylor, M., Seiwert, S., & Blatt, L. M. (2005). Global transcriptional profiling J. demonstrates the combination of type I and type II interferon enhances antiviral and immune responses at clinically relevant doses. Journal of Interferon Cytokine Research, 25, 632–649.

Taub, D. D., Sayers, T. J., Carter, C. R. D., & Ortaldo, J. R. (1995). α and β chemokines induce NK cell migration and enhance NK-mediated cytolysis. Journal of Immunology, 155, 3877-3888.

Tilg, H. (1997). New insights into the mechanisms of interferon alpha: an immunoregulatory and anti-inflammatory cytokine. Gastroenterology, 112, 1017-1021.

Toka, F. N., Nfon, C. K. Dawson, H., Estes, D., & Golde, W. T. (2009). Activation of porcine natural killer cells and lysis of foot-and-mouth disease virus infected cells. Journal of Interferon Cytokine Research, 29, 179-192.

Toka, F. N., Nfon, C. K. Dawson, H. & Golde, W. T. (2009). Accessory-cell-mediated activation of porcine NK cells by toll-like receptor 7 (TLR7) and TLR8 agonists. Clinical Vaccine Immunology, 16, 866-878.

Toka, F. N., Nfon, C. K. Dawson, H., & Golde, W. T. (2009). Natural killer cell dysfunction during acute infection with foot-and-mouth disease virus. Clinical Vaccine Immunology, 16, 1738-1749.

Trifilo, M. J., Montalto-Morrison, C., Stiles, L. N., Hurst, K. R., Hardison, J. L., Manning, J. E., Masters, P. S., & Lane, T. E. (2004). CXC chemokine ligand 10 controls viral infection in the central nervous system: evidence for a role in innate immune response through recruitment and activation of natural killer cells. Journal of Virology, 78, 585-594.

Trinchieri, G,, & Sher, A. (2007). Cooperation of Toll-like receptor signals in innate immune defense. Nature Reviews on Immunology, 7, 179-190.

Tsunoda, I., Lane, T. E., Blackett, J., & Fujinami, R. S. (2004). Distinct roles for IP-10/CXCL10 in three animal models, Theiler's virus infection, EAE, and MHV infection, for multiple sclerosis: implication of differing roles for IP-10. Multiple Sclerosis, 10, 26-34.

Valladeau, J., Ravel, O., Dezutter-Dambuyant, C., Moore, K., Kleijmeer, M., Liu, Y., Duvert-Frances, V., Vincent, C., Schmitt, D., Davoust, J., Caux, C., Lebecque, S., & Saeland, S. (2000). Langerin, a novel C-type lectin specific to Langerhans cells, is an endocytic receptor that induces the formation of Birbeck granules. Immunity, 12, 71-81.

Vakharia, V. N., Devaney, M. A., Moore, D. M., Dunn, J. J., & Grubman, M. J. (1987). Proteolytic processing of foot and mouth disease virus polyproteins expressed in a cell free system from clone derived transcripts. Journal of Virology, 61, 3199-31207.

Vivier, E., Raulet, D. H., Moretta, A., Caligiuri, M. A., Zitvogel, L., Lanier, L. L., Yokoyamal, W. M. & Ugolini, S. (2011). Innate or adaptive immunity? The example of natural killer cells. Science, 331, 44-49.

Wang, D., Fang, L. Luo, R., Ye, R., Fang, Y., Xie, L., Chen, H., & Xiao, S. (2010). Foot-and-mouth disease virus leader proteinase inhibits dsRNA-induced type I interferon transcription by decreasing interferon regulatory factor 3/7 in protein levels. Biochemical and Biophysical Research Communication, 399, 72-78.

Wang, D., Fang, L., Li, K., Zhong, H., Fan, J., Ouyang, C., Zhang, H., Duan, E., Luo, R., Zhang, Z., Liu, X., Chen, H., & Xiao, S. (2012). Foot-and-mouth disease virus 3C protease cleaves NEMO to impair innate immune signalling. Journal of Virology, 86, 9311-9322.

Wang, D., Fang, L., Liu, L., Zhong, H., Chen, Q., Luo, R., Liu, X., Zhang, Z., Chen, H., & Xiao, S. (2011). Foot-and-mouth disease virus (FMDV) leader proteinase negatively regulates the porcine interferon-λ1 pathway. Molecular Immunology, 49, 407-412.

Schoenborn, J. R., & Wilson, C. B. (2007). Regulation of interferon-gamma during innate and adaptive immune responses. Advances Immunology, 96, 41-101.

Wu, Q., Brum, M. C. S., Caron, L., Koster, M., & Grubman, M. J. (2003). Adenovirus-mediated type I interferon expression partially protects cattle from foot-and-mouth disease. Journal of Interferon Cytokine Research, 23, 371-380.

Wykes, M., Pombo, A., Jenkins, C. & MacPherson, G. G. (1998). Dendritic cells interact directly with Naive B lymphocytes to transfer antigen and initiate class switching in a primary T-dependent response. Journal of Immunology, 161, 1313–1319.

Yuan, J., Liu, Z., Lim, T., Zhang, H., He, J., Walker, E., Shier, C., Wang, Y., Su, Y., Sall, A., McManus, B., & Yang, D. (2009). CXCL10 inhibits viral replication through recruitment of natural killer cells in coxsackievirus B3-induced myocarditis. Circulation Research, 104, 628-638.

Protective Immunity vs. Immunopathogenesis: Recognition of the Structural form of the PCV2 Capsid Determines the Outcome

Benjamin R. Trible
Department of Diagnostic Medicine and Pathobiology
Kansas State University, USA

Raymond R. R. Rowland
Department of Diagnostic Medicine and Pathobiology
Kansas State University, USA

1   Introduction

Pathogens employ multiple strategies to evade host defenses. One strategy involves deploying epitopes that are immunodominant, but not protective, also known as "decoy" epitopes. Infection with porcine circovirus type 2 (PCV2), the smallest known virus to autonomously replicate, contributes to a wide variety of syndromes, which are collectively termed porcine circovirus associated disease (PCVAD). One hallmark of PCVAD is dysregulation of host immunity, including the production of large quantities of non-neutralizing antibody. The limitations placed on a small genome, with a limited number of genes, means that PCV2 and other small viruses must employ unique strategies to subvert innate and acquired immune responses.

2   Porcine Circovirus Associated Disease

PCVAD forms a group of complex multi-factorial syndromes, which can include respiratory distress, diarrhea, reproductive failure, wasting, and dermatitis (reviewed in Segales, 2012). Common syndromes include porcine multi-systemic wasting syndrome (PMWS), porcine dermatitis and nephropathy syndrome (PDNS), poor growth performance, and acute pulmonary edema (APE). Even though these and other PCV2-associated syndromes can be mimicked by other types of infections, for the purpose of this review we describe those syndromes that are linked with PCV2. Under some circumstances, mortality can reach 50%. The common component of all syndromes is a large quantity of PCV2 and/or anti-PCV2 antibody (Meehan *et al.*, 1998; Rossell *et al.*, 2000; Wellenberg *et al.*, 2004). Infection with PCV2 alone results in detectable viremia, but without overt clinical signs. The etiology of PCVAD, is linked to co-infection with viral or bacterial pathogens, such as porcine reproductive and respiratory syndrome virus (PRRSV), swine influenza virus (SIV), porcine parvovirus (PPV), *Haemophilus parasuis, Streptococcus suis, Mycoplasma hypopneumoniae, Actinobacillus pleuropneumoniae,* and others (reviewed by Opriessnig and Halbur, 2012). While the exact mechanistic basis for how co-infection contributes to PCVAD is unclear, experimental studies involving the co-infection of PCV2 with PRRSV, show increased PCV2 viremia and deposition of PCV2 antigen in lymph nodes in pigs infected with PCV2 and PRRSV (Allan *et al.*, 2000; Rovira *et al.*, 2002; Sinha *et al.*, 2011; Trible *et al.*, 2012a). However, PCV2 infection does not result in a corresponding increase in PRRSV replication. Co-infecting pathogens may function to alter the overall immune responsiveness of the host, thus preventing the induction of an effective anti-PCV2 response. Another possibility is that lymphoproliferation, in response to the co-infecting pathogen, may result in increased numbers of dividing lymphocytes, the primary targets of PCV2 replication (Darwich, *et al.*, 2004).

2.1   Porcine Multi-systemic Wasting Syndrome (PMWS)

The most common PCVAD syndrome, PMWS, was first described in high health swine herds in Canada in the early 1990's (Clark, 1997; Harding, 1997). The syndrome primarily affects pigs between 5-16 weeks of age with the greatest frequency of onset at 8-12 weeks. Mortality typically ranges between 10 and 25% (Harding & Clark, 1997; Horlen *et al.*, 2007). Clinical signs can include lethargy, diarrhea, lymphadenopathy, discoloring of the skin, jaundice, and progressive weight loss (Harding and Clark, 1997). Gross histopathology shows enlargement of the submandibular, inguinal, and bronchial lymph nodes, as well as lungs that are non-collapsed and wet. At the microscopic level, lymph nodes show granulomatious inflammation and the presence of intracytoplasmic inclusion bodies characterized by multinucleated giant cells. By the end stage of the disease, lymphoid cells in tissues are depleted and replaced by macrophages and multinucleated giant cells along with a large accumulation of PCV2 antigen (Harding and Clark, 1997).

2.2   Porcine Dermatitis and Nephropathy Syndrome (PDNS)

PDNS was first described in the United Kingdom in 1993 (Smith *et al.*, 1993). The syndrome primarily affects pigs 12-14 weeks of age (Smith *et al.*, 1993, Helie *et al.*, 1995; Horlen *et al.*, 2007). The predominant clinical sign is the presence of skin lesions, ranging in color from red to black, which primarily cover the hind legs (Smith *et al.*, 1993; Helie *et al.*, 1995; Horlen *et al.*, 2007). Gross pathology is characterized by enlarged and hemorrhagic renal and inguinal lymph nodes with increased fluid in the pleural and peritoneal cavities. Kidneys appear wet and enlarged with pinpoint hemorrhages along the capsule (Smith *et al.*, 1993; Helie *et al.*, 1995; Horlen *et al.*, 2007). Microscopically, PDNS is characterized by dermal/epidermal necrosis, fibrinous glomerulonephritis and systemic vasculitis. PDNS includes features characteristic of a type 3 hypersensitivity reaction, including the deposition of antigen-antibody complexes within capillary glomerular and vascular walls (Wellenberg *et al.*, 2004).

Even though PDNS is characterized by large quantities of anti-PCV2 antibodies, the exact etiology of the syndrome remains unclear. PDNS was successfully reproduced after the dual challenge of gnotobiotic pigs with only porcine reproductive and respiratory syndrome virus (PRRSV) and group 1 toque teno virus (TTV; Krakowka *et al.*, 2008). However, cases of PDNS in the field are linked with PCV2 infection.

2.3   Poor Growth Performance

One of the first field studies to evaluate the efficacy of a baculovirus-expressed PCV2 capsid-based vaccine is described in Horlen *et al.* (2008). The herd had a previous history of PMWS and PDNS; however, at the time of vaccination, clinical PCVAD was no longer present. The study design involved 485 pigs, which were randomly assigned to vaccine or non-vaccine groups. Pigs were vaccinated at three weeks of age and boosted three weeks later. In addition to significant decreases in mortality and PCV2 viremia, vaccination resulted in a higher average daily weight gain. The average increase in weight at market was approximately 8.8 kg. The results demonstrated increased weight gain as a benefit in the vaccination of herds that did not possess overt clinical signs of PCVAD. Other vaccine studies have reported similar findings (Fachinger *et al.*, 2008; Fort *et al.*, 2008, 2009; Kixmöller *et al.*, 2008; Martelli *et al.*, 2011; Opriessnig *et al.*, 2008, 2011).

2.4   Acute Pulmonary Edema (APE)

Typically, PCVAD syndromes, such as wasting, are slow and progressive. In 2009, a peracute syndrome, termed APE, was reported in PCV2-vaccinated herds (Cino-Ozuna *et al.*, 2011). The principal clinical feature is the rapid onset of respiratory distress in apparently healthy pigs followed by death. Gross pathology shows diffusely wet and heavy lungs and a large volume of clear fluid in the thoracic cavity. Microscopically, APE is characterized by diffuse distension of intralobular septa, and diffuse interstitial infiltration of macrophages and lymphocytes. Blood vessel walls show fibrinoid necrosis with pulmonary edema in the surrounding areas. Similar to other PCVAD syndromes, APE is associated with a large amount of PCV2 virus in blood, lymphoid depletion, and the deposition of viral antigen in lung and lymphoid tissues. The association between APE with PCV2 vaccination remains unclear.

3   Porcine Circovirus Type 2 (PCV2)

In the early 1970's, a viral contaminant of a PK-15 cell line was first described (Tischer *et al.*, 1974). Electron microscopy revealed virus particles with picornavirus-like morphology. However, based on the presence of a circular ssDNA genome, the virus was classified as a porcine circovirus (PCV). Serology identified pigs as the natural host of the virus, but infection with PCV could not be linked to clinical disease (Tischer *et al.*, 1982; Tischer *et al.* 1986). In the early 1990's, a new wasting syndrome, termed PMWS, was reported in high-health pigs in western Canada (Clark, 1997; Harding, 1997). Analysis of viral antigens and DNA from North American and European isolates revealed a new PCV, which was only 70% identical at the nucleotide level to the PK-15 contaminant (Meehan *et al.*, 1998). The terminology, PCV1 and PCV2, were used to distinguish the PK-15 contaminant from the virus linked with PMWS. PCV2 isolates are further grouped into two main genotypes, termed PCV2a (GenBank accession #AF055392 as a prototype sequence) and PCV2b (GenBank accession #AF055394 as a prototype sequence; Mehann *et al.*, 1998). A third genotype, termed PCV2c (GenBank accession #EU148503), was identified in archived pig tissues collected in Denmark during the 1980's (Dupont *et al.*, 2008). Initially, PCV2a and PCV2b were linked with disease outbreaks in North America and Europe, respectively (Segalés *et al.*, 2008). However, outbreaks of PCVAD in Canada and the U.S. in 2005 were associated with the first appearance of PCV2b in the U.S. (Horlen *et al.*, 2007). Since then, both genotypes circulate worldwide. Pigs can be co-infected with both genotypes and viruses composed of sequences from both PCV2a and PCV2b are present in the field (Hesse *et al.*, 2008).

PCV possesses an ambisense ss-DNA genome in the form of a covalently closed circle. The PCV1 genome is 1,759 nucleotides (nt) in length; whereas; genomes of PCV2a, PCV2b, and PCV2c are 1,768, 1,767 and 1,767 nt, respectively. The genome sequences of PCV1 and PCV2 share an identity of 68-76%. Sequences of PCV2a, PCV2b, and PCV2c share an identity of approximately 95% (Fenaux *et al.*, 2004). The genome possesses at least three open reading frames (ORFs; Figure 1). The largest open reading frame, ORF1, codes for two proteins termed Rep and Rep'. Rep and Rep' are translated from differentially spliced transcripts. The replicase proteins are essential for rolling circle replication (Mankertz & Hillenbrand, 2001). Oriented in the opposite direction, ORF2 is translated into a 233 or 234 amino acid capsid protein (CP; Nawagitgul *et al.*, 2000). The PCV2 virus-like particle (VLP) contains 60 CP monomers, which forms an icosahedral capsid (Khayat *et al.*, 2011). CP is essential for viral attachment and entry of the virion into cell. The basic amino acids on the N-terminus of CP are involved in shuttling the viral genome into the nucleus; the site of virus replication (Liu *et al.*, 2001; Misinzo *et al.*, 2006; Shuai *et al.*, 2008). A third gene, ORF3, is in a different reading frame embedded within ORF1 and codes for a protein associated with apoptosis (Liu *et al.*, 2005). The contribution of ORF3 to PCV2 pathogenesis remains controversial (Chaiyakul *et al.*, 2010).

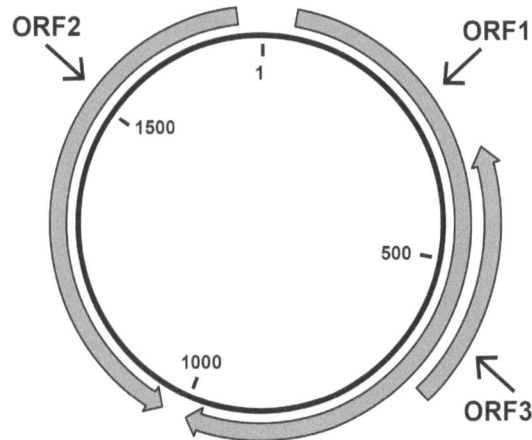

Figure 1: The PCV2 genome. The ambisense genome of PCV2 codes for at least three open reading frames (grey arrows). ORF1 codes for the replicase proteins. ORF2 codes for the capsid protein (CP) and ORF3 codes for a non-structural protein putatively linked with apoptosis.

4   Humoral Immunity

4.1   PCV2 Vaccines

PCV2 vaccination is the most effective strategy for the control and prevention of PCVAD. Currently, four commercial vaccines, based on the expression of an ORF2 antigen from PCV2a, are available for use in the field. Circumvent PCV (Intervet/Merck) and Ingelvac CircoFLEX, (Boehringer Ingelheim) consist of CP expressed by baculovirus. A third vaccine, Fostera PCV (Pfizer Animal Health), is composed of a virus prepared from a PCV1 backbone that expresses ORF2 from PCV2. The fourth vaccine, Circovac (Merial), contains inactivated whole PCV2a as the antigen. The primary mechanism for vaccine protection is the production of PCV2 neutralizing antibodies (reviewed in Kekarainen *et al.*, 2010; Trible *et al.*, 2012c).

4.2   Epitope Mapping Studies

Studies to identify antibody epitopes within CP were originally performed by Lekcharoensuk *et al.* (2004) and Mahe *et al.* (2000). Mahe *et al.* (2000) identified linear epitopes by reacting sera from infected and immunized pigs and hyperimmunized rabbits with overlapping 12-mer oligopeptides covering all of CP. Antibody reactive regions were identified between amino acids 23-43, 71-85, 117-131, and 171-202 in PCV2b CP. Using a different approach, Lekcharoensuk *et al.* (2004) identified conformational epitopes by reacting seven anti-CP monoclonal antibodies (mAb's) with cells transfected with infectious PCV chimeric DNA clones comprised of different combinations of PCV1 and PCV2a ORF2 sequences. The results showed immunoreactive regions between residues 47-85, 165-200, and 200-233. The results of both studies were combined to identify four immunoreactive regions, termed epitopes A-D (Trible *et al.*, 2011), which are illustrated in Figure 2.

```
            1          11         21         31         41         51
PCV2a MTYPRRRYRR RRHRPRSHLG QILRRRPWLV HPRHRYRWRR KNGIFNTRLS RTFGYTVKAT
PCV2b ..........  .......... .......... .......... .......... ........R.
PCV2c ..........  .......... H......... .......... .....A.... .S.V...N.S

               A
            61         71         81         91        101        111
PCV2a TVRTPSWAVD MMRFNIDDFV PPGGGTNKIS IPFEYYRIKK VKVEFWPCSP ITQGDRGVGS
PCV2b ..........  ......N..L .....S.PR. V.......R. .......... ..........
PCV2c Q.SP......  ......NQ.L .....S.PLT V.......R. .....FAR.. ..........

               B
           121        131        141        151        161        171
PCV2a TAVILDDNFV TKATALTYDP YVNYSSRHTI PQPFSYHSRY STPKPVLDST IDYFQPNNKR
PCV2b S.........  .......... .......... T......... .......F. ..........
PCV2c .....N....  .......... .......... T......... .......... ..........

               C                                              D
          181         191        201        210        220        231
PCV2a NQLWLRLQTS RNVDHVGLGT AFENSIYDQD YNIRVTMYVQ FREFNLKDPP LKP-
PCV2b .........A G.......... .........E .......... .....F.... .N.-
PCV2c ....M...T .........H ..Q..TNA.A ..V....... .......... .N.K
```

Figure 2: Alignment of PCV2 CP peptide sequences from representative PCV2 genotypes. The underlined regions within PCV2a and PCV2b represent immunoreactive regions reported by Lekcharoensuk *et al.* (2004) and Mahe *et al.* (2000), respectively. Results from both studies were combined to identify four antibody immunoreactive epitopes, termed epitopes A-D (grey boxes).

4.3   Immunondominant CP Epitopes Following Vaccination, Infection, or PCVAD

In order to characterize immunodominant epitopes within CP, sera from experimentally PCV2-infected, PCV2 vaccinated, or PCVAD pigs were reacted with CP polypeptides expressed in *E. coli* (Trible *et al.*, 2011). As summarized in Table 1, sera from vaccinated pigs recognized only the largest polypeptide, CP(43-233). In contrast, PCVAD or experimentally infected pigs showed reactivity to the largest poly-peptide, as well as reactivity against smaller fragments located in the C-terminal region. All reactive polypeptides contained the epitope C region.

To finer map the immunodominant epitope within the C region, sera from experimentally infected and PCVAD pigs were reacted with overlapping 15mer oligopeptides covering the epitope C region. As depicted in Figure 3, CP(169-180) was identified as the smallest immunoreactive oligopeptide. Further analysis incorporating alanine scanning mutagenesis identified amino acid residues 173-tyrosine, 174-phenylalanine, 175-glutamine, and 179-lysine as important for antibody recognition. Peptide sequence analysis of 462 PCV2 sequences from GenBank and other sources showed that this region is highly conserved among all PCV2 isolates.

As illustrated in Figure 4, the x-ray structure of CP shows that the CP(169-180) domain forms an external loop structure, which protrudes from the outer surface of the CP subunit (panel A and B). The key antibody binding residues, 173-Tyr, 174-Phe and 175-Glu, are located in the middle of a connecting loop domain and lie in a similar plane. This provides a structural basis for the accessibility of CP(169-180) to antibody, as well as its immunodominance. However, within the context of the virus-like particle, CP(169-180) is located near the interface of the icosahedral 3-fold axis with most of the key residues no longer exposed on the virion surface. Only 173-Tyr (blue residue in Figure 3C) is visible on the surface

Name	Epitope Regions				PC[a]	Vx	PM	PD
43-233	A	B	C	D	++++[b]	++++	++	+++
43-135					+	-	-	++
43-160					+	-	-	+
91-160					+	-	+	+++
43-180					++	+	+	+++
160-233					+++	-	+	+++
135-233					++	-	+	+++
91-233					++	-	+	+++

[a]Key: PC = PCV2-infected; Vx = vaccinated; PM = PMWS; PD = PDNS.
[b]Relative binding activity. Key: (-) no measureable binding activity; (+) low binding activity; (++) intermediate binding activity; (+++) high binding activity ; (++++) very high binding activity

Copyright © American Society for Microbiology, Clinical and Vaccine Immunology, 18(5), 2011, 749-757.

Table 1: Summary of antibody responses to PCV2 capsid polypeptides.

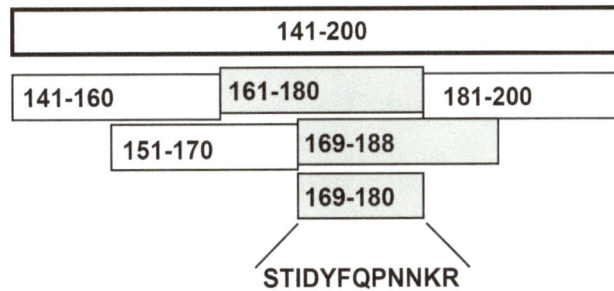

Figure 3: Summary of PEPSCAN analysis of the epitope C region. As illustrated above, overlapping oligopeptides were reacted with sera from pigs experimentally infected with PCV2 and from pigs with PCVAD. The grey rectangles show oligopeptides with positive reactivity. The results from alanine scanning mutagenesis identified key residues (underlined) as important for antibody recognition.

of the VLP, but is located at the bottom of a cleft formed by the junction of three CP monomers. Therefore, in the context of the VLP, CP(169-180) is not accessible to antibody.

To further characterize the properties of CP(169-180), immune responses and protection after virus challenge were studied in pigs immunized with a monomeric form of CP (Trible *et al.*, 2012c). To prevent assembly into VLP, CP was maintained in a stable monomer form by expressing CP as a ubiquitin (Ub) fusion protein, Ub-CP. For the purpose of comparison, pigs were immunized with baculovirus-expressed CP (Bac-CP). Baculovirus and bacteria-expressed CP spontaneously assemble to form VLP (Khayat *et al.*, 2011). As predicted, immunization of pigs with Bac-CP resulted in high levels of anti-PCV2 antibodies, including high levels of PCV2 neutralizing activity, and low amounts of antibodies against CP(169-180). After challenge with PCV2, no virus was detected in the serum. In contrast, immunization with the CP monomer, Ub-CP, also induced high levels of antibody against PCV2, including

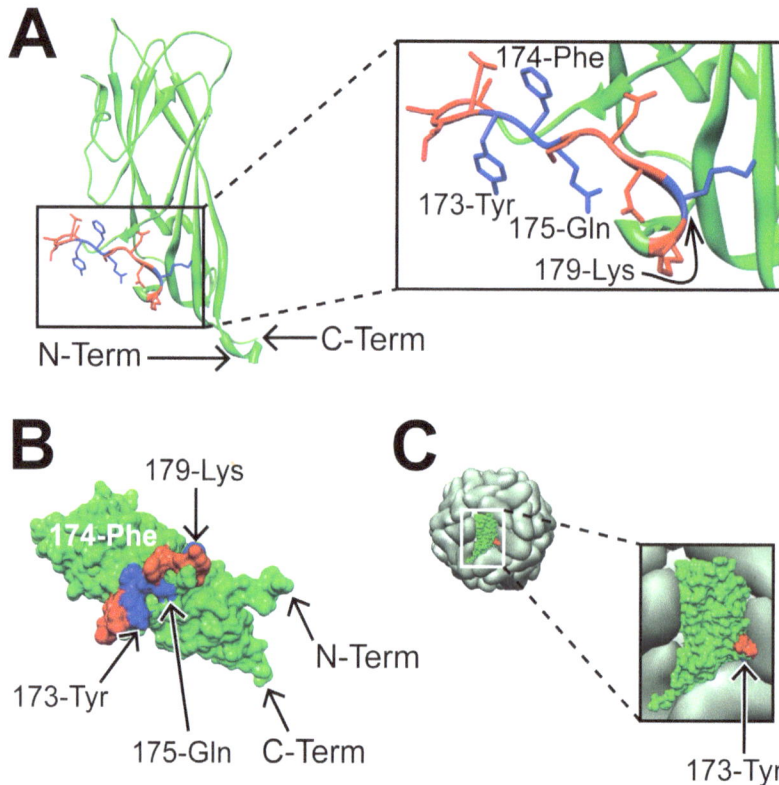

Figure 4: Location of the CP(169-180) epitope within a single CP subunit and VLP. Depicted are the ribbon (A) and surface (B) maps of a single CP subunit. The blue and red residues form the immunodominant epitope, CP(169-180). The blue residues are important for antibody recognition. The VLP (C) shows the surface of the VLP with a single CP shown in green, red, and blue. The red and blue regions correspond to the same residues in (A). Coordinates for the PCV2 CP(41-233) subunit and VLP were accessed through the RCSB Protein Data Bank (PDB ID 3R0R: (Berman *et al.*, 2000; Khayat *et al.*, 2011) and loaded into the open source molecular visual program, Chimera (Pettersen *et al.*, 2004).

significant amounts of antibody directed against CP(169-180). PCV2 neutralizing activity was not detected. Furthermore, after virus challenge, the level of viremia was no different from pigs infected with virus alone. High levels of anti-CP(169-180) without the control of virus replication reproduced the antibody response observed in pigs with PCVAD.

5   The Role of PCV2 CP Epitope C as An Immunological Decoy

A common feature of many pathogens, which establish a prolonged infection, is the ability to evade the host's immune response by deploying immunodominant, non-protective epitopes, which are termed decoy epitopes. For viruses, the most common method for diverting immunity involves antigenic variation. A classic example is glycoprotein (gp) 120, one of the major structural proteins of

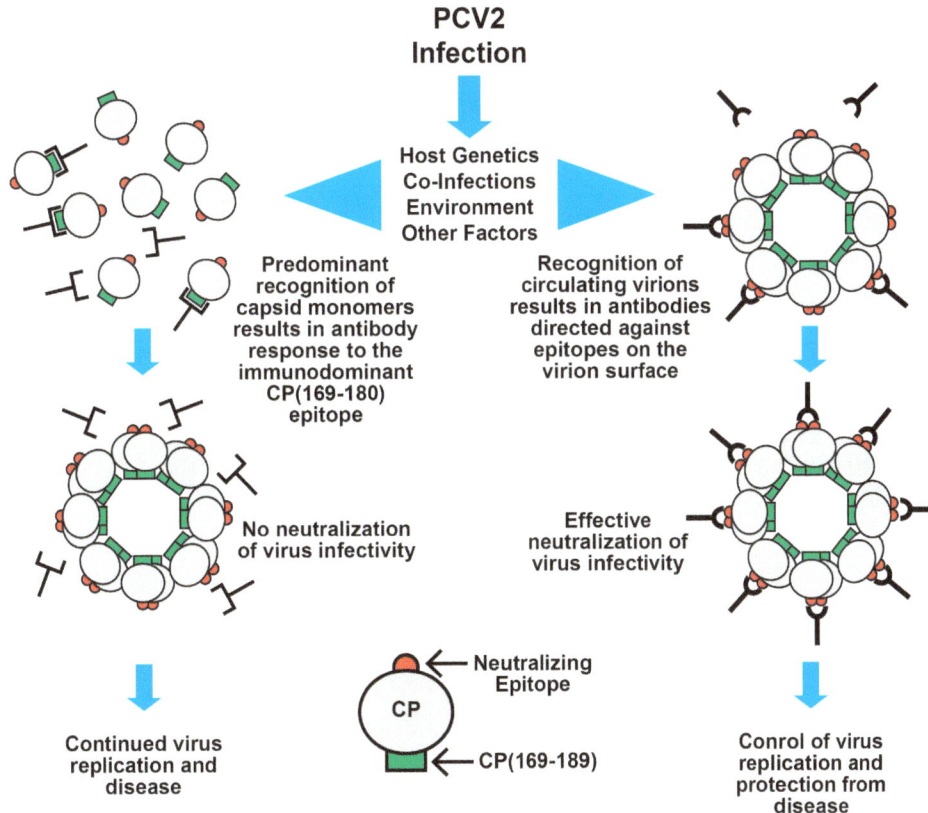

Figure 5: Structural form of PCV2 immunogen recognized by the host and relationship to outcome.

human and feline immunodeficiency viruses (Garrity *et al.*, 1997; Hosie *et al.*, 2011). Gp120 of HIV possesses five conserved (C1-C5) and five hypervariable (V1-V5) regions. V3 is immunodominant and possesses a neutralizing epitope. However, over the course of infection, peptide sequence hypervariability allows the continuous escape from antibody. Antigenic variation results in the continued recruitment, activation, and proliferation of new B-cells. The overall down-regulation of antibody production in response to continuous B cell activation results in fewer antibodies directed against conserved neutralizing epitopes. Another decoy strategy involves directing host immunity towards immunodominant, but non-essential proteins. For example, during murine gammaherpesvirus-68 (MHV-68) infection establishes a persistent infection despite a robust antibody response. The primary target of the humoral immune response is gp150, a protein dispensable for virus replication (Gillet *et al.*, 2007).

   PCV2 possesses one of the smallest known viral genomes, which limits the number and size of viral genes. As a result, all peptide sequence domains in CP are likely required to maintain the structure and function of CP necessary for virus replication and virion integrity. Conservation of structure and function places constraints on the extent of peptide sequence hypervariability. We propose a unique decoy mechanism for PCV2, which is based on the recognition of the different structural forms of CP. As illustrated in the model, presented in Figure 5, the outcome following infection can follow two pathways. Under normal circumstances antibodies are directed against the whole virion, which results in the production of neutralizing antibody. The immunodominant epitope, CP(169-180) is buried and inaccessible to recognition by antibody. The outcome is the control of virus replication and the generation of protective immunity. In contrast, the recognition of free CP and CP fragments, likely produced by infected cells, results in the production of antibodies against the immunodominant epitope, CP(169-180). Cofactors, such as co-infecting pathogens increase PCV2 replication and the production of CP monomers and fragments by infected cells. The genetics of the host and other co-factors may further skew immunity towards the recognition of CP(169-180). Recognition of the CP(169-180) results in the production of non-neutralizing antibodies, thus allowing for continue PCV2 replication, release of more monomer CP, and the progression towards disease. Overall, the model explains why the amount of circulating antibody fails to correlate with the outcome following PCV2 infection and provides a model for understanding the immunopathogenesis caused by viruses with small genomes.

References

Allan, G. M., McNeilly, F., Ellis, J., Krakowka, S., Meehan, B., McNair, I., Walker, I., et al. (2000). *Experimental infection of colostrum deprived piglets with porcine circovirus 2 (PCV2) and porcine reproductive and respiratory syndrome virus (PRRSV) potentiates PCV2 replication. Archives of Virology, 145(11), 2421–2429.*

Berman, H. M., Westbrook, J., Feng, Z., Gilliland, G., Bhat, T. N., Weissig, H., Shindyalov, I. N., et al. (2000). *The Protein Data Bank. Nucleic Acids Research, 28(1), 235–242.*

Chaiyakul, M., Hsu, K., Dardari, R., Marshall, F., & Czub, M. (2010). *Cytotoxicity of ORF3 proteins from a nonpathogenic and a pathogenic porcine circovirus. Journal of Virology, 84(21), 11440–11447.*

Cino-Ozuna, A. G., Henry, S., Hesse, R., Nietfeld, J. C., Bai, J., Scott, H. M., & Rowland, R. R. R. (2011). *Characterization of a new disease syndrome associated with porcine circovirus type 2 (PCV2) in previously vaccinated herds. Journal of Clinical Microbiology, 49(5), 2012-2016.*

Clark, E. G. (1997). *Post-weaning wasting syndrome. Proceedings of the American Association of Swine Practitioners, 28, 499–501.*

Darwich, L., Segalés, J., & Mateu, E. (2004). *Pathogenesis of postweaning multisystemic wasting syndrome caused by Porcine circovirus 2: An immune riddle. Archives of Virology, 149(5), 857–874.*

Dupont, K., Nielsen, E. O., Baekbo, P., & Larsen, L. E. (2008). *Genomic analysis of PCV2 isolates from Danish archives and a current PMWS case-control study supports a shift in genotypes with time. Veterinary Microbiology, 128(1-2), 56–64.*

Fachinger, V., Bischoff, R., Jedidia, S. B., Saalmüller, A., & Elbers, K. (2008). *The effect of vaccination against porcine circovirus type 2 in pigs suffering from porcine respiratory disease complex. Vaccine, 26(11), 1488–1499.*

Fenaux, M., Opriessnig, T., Halbur, P. G., Xu, Y., Potts, B., & Meng, X.-J. (2004). *Detection and in vitro and in vivo characterization of porcine circovirus DNA from a porcine-derived commercial pepsin product. The Journal of General Virology, 85(Pt 11), 3377–3382.*

Fort, M., Sibila, M., Allepuz, A., Mateu, E., Roerink, F., & Segalés, J. (2008). *Porcine circovirus type 2 (PCV2) vaccination of conventional pigs prevents viremia against PCV2 isolates of different genotypes and geographic origins. Vaccine, 26(8), 1063–1071.*

Fort, M., Sibila, M., Pérez-Martín, E., Nofrarías, M., Mateu, E., & Segalés, J. (2009). *One dose of a porcine circovirus 2 (PCV2) sub-unit vaccine administered to 3-week-old conventional piglets elicits cell-mediated immunity and significantly reduces PCV2 viremia in an experimental model. Vaccine, 27(30), 4031–4037.*

Garrity, R. R., Rimmelzwaan, G., Minassian, A., Tsai, W. P., Lin, G., de Jong, J. J., Goudsmit, J., et al. (1997). Refocusing neutralizing antibody response by targeted dampening of an immunodominant epitope. Journal of immunology (Baltimore, Md.: 1950), 159(1), 279–289.

Gillet, L., May, J. S., Colaco, S., & Stevenson, P. G. (2007). The murine gammaherpesvirus-68 gp150 acts as an immunogenic decoy to limit virion neutralization. PloS one, 2(8), e705.

Harding, J. C. S. (1997). Post-weaning multisystemic wasting syndrome (PMWS): Preliminary epidemiology and clinical presentation. Proceedings of the American Association of Swine Practitioners, 28, 503.

Harding, J. C. S., & Clark, E. G. (2007). Recognizing and diagnosing postweaning multisystemic wasting syndrome (PMWS). J Swine Health Prod, 5(5), 201–203.

Helie, P., Drolet, R., Germain, M-C., Bourgault, A. (1995). Systemic necrotizing vasculitis and glomerulonephritis in grower pigs in southwestern Quebec. Can. Vet. J., 36, 150-154.

Hesse, R., Kerrigan, M., & Rowland, R. R. R. (2008). Evidence for recombination between PCV2a and PCV2b in the field. Virus Research, 132(1-2), 201–207.

Horlen, K. P., Dritz, S. S., Nietfeld, J. C., Henry, S. C., Hesse, R. A., Oberst, R., Hays, M., et al. (2008). A field evaluation of mortality rate and growth performance in pigs vaccinated against porcine circovirus type 2. Journal of the American Veterinary Medical Association, 232(6), 906–912.

Horlen, K. P., Schneider, P., Anderson, J., Nietfeld, J. C., Henry, S. C., Tokach, L. M., & Rowland, R. R. R. (2007). A cluster of farms experiencing severe porcine circovirus associated disease: Clinical features and association with the PCV2b genotype. Journal of Swine Health and Production, 15(5), 270–278.

Hosie, M. J., Pajek, D., Samman, A., & Willett, B. J. (2011). Feline immunodeficiency virus (FIV) neutralization: a review. Viruses, 3(10), 1870–1890.

Khayat, R., Brunn, N., Speir, J. A., Hardham, J. M., Ankenbauer, R. G., Schneemann, A., & Johnson, J. E. (2011). The 2.3 A Structure of Porcine Circovirus 2. Journal of Virology, 85(15), 7856-7862.

Kixmöller, M., Ritzmann, M., Eddicks, M., Saalmüller, A., Elbers, K., & Fachinger, V. (2008). Reduction of PMWS-associated clinical signs and co-infections by vaccination against PCV2. Vaccine, 26(27-28), 3443–3451.

Kekarainen, T., McCullough, K., Fort, M., Fossum, C., Segales, J., Allen, G., (2010). Immune responses and vaccine-induced immunity against Porcine circovirus type 2. Veterinary Immunology and Immunopathology, 136, 185-193.

Krakowka, Steven, Hartunian, C., Hamberg, A., Shoup, D., Rings, M., Zhang, Y., Allan, G., et al. (2008). Evaluation of induction of porcine dermatitis and nephropathy syndrome in gnotobiotic pigs with negative results for porcine circovirus type 2. American Journal of Veterinary Research, 69(12), 1615–1622.

Lekcharoensuk, P., Morozov, I., Paul, P. S., Thangthumniyom, N., Wajjawalku, W., & Meng, X. J. (2004). Epitope mapping of the major capsid protein of type 2 porcine circovirus (PCV2) by using chimeric PCV1 and PCV2. Journal of Virology, 78(15), 8135–8145.

Liu, J., Chen, I., & Kwang, J. (2005). Characterization of a previously unidentified viral protein in porcine circovirus type 2-infected cells and its role in virus-induced apoptosis. Journal of Virology, 79(13), 8262–8274.

Liu, Q., Tikoo, S. K., & Babiuk, L. A. (2001). Nuclear localization of the ORF2 protein encoded by porcine circovirus type 2. Virology, 285(1), 91–99.

Mahé, D., Blanchard, P., Truong, C., Arnauld, C., Le Cann, P., Cariolet, R., Madec, F., et al. (2000). Differential recognition of ORF2 protein from type 1 and type 2 porcine circoviruses and identification of immunorelevant epitopes. The Journal of General Virology, 81(Pt 7), 1815–1824.

Mankertz, A., & Hillenbrand, B. (2001). Replication of porcine circovirus type 1 requires two proteins encoded by the viral rep gene. Virology, 279(2), 429–438.

Martelli, P., Ferrari, L., Morganti, M., De Angelis, E., Bonilauri, P., Guazzetti, S., Caleffi, A., et al. (2011). One dose of a porcine circovirus 2 subunit vaccine induces humoral and cell-mediated immunity and protects against porcine circovirus-associated disease under field conditions. Veterinary Microbiology, 149(3-4), 339–351.

Meehan, B. M., McNeilly, F., Todd, D., Kennedy, S., Jewhurst, V. A., Ellis, J. A., Hassard, L. E., et al. (1998). Characterization of novel circovirus DNAs associated with wasting syndromes in pigs. The Journal of General Virology, 79 (Pt 9), 2171–2179.

Misinzo, G., Delputte, P. L., Meerts, P., Lefebvre, D. J., & Nauwynck, H. J. (2006). Porcine circovirus 2 uses heparan sulfate and chondroitin sulfate B glycosaminoglycans as receptors for its attachment to host cells. Journal of Virology, 80(7), 3487–3494.

Nawagitgul, P., Morozov, I., Bolin, S. R., Harms, P. A., Sorden, S. D., & Paul, P. S. (2000). Open reading frame 2 of porcine circovirus type 2 encodes a major capsid protein. The Journal of General Virology, 81(Pt 9), 2281–2287.

Opriessnig, T. & Halbur, P. G. (2012). Concurrent infections are important for expression of porcine circovirusassociated disease. Virus Research, 164, 20-32.

Opriessnig, T, Madson, D. M., Prickett, J. R., Kuhar, D., Lunney, J. K., Elsener, J., & Halbur, P. G. (2008). Effect of porcine circovirus type 2 (PCV2) vaccination on porcine reproductive and respiratory syndrome virus (PRRSV) and PCV2 coinfection. Veterinary Microbiology, 131(1-2), 103–114.

Opriessnig, T, Madson, D. M., Schalk, S., Brockmeier, S., Shen, H. G., Beach, N. M., Meng, X. J., et al. (2011). Porcine circovirus type 2 (PCV2) vaccination is effective in reducing disease and PCV2 shedding in semen of boars concurrently infected with PCV2 and Mycoplasma hyopneumoniae. Theriogenology, 76(2), 351–360.

Pettersen, E. F., Goddard, T. D., Huang, C. C., Couch, G. S., Greenblatt, D. M., Meng, E. C., & Ferrin, T. E. (2004). UCSF Chimera--a visualization system for exploratory research and analysis. Journal of Computational Chemistry, 25(13), 1605–1612.

Rosell, C., Segalés, J., Ramos-Vara, J. A., Folch, J. M., Rodríguez-Arrioja, G. M., Duran, C. O., Balasch, M., et al. (2000). Identification of porcine circovirus in tissues of pigs with porcine dermatitis and nephropathy syndrome. The Veterinary Record, 146(2), 40–43.

Rovira, A., Balasch, M., Segalés, J., García, L., Plana-Durán, J., Rosell, C., Ellerbrok, H., et al. (2002). Experimental inoculation of conventional pigs with porcine reproductive and respiratory syndrome virus and porcine circovirus 2. Journal of Virology, 76(7), 3232–3239.

Segales J. (2012). Porcine circovirus type 2 (PCV2) infection: Clinical signs, pathology and laboratory diagnosis. Virus research, 164(1-2), 10-19.

Segalés, J., Olvera, A., Grau-Roma, L., Charreyre, C., Nauwynck, H., Larsen, L., Dupont, K., et al. (2008). PCV-2 genotype definition and nomenclature. The Veterinary Record, 162(26), 867–868.

Shuai, J., Wei, W., Jiang, L., Li, X., Chen, N., & Fang, W. (2008). Mapping of the nuclear localization signals in open reading frame 2 protein from porcine circovirus type 1. Acta Biochimica Et Biophysica Sinica, 40(1), 71–77.

Sinha, A., Shen, H. G., Schalk, S., Beach, N. M., Huang, Y. W., Meng, X. J., Halbur, P. G., et al. (2011). Porcine reproductive and respiratory syndrome virus (PRRSV) influences infection dynamics of porcine circovirus type 2 (PCV2) subtypes PCV2a and PCV2b by prolonging PCV2 viremia and shedding. Veterinary Microbiology, 152(3-4), 235–246.

Smith, W. J., Thomson, J. R., & Done, S. (1993). Dermatitis/nephropathy syndrome of pigs. The Veterinary Record, 132(2), 47.

Tischer, I., Gelderblom, H., Vettermann, W., & Koch, M. A. (1982). A very small porcine virus with circular single-stranded DNA. Nature, 295(5844), 64–66.

Tischer, I., Mields, W., Wolff, D., Vagt, M., & Griem, W. (1986). Studies on epidemiology and pathogenicity of porcine circovirus. Archives of Virology, 91(3-4), 271–276.

Tischer, I., Rasch, R., & Tochtermann, G. (1974). Characterization of papovavirus-and picornavirus-like particles in permanent pig kidney cell lines. Zentralblatt Für Bakteriologie, Parasitenkunde, Infektionskrankheiten Und Hygiene. Erste Abteilung Originale. Reihe A: Medizinische Mikrobiologie Und Parasitologie, 226(2), 153–167.

Trible, B. R., Kerrigan, M., Crossland, N., Potter, M., Faaberg, K., Hesse, R., & Rowland, R. R. R. (2011). Antibody recognition of porcine circovirus type 2 capsid protein epitopes after vaccination, infection, and disease. Clinical and Vaccine Immunology: CVI, 18(5), 749–757.

Trible, B. R., Ramirez, A., Suddith, A., Fuller, A., Kerrigan, M., Hesse, R., Nietfeld, J., et al. (2012a). Antibody responses following vaccination versus infection in a porcine circovirus-type 2 (PCV2) disease model show distinct differences in virus neutralization and epitope recognition. Vaccine, 30(27), 4079–4085.

Trible, B. R., & Rowland, R. R. R. (2012b). Genetic variation of porcine circovirus type 2 (PCV2) and its relevance to vaccination, pathogenesis and diagnosis. Virus research, 164(1-2), 68–77.

Trible, B. R., Suddith, A., Kerrigan, M. A., Cino-Ozuna, A. G., Hesse, R., & Rowland, R. R. R. (2012c). Recognition of the different structural forms of the capsid protein (CP) determines the outcome following infection with porcine circovirus type 2 (PCV2). Journal of virology, 86, 13508-13514.

Wellenberg, G. J., Stockhofe-Zurwieden, N., de Jong, M. F., Boersma, W. J. A., & Elbers, A. R. W. (2004). Excessive porcine circovirus type 2 antibody titres may trigger the development of porcine dermatitis and nephropathy syndrome: a case-control study. Veterinary Microbiology, 99(3-4), 203–214.

Innate Immunity in the Airways to Respiratory Viruses

Alan C-Y. Hsu
Centre for Asthma and Respiratory Disease
University of Newcastle, Australia

Heng Zhong
Centre for Asthma and Respiratory Disease
University of Newcastle, Australia

Philip M. Hansbro
Centre for Asthma and Respiratory Disease
University of Newcastle, Australia

Peter AB. Wark
Centre for Asthma and Respiratory Disease
University of Newcastle, Australia

1   Introduction

The human airways are vital to respiration, allowing access of the atmosphere to the delicate gas exchange interface of the alveoli. However in doing so they also act as a gateway for a wide range of noxious particulates and micro-organisms to enter into the lungs. Respiratory viruses are the most common cause of infection in humans worldwide and some of the most clinically important respiratory viruses are listed in Table 1. Many of these viruses have been recognised as human pathogens for some time, others such as the human SARS coronavirus (SARS-CoV) have only recently emerged with devastating though brief consequences in 2003, while viruses like influenza and respiratory syncytial virus (RSV) result in marked morbidity, mortality and socio-economic burden annually. Respiratory viral infection often causes a wide range of diseases from mild symptoms such as cough and sore throat to severe life-threatening pneumonia. The consequences of infection are the result of a complex interplay between the virulence of the pathogen and the ability of the host to resist and mount an effective immune response.

Human immune system is a complicated and yet structured biological process that protects the host from infection. Advances in molecular immunology have provided valuable insight into the functional characterization of novel signalling proteins and cytokines that are involved in human immunity. The innate arm of human immune system has become a major research focus since the discovery of pattern recognition receptors, overthrowing the theory of non-discriminative innate immune responses against self and non-self entities. The ability of innate immune system to recognize different foreign pathogens further identifies innate immunity as the most important first line of defence that not only limits viral replication and spread, but also directs appropriate pathogen-specific adaptive immune activation for efficient clearance of viruses.

Similarly, over the course of virus-human co-evolution numerous respiratory viruses have also developed immune evasion strategies for efficient infection in the host. Advances in reverse genetic engineering has discovered novel viral virulence factors, and characterized their function and interaction with immune cells, thereby further delineating the mechanism of viral infection and uncovering novel therapeutic strategies. Although innate immune signalling networks have been extensively investigated, there are still numerous signalling proteins, regulatory and intercepting pathways, and transcriptional mechanisms that are still poorly defined. This review will therefore explore current understandings of innate immune responses to respiratory viruses in the human airways, and how these responses can be altered by the invading viruses. In addition, in the context of virus infection the host immune response can also be as damaging as the direct effects of infection. This is highlighted particularly in the case of those with chronic airways diseases such as asthma and chronic obstructive pulmonary disease (COPD), whom not only have abnormal regulations of immune responses but also are more susceptible to viral infection and suffer more severe symptoms and exacerbation of their pre-existing conditions following infection. The molecular mechanisms underlying the increased susceptibility and severe infection outcome in those with chronic airways diseases are largely unknown, this review will also discuss potential abnormalities in the innate immunity and how respiratory viral infection can further worsen the infection outcome in these individuals.

Family	Virus name	Strandedness
Adenoviridae*	Human adenovirus	dsRNA
Bunyaviridae	Hentavirus	ssRNA
Coronaviridae*	Human coronavirus (SARS-CoV)	ssRNA
Herpesviridae	Cytomegalovirus or human herpes virus type 5	dsDNA
	Epstein-Barr virus or human herpes virus type 4	dsDNA
	Vericella-zoster virus or human herpes virus type 3	dsDNA
Orthomyxoviridae*	Influenza virus A and B	ssRNA
Paramyxoviridae*	Human metapneumovirus 1 – 4	ssRNA
	Human parainfluenza virus 1 – 4	ssRNA
	Human respiratory syncytial virus (RSV) A and B	ssRNA
Picornaviridae*	Human rhinovirus A, B, or C	ssRNA
	Human enterovirus A – D	ssRNA

Table 1: Viruses that are known to cause diseases in the human airways. * indicates clinically important respiratory viruses.

2   Viral Infection and Innate Immunity in the Airways

2.1   Airway Epithelium

As the portal to the external environment, the mucosal epithelium that lines the respiratory system is an important barrier that defends against foreign pathogens. As the first point to contact, respiratory viruses therefore primarily infect and replicate in the airway epithelial cells (AECs).

Before infection can be established a virus must bind to glycoproteins on the host cell surface, tricking host cells to initiate receptor-mediated endocytosis. The specific host cell receptors to which viruses attach vary greatly, however these host receptors are usually ubiquitously expressed on human cells. For example, SARS-CoV binds to angiotensin-converting enzyme 2 (ACE2) to be endocytosed into the cells (W. Li *et al.*, 2003), while influenza viruses bind to glycoproteins with terminal sialic acid (SA) residues of specific configurations. Human rhinoviruses of major group receptor bind to intracellular adhesion molecule (ICAM) -1 and that of minor group bind to low-density lipoproteins (LDLs), all of which are expressed on airway epithelial cells (Papi & Johnston, 1999; Suzuki *et al.*, 2001).

Binding diversity within the same virus family has been most thoroughly studied in influenza, as different strains of which may bind with its surface protein haemagglutinin (HA) to SA residues of different modifications, and will be discussed here. SA are monosaccharide molecules found ubiquitously as terminal residues on the glycan chain of many polysaccharide and glycoproteins on human epithelial cell surface, secreted glycoproteins, as well as surface glycolipids (Suzuki *et al.*, 2005). Diversity in SA presentation includes the position of SA branching from the carbon backbone of glycoproteins, modification of hydroxyl group, and different α-linkages from the 2-carbon to the sugar chain. Different strains of influenza bind to SA residues with different linkage to the carbon backbone of glycoproteins. Human influenza viruses preferentially bind to SAα2,6Gal terminal linkages, which are predominantly found on epithelial cells of the upper respiratory tract, whereas avian influenza viruses bind to terminal SAα2,3Gal linkages in the lower airways (Baum & Paulson, 1990; T. Ito et al., 1997; Rogers & Paulson, 1983; Ryan-Poirier et al., 1998). The difference in their binding specificities are partly attributed to the amino acid residue at position 226 and 228 of the HA glycoprotein. The HA of human influenza viruses contains a 226Leu and 228Ser that results in the preferential binding to SAα2,6Gal residues. In contrast, the HA of avian influenza viruses have a 226Gln and 228Gly, which binds to SAα2,3Gal linkages (Connor et al., 1994; Rogers & D'Souza, 1989). This difference in amino acid residues and distribution of SA residues in the airways may explain why highly pathogenic avian influenza virus H5N1 is currently incapable of sustainable human-to-human transmission, as mutations at neither sites were found in H5N1 strain isolated from infected individuals (Yamada et al., 2006).

Two recent studies further investigated the molecular changes required for H5N1 to become efficiently transmissible amongst humans, and identified a number of mutations that transformed SAα2,3Gal binding property of H5 HA protein to SAα2,6Gal binding. One study found that Gln226Leu/Gly228Ser mutations increased the binding of H5 HA to SAα2,6Gal while retaining the binding capacity to SAα2,3Gal. However together with mutations at Asn158Asp/Asn224Lys/ Gln226Leu/Thr318Ile this fully converted the virus with mutant H5 HA in a 2009 pandemic H1N1 backbone to become efficient in aerosol transmission in ferret model, a standard and widely accepted animal model for influenza transmissibility studies (Imai et al., 2012). Another study identified another set of mutations in H5N1 that transformed this highly pathogenic avian influenza with inefficient human-to-human transmission to sustainable airborne transmission (Herfst et al., 2012). Herfst et al. showed that mutant H5N1 virus with mutations at Gln222Leu, Gly224Ser, His103Tyr, and Thr156Ala in H5N1 HA protein, and Glu627Lys in the viral polymerase protein PB2 were able to transmit efficiently between ferret models via aerosols. This clearly illustrates the importance of these mutations in HA and PB2 protein for efficient transmission and spread amongst humans, although it remains unclear if any influenza viruses can become airborne with these mutations. These results provide valuable insight into new vaccine design strategies, and current and future avian influenza surveillance network.

While the binding specificities of influenza viruses have been well established using various techniques such as structural biology and glycan microarray, the viruses can still cause infection in the absence of their respective receptors. This therefore raises questions as to whether viruses can enter into airway epithelial cells via other mechanisms. Supporting this hypothesis, a study showed that human influenza virus was able to infect and replicate to a similar titre in the lungs of mice lacking SAα2,6Gal linkage receptors compared to wild type mice (Glaser et al., 2007). In addition, we have also recently shown that despite low levels of SAα2,3Gal linkage on BECs, a low pathogenic avian influenza virus H11N9 was still able to endocytose into the BECs at similar efficiency as human strain and replicated to high viral titre (A. C. Hsu et al., 2011). The highly pathogenic avian influenza H5N1 was also able to replicate to even higher extent compared to H3N2 and H11N9 (A. C. Hsu, Parsons, K., Barr, I., Lowther, S., Middleton, D., Hansbro, PM., Wark, PAB. , 2012).

There are several potential host surface glycoproteins with other modifications such as fucosylation that have been shown to be bound by influenza HA proteins (Rapoport et al., 2006), however recent evidence suggests that phosphotidylinositol-3-kinase (PI3K) signalling pathway is heavily involved in viral endocytosis. PI3K is a ubiquitous signalling pathway that controls cellular metabolism and proliferation [26], and also highly regulates an internalization process called macropinocytosis (Araki *et al.*, 1996; Hewlett *et al.*, 1994; West *et al.*, 2000). Macropinocytosis is a non-specific, receptor-independent internalization process that forms endocytic vesicles and brings the attaching virus into the host cells, though the mechanisms of how viruses activate this process remain unknown. Nevertheless a number of respiratory viruses have been shown to utilize the PI3K pathway for viral entry, including influenza and rhinoviruses. Influenza is able to activate PI3K pathway that facilitates viral endocytosis into BECs, while inhibition of PI3K results in reduced viral endocytosis and viral replication (de Vries *et al.*, 2011; Ehrhardt *et al.*, 2006). This PI3K activation was shown to be due to the influenza non-structural (NS) 1 protein that binds and activate PI3K for efficient viral endocytosis and infection. There is also evidence of PI3K-mediated viral entry of human rhinovirus and adenovirus into the host cells, although the exact mechanism of this viral-PI3K-mediated macropinocytosis is still unclear (Lau *et al.*, 2008; E. Li *et al.*, 1998). This indicates that viral entry into host cells is not completely dependent on the receptor-mediated endocytosis, but also involves receptor-independent macropinocytosis, and PI3K signalling appears to be important in this process. Receptor blocking therapeutics already exist on the market, such as oseltamivir that inhibits the influenza surface protein neuraminidase (NA) which cleaves HA-SA interaction and releases the newly made virions. Although drug resistance is rapidly emerging, investigation in the molecular mechanisms of virus-induced macropinocytosis may reveal potential therapeutic targets for respiratory viral infections, particularly for influenza.

Following successful endocytosis viruses must utilize the host cells to replicate and then spread to neighbouring cells. As BECs are the primary site of infection for respiratory viruses, they often initiate the early immune response to infection, which is likely to have a profound effect on the subsequent inflammatory and immune response. Innate immunity is an evolutionary conserved first line of defence that is initiated in infected cells in an attempt to limit viral replication and spread, concomitantly induce the development of pathogen-specific adaptive immunity for viral clearance. During infection, replicating viruses produce RNA or DNA intermediate products, which can be recognized by host intracellular pattern recognition receptors (PRRs), and then initiate early innate immune responses to contain viral infection at the site of infection. Toll-like receptors (TLRs) are a family of membrane-spanning PRRs that recognize components that are broadly shared by pathogens but are distinctive from host molecules, and are collectively called pathogen associated molecular patterns (PAMPs). There are currently 12 members of TLRs identified in mammals, three of which play an important role in viral innate immunity and viral pathogenesis.

Most respiratory viruses are ssRNA viruses, though they also produce dsRNA intermediates during replication. Viral ssRNA and dsRNA are recognised as foreign entity by different families of PRRs (Figure 1). TLR3 is a membrane spanning PRR located in the endosomal membrane that recognizes viral dsRNA and predominantly initiates inflammatory response (Alexopoulou *et al.*, 2001). Upon binding TLR3 initiates a signalling cascade that activates cytoplasmic nuclear factor κB (NF-κB), which is then translocated to the nucleus where it induces the expression of pro-inflammatory cytokines such as CXCL-8 and tumour necrosis factor (TNF) -α, leading to acute inflammation including the infiltration and activation of neutrophils (Chaouat *et al.*, 2009). Viral-mediated activation of NF-κB also drives the expression and release of another class of innate immune protein called human defensins, which is classified into α and β sub-family. Human α defensins (HDs) are mainly induced by blood immune cells such as neutrophils (Ganz, 2003; Rehaume & Hancock, 2008), whereas human β defensins (HBDs) are mainly produced by lung epithelial cells and immune cells (Ganz, 2003; Yang *et al.*, 2004). Respiratory viruses including rhinovirus, influenza viruses, and RSV have all been shown to induce HBD2 and HBD3 in a NF-κB and TNF-α-dependent manner (Duits *et al.*, 2003; Kota *et al.*, 2008; Leikina *et al.*, 2005; Proud *et al.*, 2004), and their functions are mainly involved in the inhibition of viral entry and disruption of viral envelope. HBD2 has been shown to bind and disintegrate RSV envelope under electron microscopy, leading to the fragmentation of the virus (Kota, *et al.*, 2008). Similarly HBD3 was shown to inhibit viral-host membrane fusion during influenza infection leading to reduced viral entry (Leikina, *et al.*, 2005). Together with other HDs and HBDs such as HD5 that also inhibits viral entry step of another virus family herpes simplex virus (HSVs) (Hazrati *et al.*, 2006), this indicates that the defensins may be broadly involved in the antiviral responses to invading viruses at the early phase of infection.

The second set of PRRs that also recognizes foreign pathogens are the nucleotide-binding domain and leucine-rich-repeat-containing (NLR) family. NLR protein 3 (NLRP3) can recognize dsRNAs and ssRNA, and can be induced by viral infection including influenza (Allen *et al.*, 2009) and rhinovirus (Schneider *et al.*, 2010) (Figure 1). Upon binding to viral RNAs, NLRP3 interacts with an adaptor protein Apoptotic Speck protein containing caspase activation and recruitment domain (CARD) (ASC) and forms a complex known as the NLRP3 inflammasome. This complex then activates pro-caspase 1 into functional caspase 1, which in turn activate pro-IL-1 into its biological active form IL-1β, which binds to toll/IL-1 receptor (TIR) that shares signalling with TLRs and upregulates inflammatory cytokines (Takeda *et al.*, 2003). IL-1β also recruits neutrophils to the site of infection and further promotes inflammatory mediators (Akira *et al.*, 2006; Allen, *et al.*, 2009; Ting *et al.*, 2008).

The third family of PRRs called retinoic acid-inducible gene-I (RIG-I)-like receptors (RLRs), including RIG-I, melanoma-differentiation-associated gene-5 (MDA-5), and laboratory of genetics and physiology 2 (LGP2), are also able to recognize different forms of viral RNAs, and are primarily responsible for the induction of type I and type III interferons (IFNs), a critical component of the innate antiviral responses that limit viral replication (Figure 1). RIG-I preferentially recognizes ssRNAs with 5` triphosphate (5`ppp ssRNA) that are only generated during influenza, RSV, and human metapneumovirus replication (Le Goffic *et al.*, 2007; Loo *et al.*, 2008; Pichlmair *et al.*, 2006; Saito & Gale, 2008). In contrast MDA-5 is critical in the detection of dsRNA viruses or those with dsRNA intermediates including human rhinoviruses (Kato *et al.*, 2006; Satoh *et al.*). LGP2 is a positive regulator that aids the viral RNA binding by RIG-I and MDA-5 (Satoh, *et al.*). After initial binding to viral RNAs by RIG-I/MDA-5/LGP2, the adaptor protein tripartite motif protein 25 (TRIM25) ubiquitinates the first CARD domain of RIG-I/MDA-5. This results in a conformational change that allows the second CARD domain to associate with the adaptor protein IFN-β promoter stimulator 1 (IPS-1; also known as MAVS, VISA or CARDIF) on the mitochondrial membrane. Tumour Necrosis Factor (TNF)-receptor-associated factor (TRAF3) then associates with this complex and activates TRAF family member-associated NF-κB activator (TANK)-binding kinase 1

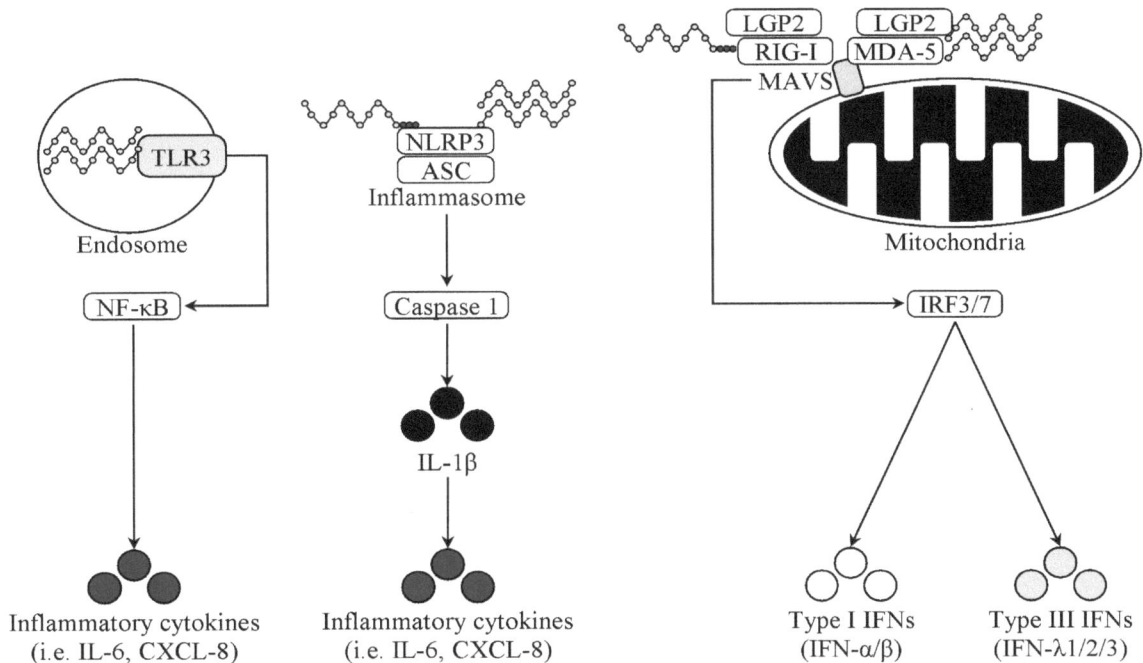

Figure 1: RIG-I/MDA-5/LGP2, TLR3 and NLRP3 inflammasome pathway leading to the expression and release of type I/III IFNs and inflammatory cytokines in epithelial cells.

(TBK1) and inducible IκB kinase (Oganesyan *et al.*, 2006). These kinases phosphorylate interferon regulatory factor 3 (IRF3) and IRF7, which then translocate to the nucleus where they initiate the expression of type I and type III IFNs (Doyle *et al.*, 2006; Fitzgerald *et al.*, 2003; Kotenko *et al.*, 2003).

Type I (IFN-α/-β) and type III (IFN-λ1/2/3) IFNs are potent innate antiviral mediators that are released by epithelial cells upon viral infection. These secreted IFNs then bind to type I IFN (IFNAR1/2) and type III IFN (IL28Rα/IL-10Rβ) receptor on the same or neighbouring cells (Kotenko, *et al.*, 2003; Pestka *et al.*, 1987; Sheppard *et al.*, 2003), and induce the expression of over 300 IFN-stimulated genes (ISGs), through the activation of signal transducer and activator of transcription (STAT)-1 and -2 (Figure 2) (Levy & Garcia-Sastre, 2001; G. R. Stark *et al.*, 1998). This promotes the establishment of the full antiviral responses of epithelial cells and provides positive reinforcement of IFN responses.

Many ISGs have been identified to have roles in host defence against viral infection. Protein kinase RNA-activated (PKR) is a dsRNA-activated cellular enzyme that not only induces a rapid and potent expression of IFN proteins (Kujime *et al.*, 2000; Kumar *et al.*, 1994), but also induces apoptosis upon viral infection, thus preventing virus replication (Garcia *et al.*, 2006; Gil & Esteban, 2000; Zhang & Samuel, 2007). PKR also phosphorylates the elongation initiation factor eIF2, which results in a rapid inhibition of viral mRNA translation (G. R. Stark, *et al.*, 1998). Proteins such as 2', 5' – oligoadenylate synthetase (OAS) and MxA protein elicit an antiviral state in the infected cells by inhibiting the viral replication. OAS can be activated by viral RNA, which in turn activates an endoribonuclease RNase L that

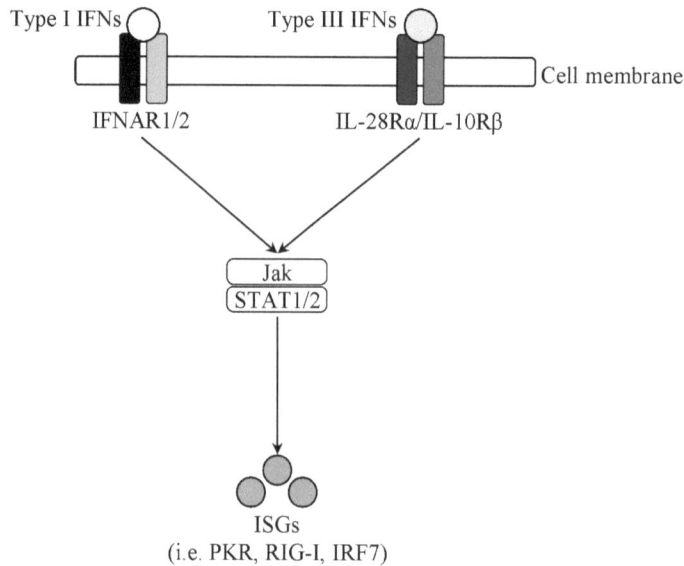

Figure 2: Type I and type III IFNs mediated induction of ISGs expression in epithelial cells.

can cleave extensively viral RNA (Chen *et al.*, 1999). MxA also interferes with viral protein synthesis and inhibits viral replication by promoting host cell apoptosis (Mibayashi *et al.*, 2002; Pavlovic *et al.*, 1992; Zhou *et al.*, 1997; Zurcher *et al.*, 2000). Positive regulators such as RIG-I, MDA-5, and IRF7 further amplify the antiviral responses (Garcia, *et al.*, 2006; Kujime, *et al.*, 2000; Pavlovic, *et al.*, 1992; Slater *et al.*, 2010).

Despite the distinctive viral recognition and signalling outcomes of TLRs and RLRs, recent characterization of these PRRs also revealed cross-regulation of these signalling pathways. Human rhinovirus is a ssRNA virus that generates dsRNAs during replication, which can be recognized by TLR3 and MDA-5, stimulating an inflammatory and antiviral response. In contrast influenza, also a ssRNA virus, only produces ssRNAs with 5' triphosphate (5'ppp-ssRNAs), which is recognized by RIG-I, and not dsRNAs during replication (Pichlmair, *et al.*, 2006). Although influenza has been demonstrated to induce inflammatory response via TLR3 signalling, it is questionable as how influenza 3'ppp-ssRNAs are recognized by TLR3, and may possibly involve other pathways such as NLRP3. NLRP3 has been shown to recognize influenza RNAs and induce inflammatory response, although the specific RNA configurations that NLRP3 binds are yet to be characterized. TLR3 and NLRP3 may therefore both contribute to the inflammation in the lung of infected individuals (Jiang *et al.*, 2004; Le Goffic, *et al.*, 2007). This is especially true with the highly pathogenic avian influenza H5N1. A hallmark feature of H5N1 infection in the infected individuals is a massive pro-inflammatory cytokine storm, leading to severe toxic shock and multi-organ failure with a fatality rate of approximately 60% (Chotpitayasunondh *et al.*, 2005; Tran *et al.*, 2004).

Although the PRRs that results in this inflammatory cytokines release in H5N1 infection are not known, NF-κB has been shown to play a critical role, while inhibition of NF-κB has resulted in a marked reduction in the production of these cytokines (Schmolke *et al.*, 2009). Interestingly preventing this cytokine storm in H5N1-infected knockout mice model did not lead to reduced pathogenicity or improved mortality (Droebner *et al.*, 2008; Salomon *et al.*, 2007). It then appears that that the removal of damaging effects of inflammatory cytokines is not enough to reduce high mortality associated with H5N1 infection.

TLR3 signalling pathway, typically involved in the inflammatory responses, has also been shown to regulate the expression of antiviral proteins via NF-κB. This transcription factor downstream of TLR3 is normally involved in the induction of inflammatory cytokines, however Thomson, *et al.* identified a cluster of NF-κB binding sites on human IFN-λ1 promoter, demonstrated that NF-κB was critical in IFN-λ1 induction (Thomson *et al.*, 2009). IFN-β on the other hand can also be up-regulated by a complex of transcriptional factors. IFN-β gene enhancer can be recognized by three major transcription factors, nuclear factor (NF) -κB, interferon-regulatory factors (IRFs), and activating transcription factor (ATF) -2. These three factors then bind to a structural protein called high mobility group (HMG) -I protein, forming a multi-component transcription factor-enhancer complex named the IFN-β enhanceosome. HMG-I promotes and stabilizes of the binding to transcription co-activator cAMP response element-binding (CREB) binding protein (CBP)/p300, and increases the formation of another complex called transcription pre-initiation complex (PIC) that facilitates the positioning of RNA polymerase II over the gene transcription start site, denatures DNA thereby initiating the transcription of IFN-β gene (Kim & Maniatis, 1997; Yie *et al.*, 1999) (Figure 3). Although the formation kinetics of IFN-β enhanceosome during respiratory viral infections is still unclear, the formation of IFN-β enhanceosome is critical in the induction of IFN-β during viral infection.

This differential binding of transcription factors therefore ensures dynamic up-regulation of these important antiviral proteins following viral infection, especially when the invading viruses such as influenza possess antiviral evasion strategies to maximize replication. The multiple layers of host innate defences attempt to restrict replicating viruses, and at the same time signal for other important immune cells to the site of infection for further clearance of viruses.

2.2   Airway immune cells

Neutrophils are important innate immune cells that respond to signals of tissue damage and infection (Cowburn *et al.*, 2008). These effector cells express the surface receptor CXC Chemokine Receptor 1 and 2 (CXCR1 and 2), which are attracted by CXCL-8 produced by the infected BECs and recruited to the site of infection down a chemokine-induced gradient (Woolhouse *et al.*, 2002). Respiratory viral infections result in a rapid infiltration of neutrophils into the lung, and once at the site of infection neutrophils, via cluster of differentiation (CD) 11a/CD18, adhere to ICAM-1 on BECs, and phagocytose infected and/or damaged cells, resulting in the formation of phagosome (Tate *et al.*, 2008; Tate *et al.*, 2011). Within which toxic proteases (including neutrophil elastases, matrix metalloproteases (MMPs), and myeloperoxidase (MPO) are produced to convert reactive oxygen species (ROS) such as hydrogen peroxide into hypochlorous acid that then degrades ingested viral proteins (Lambeth, 2004; Yamamoto *et al.*, 1991). This event is called neutrophil oxidative burst and provides a secondary defence against foreign pathogens. Neutrophils therefore play a critical role in the clearance of replicating virus, and this importance was further demonstrated in the reduced survival to influenza infection in mice that had been depleted of neutrophils (Tate, *et al.*, 2008). Furthermore, BECs infected by influenza, parainfluenza, rhinovirus and RSV have been shown to increase ICAM-1 expression that allows enhanced neutrophil adherence to the infected cells, thereby further enhancing viral clearance (Ratcliffe *et al.*, 1988; J. M. Stark *et al.*, 1992; S. Z. Wang *et al.*, 1998). Concomitantly neutrophils themselves are also capable of inducing

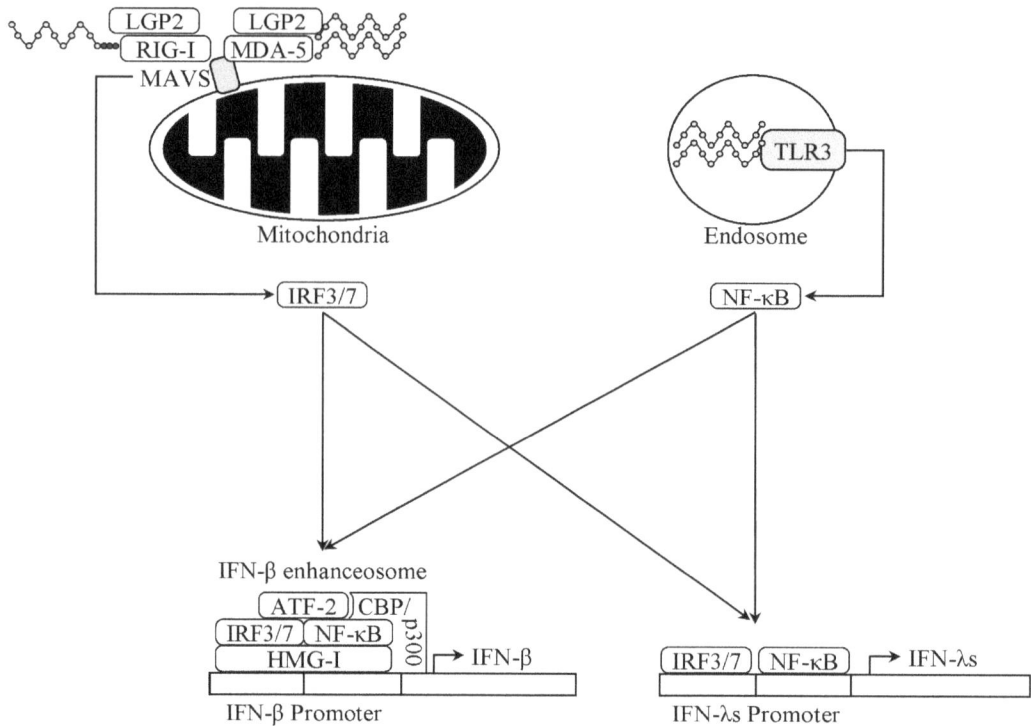

Figure 3: Formation of IFN-β enhanceosome in IFN-β induction and IRF3/7 and NF-κB co-regulation of IFN-λs induction. Transcriptional factor IRF3/7, NF-κB, and ATF-2 forms a large complex with HMG-I, which then binds to CBP/p300 and drives the transcription of IFN-β. The IRF-3/7 and NF-κB binding site on the IFN-λ promoter allows for IFN-λs gene transcription.

inflammatory cytokines including CXL-8, TNF-α, and IL-1β that further amplify the inflammatory response to respiratory viral infection (Cassatella, 1999; Ochiai *et al.*, 1993; J. P. Wang *et al.*, 2008). In addition, neutrophils also produce human α defensins known as human neutrophil peptides (HNPs) 1 and 2, which interfere with influenza virus and adenovirus replication and enhance viral clearance by neutrophils. HNP1 and 2 was found to bind to surfactant protein (SP) D, a protein that binds to the carbohydrate side chain of influenza HA and NA, and promote neutrophil uptake of influenza virus (Hartshorn *et al.*, 2006; LeVine *et al.*, 2001; Tecle *et al.*, 2007). HNP1 was also demonstrated to bind to the capsid protein of adenovirus and inhibited viral entry (Bastian & Schafer, 2001; Smith & Nemerow, 2008).

Macrophages are another type of phagocytic cells that scavenge foreign pathogens and dead cellular debris in the lung, while also participate in inflammation. These scavenger immune cells are of haemopoietic origin and migrate to the respiratory tract via blood and lymphatic vessels. Pro-monocytes migrate from bone marrow into the circulation and mature into monocytes, which then differentiate into macrophages when they reach their destined organs. In the lungs, alveolar macrophages are also an important component of pulmonary defence that are recruited to the site of infection by chemokines including chemokine (C-C motif) ligand (CCL3, also known as Macrophage Inflammatory Protein (MIP) -1α) and CCL5 (also known as Regulated And Normal T cell Expressed and Secreted (RANTES)) released from virus-infected cells. They are then capable of recognizing externalized phospholipid phosphatidylserine, a hallmark feature of apoptosis, on the surface of infected cells and initiate phagocytosis (Hashimoto *et al.*, 2007; Piccolo *et al.*, 1999; Shiratsuchi *et al.*, 2000; Shukaliak & Dorovini-Zis, 2000). CCL2 (or Monocyte Chemotactic Protein (MCP) -1) can also be induced by macrophages to recruit monocytes, and DCs to the site of inflammation (Xu *et al.*, 1996). The inductions of these chemokines are dependent on the activation of NF-κB (Qin *et al.*, 2012; Rimbach *et al.*, 2000; Werts *et al.*, 2007). Macrophages also appear to have similar innate immune signalling system, and many respiratory viruses such as influenza, rhinoviruses, and RSV are able to infect and replicate in macrophages and induce similar innate immune responses as that found in BECs. Infection of macrophages with these respiratory viruses has been shown to induce TLR3 and NF-κB with up-regulated pro-inflammatory cytokines such as CXCL-8 and TNF-α. RIG-I/MDA-5 was also induced and led to increased type I IFN responses after infection (Cheung *et al.*, 2002; Laza-Stanca *et al.*, 2006; Senft *et al.*, 2010; J. Wang *et al.*, 2012). Macrophages also produce SP-A that binds to influenza HA and NA, RSV F (fusion) and G (attachment) protein that results in enhanced viral uptake and phagocytosis by the macrophages (Barr *et al.*, 2000; Ghildyal *et al.*, 1999; Malhotra *et al.*, 1994).

Natural Killer (NK) cells are a class of cytotoxic lymphocytes that play a crucial role in innate antiviral responses to viral infections. NK cells can be activated by cytokines including type I IFNs, CCL2, CCL3, and CCL5 induced by viral infection. At the site of infection NK cells are able to recognize the natural cytotoxicity receptor such as NKp46 on the virus-infected cells and release intracellular proteases including perforin and granzymes, leading to the induction of apoptosis of infected cells (Biron *et al.*, 1999; Mandelboim *et al.*, 2001). NK cells are also capable of secreting cytokines such as TNF-α, further contributing to the inflammatory response after viral infection. While NK cells appears to be an important effector immune cells against viruses such as and parainfluenza virus and RSV, influenza viruses have been shown to infect and replicate in NK cells, after which kills the infected NK cells by inducing apoptosis *via* unknown mechanism (Anderson *et al.*, 1989; Mao *et al.*, 2009).

Another important class of immune cells are the dendritic cells (DCs), which play a pivotal role in both the innate response to infection, as well as initiating the adaptive immune response in response to infection. There are several phenotypes of DCs in the lung with varying immune functions. Plasmocytoid (p)DCs, on the other hand, are potent IFN producers against viral infection. pDCs share similar immune signalling pathways as BECs, however RIG-I appears to be dispensable during viral infection and instead rely on TLR7/8 and 9 in the endosome to recognize viral RNAs and initiate IFN responses via IRF7 and inflammatory response via NF-κB (Honda & Taniguchi, 2006; Takeda & Akira, 2005). Interestingly, human influenza H3N2 and H1N1, human rhinovirus, RSV, and human metapneumovirus have all been shown to have restricted replication due to potent type I IFN responses in pDCs (Boogaard *et al.*, 2007; Fonteneau *et al.*, 2003; Schrauf *et al.*, 2009; Smed-Sorensen *et al.*, 2012). It is possible that the high antiviral responses exerted in the pDCs circumvent the need for cytoplasmic PRRs such as RIG-I. High pathogenic avian influenza H5N1 on the other hand was able to replicate efficiently by heavily suppressing this type I IFN responses in the infected pDCs (Thitithanyanont *et al.*, 2007). The IFNs produced by BECs and pDCs not only establish antiviral responses and contain viral replication, but can also promote DC maturation and their ability to stimulate virus-specific cytotoxic T cells response for efficient viral clearance (Luft *et al.*, 1998; Spadaro *et al.*, 2012). Myeloid (m)DCs, as well as macrophages, are the sentinel cells that capture viral antigens that are released from infected BECs, and present the antigens to naïve T cells in the lymph node, leading to an virus-specific cytotoxic T cell response to efficiently clear the invading virus and memory T cell response in preparation for future re-infection (Cerwenka *et al.*,

1999). DCs have also been discovered to interact with unique subsets of T lymphocytes called invariant natural killer T (iNKT) and Th17 cells, which have been shown to contribute to innate inflammatory response to viral infections. For example, influenza infection has been shown to induce IL-1β via RIG-I, TLR7 and NF-κB in DCs, which then binds to IL-1 receptor (IL-1R) on DCs and can up-regulate the expression of IL-6 and TNF-α via NF-κB, further driving inflammatory response to infection (Boehm *et al.*, 1997; Cogswell *et al.*, 1994; Ho *et al.*, 2008; Paget *et al.*, 2012). IL-1β can also activate iNKT cells to release immune-modulatory cytokines via NF-κB, including type II IFN, IFN-γ, that further stimulate BECs and DCs to produce inflammatory cytokines that recruit macrophages and neutrophils to the site of infection and inflammation (Boehm, *et al.*, 1997; Ho, *et al.*, 2008; Paget, *et al.*, 2012). Influenza infected DCs also release IL-1β, IL-6, TNF-α, IL-10, and IL-23, which differentiate and expand Th17 population that then release IL-17 and IL-22, also via NF-κB, and further enhance the inflammatory responses in DCs and BECs (Cho *et al.*, 2006; Dong, 2008; Hamada *et al.*, 2009; Laan *et al.*, 2001; Manel *et al.*, 2008; Yao *et al.*, 1995). This plethora of innate immune cytokines and complex innate immune network therefore contribute to the efficient viral clearance, nevertheless most viruses have also developed strategies to either evade or suppress host immune systems.

3   Viral Evasion of Innate Immunity

Co-evolution of viruses and animals has resulted in the development of multiple layers to the innate defensive response with the aim of containing invading viruses at the initial site of infection. On the other hand respiratory viruses have also evolved abilities to evade and inhibit host immune responses to promote survival.

Amongst the respiratory viruses, influenza is one of the best characterized viruses in their immune evasion capabilities and is therefore discussed here. Influenza viruses undergo frequent mutations ($\sim 1/10^4$ bases per replication cycle) due to the relatively low proof-reading property of the influenza RNA-dependent RNA polymerase (Zambon, 2001). These genetic changes often occur in the gene encoding for the HA and NA, resulting in a new strain that is able to evade host antibodies generated from previous infection or vaccination. This phenomenon, known as antigenic drift, is the reason for annual update to influenza vaccine (Webster *et al.*, 1992). A more significant antigenic change occurs when different virus strains from two or more host species co-infect a single host, allowing genetic reassortment to occur in the infected host and generate a new strain of influenza virus to which the population may have little or no immune memory (Webster, *et al.*, 1992). This process, known as antigenic shift, may result in a viral strain with pandemic potential due to it un-predictable pathogenicity (Zambon, 1999). Antiviral drugs such as influenza M2 ion channel blockers (adamantine and rimantadine) and NA inhibitors (oseltamivir and zanamivir) are also available. M2 ion channel is critical in driving the uncoating of the virus after entry into the host cell, and M2 blockers therefore inhibits early step of the replication cycle. NA inhibitors block the detachment of newly made influenza virions from the host cell surface. These drugs have similar efficacy when given in season prophylaxis and post-exposure against influenza infection (Hayden *et al.*, 1999; Jefferson *et al.*, 2006; Monto *et al.*, 1999). Due to the high use of antiviral drugs and fast mutation rate of influenza these viruses have acquired resistance to current drugs (de Jong *et al.*, 2005; Kiso *et al.*, 2004; Monto *et al.*, 2006; Ward *et al.*, 2005). Our recent report of the rapid emergence of oseltamivir-resistant 2009 H1N1 pandemic virus (A/Newcastle/89/2011) in Australia further highlights the danger of a heavy reliance on current antiviral drugs and discovery of novel therapeutic options (Hurt *et al.*, 2011; Hurt *et al.*, 2012).

Influenza viruses also encode proteins that suppress the transcription and function of important antiviral proteins including type I and III IFNs. The non-structural (NS) 1 protein of influenza is a protein with molecular mass of approximately 26,000, and is a multi-functional protein expressed very rapidly to help the establishment of viral infection by interfering with host mRNA processing and translation, as well as inhibiting host immune responses, especially the antiviral system. Influenza NS1 protein is able to bind, with its effector domain, to essential host mRNA processing and translation protein, cleavage and polyadenylation specificity factor subunit 30 (CPSF30) and poly A binding protein (PAB) II, shutting down the host protein synthesis to gain control of the host machinery required for viral protein synthesis (Figure 4).

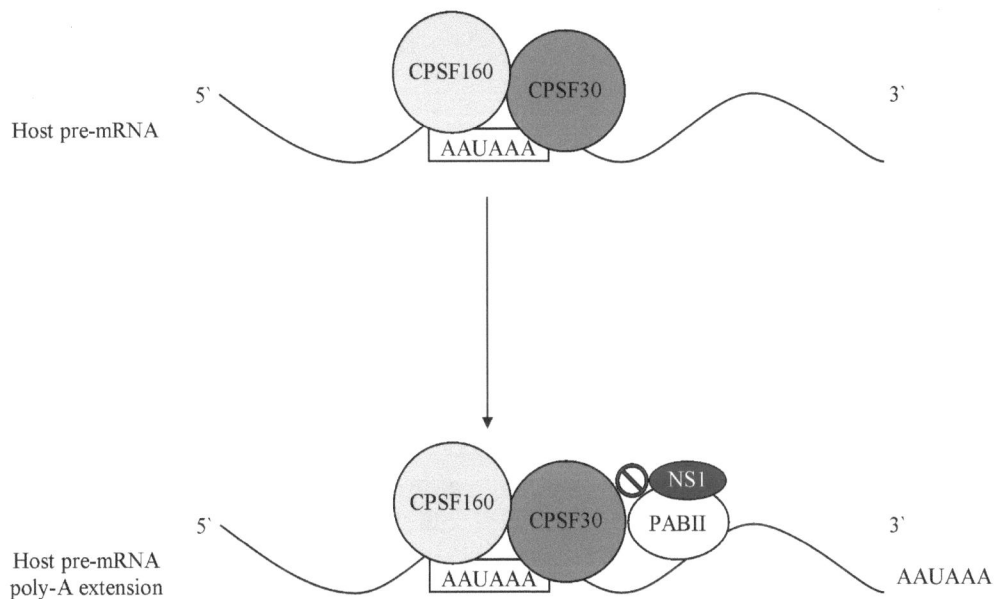

Figure 4: Influenza NS1 inhibition of host mRNA processing.

The IFN antagonistic property of NS1 occurs at multiple stages of the IFN signalling cascade. NS1 interacts with the viral sensor RIG-I, and can also inhibit the downstream activation of MAVS and nuclear translocation of IRF3, thereby inhibiting IFNs response (Mibayashi *et al.*, 2007; Talon *et al.*, 2000). The NS1 protein specifically inhibits TRIM25-mediated RIG-I ubiquitination, which is crucial for maximal IFNs expression during viral infection (Gack *et al.*, 2009). This NS1-TRIM25 binding event is dependent on the arginine and lysine at position 38 and 41 respectively in the RNA binding domain, and glutamic acid at position 96 and 97 in the effector domain of NS1 (Bornholdt & Prasad, 2008; X. Wang *et al.*, 2002). Beside the inhibitory role in IFNs expression, NS1 protein also inhibits cellular proteins that establish the antiviral state of infected cells. The RNA-binding domain of NS1 can bind to viral RNA to prevent detection by PKR (Y. Lu *et al.*, 1995). It also binds to PKR itself via the effector domain (residue

123 – 127) and inhibits PKR-mediated viral mRNA suppression and PKR-induced apoptosis (Figure 5) (Bergmann *et al.*, 2000; Dauber *et al.*, 2006; S. Li *et al.*, 2006; Min *et al.*, 2007).

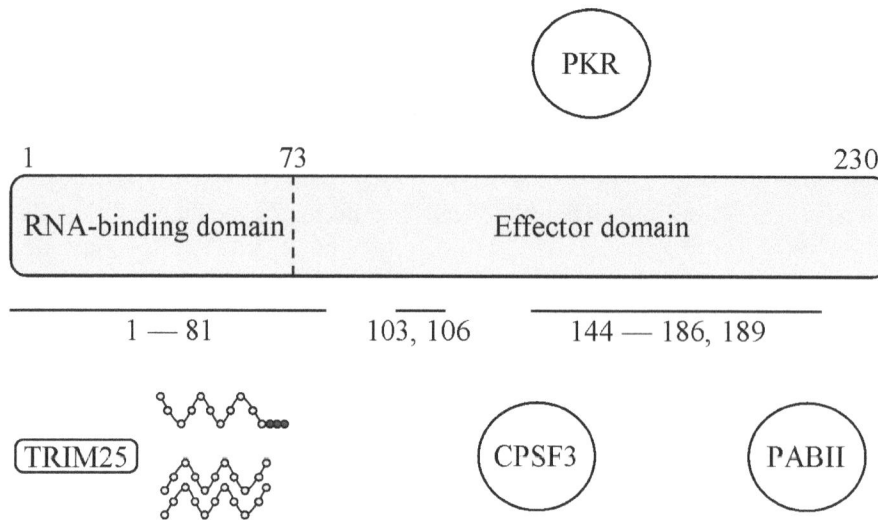

Figure 5: Known binding targets of influenza NS1 protein in relations to amino acids involved.

The frequent mutations of the influenza genome often generate variant strains with different pathogenesis, and therefore the strength of NS1-mediated antiviral inhibition also varies with different strains of influenza. We have shown that primary BECs (pBECs) elicited reduced type I and III IFNs responses to a human influenza virus H3N2, when compared to a low pathogenic avian influenza H11N9 (A. C. Hsu, *et al.*, 2011). This differential response observed with these two strains was due to the more effective NS1 of H3N2 that effectively inhibited the IFN responses, while the NS-1 of H11N9 was relatively weak in this inhibition. This is likely to represent another example of the adaptation of the H3N2 to its human host, in which it had been circulating for approximately 50 years. The high pathogenic avian influenza H5N1 on the other hand completely abolished the type I and III IFN responses, resulting in higher viral replication compared to H3N2 infection and cell death (A. C. Hsu, Parsons, K., Barr, I., Lowther, S., Middleton, D., Hansbro, PM., Wark, PAB. , 2012). A number of studies have identified that the NS1 of H5N1 is a very potent inhibitor of RIG-I-mediated signalling and type I and III IFN responses (Bornholdt & Prasad, 2008; Jackson *et al.*, 2008; Jiao *et al.*, 2008). Further studies revealed that while human influenza is sensitive to exogenous treatment of type I and III IFNs regardless of the inhibition by NS1, the H5N1 strain was able to survive regardless of IFNs treatment (A. C. Hsu, *et al.*, 2011; Hyland *et al.*, 2006). Normally IFN-induced antiviral proteins including PKR can degrade NS and other viral genes, but NS1 of H5N1 is able to bind to and effectively inactivate these antiviral proteins (Seo *et al.*, 2002). This antiviral resistance of NS1 was found to require a glutamic acid at position 92. Human influenza engineered with NS1 of H5N1 showed an enhanced replication in the presence of IFNs, whereas the wild type and the mutant virus containing a mutation at residue 92 failed to replicate under the same condition (Seo, *et al.*, 2002).

While similar NS1-mediated antiviral inhibition was also observed in immune cells including macrophages and pDCs, especially with high pathogenic avian H5N1 virus (Fernandez-Sesma *et al.*, 2006; Jia *et al.*, 2010), other respiratory viruses also have developed similar antiviral inhibitory capability. For example, adenovirus contains an early region 4 (E4) that encodes proteins involved in efficient viral replication, and E4 open reading frame 3 (E4 ORF3) specifically inhibits type I IFN responses and enhances viral replication (Ullman *et al.*, 2007). RSV has been shown to utilize its NS1/2 protein to degrade STAT2 and impair the type I IFNs mediated antiviral response in tracheobronchial epithelial cells (Elliott *et al.*, 2007; Ramaswamy *et al.*, 2004; Ramaswamy *et al.*, 2006). Similarly SARS-CoV was recently found to encode a highly basic nucleocapsid (N) protein that inhibits the synthesis of type I IFN response, although the mechanism of this suppression remains unclear (X. Lu *et al.*, 2011). As immune cells such as pDCs have similar innate immune signalling system as BECs, respiratory viruses would exert IFN inhibition in a similar fashion as that in BECs. This demonstrates the importance of early innate immune evasion strategies in viruses that are successful as human respiratory pathogens.

Type I IFNs are an important antiviral cytokines that are induced by viral infection and amplify antiviral responses through type I IFN receptors and Jak/STAT pathway and eradicate replicating viruses. One would assume that these potent IFNs are only induced upon viral infection (inducible IFNs) and subside once infection is resolved. However several studies, including our recent findings, have found the expression of constitutive IFN-β, which played a pivotal role in containing viral replication, even when faced with potent IFN suppressive effect of viral virulence factors such as influenza NS1 (Bocci, Muscettola, *et al.*, 1985; Bocci, Paulesu, *et al.*, 1985; De Maeyer-Guignard *et al.*, 1988; A. C. Hsu, *et al.*, 2011; A. C. Hsu, Parsons, K., Barr, I., Lowther, S., Middleton, D., Hansbro, PM., Wark, PAB. , 2012; Sato *et al.*, 2000; Taniguchi & Takaoka, 2001).

Bocci (1980) first observed the presence of IFN-β in un-infected tissues and this low levels of IFN-β exerted antiviral activities (Bocci, 1980), and later IFN-β mRNA and protein was also found in tissues of healthy mice maintained in specific pathogen-free conditions (Gresser, 1990; Tovey *et al.*, 1987). We also found that BECs secrete low levels of IFN-β when viral infection is absent, and when host protein synthesis was inhibited at translational step with an inhibitor cycloheximide, to determine if IFN-β could still be made and secreted, an enhanced release of IFN-β was observed with and without influenza infection (A. C. Hsu, Parsons, K., Barr, I., Lowther, S., Middleton, D., Hansbro, PM., Wark, PAB. , 2012). This increased IFN-β was then found to be due to the release of pre-formed IFN-β from within the cytosol. While blocking of the IFN-β receptor IFNAR2 reduced the effect of this enhanced IFN-β and led to increased influenza replication.

The mechanism of the production of constitutive IFN-β is yet to be fully elucidated, however Hata *et al.* (2001) found that deletion of IRF3/7 did not affect constitutive IFN-β production, and this IFN-β release would then stimulate the expression of IRF7 and further induce the ISGs expression following viral infection. The transcription factor NF-κB has also been implicated in the induction of constitutive IFN-β. NF-κB is composed of dimerized subunits of p50, p52, p65, and RelB, and this complex is normally under inhibition by IκB kinase. Once stimulated by various factors including viral infection, IκB kinase is degraded by ubiquitination, allowing the NF-κB complex to translocate into the nucleus and induce the expression of inflammatory and type I IFNs (Chaouat, *et al.*, 2009; Jacobs & Harrison, 1998). The subunit p65 has recently been demonstrated to drive the constitutive production of IFN-β, and when p65 was absent in murine embryo fibroblasts, this constitutive IFN-β was significantly diminished, and subsequently failed to induce efficient antiviral response to vesicular stomatitis virus (VSV) infection

(Basagoudanavar *et al.*, 2011). These findings provide novel insights into the possible mechanisms of constitutive IFN-β production, which is able to counter-act some of the suppressive effects by influenza NS1 protein via IFN-β-IFNAR2 signalling and induce early antiviral responses following infection. While our observation of pre-formed IFN-β protein that is stored within the cells is also novel, the exact mechanism by which IFN-β is released when host protein synthesis was blocked at a translational level is unclear. The enhanced IFN-β production associated with cycloheximide may reflect that influenza-induced inhibition of host protein synthesis is a potential trigger for this constitutive release of IFN-β via a novel pathway.

These observations are in agreement with the notion of a "revving up model" first proposed by Taniguchi and Takaoka (Bocci, Muscettola, *et al.*, 1985; Bocci, Paulesu, *et al.*, 1985; De Maeyer-Guignard, *et al.*, 1988; Sato, *et al.*, 2000). Constitutive IFN-β and its downstream signalling primes BECs to exert a more robust antiviral response to viral infection, whereas in the absence of this signal epithelial cells become hypo-responsive to this IFN stimulus (Sato, *et al.*, 2000; Taniguchi & Takaoka, 2001) (Figure 6). Nevertheless it is currently unknown if type III IFNs are also constitutively expressed with type I IFNs for synergistic antiviral effects.

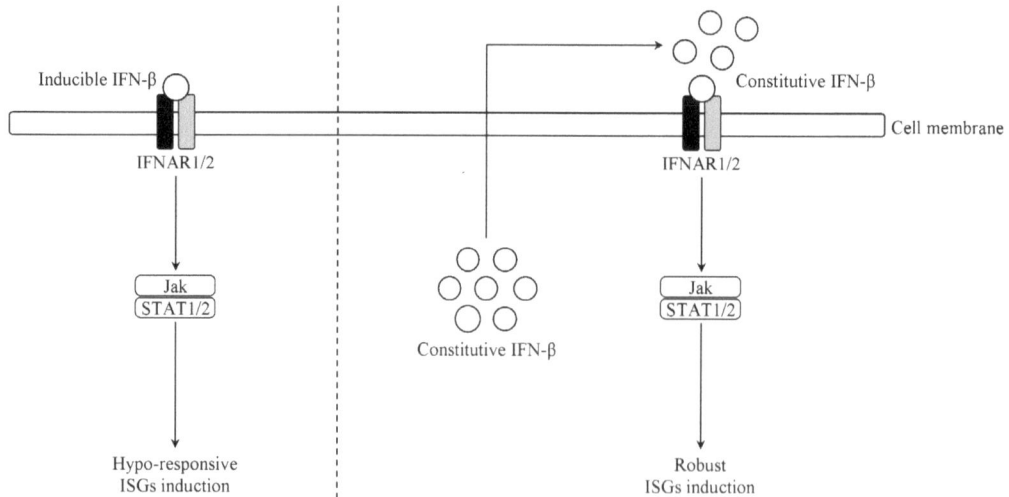

Figure 6: Constitutive release of IFN-β leads to a robust antiviral response via IFNAR1/2 receptor and Jak/STAT1/2.

4   Virus Infection in Chronic Airways Diseases

Respiratory viral infections in healthy individuals usually results in symptoms that normally subside within seven days, those with chronic airways diseases including asthma and chronic obstructive pulmonary disease (COPD) are more susceptible to the effect of infection, leading to more severe symptoms following infection.

Asthma and COPD are both characterized by airflow obstruction, which is reversible in asthma but is progressive and not fully reversible in COPD. These diseases are associated with an increase in sensitivity of the lung to a variety of stimuli, for asthma these include allergens such as house dust mite and air pollutions. COPD is primarily caused by chronic cigarette smoke, however inhaling of industrial toxins, fumes, and chemicals as well as prolonged exposure to air pollution and second hand smoke can also lead to this disease. This high sensitivity to foreign pathogens and particulates then leads to heightened inflammation in the airways of those with chronic airways diseases. Despite the similarities in the clinical features of asthma and COPD, there are also differences in these diseases. Inflammation in asthma is primarily observed in the large and small airways, whereas in COPD inflammation mainly affects small airways and lung parenchyma leading to emphysema, although large airways may also be affected (chronic bronchitis) (Jeffery, 2000). The heightened inflammation is thought to lead to a cycle of continuous airway injury and repair, leading to a vicious cycle that further enhances inflammation. The enhanced inflammatory cytokines including CXCL-8 from the BECs and neutrophils can release these inflammatory mediators and further drive excessive inflammation. This results in symptoms of shortness of breath, persistent cough, sputum production, wheezing, chest tightening, which are often worsened by recurring respiratory viral infection.

Respiratory tract viral infections are associated with the majority (40% - 60%) of the acute exacerbations in asthma (Johnston et al., 1995) and COPD subjects (Seemungal et al., 2001). They lead to more severe lower airway symptoms and are associated with increased hospitalizations (Johnston et al., 1996). A recent study demonstrated that asthmatic children are more susceptible to 2009 H1N1 influenza virus compared to non-asthmatics, and suffered loss of asthma control during infection (Kloepfer et al., 2012). Interestingly, another recent study showed that while individuals with asthma had greater respiratory symptoms due to influenza infection compared to non-asthmatics at the time of hospital admission, asthmatics were not more likely to have severe outcome of infection (Myles et al., 2012). Management of asthma condition with corticosteroid use correlated with this decreased likelihood of severe symptoms. However influenza vaccination status of the recruited subjects in the study was not recorded and may explain this decreased infection outcome in the asthmatics.

The specific pathways that lead to this susceptibility to viral infection and the severe outcomes in these individuals, though are still poorly defined, may be attributed to the abnormal innate immune responses in the lungs of those with chronic airways diseases. Viral infection in asthma and COPD results in heightened airway inflammation with the release of inflammatory cytokines including TNF-α and CXCL-8 from the infected cells and further recruits neutrophils and other immune cells to the site of infection. IL-17 has also been shown to induce the release of CXCL-8 from the infected cells, contributing to the already exaggerated inflammation in the airways and resulting in destructive changes in those with asthma and COPD (Wiehler & Proud, 2007). This therefore indicates that while inflammation may be protective against viral infections, in those with chronic airways diseases this does not appear to efficiently clear the replicating virus and instead cause severe complications that increase mortality.

As antiviral responses are critical in controlling viral infections at the site of infection, the early innate antiviral response to viral infection therefore may also be altered in asthma and COPD. Recent studies have demonstrated that subjects with chronic airways diseases have an impaired antiviral response to infection with rhinovirus, which leads to increased susceptibility to infection and more severe clinical disease. Rhinovirus-infected primary BECs (pBECs) from those with asthma and COPD induced heightened inflammatory cytokines such as CXCL-8 and a lower level of IFN-β and IFN-λ1 response compared to healthy controls (Contoli et al., 2006; Mallia et al., 2011; Uller et al., 2010; Wark et al., 2005). This directly impaired the ability of the infected host cells to undergo early apoptosis, leading to increased virus replication and ultimately cytolysis of the infected cells (Contoli, et al., 2006; Wark, et al., 2005).

This impaired type I and type III IFN responses appear to be a common feature in those with chronic airways diseases, as pBECs from subjects with cystic fibrosis, a genetic disorder that mostly affect the lung, have also been shown to have reduced antiviral IFN responses to rhinovirus infection (Vareille et al., 2012). The early innate IFN response to respiratory viral infection is therefore crucial in limiting the severity of infection. This was further shown in STAT1 knockout mice, which are unable to respond to virus infection with type I IFNs, consequently these mice were 100 times more sensitive to influenza infection and developed disseminated infection, while wild type mice had infection confined to the lungs and more mild clinical disease (Garcia-Sastre et al., 1998).

As those with COPD also share an exaggerated inflammatory response in the airways with asthma, it is plausible that those with COPD may also have reduced antiviral responses to respiratory viral infection, leading to severe complications following infection with respiratory viruses. Indeed, a recent study experimentally infected individuals with COPD with human rhinovirus, and showed impaired antiviral responses compared to healthy subjects (Mallia, et al., 2011). Rhinovirus infection in those with COPD resulted in an intense inflammatory CXCL-8 response in the lungs, with deficient IFN-β protein production compared to the infected healthy individuals. This finding therefore provide important insight into the mechanisms underpinning the high susceptibility to the effect of viral infection in those with chronic airways diseases, and the specific pathways leading to this impaired antiviral response in asthmatics and those with COPD is currently under intense investigation.

The increased susceptibility and severe outcomes of infection in asthma and COPD may be attributed in part to the chronic exposure to chronic inflammation in the airways. Chronic inflammation is known to alter the epigenetics within the cells and tissues, resulting in DNA hyper-methylation and gene silencing, and often precedes the development of many types of cancer (Brower, 2011). In fact, COPD is associated with reduced expression and activity of histone deacetylase 2 (HDAC2) that suppresses inflammatory gene expression (Cosio et al., 2004; K. Ito et al., 2000; K. Ito et al., 2005). HDAC is a family of nuclear enzymes that tightly modulate gene transcription by regulating the "tightness" of chromatins that are wrapped around the histones, and HDAC2 was found to be reduced in the lung tissues of those with COPD, and led to uncontrolled expression of inflammatory cytokines (K. Ito, et al., 2005), which may be further enhanced during infection with respiratory viruses. Similar epigenetic controls such as HDAC1 that regulate antiviral responses may also be abnormal in those with chronic airways diseases (Nusinzon & Horvath, 2003; Roger et al., 2011). In addition, cigarette smoke, the primary cause of COPD, has been shown to impair RIG-I and JAK/STAT pathway, leading to reduced type I IFN response after influenza and RSV infection in human epithelial cells (Modestou et al., 2010; Proud et al., 2012; Wu et al., 2011). The chronic cigarette smoke exposure in the airways may therefore be progressively driving continuous inflammation, tissue damage/repair, while altering the innate antiviral responses to viral infection. Inflammation, viral infection, and cigarette smoke can also independently lead to the generation of oxidative stress in the airways. The level of reactive oxygen species (ROS), have been found to be higher in the lungs of those with chronic airways diseases (Morcillo et al., 1999; Rahman et al., 1996). Acute and/or chronic inflammation resulted from viral infection and/or cigarette smoke can generate ROS, such as superoxide anion, at a rate that outpaces the effect of endogenous antioxidants, leading to oxidative stress (Fridovich, 1999). Oxidative stress itself can also activate NF-κB and enhance the induction of inflammatory response (Rahman et al., 2001), and also inhibit Jak/STAT1/2 signalling, leading to reduced type I IFN-mediated ISGs response (Di Bona et al., 2006).

Furthermore respiratory viruses such as influenza have also developed strategies to evade and suppress host antiviral responses. The combined level of ROS generated from infection, chronic inflammation and cigarette smoke exposure therefore worsens the symptoms by heightening inflammation and reducing antiviral immunity, and ultimately leading to increased mortality.

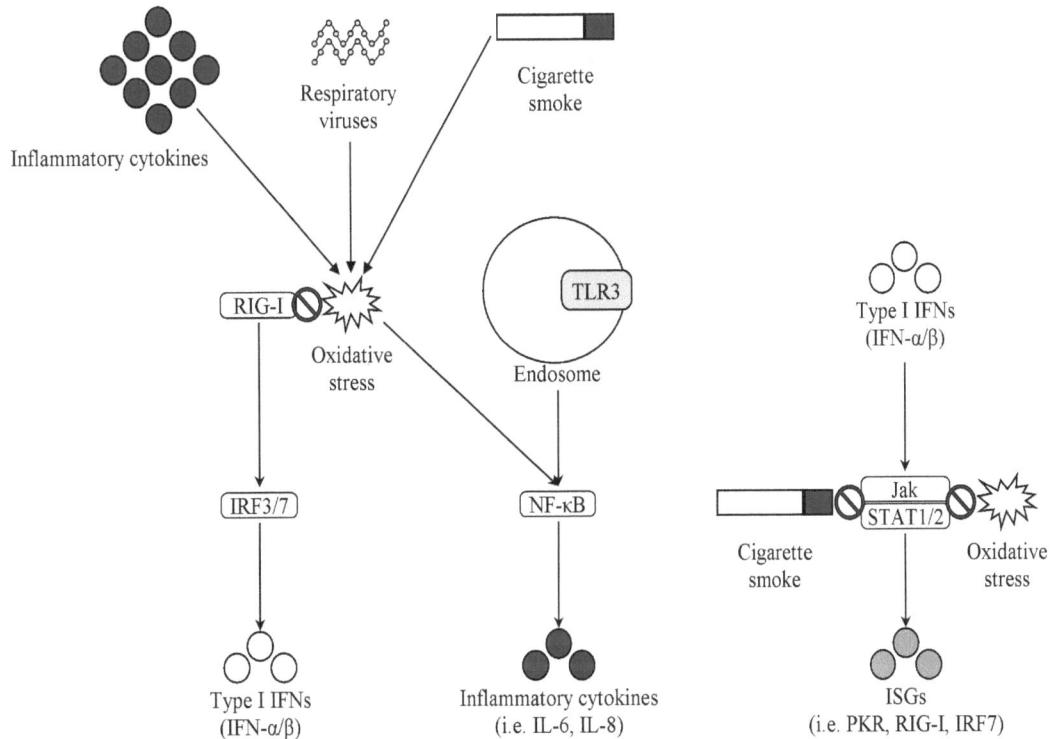

Figure 7: Oxidative stress from high inflammation, respiratory viral infection, and cigarette smoke enhances the induction of inflammatory cytokines, and inhibits antiviral signalling proteins and response.

5   Concluding remarks

Innate immunity is crucial in the defence against respiratory viral infections, especially influenza viruses, and abnormalities in these early immune responses have an important impact on the outcome of infection. Different respiratory viruses have different binding target for efficient endocytosis, however PI3K-mediated macropinocytosis appears to be an evolutionary conserved path into the host cells used by several viruses, signifying a potential therapeutics exploration, especially for viruses with pandemic potential.

The human innate immunity is a complex system that includes the detection of conserved pathogen associated molecules that then result in an immediate inflammatory and antiviral response that ensures the clearance of invading viruses. Conversely viruses have evolved highly effective strategies to compromise this response, allow the establishment of infection and the consequent development of inflammation. Substantial research is being performed to elucidate the complex interactions of the human immune system with respiratory viruses, including exploration of additional antiviral signalling pathways and functional studies of un-characterized ISGs. Reverse genetic engineering and profiling of other additional functions and binding targets of viral virulence factors may also reveal previously un-identified host antiviral proteins. The use of more relevant cells such as primary airways cells or more suitable animal models to further understand host immunity and viral infection and pathogenesis, identifying novel and potentially viable therapeutic strategies that can be used to fight against drug-resistant viruses and those with pandemic potentials.

Furthermore subjects with chronic airways diseases such as asthma and COPD have chronically inflamed airways, and are more susceptible to respiratory viral infections, particularly with seasonal and pandemic influenza. Viral infection further exacerbates the pre-existent chronic inflammation and lead to more severe complications following infections with increased mortality. Although studies have uncovered the reduced antiviral immunity in pBECs of those with asthma and COPD, the molecular mechanisms underlying this impaired antiviral response are currently being investigated intensely in hope to identify novel therapeutic targets that may calm the inflammation and enhance the antiviral responses to respiratory viral infection.

Acknowledgement

This work was supported by National Health and Medical Research Council (Grant No. 510762 and 401314

References

Akira, S., Uematsu, S., & Takeuchi, O. (2006). Pathogen recognition and innate immunity. Cell, 124(4), 783-801.

Alexopoulou, L., Holt, A. C., Medzhitov, R., & Flavell, R. A. (2001). Recognition of double-stranded RNA and activation of NF-kappaB by Toll-like receptor 3. Nature, 413(6857), 732-738.

Allen, I. C., Scull, M. A., Moore, C. B., Holl, E. K., McElvania-TeKippe, E., Taxman, D. J., Guthrie, E. H., Pickles, R. J., & Ting, J. P. (2009). The NLRP3 inflammasome mediates in vivo innate immunity to influenza A virus through recognition of viral RNA. Immunity, 30(4), 556-565.

Anderson, J. J., Serin, M., Harrop, J., Amin, S., Toms, G. L., & Scott, R. (1989). Natural killer cell response to respiratory syncytial virus in the Balb/c mouse model. Adv Exp Med Biol, 257, 211-220.

Araki, N., Johnson, M. T., & Swanson, J. A. (1996). A role for phosphoinositide 3-kinase in the completion of macropinocytosis and phagocytosis by macrophages. J Cell Biol, 135(5), 1249-1260.

Barr, F. E., Pedigo, H., Johnson, T. R., & Shepherd, V. L. (2000). Surfactant protein-A enhances uptake of respiratory syncytial virus by monocytes and U937 macrophages. Am J Respir Cell Mol Biol, 23(5), 586-592.

Basagoudanavar, S. H., Thapa, R. J., Nogusa, S., Wang, J., Beg, A. A., & Balachandran, S. (2011). Distinct roles for the NF-kappa B RelA subunit during antiviral innate immune responses. Journal of Virology, 85(6), 2599-2610.

Bastian, A., & Schafer, H. (2001). Human alpha-defensin 1 (HNP-1) inhibits adenoviral infection in vitro. Regulatory Peptides, 101(1-3), 157-161.

Baum, L. G., & Paulson, J. C. (1990). Sialyloligosaccharides of the respiratory epithelium in the selection of human influenza virus receptor specificity. Acta Histochem Suppl, 40, 35-38.

Bergmann, M., Garcia-Sastre, A., Carnero, E., Pehamberger, H., Wolff, K., Palese, P., & Muster, T. (2000). Influenza virus NS1 protein counteracts PKR-mediated inhibition of replication. J Virol, 74(13), 6203-6206.

Biron, C. A., Nguyen, K. B., Pien, G. C., Cousens, L. P., & Salazar-Mather, T. P. (1999). Natural killer cells in antiviral defense: function and regulation by innate cytokines. Annu Rev Immunol, 17, 189-220.

Bocci, V. (1980). Is interferon produced in physiologic conditions? Medical Hypotheses, 6(7), 735-745.

Bocci, V., Muscettola, M., Paulesu, L., & Grasso, G. (1985). The physiological interferon response. V. Antiviral activity present in rat lymph is neutralized by anti-mouse interferon-gamma antibodies. Microbiologica, 8(4), 405-410.

Bocci, V., Paulesu, L., Muscettola, M., & Viti, A. (1985). The physiologic interferon response. VI. Interferon activity in human plasma after a meal and drinking. Lymphokine Res, 4(2), 151-158.

Boehm, U., Klamp, T., Groot, M., & Howard, J. C. (1997). Cellular responses to interferon-gamma. Annual Review of Immunology, 15, 749-795.

Boogaard, I., van Oosten, M., van Rijt, L. S., Muskens, F., Kimman, T. G., Lambrecht, B. N., & Buisman, A. M. (2007). Respiratory syncytial virus differentially activates murine myeloid and plasmacytoid dendritic cells. Immunology, 122(1), 65-72.

Bornholdt, Z. A., & Prasad, B. V. (2008). X-ray structure of NS1 from a highly pathogenic H5N1 influenza virus. Nature.

Brower, V. (2011). Epigenetics: Unravelling the cancer code. Nature, 471(7339), S12-13.

Cassatella, M. A. (1999). Neutrophil-derived proteins: selling cytokines by the pound. Advances in Immunology, 73, 369-509.

Cerwenka, A., Morgan, T. M., & Dutton, R. W. (1999). Naive, Effector, and Memory CD8 T Cells in Protection Against Pulmonary Influenza Virus Infection: Homing Properties Rather Than Initial Frequencies Are Crucial. J Immunol, 163(10), 5535-5543.

Chaouat, A., Savale, L., Chouaid, C., Tu, L., Sztrymf, B., Canuet, M., Maitre, B., Housset, B., Brandt, C., Le Corvoisier, P., Weitzenblum, E., Eddahibi, S., & Adnot, S. (2009). Role for interleukin-6 in COPD-related pulmonary hypertension. Chest, 136(3), 678-687.

Chen, Z., Li, Y., & Krug, R. M. (1999). Influenza A virus NS1 protein targets poly(A)-binding protein II of the cellular 3'-end processing machinery. Embo J, 18(8), 2273-2283.

Cheung, C. Y., Poon, L. L., Lau, A. S., Luk, W., Lau, Y. L., Shortridge, K. F., Gordon, S., Guan, Y., & Peiris, J. S. (2002). Induction of proinflammatory cytokines in human macrophages by influenza A (H5N1) viruses: a mechanism for the unusual severity of human disease? Lancet, 360(9348), 1831-1837.

Cho, M. L., Kang, J. W., Moon, Y. M., Nam, H. J., Jhun, J. Y., Heo, S. B., Jin, H. T., Min, S. Y., Ju, J. H., Park, K. S., Cho, Y. G., Yoon, C. H., Park, S. H., Sung, Y. C., & Kim, H. Y. (2006). STAT3 and NF-kappaB signal pathway is required for IL-23-mediated IL-17 production in spontaneous arthritis animal model IL-1 receptor antagonist-deficient mice. J Immunol, 176(9), 5652-5661.

Chotpitayasunondh, T., Ungchusak, K., Hanshaoworakul, W., Chunsuthiwat, S., Sawanpanyalert, P., Kijphati, R., Lochindarat, S., Srisan, P., Suwan, P., Osotthanakorn, Y., Anantasetagoon, T., Kanjanawasri, S., Tanupattarachai, S., Weerakul, J., Chaiwirattana, R., Maneerattanaporn, M., Poolsavathitikool, R., Chokephaibulkit, K., Apisarnthanarak, A., & Dowell, S. F. (2005). Human disease from influenza A (H5N1), Thailand, 2004. Emerg Infect Dis, 11(2), 201-209.

Cogswell, J. P., Godlevski, M. M., Wisely, G. B., Clay, W. C., Leesnitzer, L. M., Ways, J. P., & Gray, J. G. (1994). NF-kappa B regulates IL-1 beta transcription through a consensus NF-kappa B binding site and a nonconsensus CRE-like site. J Immunol, 153(2), 712-723.

Connor, R. J., Kawaoka, Y., Webster, R. G., & Paulson, J. C. (1994). Receptor specificity in human, avian, and equine H2 and H3 influenza virus isolates. Virology, 205(1), 17-23.

Contoli, M., Message, S. D., Laza-Stanca, V., Edwards, M. R., Wark, P. A., Bartlett, N. W., Kebadze, T., Mallia, P., Stanciu, L. A., Parker, H. L., Slater, L., Lewis-Antes, A., Kon, O. M., Holgate, S. T., Davies, D. E., Kotenko, S. V., Papi, A., & Johnston, S. L. (2006). Role of deficient type III interferon-lambda production in asthma exacerbations. Nat Med, 12(9), 1023-1026.

Cosio, B. G., Tsaprouni, L., Ito, K., Jazrawi, E., Adcock, I. M., & Barnes, P. J. (2004). Theophylline restores histone deacetylase activity and steroid responses in COPD macrophages. J Exp Med, 200(5), 689-695.

Cowburn, A. S., Condliffe, A. M., Farahi, N., Summers, C., & Chilvers, E. R. (2008). Advances in neutrophil biology: clinical implications. Chest, 134(3), 606-612.

Dauber, B., Schneider, J., & Wolff, T. (2006). Double-stranded RNA binding of influenza B virus nonstructural NS1 protein inhibits protein kinase R but is not essential to antagonize production of alpha/beta interferon. J Virol, 80(23), 11667-11677.

de Jong, M. D., Tran, T. T., Truong, H. K., Vo, M. H., Smith, G. J., Nguyen, V. C., Bach, V. C., Phan, T. Q., Do, Q. H., Guan, Y., Peiris, J. S., Tran, T. H., & Farrar, J. (2005). Oseltamivir resistance during treatment of influenza A (H5N1) infection. N Engl J Med, 353(25), 2667-2672.

De Maeyer-Guignard, J., Marcucci, F., & De Maeyer, E. (1988). Identification by in situ hybridization of IFN-beta-producing murine macrophages obtained from high and low interferon producers. Ann Inst Pasteur Virol, 139(1), 51-57.

de Vries, E., Tscherne, D. M., Wienholts, M. J., Cobos-Jimenez, V., Scholte, F., Garcia-Sastre, A., Rottier, P. J., & de Haan, C. A. (2011). Dissection of the influenza A virus endocytic routes reveals macropinocytosis as an alternative entry pathway. PLoS Pathog, 7(3), e1001329.

Di Bona, D., Cippitelli, M., Fionda, C., Camma, C., Licata, A., Santoni, A., & Craxi, A. (2006). Oxidative stress inhibits IFN-alpha-induced antiviral gene expression by blocking the JAK-STAT pathway. Journal of Hepatology, 45(2), 271-279.

Dong, C. (2008). TH17 cells in development: an updated view of their molecular identity and genetic programming. Nature reviews. Immunology, 8(5), 337-348.

Doyle, S. E., Schreckhise, H., Khuu-Duong, K., Henderson, K., Rosler, R., Storey, H., Yao, L., Liu, H., Barahmand-pour, F., Sivakumar, P., Chan, C., Birks, C., Foster, D., Clegg, C. H., Wietzke-Braun, P., Mihm, S., & Klucher, K. M. (2006). Interleukin-29 uses a type 1 interferon-like program to promote antiviral responses in human hepatocytes. Hepatology, 44(4), 896-906.

Droebner, K., Reiling, S. J., & Planz, O. (2008). Role of hypercytokinemia in NF-kappaB p50-deficient mice after H5N1 influenza A virus infection. J Virol, 82(22), 11461-11466.

Duits, L. A., Nibbering, P. H., van Strijen, E., Vos, J. B., Mannesse-Lazeroms, S. P., van Sterkenburg, M. A., & Hiemstra, P. S. (2003). Rhinovirus increases human beta-defensin-2 and -3 mRNA expression in cultured bronchial epithelial cells. FEMS Immunol Med Microbiol, 38(1), 59-64.

Ehrhardt, C., Marjuki, H., Wolff, T., Nurnberg, B., Planz, O., Pleschka, S., & Ludwig, S. (2006). Bivalent role of the phosphatidylinositol-3-kinase (PI3K) during influenza virus infection and host cell defence. Cell Microbiol, 8(8), 1336-1348.

Elliott, J., Lynch, O. T., Suessmuth, Y., Qian, P., Boyd, C. R., Burrows, J. F., Buick, R., Stevenson, N. J., Touzelet, O., Gadina, M., Power, U. F., & Johnston, J. A. (2007). Respiratory syncytial virus NS1 protein degrades STAT2 by using the Elongin-Cullin E3 ligase. Journal of Virology, 81(7), 3428-3436.

Fernandez-Sesma, A., Marukian, S., Ebersole, B. J., Kaminski, D., Park, M. S., Yuen, T., Sealfon, S. C., Garcia-Sastre, A., & Moran, T. M. (2006). Influenza virus evades innate and adaptive immunity via the NS1 protein. J Virol, 80(13), 6295-6304.

Fitzgerald, K. A., McWhirter, S. M., Faia, K. L., Rowe, D. C., Latz, E., Golenbock, D. T., Coyle, A. J., Liao, S. M., & Maniatis, T. (2003). IKKepsilon and TBK1 are essential components of the IRF3 signaling pathway. Nat Immunol, 4(5), 491-496.

Fonteneau, J. F., Gilliet, M., Larsson, M., Dasilva, I., Munz, C., Liu, Y. J., & Bhardwaj, N. (2003). Activation of influenza virus-specific CD4+ and CD8+ T cells: a new role for plasmacytoid dendritic cells in adaptive immunity. Blood, 101(9), 3520-3526.

Fridovich, I. (1999). Fundamental aspects of reactive oxygen species, or what's the matter with oxygen? Annals of the New York Academy of Sciences, 893, 13-18.

Gack, M. U., Albrecht, R. A., Urano, T., Inn, K. S., Huang, I. C., Carnero, E., Farzan, M., Inoue, S., Jung, J. U., & Garcia-Sastre, A. (2009). Influenza A virus NS1 targets the ubiquitin ligase TRIM25 to evade recognition by the host viral RNA sensor RIG-I. Cell Host Microbe, 5(5), 439-449.

Ganz, T. (2003). Defensins: antimicrobial peptides of innate immunity. Nat Rev Immunol, 3(9), 710-720.

Garcia-Sastre, A., Durbin, R. K., Zheng, H., Palese, P., Gertner, R., Levy, D. E., & Durbin, J. E. (1998). The role of interferon in influenza virus tissue tropism. J Virol, 72(11), 8550-8558.

Garcia, M. A., Gil, J., Ventoso, I., Guerra, S., Domingo, E., Rivas, C., & Esteban, M. (2006). Impact of protein kinase PKR in cell biology: from antiviral to antiproliferative action. Microbiol Mol Biol Rev, 70(4), 1032-1060.

Ghildyal, R., Hartley, C., Varrasso, A., Meanger, J., Voelker, D. R., Anders, E. M., & Mills, J. (1999). Surfactant protein A binds to the fusion glycoprotein of respiratory syncytial virus and neutralizes virion infectivity. J Infect Dis, 180(6), 2009-2013.

Gil, J., & Esteban, M. (2000). Induction of apoptosis by the dsRNA-dependent protein kinase (PKR): mechanism of action. Apoptosis, 5(2), 107-114.

Glaser, L., Conenello, G., Paulson, J., & Palese, P. (2007). Effective replication of human influenza viruses in mice lacking a major alpha2,6 sialyltransferase. Virus Res, 126(1-2), 9-18.

Gresser, I. (1990). Biologic effects of interferons. J Invest Dermatol, 95(6 Suppl), 66S-71S.

Hamada, H., Garcia-Hernandez Mde, L., Reome, J. B., Misra, S. K., Strutt, T. M., McKinstry, K. K., Cooper, A. M., Swain, S. L., & Dutton, R. W. (2009). Tc17, a unique subset of CD8 T cells that can protect against lethal influenza challenge. Journal of Immunology, 182(6), 3469-3481.

Hartshorn, K. L., White, M. R., Tecle, T., Holmskov, U., & Crouch, E. C. (2006). Innate defense against influenza A virus: activity of human neutrophil defensins and interactions of defensins with surfactant protein D. J Immunol, 176(11), 6962-6972.

Hashimoto, Y., Moki, T., Takizawa, T., Shiratsuchi, A., & Nakanishi, Y. (2007). Evidence for phagocytosis of influenza virus-infected, apoptotic cells by neutrophils and macrophages in mice. J Immunol, 178(4), 2448-2457.

Hata, N., Sato, M., Takaoka, A., Asagiri, M., Tanaka, N., & Taniguchi, T. (2001). Constitutive IFN-alpha/beta signal for efficient IFN-alpha/beta gene induction by virus. Biochemical and Biophysical Research Communications, 285(2), 518-525.

Hayden, F. G., Treanor, J. J., Fritz, R. S., Lobo, M., Betts, R. F., Miller, M., Kinnersley, N., Mills, R. G., Ward, P., & Straus, S. E. (1999). Use of the oral neuraminidase inhibitor oseltamivir in experimental human influenza: randomized controlled trials for prevention and treatment. Jama, 282(13), 1240-1246.

Hazrati, E., Galen, B., Lu, W., Wang, W., Ouyang, Y., Keller, M. J., Lehrer, R. I., & Herold, B. C. (2006). Human alpha- and beta-defensins block multiple steps in herpes simplex virus infection. J Immunol, 177(12), 8658-8666.

Herfst, S., Schrauwen, E. J., Linster, M., Chutinimitkul, S., de Wit, E., Munster, V. J., Sorrell, E. M., Bestebroer, T. M., Burke, D. F., Smith, D. J., Rimmelzwaan, G. F., Osterhaus, A. D., & Fouchier, R. A. (2012). Airborne transmission of influenza A/H5N1 virus between ferrets. Science, 336(6088), 1534-1541.

Hewlett, L. J., Prescott, A. R., & Watts, C. (1994). The coated pit and macropinocytic pathways serve distinct endosome populations. J Cell Biol, 124(5), 689-703.

Ho, L. P., Denney, L., Luhn, K., Teoh, D., Clelland, C., & McMichael, A. J. (2008). Activation of invariant NKT cells enhances the innate immune response and improves the disease course in influenza A virus infection. European Journal of Immunology, 38(7), 1913-1922.

Honda, K., & Taniguchi, T. (2006). IRFs: master regulators of signalling by Toll-like receptors and cytosolic pattern-recognition receptors. Nature reviews. Immunology, 6(9), 644-658.

Hsu, A. C., Barr, I., Hansbro, P. M., & Wark, P. A. (2011). Human influenza is more effective than avian influenza at antiviral suppression in airway cells. American Journal of Respiratory Cell and Molecular Biology, 44(6), 906-913.

Hsu, A. C., Parsons, K., Barr, I., Lowther, S., Middleton, D., Hansbro, PM., Wark, PAB. . (2012). Critical role of type I interferon response in bronchial epithelial cell to influenza infection. PLoS ONE, 7(3), e32947.

Hurt, A. C., Hardie, K., Wilson, N. J., Deng, Y. M., Osbourn, M., Gehrig, N., & Kelso, A. (2011). Community transmission of oseltamivir-resistant A(H1N1)pdm09 influenza. N Engl J Med, 365(26), 2541-2542.

Hurt, A. C., Hardie, K., Wilson, N. J., Deng, Y. M., Osbourn, M., Leang, S. K., Lee, R. T., Iannello, P., Gehrig, N., Shaw, R., Wark, P., Caldwell, N., Givney, R. C., Xue, L., Maurer-Stroh, S., Dwyer, D. E., Wang, B., Smith, D. W., Levy, A., Booy, R., Dixit, R., Merritt, T., Kelso, A., Dalton, C., Durrheim, D., & Barr, I. G. (2012). Characteristics of a widespread community cluster of H275Y oseltamivir-resistant A(H1N1)pdm09 influenza in Australia. J Infect Dis, 206(2), 148-157.

Hyland, L., Webby, R., Sandbulte, M. R., Clarke, B., & Hou, S. (2006). Influenza virus NS1 protein protects against lymphohematopoietic pathogenesis in an in vivo mouse model. Virology, 349(1), 156-163.

Imai, M., Watanabe, T., Hatta, M., Das, S. C., Ozawa, M., Shinya, K., Zhong, G., Hanson, A., Katsura, H., Watanabe, S., Li, C., Kawakami, E., Yamada, S., Kiso, M., Suzuki, Y., Maher, E. A., Neumann, G., & Kawaoka, Y. (2012). Experimental adaptation of an influenza H5 HA confers respiratory droplet transmission to a reassortant H5 HA/H1N1 virus in ferrets. Nature, 486(7403), 420-428.

Ito, K., Barnes, P. J., & Adcock, I. M. (2000). Glucocorticoid receptor recruitment of histone deacetylase 2 inhibits interleukin-1beta-induced histone H4 acetylation on lysines 8 and 12. Molecular and Cellular Biology, 20(18), 6891-6903.

Ito, K., Ito, M., Elliott, W. M., Cosio, B., Caramori, G., Kon, O. M., Barczyk, A., Hayashi, S., Adcock, I. M., Hogg, J. C., & Barnes, P. J. (2005). Decreased histone deacetylase activity in chronic obstructive pulmonary disease. N Engl J Med, 352(19), 1967-1976.

Ito, T., Suzuki, Y., Mitnaul, L., Vines, A., Kida, H., & Kawaoka, Y. (1997). Receptor specificity of influenza A viruses correlates with the agglutination of erythrocytes from different animal species. Virology, 227(2), 493-499.

Jackson, D., Hossain, M. J., Hickman, D., Perez, D. R., & Lamb, R. A. (2008). A new influenza virus virulence determinant: the NS1 protein four C-terminal residues modulate pathogenicity. Proc Natl Acad Sci U S A, 105(11), 4381-4386.

Jacobs, M. D., & Harrison, S. C. (1998). Structure of an IkappaBalpha/NF-kappaB complex. Cell, 95(6), 749-758.

Jefferson, T., Demicheli, V., Rivetti, D., Jones, M., Di Pietrantonj, C., & Rivetti, A. (2006). Antivirals for influenza in healthy adults: systematic review. Lancet, 367(9507), 303-313.

Jeffery, P. K. (2000). Comparison of the structural and inflammatory features of COPD and asthma. Giles F. Filley Lecture. Chest, 117(5 Suppl 1), 251S-260S.

Jia, D., Rahbar, R., Chan, R. W., Lee, S. M., Chan, M. C., Wang, B. X., Baker, D. P., Sun, B., Peiris, J. S., Nicholls, J. M., & Fish, E. N. (2010). Influenza virus non-structural protein 1 (NS1) disrupts interferon signaling. PLoS ONE, 5(11), e13927.

Jiang, Z., Mak, T. W., Sen, G., & Li, X. (2004). Toll-like receptor 3-mediated activation of NF-kappaB and IRF3 diverges at Toll-IL-1 receptor domain-containing adapter inducing IFN-beta. Proc Natl Acad Sci U S A, 101(10), 3533-3538.

Jiao, P., Tian, G., Li, Y., Deng, G., Jiang, Y., Liu, C., Liu, W., Bu, Z., Kawaoka, Y., & Chen, H. (2008). A single-amino-acid substitution in the NS1 protein changes the pathogenicity of H5N1 avian influenza viruses in mice. J Virol, 82(3), 1146-1154.

Johnston, S. L., Pattemore, P. K., Sanderson, G., Smith, S., Campbell, M. J., Josephs, L. K., Cunningham, A., Robinson, B. S., Myint, S. H., Ward, M. E., Tyrrell, D. A., & Holgate, S. T. (1996). The relationship between upper respiratory infections and hospital admissions for asthma: a time-trend analysis. Am J Respir Crit Care Med, 154(3 Pt 1), 654-660.

Johnston, S. L., Pattemore, P. K., Sanderson, G., Smith, S., Lampe, F., Josephs, L., Symington, P., O'Toole, S., Myint, S. H., Tyrrell, D. A., & et al. (1995). Community study of role of viral infections in exacerbations of asthma in 9-11 year old children. Bmj, 310(6989), 1225-1229.

Kato, H., Takeuchi, O., Sato, S., Yoneyama, M., Yamamoto, M., Matsui, K., Uematsu, S., Jung, A., Kawai, T., Ishii, K. J., Yamaguchi, O., Otsu, K., Tsujimura, T., Koh, C. S., Reis e Sousa, C., Matsuura, Y., Fujita, T., & Akira, S. (2006). Differential roles of MDA5 and RIG-I helicases in the recognition of RNA viruses. Nature, 441(7089), 101-105.

Kim, T. K., & Maniatis, T. (1997). The mechanism of transcriptional synergy of an in vitro assembled interferon-beta enhanceosome. Molecular Cell, 1(1), 119-129.

Kiso, M., Mitamura, K., Sakai-Tagawa, Y., Shiraishi, K., Kawakami, C., Kimura, K., Hayden, F. G., Sugaya, N., & Kawaoka, Y. (2004). Resistant influenza A viruses in children treated with oseltamivir: descriptive study. Lancet, 364(9436), 759-765.

Kloepfer, K. M., Olenec, J. P., Lee, W. M., Liu, G., Vrtis, R. F., Roberg, K. A., Evans, M. D., Gangnon, R. E., Lemanske, R. F., Jr., & Gern, J. E. (2012). Increased H1N1 Infection Rate in Children with Asthma. American Journal of Respiratory and Critical Care Medicine, 185(12), 1275-1279.

Kota, S., Sabbah, A., Chang, T. H., Harnack, R., Xiang, Y., Meng, X., & Bose, S. (2008). Role of human beta-defensin-2 during tumor necrosis factor-alpha/NF-kappaB-mediated innate antiviral response against human respiratory syncytial virus. J Biol Chem, 283(33), 22417-22429.

Kotenko, S. V., Gallagher, G., Baurin, V. V., Lewis-Antes, A., Shen, M., Shah, N. K., Langer, J. A., Sheikh, F., Dickensheets, H., & Donnelly, R. P. (2003). IFN-lambdas mediate antiviral protection through a distinct class II cytokine receptor complex. Nat Immunol, 4(1), 69-77.

Kujime, K., Hashimoto, S., Gon, Y., Shimizu, K., & Horie, T. (2000). p38 mitogen-activated protein kinase and c-jun-NH2-terminal kinase regulate RANTES production by influenza virus-infected human bronchial epithelial cells. J Immunol, 164(6), 3222-3228.

Kumar, A., Haque, J., Lacoste, J., Hiscott, J., & Williams, B. R. (1994). Double-stranded RNA-dependent protein kinase activates transcription factor NF-kappa B by phosphorylating I kappa B. Proc Natl Acad Sci U S A, 91(14), 6288-6292.

Laan, M., Lotvall, J., Chung, K. F., & Linden, A. (2001). IL-17-induced cytokine release in human bronchial epithelial cells in vitro: role of mitogen-activated protein (MAP) kinases. British Journal of Pharmacology, 133(1), 200-206.

Lambeth, J. D. (2004). NOX enzymes and the biology of reactive oxygen. Nat Rev Immunol, 4(3), 181-189.

Lau, C., Wang, X., Song, L., North, M., Wiehler, S., Proud, D., & Chow, C. W. (2008). Syk associates with clathrin and mediates phosphatidylinositol 3-kinase activation during human rhinovirus internalization. J Immunol, 180(2), 870-880.

Laza-Stanca, V., Stanciu, L. A., Message, S. D., Edwards, M. R., Gern, J. E., & Johnston, S. L. (2006). Rhinovirus replication in human macrophages induces NF-kappaB-dependent tumor necrosis factor alpha production. Journal of Virology, 80(16), 8248-8258.

Le Goffic, R., Pothlichet, J., Vitour, D., Fujita, T., Meurs, E., Chignard, M., & Si-Tahar, M. (2007). Cutting Edge: Influenza A virus activates TLR3-dependent inflammatory and RIG-I-dependent antiviral responses in human lung epithelial cells. J Immunol, 178(6), 3368-3372.

Leikina, E., Delanoe-Ayari, H., Melikov, K., Cho, M. S., Chen, A., Waring, A. J., Wang, W., Xie, Y., Loo, J. A., Lehrer, R. I., & Chernomordik, L. V. (2005). Carbohydrate-binding molecules inhibit viral fusion and entry by crosslinking membrane glycoproteins. Nat Immunol, 6(10), 995-1001.

LeVine, A. M., Whitsett, J. A., Hartshorn, K. L., Crouch, E. C., & Korfhagen, T. R. (2001). Surfactant protein D enhances clearance of influenza A virus from the lung in vivo. J Immunol, 167(10), 5868-5873.

Levy, D. E., & Garcia-Sastre, A. (2001). The virus battles: IFN induction of the antiviral state and mechanisms of viral evasion. Cytokine Growth Factor Rev, 12(2-3), 143-156.

Li, E., Stupack, D., Klemke, R., Cheresh, D. A., & Nemerow, G. R. (1998). Adenovirus endocytosis via alpha(v) integrins requires phosphoinositide-3-OH kinase. Journal of Virology, 72(3), 2055-2061.

Li, S., Min, J. Y., Krug, R. M., & Sen, G. C. (2006). Binding of the influenza A virus NS1 protein to PKR mediates the inhibition of its activation by either PACT or double-stranded RNA. Virology, 349(1), 13-21.

Li, W., Moore, M. J., Vasilieva, N., Sui, J., Wong, S. K., Berne, M. A., Somasundaran, M., Sullivan, J. L., Luzuriaga, K., Greenough, T. C., Choe, H., & Farzan, M. (2003). Angiotensin-converting enzyme 2 is a functional receptor for the SARS coronavirus. Nature, 426(6965), 450-454.

Loo, Y. M., Fornek, J., Crochet, N., Bajwa, G., Perwitasari, O., Martinez-Sobrido, L., Akira, S., Gill, M. A., Garcia-Sastre, A., Katze, M. G., & Gale, M., Jr. (2008). Distinct RIG-I and MDA5 signaling by RNA viruses in innate immunity. J Virol, 82(1), 335-345.

Lu, X., Pan, J., Tao, J., & Guo, D. (2011). SARS-CoV nucleocapsid protein antagonizes IFN-beta response by targeting initial step of IFN-beta induction pathway, and its C-terminal region is critical for the antagonism. Virus Genes, 42(1), 37-45.

Lu, Y., Wambach, M., Katze, M. G., & Krug, R. M. (1995). Binding of the influenza virus NS1 protein to double-stranded RNA inhibits the activation of the protein kinase that phosphorylates the eIF-2 translation initiation factor. Virology, 214(1), 222-228.

Luft, T., Pang, K. C., Thomas, E., Hertzog, P., Hart, D. N., Trapani, J., & Cebon, J. (1998). Type I IFNs enhance the terminal differentiation of dendritic cells. Journal of Immunology, 161(4), 1947-1953.

Malhotra, R., Haurum, J. S., Thiel, S., & Sim, R. B. (1994). Binding of human collectins (SP-A and MBP) to influenza virus. Biochem J, 304 (Pt 2), 455-461.

Mallia, P., Message, S. D., Gielen, V., Contoli, M., Gray, K., Kebadze, T., Aniscenko, J., Laza-Stanca, V., Edwards, M. R., Slater, L., Papi, A., Stanciu, L. A., Kon, O. M., Johnson, M., & Johnston, S. L. (2011). Experimental rhinovirus infection as a human model of chronic obstructive pulmonary disease exacerbation. American Journal of Respiratory and Critical Care Medicine, 183(6), 734-742.

Mandelboim, O., Lieberman, N., Lev, M., Paul, L., Arnon, T. I., Bushkin, Y., Davis, D. M., Strominger, J. L., Yewdell, J. W., & Porgador, A. (2001). Recognition of haemagglutinins on virus-infected cells by NKp46 activates lysis by human NK cells. Nature, 409(6823), 1055-1060.

Manel, N., Unutmaz, D., & Littman, D. R. (2008). The differentiation of human T(H)-17 cells requires transforming growth factor-beta and induction of the nuclear receptor RORgammat. Nat Immunol, 9(6), 641-649.

Mao, H., Tu, W., Qin, G., Law, H. K., Sia, S. F., Chan, P. L., Liu, Y., Lam, K. T., Zheng, J., Peiris, M., & Lau, Y. L. (2009). Influenza virus directly infects human natural killer cells and induces cell apoptosis. J Virol, 83(18), 9215-9222.

Mibayashi, M., Martinez-Sobrido, L., Loo, Y. M., Cardenas, W. B., Gale, M., Jr., & Garcia-Sastre, A. (2007). Inhibition of retinoic acid-inducible gene I-mediated induction of beta interferon by the NS1 protein of influenza A virus. J Virol, 81(2), 514-524.

Mibayashi, M., Nakad, K., & Nagata, K. (2002). Promoted cell death of cells expressing human MxA by influenza virus infection. Microbiol Immunol, 46(1), 29-36.

Min, J. Y., Li, S., Sen, G. C., & Krug, R. M. (2007). A site on the influenza A virus NS1 protein mediates both inhibition of PKR activation and temporal regulation of viral RNA synthesis. Virology, 363(1), 236-243.

Modestou, M. A., Manzel, L. J., El-Mahdy, S., & Look, D. C. (2010). Inhibition of IFN-gamma-dependent antiviral airway epithelial defense by cigarette smoke. Respir Res, 11, 64.

Monto, A. S., McKimm-Breschkin, J. L., Macken, C., Hampson, A. W., Hay, A., Klimov, A., Tashiro, M., Webster, R. G., Aymard, M., Hayden, F. G., & Zambon, M. (2006). Detection of influenza viruses resistant to neuraminidase inhibitors in global surveillance during the first 3 years of their use. Antimicrob Agents Chemother, 50(7), 2395-2402.

Monto, A. S., Robinson, D. P., Herlocher, M. L., Hinson, J. M., Jr., Elliott, M. J., & Crisp, A. (1999). Zanamivir in the prevention of influenza among healthy adults: a randomized controlled trial. Jama, 282(1), 31-35.

Morcillo, E. J., Estrela, J., & Cortijo, J. (1999). Oxidative stress and pulmonary inflammation: pharmacological intervention with antioxidants. Pharmacological research : the official journal of the Italian Pharmacological Society, 40(5), 393-404.

Myles, P., Nguyen-Van-Tam, J. S., Semple, M. G., Brett, S. J., Bannister, B., Read, R. C., Taylor, B. L., McMenamin, J., Enstone, J. E., Nicholson, K. G., Openshaw, P., Lim, W. S., & Flu-Cin, I. C. (2012). Differences between asthmatics and non-asthmatics hospitalised with influenza A infection. Eur Respir J.

Nusinzon, I., & Horvath, C. M. (2003). Interferon-stimulated transcription and innate antiviral immunity require deacetylase activity and histone deacetylase 1. Proceedings of the National Academy of Sciences of the United States of America, 100(25), 14742-14747.

Ochiai, H., Ikesue, A., Kurokawa, M., Nakajima, K., & Nakagawa, H. (1993). Enhanced production of rat interleukin-8 by in vitro and in vivo infections with influenza A NWS virus. J Virol, 67(11), 6811-6814.

Oganesyan, G., Saha, S. K., Guo, B., He, J. Q., Shahangian, A., Zarnegar, B., Perry, A., & Cheng, G. (2006). Critical role of TRAF3 in the Toll-like receptor-dependent and -independent antiviral response. Nature, 439(7073), 208-211.

Paget, C., Ivanov, S., Fontaine, J., Renneson, J., Blanc, F., Pichavant, M., Dumoutier, L., Ryffel, B., Renauld, J. C., Gosset, P., Si-Tahar, M., Faveeuw, C., & Trottein, F. (2012). Interleukin-22 is produced by invariant natural killer T lymphocytes during influenza A virus infection: potential role in protection against lung epithelial damage. J Biol Chem.

Papi, A., & Johnston, S. L. (1999). Rhinovirus infection induces expression of its own receptor intercellular adhesion molecule 1 (ICAM-1) via increased NF-kappaB-mediated transcription. J Biol Chem, 274(14), 9707-9720.

Pavlovic, J., Haller, O., & Staeheli, P. (1992). Human and mouse Mx proteins inhibit different steps of the influenza virus multiplication cycle. J Virol, 66(4), 2564-2569.

Pestka, S., Langer, J. A., Zoon, K. C., & Samuel, C. E. (1987). Interferons and their actions. Annu Rev Biochem, 56, 727-777.

Piccolo, M. T., Wang, Y., Sannomiya, P., Piccolo, N. S., Piccolo, M. S., Hugli, T. E., Ward, P. A., & Till, G. O. (1999). Chemotactic mediator requirements in lung injury following skin burns in rats. Experimental and Molecular Pathology, 66(3), 220-226.

Pichlmair, A., Schulz, O., Tan, C. P., Naslund, T. I., Liljestrom, P., Weber, F., & Reis e Sousa, C. (2006). RIG-I-mediated antiviral responses to single-stranded RNA bearing 5'-phosphates. Science, 314(5801), 997-1001.

Proud, D., Hudy, M. H., Wiehler, S., Zaheer, R. S., Amin, M. A., Pelikan, J. B., Tacon, C. E., Tonsaker, T. O., Walker, B. L., Kooi, C., Traves, S. L., & Leigh, R. (2012). Cigarette smoke modulates expression of human rhinovirus-induced airway epithelial host defense genes. PLoS ONE, 7(7), e40762.

Proud, D., Sanders, S. P., & Wiehler, S. (2004). Human rhinovirus infection induces airway epithelial cell production of human beta-defensin 2 both in vitro and in vivo. J Immunol, 172(7), 4637-4645.

Qin, H., Holdbrooks, A. T., Liu, Y., Reynolds, S. L., Yanagisawa, L. L., & Benveniste, E. N. (2012). SOCS3 Deficiency Promotes M1 Macrophage Polarization and Inflammation. J Immunol, 189(7), 3439-3448.

Rahman, I., Morrison, D., Donaldson, K., & MacNee, W. (1996). Systemic oxidative stress in asthma, COPD, and smokers. American Journal of Respiratory and Critical Care Medicine, 154(4 Pt 1), 1055-1060.

Rahman, I., Mulier, B., Gilmour, P. S., Watchorn, T., Donaldson, K., Jeffery, P. K., & MacNee, W. (2001). Oxidant-mediated lung epithelial cell tolerance: the role of intracellular glutathione and nuclear factor-kappaB. Biochemical Pharmacology, 62(6), 787-794.

Ramaswamy, M., Shi, L., Monick, M. M., Hunninghake, G. W., & Look, D. C. (2004). Specific inhibition of type I interferon signal transduction by respiratory syncytial virus. American Journal of Respiratory Cell and Molecular Biology, 30(6), 893-900.

Ramaswamy, M., Shi, L., Varga, S. M., Barik, S., Behlke, M. A., & Look, D. C. (2006). Respiratory syncytial virus nonstructural protein 2 specifically inhibits type I interferon signal transduction. Virology, 344(2), 328-339.

Rapoport, E. M., Mochalova, L. V., Gabius, H. J., Romanova, J., & Bovin, N. V. (2006). Search for additional influenza virus to cell interactions. Glycoconj J, 23(1-2), 115-125.

Ratcliffe, D. R., Nolin, S. L., & Cramer, E. B. (1988). Neutrophil interaction with influenza-infected epithelial cells. Blood, 72(1), 142-149.

Rehaume, L. M., & Hancock, R. E. (2008). Neutrophil-derived defensins as modulators of innate immune function. Critical Reviews in Immunology, 28(3), 185-200.

Rimbach, G., Valacchi, G., Canali, R., & Virgili, F. (2000). Macrophages stimulated with IFN-gamma activate NF-kappa B and induce MCP-1 gene expression in primary human endothelial cells. Mol Cell Biol Res Commun, 3(4), 238-242.

Roger, T., Lugrin, J., Le Roy, D., Goy, G., Mombelli, M., Koessler, T., Ding, X. C., Chanson, A. L., Reymond, M. K., Miconnet, I., Schrenzel, J., Francois, P., & Calandra, T. (2011). Histone deacetylase inhibitors impair innate immune responses to Toll-like receptor agonists and to infection. Blood, 117(4), 1205-1217.

Rogers, G. N., & D'Souza, B. L. (1989). Receptor binding properties of human and animal H1 influenza virus isolates. Virology, 173(1), 317-322.

Rogers, G. N., & Paulson, J. C. (1983). Receptor determinants of human and animal influenza virus isolates: differences in receptor specificity of the H3 hemagglutinin based on species of origin. Virology, 127(2), 361-373.

Ryan-Poirier, K., Suzuki, Y., Bean, W. J., Kobasa, D., Takada, A., Ito, T., & Kawaoka, Y. (1998). Changes in H3 influenza A virus receptor specificity during replication in humans. Virus Res, 56(2), 169-176.

Saito, T., & Gale, M., Jr. (2008). Differential recognition of double-stranded RNA by RIG-I-like receptors in antiviral immunity. J Exp Med, 205(7), 1523-1527.

Salomon, R., Hoffmann, E., & Webster, R. G. (2007). Inhibition of the cytokine response does not protect against lethal H5N1 influenza infection. Proc Natl Acad Sci U S A, 104(30), 12479-12481.

Sato, M., Suemori, H., Hata, N., Asagiri, M., Ogasawara, K., Nakao, K., Nakaya, T., Katsuki, M., Noguchi, S., Tanaka, N., & Taniguchi, T. (2000). Distinct and essential roles of transcription factors IRF-3 and IRF-7 in response to viruses for IFN-alpha/beta gene induction. Immunity, 13(4), 539-548.

Satoh, T., Kato, H., Kumagai, Y., Yoneyama, M., Sato, S., Matsushita, K., Tsujimura, T., Fujita, T., Akira, S., & Takeuchi, O. LGP2 is a positive regulator of RIG-I- and MDA5-mediated antiviral responses. Proc Natl Acad Sci U S A, 107(4), 1512-1517.

Schmolke, M., Viemann, D., Roth, J., & Ludwig, S. (2009). Essential impact of NF-kappaB signaling on the H5N1 influenza A virus-induced transcriptome. J Immunol, 183(8), 5180-5189.

Schneider, D., Ganesan, S., Comstock, A. T., Meldrum, C. A., Mahidhara, R., Goldsmith, A. M., Curtis, J. L., Martinez, F. J., Hershenson, M. B., & Sajjan, U. (2010). Increased cytokine response of rhinovirus-infected airway epithelial cells in chronic obstructive pulmonary disease. American Journal of Respiratory and Critical Care Medicine, 182(3), 332-340.

Schrauf, C., Kirchberger, S., Majdic, O., Seyerl, M., Zlabinger, G. J., Stuhlmeier, K. M., Sachet, M., Seipelt, J., & Stockl, J. (2009). The ssRNA genome of human rhinovirus induces a type I IFN response but fails to induce maturation in human monocyte-derived dendritic cells. J Immunol, 183(7), 4440-4448.

Seemungal, T., Harper-Owen, R., Bhowmik, A., Moric, I., Sanderson, G., Message, S., Maccallum, P., Meade, T. W., Jeffries, D. J., Johnston, S. L., & Wedzicha, J. A. (2001). Respiratory viruses, symptoms, and inflammatory markers in acute exacerbations and stable chronic obstructive pulmonary disease. Am J Respir Crit Care Med, 164(9), 1618-1623.

Senft, A. P., Taylor, R. H., Lei, W., Campbell, S. A., Tipper, J. L., Martinez, M. J., Witt, T. L., Clay, C. C., & Harrod, K. S. (2010). Respiratory syncytial virus impairs macrophage IFN-alpha/beta- and IFN-gamma-stimulated transcription by distinct mechanisms. American Journal of Respiratory Cell and Molecular Biology, 42(4), 404-414.

Seo, S. H., Hoffmann, E., & Webster, R. G. (2002). Lethal H5N1 influenza viruses escape host anti-viral cytokine responses. Nat Med, 8(9), 950-954.

Sheppard, P., Kindsvogel, W., Xu, W., Henderson, K., Schlutsmeyer, S., Whitmore, T. E., Kuestner, R., Garrigues, U., Birks, C., Roraback, J., Ostrander, C., Dong, D., Shin, J., Presnell, S., Fox, B., Haldeman, B., Cooper, E., Taft, D., Gilbert, T., Grant, F. J., Tackett, M., Krivan, W., McKnight, G., Clegg, C., Foster, D., & Klucher, K. M. (2003). IL-28, IL-29 and their class II cytokine receptor IL-28R. Nat Immunol, 4(1), 63-68.

Shiratsuchi, A., Kaido, M., Takizawa, T., & Nakanishi, Y. (2000). Phosphatidylserine-mediated phagocytosis of influenza A virus-infected cells by mouse peritoneal macrophages. J Virol, 74(19), 9240-9244.

Shukaliak, J. A., & Dorovini-Zis, K. (2000). Expression of the beta-chemokines RANTES and MIP-1 beta by human brain microvessel endothelial cells in primary culture. Journal of Neuropathology and Experimental Neurology, 59(5), 339-352.

Slater, L., Bartlett, N. W., Haas, J. J., Zhu, J., Message, S. D., Walton, R. P., Sykes, A., Dahdaleh, S., Clarke, D. L., Belvisi, M. G., Kon, O. M., Fujita, T., Jeffery, P. K., Johnston, S. L., & Edwards, M. R. (2010). Co-ordinated role of TLR3, RIG-I and MDA5 in the innate response to rhinovirus in bronchial epithelium. PLoS Pathog, 6(11), e1001178.

Smed-Sorensen, A., Chalouni, C., Chatterjee, B., Cohn, L., Blattmann, P., Nakamura, N., Delamarre, L., & Mellman, I. (2012). Influenza A virus infection of human primary dendritic cells impairs their ability to cross-present antigen to CD8 T cells. PLoS Pathog, 8(3), e1002572.

Smith, J. G., & Nemerow, G. R. (2008). Mechanism of adenovirus neutralization by Human alpha-defensins. Cell Host Microbe, 3(1), 11-19.

Spadaro, F., Lapenta, C., Donati, S., Abalsamo, L., Barnaba, V., Belardelli, F., Santini, S. M., & Ferrantini, M. (2012). IFN-alpha enhances cross-presentation in human dendritic cells by modulating antigen survival, endocytic routing, and processing. Blood, 119(6), 1407-1417.

Stark, G. R., Kerr, I. M., Williams, B. R., Silverman, R. H., & Schreiber, R. D. (1998). How cells respond to interferons. Annu Rev Biochem, 67, 227-264.

Stark, J. M., van Egmond, A. W., Zimmerman, J. J., Carabell, S. K., & Tosi, M. F. (1992). Detection of enhanced neutrophil adhesion to parainfluenza-infected airway epithelial cells using a modified myeloperoxidase assay in a microtiter format. J Virol Methods, 40(2), 225-242.

Suzuki, T., Takahashi, T., Guo, C. T., Hidari, K. I., Miyamoto, D., Goto, H., Kawaoka, Y., & Suzuki, Y. (2005). Sialidase activity of influenza A virus in an endocytic pathway enhances viral replication. J Virol, 79(18), 11705-11715.

Suzuki, T., Yamaya, M., Kamanaka, M., Jia, Y. X., Nakayama, K., Hosoda, M., Yamada, N., Nishimura, H., Sekizawa, K., & Sasaki, H. (2001). Type 2 rhinovirus infection of cultured human tracheal epithelial cells: role of LDL receptor. American journal of physiology. Lung cellular and molecular physiology, 280(3), L409-420.

Takeda, K., & Akira, S. (2005). Toll-like receptors in innate immunity. International Immunology, 17(1), 1-14.

Takeda, K., Kaisho, T., & Akira, S. (2003). Toll-like receptors. Annual Review of Immunology, 21, 335-376.

Talon, J., Horvath, C. M., Polley, R., Basler, C. F., Muster, T., Palese, P., & Garcia-Sastre, A. (2000). Activation of interferon regulatory factor 3 is inhibited by the influenza A virus NS1 protein. J Virol, 74(17), 7989-7996.

Taniguchi, T., & Takaoka, A. (2001). A weak signal for strong responses: interferon-alpha/beta revisited. Nat Rev Mol Cell Biol, 2(5), 378-386.

Tate, M. D., Brooks, A. G., & Reading, P. C. (2008). The role of neutrophils in the upper and lower respiratory tract during influenza virus infection of mice. Respir Res, 9, 57.

Tate, M. D., Ioannidis, L. J., Croker, B., Brown, L. E., Brooks, A. G., & Reading, P. C. (2011). The role of neutrophils during mild and severe influenza virus infections of mice. PLoS ONE, 6(3), e17618.

Tecle, T., White, M. R., Gantz, D., Crouch, E. C., & Hartshorn, K. L. (2007). Human neutrophil defensins increase neutrophil uptake of influenza A virus and bacteria and modify virus-induced respiratory burst responses. J Immunol, 178(12), 8046-8052.

Thitithanyanont, A., Engering, A., Ekchariyawat, P., Wiboon-ut, S., Limsalakpetch, A., Yongvanitchit, K., Kum-Arb, U., Kanchongkittiphon, W., Utaisincharoen, P., Sirisinha, S., Puthavathana, P., Fukuda, M. M., & Pichyangkul, S. (2007). High susceptibility of human dendritic cells to avian influenza H5N1 virus infection and protection by IFN-alpha and TLR ligands. J Immunol, 179(8), 5220-5227.

Thomson, S. J., Goh, F. G., Banks, H., Krausgruber, T., Kotenko, S. V., Foxwell, B. M., & Udalova, I. A. (2009). The role of transposable elements in the regulation of IFN-lambda1 gene expression. Proceedings of the National Academy of Sciences of the United States of America, 106(28), 11564-11569.

Ting, J. P., Lovering, R. C., Alnemri, E. S., Bertin, J., Boss, J. M., Davis, B. K., Flavell, R. A., Girardin, S. E., Godzik, A., Harton, J. A., Hoffman, H. M., Hugot, J. P., Inohara, N., Mackenzie, A., Maltais, L. J., Nunez, G., Ogura, Y., Otten, L. A., Philpott, D., Reed, J. C., Reith, W., Schreiber, S., Steimle, V., & Ward, P. A. (2008). The NLR gene family: a standard nomenclature. Immunity, 28(3), 285-287.

Tovey, M. G., Streuli, M., Gresser, I., Gugenheim, J., Blanchard, B., Guymarho, J., Vignaux, F., & Gigou, M. (1987). Interferon messenger RNA is produced constitutively in the organs of normal individuals. Proceedings of the National Academy of Sciences of the United States of America, 84(14), 5038-5042.

Tran, T. H., Nguyen, T. L., Nguyen, T. D., Luong, T. S., Pham, P. M., Nguyen, V. C., Pham, T. S., Vo, C. D., Le, T. Q., Ngo, T. T., Dao, B. K., Le, P. P., Nguyen, T. T., Hoang, T. L., Cao, V. T., Le, T. G., Nguyen, D. T., Le, H. N., Nguyen, K. T., Le, H. S., Le, V. T., Christiane, D., Tran, T. T., Menno de, J., Schultsz, C., Cheng, P., Lim, W., Horby, P., & Farrar, J. (2004). Avian influenza A (H5N1) in 10 patients in Vietnam. N Engl J Med, 350(12), 1179-1188.

Uller, L., Leino, M., Bedke, N., Sammut, D., Green, B., Lau, L., Howarth, P. H., Holgate, S. T., & Davies, D. E. (2010). Double-stranded RNA induces disproportionate expression of thymic stromal lymphopoietin versus interferon-beta in bronchial epithelial cells from donors with asthma. Thorax, 65(7), 626-632.

Ullman, A. J., Reich, N. C., & Hearing, P. (2007). Adenovirus E4 ORF3 protein inhibits the interferon-mediated antiviral response. Journal of Virology, 81(9), 4744-4752.

Vareille, M., Kieninger, E., Alves, M. P., Kopf, B. S., Moller, A., Geiser, T., Johnston, S. L., Edwards, M. R., & Regamey, N. (2012). Impaired type I and type III interferon induction and rhinovirus control in human cystic fibrosis airway epithelial cells. Thorax, 67(6), 517-525.

Wang, J., Nikrad, M. P., Travanty, E. A., Zhou, B., Phang, T., Gao, B., Alford, T., Ito, Y., Nahreini, P., Hartshorn, K., Wentworth, D., Dinarello, C. A., & Mason, R. J. (2012). Innate immune response of human alveolar macrophages during influenza A infection. PLoS ONE, 7(3), e29879.

Wang, J. P., Bowen, G. N., Padden, C., Cerny, A., Finberg, R. W., Newburger, P. E., & Kurt-Jones, E. A. (2008). Toll-like receptor-mediated activation of neutrophils by influenza A virus. Blood, 112(5), 2028-2034.

Wang, S. Z., Xu, H., Wraith, A., Bowden, J. J., Alpers, J. H., & Forsyth, K. D. (1998). Neutrophils induce damage to respiratory epithelial cells infected with respiratory syncytial virus. Eur Respir J, 12(3), 612-618.

Wang, X., Basler, C. F., Williams, B. R., Silverman, R. H., Palese, P., & Garcia-Sastre, A. (2002). Functional replacement of the carboxy-terminal two-thirds of the influenza A virus NS1 protein with short heterologous dimerization domains. J Virol, 76(24), 12951-12962.

Ward, P., Small, I., Smith, J., Suter, P., & Dutkowski, R. (2005). Oseltamivir (Tamiflu) and its potential for use in the event of an influenza pandemic. J Antimicrob Chemother, 55 Suppl 1, i5-i21.

Wark, P. A., Johnston, S. L., Bucchieri, F., Powell, R., Puddicombe, S., Laza-Stanca, V., Holgate, S. T., & Davies, D. E. (2005). Asthmatic bronchial epithelial cells have a deficient innate immune response to infection with rhinovirus. J Exp Med, 201(6), 937-947.

Webster, R. G., Bean, W. J., Gorman, O. T., Chambers, T. M., & Kawaoka, Y. (1992). Evolution and ecology of influenza A viruses. Microbiol Rev, 56(1), 152-179.

Werts, C., le Bourhis, L., Liu, J., Magalhaes, J. G., Carneiro, L. A., Fritz, J. H., Stockinger, S., Balloy, V., Chignard, M., Decker, T., Philpott, D. J., Ma, X., & Girardin, S. E. (2007). Nod1 and Nod2 induce CCL5/RANTES through the NF-kappaB pathway. Eur J Immunol, 37(9), 2499-2508.

West, M. A., Prescott, A. R., Eskelinen, E. L., Ridley, A. J., & Watts, C. (2000). Rac is required for constitutive macropinocytosis by dendritic cells but does not control its downregulation. Curr Biol, 10(14), 839-848.

Wiehler, S., & Proud, D. (2007). Interleukin-17A modulates human airway epithelial responses to human rhinovirus infection. American journal of physiology. Lung cellular and molecular physiology, 293(2), L505-515.

Woolhouse, I. S., Bayley, D. L., & Stockley, R. A. (2002). Sputum chemotactic activity in chronic obstructive pulmonary disease: effect of alpha(1)-antitrypsin deficiency and the role of leukotriene B(4) and interleukin 8. Thorax, 57(8), 709-714.

Wu, W., Patel, K. B., Booth, J. L., Zhang, W., & Metcalf, J. P. (2011). Cigarette smoke extract suppresses the RIG-I-initiated innate immune response to influenza virus in the human lung. American journal of physiology. Lung cellular and molecular physiology, 300(6), L821-830.

Xu, L. L., Warren, M. K., Rose, W. L., Gong, W., & Wang, J. M. (1996). Human recombinant monocyte chemotactic protein and other C-C chemokines bind and induce directional migration of dendritic cells in vitro. J Leukoc Biol, 60(3), 365-371.

Yamada, S., Suzuki, Y., Suzuki, T., Le, M. Q., Nidom, C. A., Sakai-Tagawa, Y., Muramoto, Y., Ito, M., Kiso, M., Horimoto, T., Shinya, K., Sawada, T., Usui, T., Murata, T., Lin, Y., Hay, A., Haire, L. F., Stevens, D. J., Russell, R. J., Gamblin, S. J., Skehel, J. J., & Kawaoka, Y. (2006). Haemagglutinin mutations responsible for the binding of H5N1 influenza A viruses to human-type receptors. Nature, 444(7117), 378-382.

Yamamoto, K., Miyoshi-Koshio, T., Utsuki, Y., Mizuno, S., & Suzuki, K. (1991). Virucidal activity and viral protein modification by myeloperoxidase: a candidate for defense factor of human polymorphonuclear leukocytes against influenza virus infection. J Infect Dis, 164(1), 8-14.

Yang, D., Biragyn, A., Hoover, D. M., Lubkowski, J., & Oppenheim, J. J. (2004). Multiple roles of antimicrobial defensins, cathelicidins, and eosinophil-derived neurotoxin in host defense. Annu Rev Immunol, 22, 181-215.

Yao, Z., Painter, S. L., Fanslow, W. C., Ulrich, D., Macduff, B. M., Spriggs, M. K., & Armitage, R. J. (1995). Human IL-17: a novel cytokine derived from T cells. Journal of Immunology, 155(12), 5483-5486.

Yie, J., Senger, K., & Thanos, D. (1999). Mechanism by which the IFN-beta enhanceosome activates transcription. Proceedings of the National Academy of Sciences of the United States of America, 96(23), 13108-13113.

Zambon, M. C. (1999). Epidemiology and pathogenesis of influenza. J Antimicrob Chemother, 44 Suppl B, 3-9.

Zambon, M. C. (2001). *The pathogenesis of influenza in humans. Rev Med Virol, 11(4), 227-241.*

Zhang, P., & Samuel, C. E. (2007). *Protein kinase PKR plays a stimulus- and virus-dependent role in apoptotic death and virus multiplication in human cells. J Virol, 81(15), 8192-8200.*

Zhou, A., Paranjape, J., Brown, T. L., Nie, H., Naik, S., Dong, B., Chang, A., Trapp, B., Fairchild, R., Colmenares, C., & Silverman, R. H. (1997). *Interferon action and apoptosis are defective in mice devoid of 2',5'-oligoadenylate-dependent RNase L. Embo J, 16(21), 6355-6363.*

Zurcher, T., Marion, R. M., & Ortin, J. (2000). *Protein synthesis shut-off induced by influenza virus infection is independent of PKR activity. J Virol, 74(18), 8781-8784.*

Double Rolling Circle Replication (DRCR): Involvement in Gene Amplification and Genome Replication including HSV

Takashi Horiuchi
Department of Molecular Life Science
Division of Basic Medical Science and Molecular Medicine
Tokai University, Kanagawa Japan

Taka-aki Watanabe
Department of Molecular Genetics
Cleveland Clinic Lerner Research Institute, Cleveland, USA

1   Introduction

The phenomenon known as 'gene amplification' occurs in many different organisms (Cowell, 1982; Stark and Wahl, 1984; Schimke, 1984; Devonshire and Field, 1991). Much work has been done on gene amplification because of its importance in biology and evolution, and from the practical medical standpoint. However, until very recently, the mechanisms responsible for this process had remained unresolved. In general, there are two types of gene amplification, ribosomal RNA gene (rDNA)-type and oncogene or drug-resistant gene-type. After we had determined the mechanism of rDNA-type gene amplification (Kobayashi and Horiuchi, 1996; Kobayashi et al., 1998; Kobayashi et al., 2001), we addressed the mechanism of oncogene-type amplification. Assuming that a central reaction in oncogene-type amplification was double rolling circle replication (DRCR), we constructed a DRCR-inducing system in yeast and found that two types of amplification products were obtained (Watanabe and Horiuchi, 2005). One product corresponded to HSR (homogeneous staining region)-type products and the other to DM (double-minutes)-type products in cultured cells.

Interestingly, from structural analysis of the HSR-type product, we found that sequences flanked by inverted repeats (IR) were freely inverted. Although this type of free IR recombination is known to occur in HSV-1 DNA (Roizman, 1979; Figure 1(B)), chloroplast DNA (Palmer, 1983; Figure 1(A)) and in 2μ plasmids (Broach and Volkert, 1991; Figure 1(C)), the mechanism(s) remained unresolved. Interestingly, in these cases, the DNA is circular, and has a pair of IR structures when in the host cell. Furthermore, the 2μ plasmid is unique because it replicates in both normal and DRCR mode and is known to be recombinogenic under physiological conditions (Jayaram and Broach, 1983; Figure 1(D)). From these observations, we proposed that DRCR itself markedly activates recombination, as determined using 2μ plasmids. We were able to ascertain that DRCR itself does indeed activate recombination extensively.

When drug-resistant gene amplification is engendered in tissue culture, it is well-established that an initial amplification unit (called an amplicon) has a giant inverted repeated structure. Later, under increasing concentrations of the drug, whereas amplicon gradually shorten, their copy number increases. Although the reason for these changing amplicon processes (called evolution) remained unresolved, we inferred that the following events would be occurring in the initial stage, two pairs of inverted repeats (——▶◀—— ——▶◀——) are formed spontaneously in the Break-Fusion-Bridge (BFB) cycle, discovered and named by McClintock (1941). We confirmed experimentally that DRCR can initiate from the two pairs of inverted repeats and represents a clear oncogene amplifying mechanism (in preparation). Regarding the shortening and increasing copy number of amplicon during this process, we propose the following. Because there is a large number of repeated sequences, transposable elements and retrotransposons in higher eukaryotes' (about 50% of the whole genome), highly activated recombination (deletion, inversion and duplication) by DRCR randomly occurs between these repeated sequences under selective conditions. This would result in amplification of advantageous genes, whereas disadvantageous or neutral genes would be lost. This is one aspect of gene evolution. Finally, we propose a model for DRCR-dependent activation of recombination.

2   Gene amplification- Induction of DRCR on Linear Chromosomes

In rDNA amplification, we found that DNA replication fork blocking events at replication fork barriers (RFB) trigger an increase or a decrease in rDNA copy number (Kobayashi and Horiuchi, 1996; Kobayashi et al., 1998; Kobayashi et al., 2001; Kobayashi et al., 2004). On the other hand, for the oncogene amplification mechanisms studied up to that date, although several models deduced from the experiments using cultured cells had been proposed, they had only been able to partly explain the amplification mechanisms (Hyrien *et al.*, 1988; Ma *et al.*, 1993; Smith *et al.*, 1992; Toledo *et al.*, 1992,). Currently, detailed molecular mechanisms responsible for gene amplification remain to be determined (Debatisse and Malfor, 2005; Tanaka and Yao, 2009; Mondello *et al.*, 2010). Furthermore, although several attempts have been made to artificially induce even partial oncogene-type amplification processes using cultured cells or yeast; these have remained unsuccessful (Ruiz *et al.*, 1988; Butler *et al.*, 1996; Pipiras *et al.*, 1998; Tanaka *et al.*, 2002).

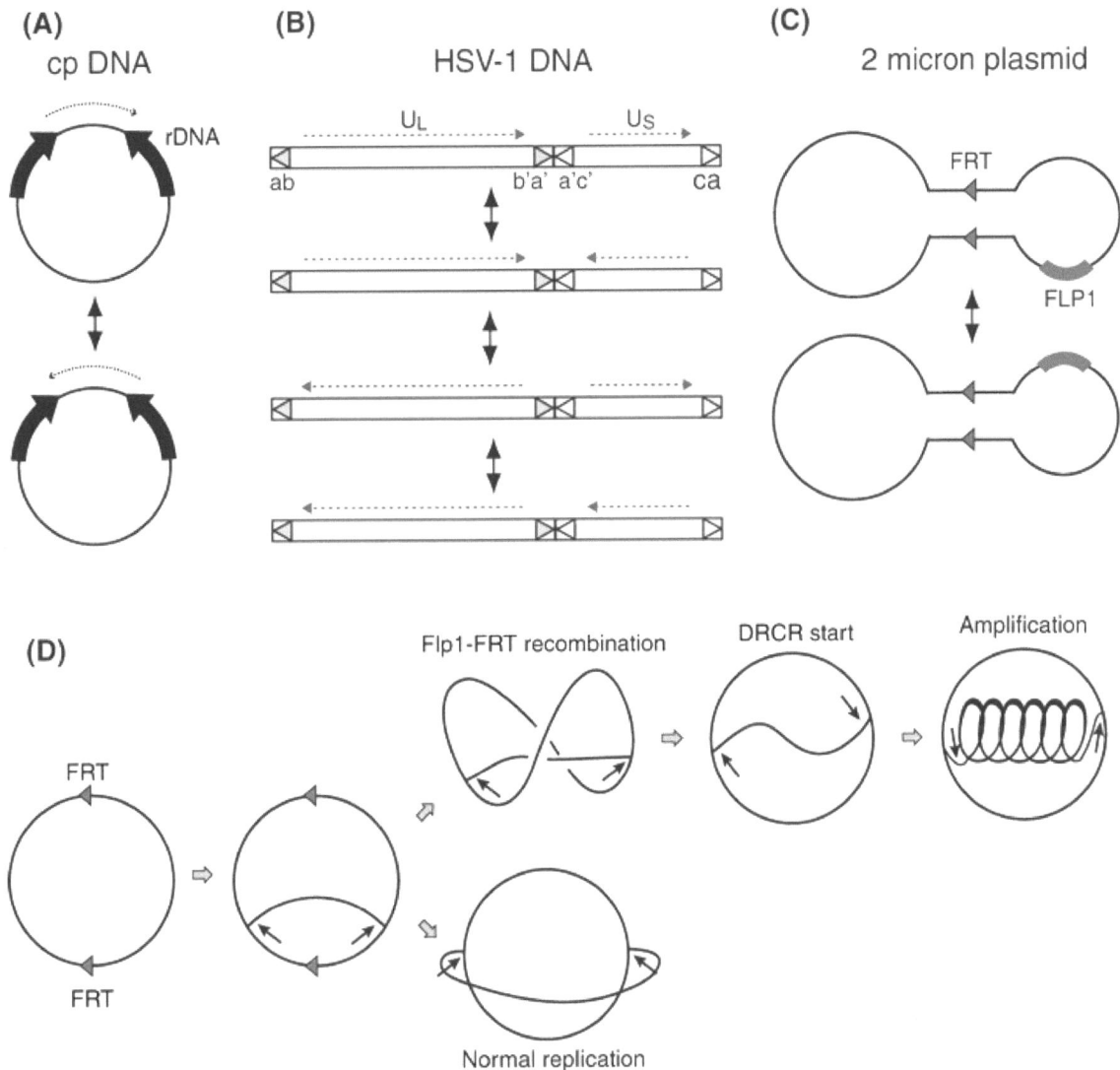

Figure 1: Isomeric structures of chloroplast (cp) DNA, HSV-1 DNA, 2-μm plasmid DNA and two modes (normal and DRCR) of replication in 2-μm plasmids. (A) Two isoform structures of chloroplast (cp)DNA, (B) four isoform structures of HSV-1 DNA, (C), two isoform structures of yeast 2-μm plasmid, (D) two modes of replication of 2-μm plasmids, normal and double rolling circle replication (DRCR).

Our hypothesis concerning oncogene-type amplification mechanisms is as follows: oncogene-type amplification occurs through DRCR (Figures 2A and 5), because it produces products with an inverted repeat (IR) structure. We chose budding yeast as a model system, and tried to induce DRCR using three different recombination systems: (1) break-induced replication (BIR) (Kraus *et al.*, 2001), (2) site-specific Cre-*lox* recombination (Stark *et al.*, 1992) and (3) homologous recombination. Although DRCR had been proposed as one of several models to explain oncogene-type amplification (Hyrien *et al.*, 1988), the initiation of DRCR is different from ours and to the best of our knowledge, the hypothesis has not yet been put to the test.

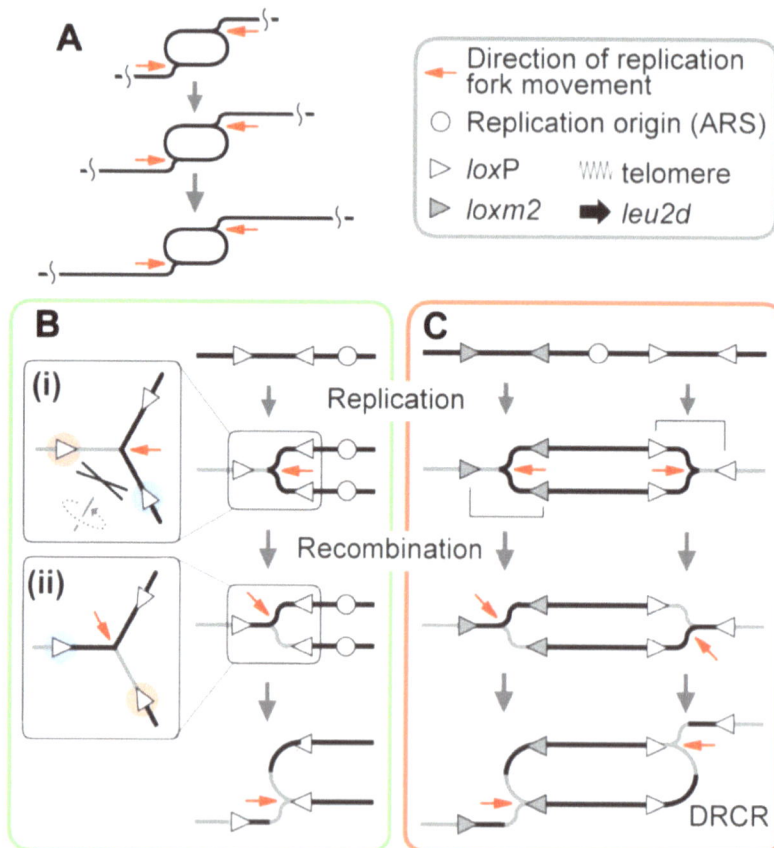

Figure 2: Recombinational process coupled with replication. (A) DRCR. Two replication forks chase each other. One replication forks chase each other. (B) Recombinational process coupled with replication. The gray and black lines indicate the un-replicated and recently replicated regions at the time of recombination, respectively. If recombination occurs between *loxP* sites marked red and blue (i), the replication template is switched and thereafter the replicated region is replicated again(ii). (C) DRCR induction. If both bidirectional DNA replications undergo the processes as described in (B), DRCR can be induced.

Although DRCR induction is accomplished by all three methods, here we illustrate how Cre-*lox* recombination initiates DRCR, as this is the easiest to understand. DRCR in linear genomes is illustrated in Figure 2A. Two replication forks follow each other around a circle of DNA, from which two linear

DNA double strands elongate continuously in opposite directions. In order to induce DRCR, first, as shown in Figure 2B, a pair of inverted *lox* sequences is arranged at the left side of a replication origin (O). When a replication fork initiated from the replication origin advances left and arrives at the region between a pair of *lox*, recombination between inverted *lox* sites changes the direction of the fork (in Figure 2B(i) to (ii)), and one DRCR-type replication fork is formed. If another recombination event occurs rotationally symmetrically to the right of the replication origin (Figure 2C), two replication forks should follow each other and initiate DRCR. To terminate DRCR, two reverse recombinations change the replication forks from following one another to bi-directional forks, although a large number of inverted repeats remain behind.

3   Gene amplification: Two Types of Amplification Depending on Initial Recombination of DRCR

If an alternative type of recombination occurs not rotationally symmetrically, but plane symmetrically (Figure 3, on the right), two replication forks should meet, producing an acentric circular genome with a pair of large IR structures, with retention of the original linear genome. Thus, in a linear genome, DRCR is expected to produce the two kinds of products shown in Figure 3, one being an HSR-type product (the linear genome with a large number of inverted repeats) and the other DM-type products (the acentric multi-copy circular mini-chromosome with a pair of inverted structures). In fact, we carried out DRCR gene amplification experiments using the Cre-*lox* system (Stark *et al.*, 1992) in yeast and did indeed obtain two kinds of products: one being a chromosome with a large number of genes in inverted repeats, and the other a high copy number of linear not circular mini-chromosomes with an inverted structure. The reason why we obtained linear but not circular mini-chromosomes is because we inserted the *lox* sequences into the terminus region of chromosome VI (Watanabe and Horiuchi, 2005; Watanabe *et al*, 2011).

When DRCR initiates or terminates, if recombination occurs asymmetrically at initiation, a chromosome with a giant IR structure should be produced and at termination, a similar chromosome with a giant IR structure should be produced, but at the center of the chromosome, amplified region should be inserted.

What is the mechanism for gene amplification under natural conditions? Around 1990, several groups (Ruiz and Wahl, 1988; Smith et al., 1992; Ma et al., 1993) reported that the initial step of gene amplification can occur via the BFB cycle, a process first described by McClintock (1941). She reported that double strand breaks occur at a site into which a transposable element is inserted, and this initiates the BFB cycle. In addition, we speculate that TS (temperate switching; see Figure 4A) is another trigger for the BFB cycle. Our artificial chromosomal structures are shown in Fig. 4B (one is the Cre-*lox* system and the other consists of the two pairs of inverted structures). Figures 4C and 4D show that two types of gene amplification, DRCR and CR (convergent replication) produce HSR type and DMs products, respectively.

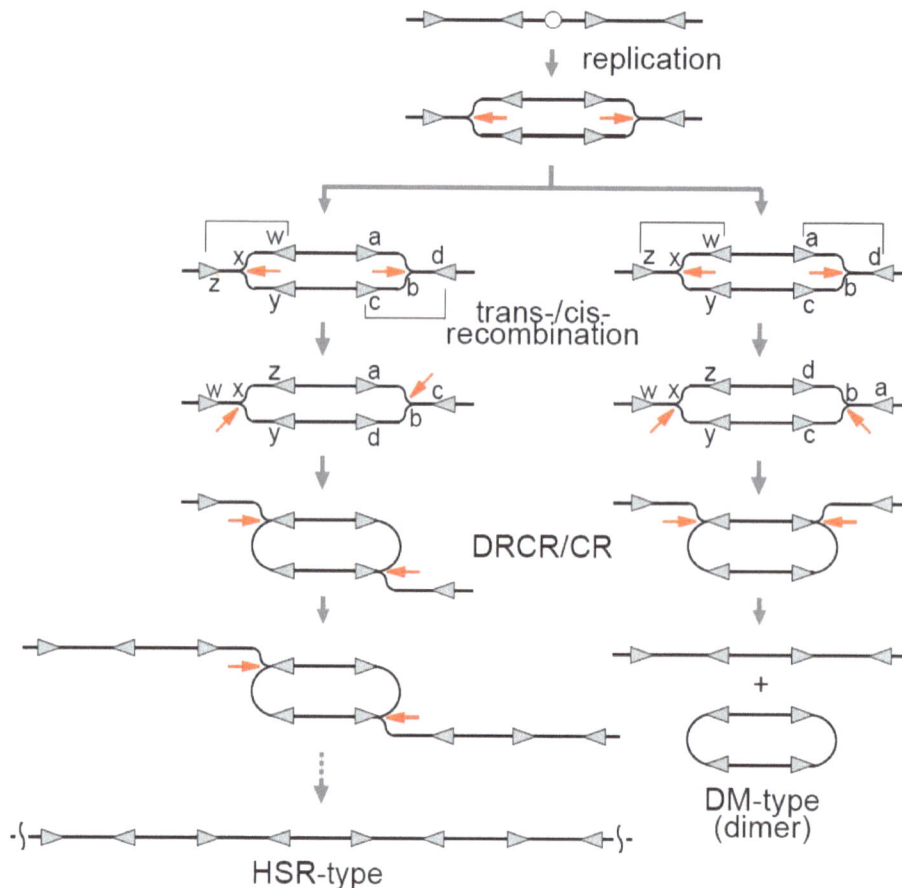

Figure 3: A model for the HSR amplification and DMs production by Cre recombination couple with replication. (CR: convergent replication)

4   Extreme of DRCR and its Consequences: Evolution of Amplicon under DRCR

A key question remains. From the microscopic observation of the process of gene amplification in cultured cells, as we have seen above, the amplification unit (amplicon) gradually shortens and the copy number increases with increasing drug concentration. This phenomenon is called 'evolution'. Such evolutionary changes remain to be accounted for. We may regard this phenomenon as gene evolution, because the cell possesses mechanisms to select and amplify genes that are advantageous for the cell itself. How does such a complex change come about? A key to solving the mystery was found in the first successful experiment, in which gene amplification was achieved by DRCR initiated by the BIR method (Watanabe and Horiuchi, 2005). When we analyzed the structure of amplified HSR-type products with restriction enzymes, we found that, in addition to the products with the expected structure, those with an unexpected structure also emerged. To our surprise, the ratio of expected to unexpected products was 1:1.

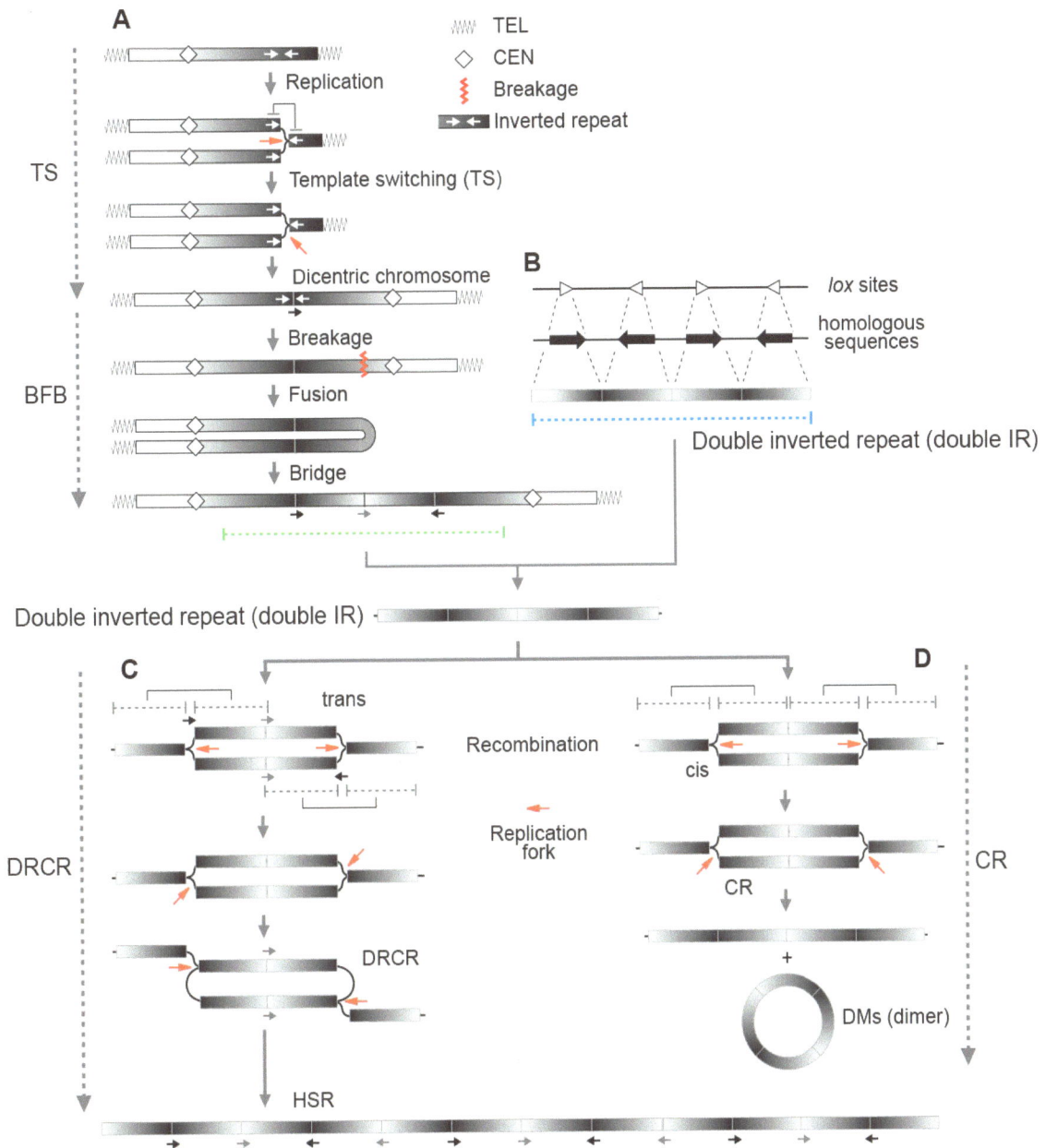

Figure 4: Initiation mechanism of DRCR under natural conditions; Involvement of BFB (Break-Fusion-Bridge) cycle A. Template switching (TS); When DNA replication proceeds to a center of a pair of IR structure, recombination occurs between the pair of IR and the direction of the replication fork is changed as shown in Figure 4A, producing a di-centromeric chromosome. Thus, in mitosis, chromosomal breaking occurs, after replication of the breaking sister-chromatid, the two sister-chromatids are fused, producing a dicentromeric chromosome. Because this chromosome structure is corresponding to structure of four *lox* sites, shown in B, and thus this (Double inverted repeat; double IR) is a starting structure of DRCR. From this structure, two alternate processes initiates; C is DRCR, producing HSR structure, or D is circle replication, producing a circle molecule with IR structure.

If DRCR proceeds as expected, the structure of the products should be as shown in the upper line in Figure 5, with two major bands of 4.4 kb and 10.3 kb produced by *Xho*I digestion. However, the observed gel pattern was unexpected, in that two other dense bands of 8.2 kb and 6.4 kb were produced, as shown on the left of Figure 5. This pattern can only be explained by assuming that a pair of fixed IR leu2d gene structures is freely inverted. The amounts of these unexpected fragments were so large that all four DNA bands could be detected not only by southern hybridization, but also by EtBr (ethidium bromide) staining. The same results were obtained not only for DRCR induced by Cre-*lox*, but also homologous recombination, thereby strongly suggesting that the DRCR process itself may be recombinogenic. To test this hypothesis more rigorously, we investigated recombinogenic properties using the 2μ plasmid system.

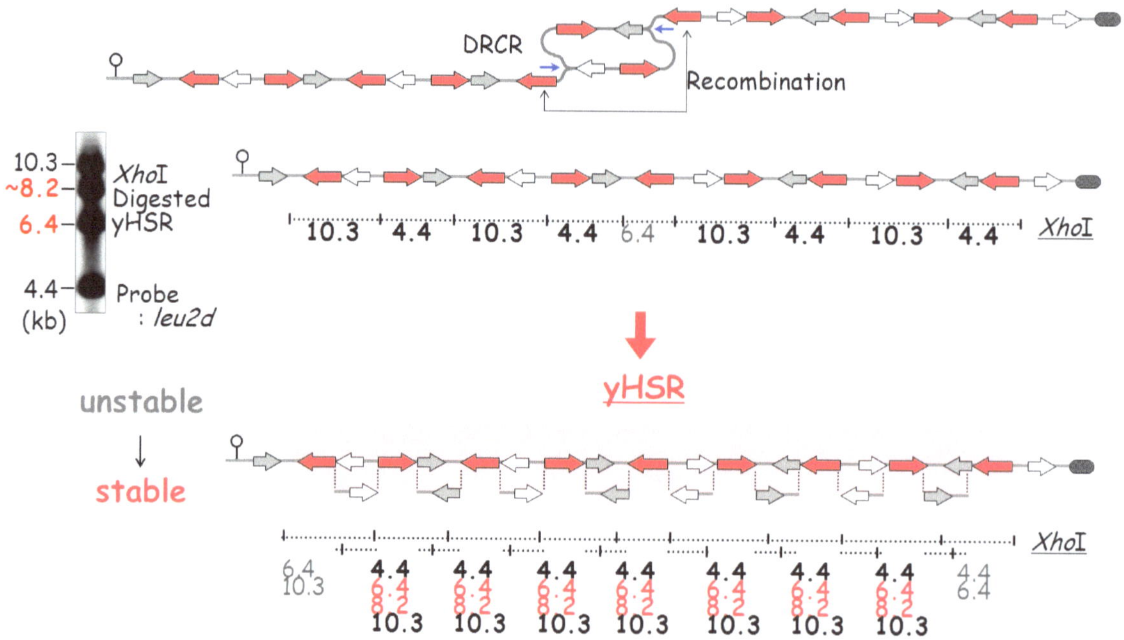

Figure 5: DRCR-dependent free inversion. DRCR is expected to produces the product whose structure is shown in the upper line and its XhoI digestion products is expected to be two main DNA fragments, 10.3 kb and 4.4 kb in length. However, the actual digestion pattern, shown in left side, shows four DNA fragments, 8.2 kb and 6.4 kb in addition to 10.3 kb and 4.4 kb. Thus, these results indicate that free inversion occurs between red regions occurs.

The 2μ plasmid is the only known example of a replicon which replicates in DRCR mode under natural conditions. It is a double stranded circular DNA (~ 6.3 kb) found in budding yeast. Interestingly, it can be maintained by normal replication, but depending on circumstances, for example, when the copy number is decreased, it replicates in DRCR mode to recover copy number quickly (Volkert and Broach, 1986). The reason that the 2μ plasmid can replicate by DRCR is that it has a site-specific recombination system, like Cre-*lox* (Broach, *et al.*, 1982). The plasmid has a pair of IR (0.6 kb), where a site-specific recombinational sequence (*FRT* sequence) is located and a site-specific recombinase (Flp protein) is encoded on the plasmid. Thus, as shown in Figure 1, normal replication starts bi-directionally from the replication origin, but a recombination occurs between two FRT sites mediated by the Flp protein, and the replication mode changes from bi-directional replication forks to those following one another. This recombination initiates DRCR and the plasmid copy number increases rapidly (Volkert & Broach, 1986). This DRCR ability of the 2μ plasmid was first deduced theoretically from the genome structure by lication origin, but a recombination occurs between two FRT sites mediated by the Flp protein, and the replication mode changes from bi-directional replication forks to those following one another. This recombination initiates DRCR and the plasmid copy number increases rapidly (Volkert & Broach, 1986).

This DRCR ability of the 2μ plasmid was first deduced theoretically from the genome structure by Futcher (1986) and soon afterwards Broach's group confirmed experimentally that the plasmid can replicate in two replication modes, one normal and the other DRCR. Under natural conditions, two structural isomers are present in equal amounts. Thus, it is to be expected that other plasmids or virus DNAs exist, with a pair of IR structures, like the 2μ plasmid DNA, and which could also replicate in DRCR mode. Furthermore, if the length of the IR is substantial, homologous recombination should initiate DRCR.

Interestingly, Broach's group previously reported that recombination was enhanced in 2μ plasmids (Jayaram and Broach, 1983). Therefore, we postulated that DRCR itself is recombinogenic and we repeated their experiments. We used 2μ plasmid DNA into which transposon Tn5 (IR) was transposed. Tn5 (IR) consists of three parts, the center region containing a kanamycin-resistance gene, and two inverted arms. We then introduced the Tn5-transposed 2μ plasmid DNA into yeast, cultured them, and then extracted DNA. We reconfirmed Broach's results that Tn5 is frequently inverted, but in the site-specific FLP recombinase-defective plasmid, it could only undergo normal replication and Tn5 (IR) inversion was not observed. Next, we changed the structure of Tn5 from a form with the arms inverted to directly repeated arms [Tn5 (DR)]. We found that in the 2μ plasmid with the Tn5 (DR), duplication and deletion of directly repeated arms occurs frequently. However, no structural changes were seen in the site-specific recombination-defective plasmid. Finally, we inserted Tn5 (DR) into the DRCR amplifying unit of the yeast chromosome, induced DRCR and examined the structure of the amplified products. In the amplified region, we found that deletion and duplication of Tn5 (DR) occurred frequently. From these results, we concluded that, regardless of whether the genome was linear or circular, DRCR itself is highly recombinogenic (Okamoto et al., 2011).

So how is DRCR recombinogenic? Actually, when DRCR was induced in yeast, recombination is saturated, that is, the amount of substrate for recombination equaled the amount of recombination product. We propose a model, in Figure 6, which explains how DRCR becomes so recombinogenic. Normal replication proceeds simultaneously with the production of a pair of sister chromatids, held together by a protein complex, "cohesin". However, unlike in normal replication, as shown in Figure 6, in either circular or linear genomes, the DRCR replication fork is expected to forcibly separate the chromatids, thus freeing them from one another, resulting in what we termed 'a single daughter chromatid', which is expected to be recombinogenic. This model is supported by two studies, one of which was by us (Grossenbacher-Grunder and Thuriaux, 1981; Kobayashi et al., 2004). Both reported that homologous recombination is enhanced in mutants partially defective in cohesion. If this model is correct, cohesin should have an additional function as an anti-recombinogenic.

To return to our question, what is the relationship between recombinogenic DRCR and evolution of amplicon, we suggest that there are two mechanisms responsible for the recombinogenic properties of DRCR. One is the disarrangement of regularly repeated sequences. Regularly repeated sequences should render the amplified region unstable, but randomization of the orientation of inverted repeats by DRCR stabilizes the amplified region. The second is that, in the higher eukaryote genome, there are a very large

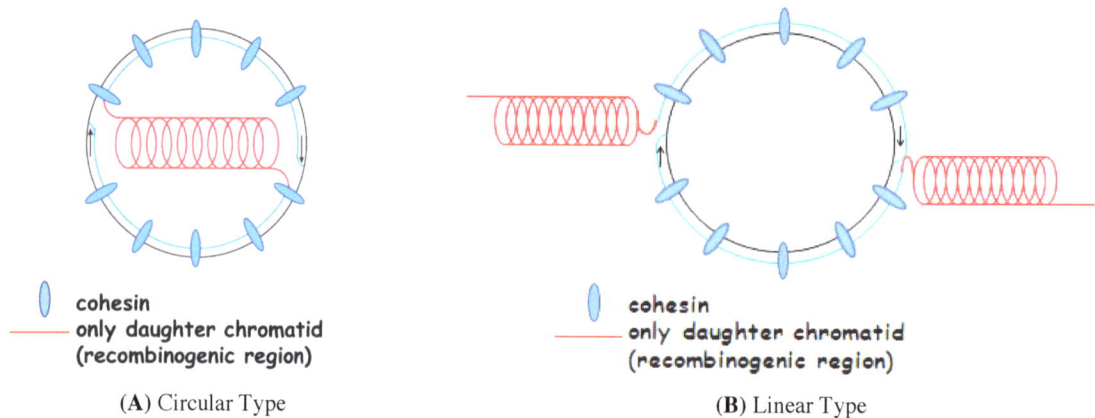

(A) Circular Type   **(B)** Linear Type

Figure 6: Double rolling circle replication (DRCR)-dependent recombinogenic model. (A) 2 micron plasmid-type DRCR, (B) linear-type DRCR. Arrow indicate replication fork, and blue oval structure indicates cohesin that bundles sister chromatids soon after replication. Red line indicates cohesin-free sister chromatid, which we designate the 'only-daughter' chromatid. This model suggests cohesin play a role in anti-recombinational factor.

number of repeated sequences, including transposons, insertion sequences, retro-transposons, etc. The total amount of these repeated sequences is estimated at about 50% of the entire human genome. If re-combinogenic DRCR acts on such chromosomes containing these repeated sequences, a large number of recombination events, including deletion, inversion, and duplication, should often occur between repeated sequences, during the amplification of different regions. As a result, under conditions selecting for drug resistance, only clones with a large number of amplified resistance genes will survive. In contrast, clones with amplified unnecessary or disadvantageous regions or genes will be eliminated. This is the evolution of gene amplification. Interestingly, in our gene amplification experiments using yeast, this kind of evolution of gene amplification in cultured cells has not been observed. This can be explained by the very low amount of repeated sequences (about 2%) in the yeast genome relative to the higher eukaryote genome.

To return to our question, what is the relationship between recombinogenic DRCR and evolution of amplicon, we suggest that there are two mechanisms responsible for the recombinogenic properties of DRCR. One is the disarrangement of regularly repeated sequences. Regularly repeated sequences should render the amplified region unstable, but randomization of the orientation of inverted repeats by DRCR stabilizes the amplified region. The second is that, in the higher eukaryote genome, there are a very large number of repeated sequences, including transposons, insertion sequences, retro-transposons, etc. The total amount of these repeated sequences is estimated at about 50% of the entire human genome. If re-combinogenic DRCR acts on such chromosomes containing these repeated sequences, a large number of recombination events, including deletion, inversion, and duplication, should often occur between repeated sequences, during the amplification of different regions. As a result, under conditions selecting for drug resistance, only clones with a large number of amplified resistance genes will survive. In contrast, clones with amplified unnecessary or disadvantageous regions or genes will be eliminated. This is the evolution of gene amplification. Interestingly, in our gene amplification experiments using yeast, this kind of evolution of gene amplification in cultured cells has not been observed. This can be explained by the very low amount of repeated sequences (about 2%) in the yeast genome relative to the higher eukaryote genome.

5   Involvement of DRCR in Natural Genome Replication: A Model for HSV-1 and Chloroplasts

As described above, because the 2μ plasmid DNA is replicated (amplified) by DRCR, it would not be surprising if other plasmids or viruses also replicated their DNA by DRCR. Even today, there remain many plasmids and virus whose DNA replication modes are still unknown. Here, we consider Herpes Simplex Virus (HSV) and chloroplast DNA. Their DNAs are both double stranded, but the former is linear and the latter circular. Chloroplast and 2μ plasmid DNA are structurally very similar in that both contain a pair of IR structures (Tobacco chloroplast 25.3kb each IR/156 kb total length (Kolodner and Tewari, 1979); 2μ 0.6 kb each IR/6.3 kb total length (Broach and Volkert, 1991)) and both consist of equal amounts of two structural isomers, suggesting frequent inversion occurring between IRs. Moreover, several mitochondrial DNAs (mtDNA) also have this type of structure (for example, mtDNA of Achlya (Hudspeth et al., 1983)). Furthermore, when HSV-1 infects cultured cells, its DNA is immediately circularized, which makes its structure very similar to chloroplast and the 2μ plasmid DNA (15.5kb each IR/152kb total HSV-1 length). Their replication intermediates possess a large number of branched structures and are very complicated (Zhang et al., 1994; Severini et al., 1996). For example, even if HSV-1 replication intermediates are treated by a restriction enzyme, which can digest one cut per single HSV-1 DNA unit, structural analysis using PFGE or Field Inversion techniques reveals that the majority of the sample DNA remains in the original well (Severini et al., 1994; Zhang et al., 1994). During DNA replication, homologous recombination between two IRs is expected to occur so frequently that two or four structural isomers are produced at a 1:1 ratio in chloroplasts and 1:1:1:1 in HSV, suggesting a significant association between replication and recombination (Roizman, 1979; Bataille and Epstein, 1995; Umene, 1999; Wilkinson and Weller, 2003). DRCR, which is a highly recombinogenic process, accounts for all these properties.

However, there are several exceptions to this rule for both chloroplast DNA and HSV. For example, chloroplast DNA in allied species in the subfamily Papilonoidea of the legume family (Fabaceae) and Douglas-fir and radiata pine do not have an IR structure but rather a single rDNA gene. Thus, they must be unable to replicate by DRCR. However, Bendich reported that replication intermediate of pea chloroplast DNA with only one rDNA has a complex structure like chloroplast DNAs with IR (Bendich 2004; Bendich 1991). The replication intermediate structure is currently still unresolved. A likely explanation is that they may replicate in the same manner as mtDNA type in organisms that are not animals, but this mechanism remains to be determined.

In HSV-1, it has been well established that replication is associated with recombination. We mentioned above that an equal number of viruses with four different structural isomers are produced by recombination associated with replication. Furthermore, when Tn5-transposed HSV-1 DNA replicated it inverted at high frequency, in the same manner as Tn5-transposed 2μ plasmid (Weber et al., 1988). These observations can be explained well by DRCR–dependent recombination. Here, we have presented a DRCR-dependent HSV-1 replication model. Previously, we proposed the model illustrated in Figure 7-1 (Okamoto et al., 2011) on the basis of the report that after HSV-1 infection, the viral DNA does not circularize, but remains linear (Jackson & DeLuca, 2003). However, a later paper from a different group reported findings completely opposite from those of Jackson & DeLuca (Strang & Stow, 2005). Taking this into account, here we present two models, one of which is a linear model (Figure 7-1) and the other circular (Figure7-2). In the latter model, DNA is contiguous and some replicates normally, while some does so in DRCR mode.

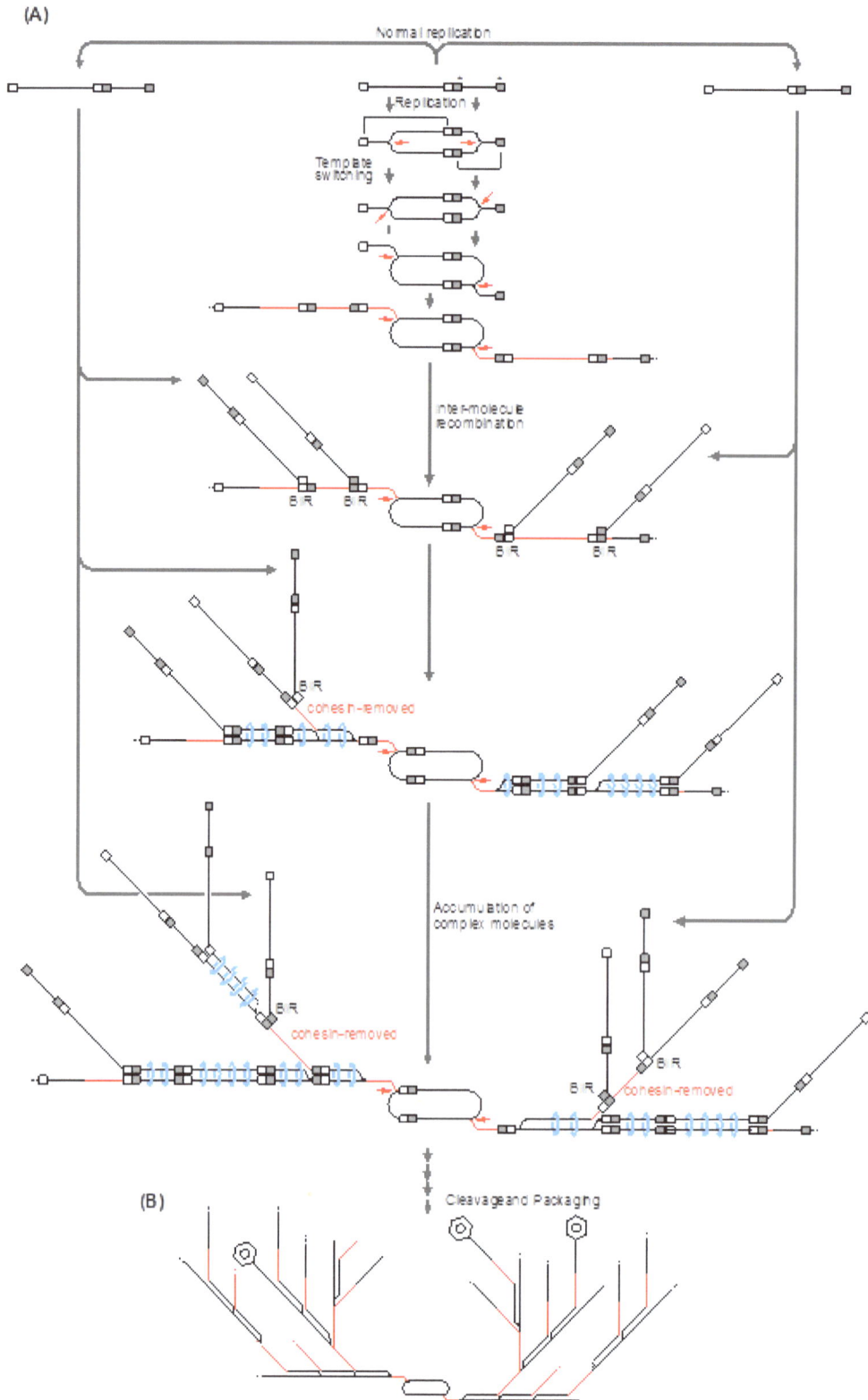

Figure 7 (1): HSV-1 DNA replication model (Linear model). Red lines indicate single daughter chromatid.

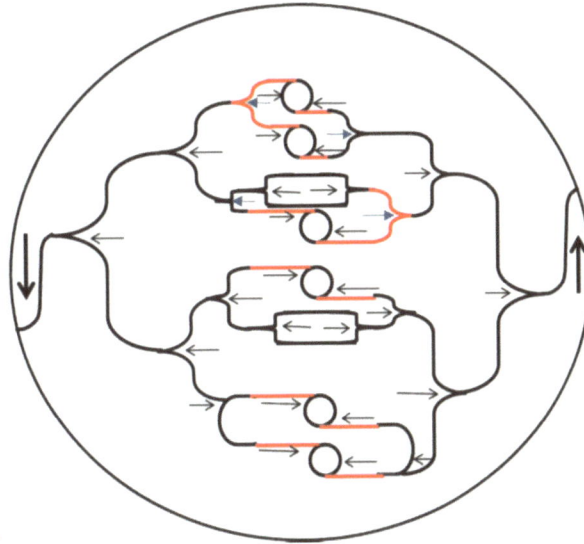

Figure 7 (2): HSV-1 DNA replication model (Circular model). Red lines indicate single daughter chromatid.

On the other hand, it has been generally thought that rolling circle replication (RCR) is involved in DNA replication of HSV-1 (Roizman, 1979; Lehman and Boehmer, 1999; Weller and Coen, 2012). However, as described above, replication intermediates have highly complex structure with a large number of DNA branches. HSV-1 DNA has three replication origins (one OriL and two OriS), to which the viral coded protein, UL9 (or OBP), binds (Elias *et al.*, 1986) and initiates DNA replication. By using the temperature sensitive UL9 mutant viruses, UL9-dependent DNA replication was found to be limited to the first 6 hours after infection. Subsequently, UL9-independent replication occurs and the huge mass of viral DNA accumulates (Blümel and Matz, 1995; Schildgen *et al.*, 2005). These results suggest that HSV-1 replication is not so simple like RCR, but more complex and recombinogenic, producing equal number of four types of genomic isomers. Thus, so far, there have been several reports alluding to the possibility that replication of HSV DNA might be by DRCR. However, they did not refer to potential recombinogenic properties of DRCR (Hammerschmidt and Mankertz, 1991; Zhang *et al.*, 1994; Grossenbacher-Grunder and Thuriaux, 1981, Severini *et al.*, 1996).

There is another piece of evidence that HSV-1 replicates in DRCR mode. The herpes virus family contains a large number of members, some with a DNA structure quite different from HSV-1. One of them, HHV-6, has DNA with only a 10 kb DR structure at two terminus ends; after infection, virus DNA is thought to be circularized but lacks any other homologous regions required for DRCR. Investigations on HHV-6 replication intermediates after virus infection showed that DNA was circularized but its replication intermediates were only simple linear-multimer, circular-monomer, and -oligomer forms, with no branched structures (Severini *et al.*, 2003). These data strongly suggest that HHV-6 replication is not by DRCR, but solely normal.

EHV (Equine Herpes Virus) and VZV (Varicella Zoster Virus) are further members of the herpesviridiae, but although their DNA structures are similar to HSV-1, they have only two or four structural isomers. However, when there are four isomers two are major and the other two minor. After infection, if these genomes are circularized and replicate in DRCR mode, such unbalanced isomer formation could not be explained. However, further subsequent reports revealed that in the replication step of virus DNA, although equal amounts of the four structural isomers are present, in the packaging step, different distributions of major and minor virus DNA isomers appear. This suggests that the unbalance is not relevant for DNA replication (Slobedman and Simmons, 1997; Schynts *et al.*, 2003).

In HSV-1 and closely related viruses, several mutants have been isolated in which a common region between UL and Us is deleted. According to our model, these mutants would be predicted to be unable to replicate in DRCR mode. Unexpectedly, however, when these viruses infect cultured cells, there is a slight drop in productivity, but growth is little affected (Sauer *et al.*, 2010). However, similar experiments using a mutant Equine Herpes Virus (which is closely-related to HSV-1) with a similar common region deletion resulted in a smaller plaque size and delayed growth kinetics. On the other hand, when animals infected directly with these viruses, growth rates of the mutants were significantly lower than seen for wild-type viruses, and pathogenicity was also decreased (Jenkins and Roizman, 1986; Poffenberger and Roizman, 1985; Poffenberger *et al.*, 1983). These results suggest that DRCR might play an important role in vivo, but in vitro HHV-6 type replication described above might occur.

6   Conclusion

Until now there are some amplification whose mechanisms have yet to be elucidated. One is the gene amplification occurred in H region of genome in *Leishmania* protozoa (Olmo *et al.*, 1995) and the other is 'palindrome' type amplification of petite (*rho⁻*) mutants of budding yeast (Rayko and Goursot, 1996). The formers are two types, circle and linear, circle type can be produced by DMs type reaction (see DM production in Figure 3), linear type can be done by giant palindrome formation (see page 9, lines 2-4). The latter type of amplification unit coincides with that of DRCR amplification unit. Thus, *rho⁻* palindrome type amplification is very likely to be produced by DRCR. The characteristic of this inverted repeat is short unit (1~2kb).

DRCR has long been believed to be an exceptional DNA synthetic mechanism unique to the yeast 2μ plasmid. As we discussed in this review, however, DRCR have more extensive roles in other biological systems. We predicted and subsequently found, for example, that DRCR is involved in oncogene-type gene amplification. Importantly, DRCR appears to be intrinsically recombinogenic, and this characteristic must be important in stabilizing repeated structure of amplified products in lower eukaryotes, and in "evolution" of highly repeated short amplicon from a small number of long amplicon in higher eukaryotes. In a fashion similar to our model system, DRCR may have been involved in natural gene evolution.

In addition to well-documented DRCR involvement in 2 micron replication, we speculate that DRCR is also important in replication of other natural replicons such as chloroplasts, mitochondria and HSV. In the case of mitochondria, many types of replicons, some circular and others linear have been documented. In this case, DRCR involvement may not be universal. In contrast, most if not all chloroplast DNA has a pair of inverted repeat structure. It is therefore possible that chloroplast DNA is exclusively replicated through DRCR because of yet unknown advantages in chloroplast function.

We described that combination of amplification and recombination, expected for DRCR, can explain extreme complexity of HSV-1 DNA structure. It should be noted that amplified products here also contain replication origins, from which further replication can initiate. Explosive increase in viral DNA and particles could be the result of these processes, which are quite different from more classical and extensively studied cellular genome replication.

HSR-type DRCR amplification produces highly repeated sequences. It has been generally postulated that multiplication of genes has a major role in evolution partly because it generates functional redundancy. In the case of *Neurospora crassa*, a phenomenon referred to as RIP (repeat-induced point mutation) is documented (Galagan and Selker, 2004). RIP, which is induced only after fertilization but before DNA synthesis or nuclear fusion, results in extremely abundant mutations restricted on repeated DNA. By combining DRCR with RIP, we imagine that it may be possible to device a bio machine for artificial gene evolution, in which highly repeated and rapidly mutated genes can evolve rapidly. Furthermore, RIP may not be unique to *Neurospora crassa*; mutations may be induced on repeated DNA in other organisms also, although may not be as extensive as in *Neurospora crassa*. If that is the case, repeated genes, such as those generated though DRCR, could have been important in evolution not only because the functional redundancy but also because of their high mutation rates.

Acknowledgement

In writing this review, we thank a lot of members for helping and encouraging us. Especially, we would like to thank Dr. Haruko Oksmoto (Toyota Central R & D Labs. Inc.) for carrying out experimental work on recombinogenic property of DRCR, Dr. A. J. Bendich (Univ. Washington) for giving us information of replication of chloroplast DNA and Dr. K. Umene (Fukuoka Woman's University) for discussing about HSV DNA replication. Furthermore, we give a special thanks Dr. M. Tanaka (Tokai Univ.) for critically reading the manuscript and giving invaluable advice, Dr. M. Kimura (Tokai Univ.) and Dr. H. Inoko (Tokai Univ.) for continuous supporting and encouraging us.

References

Bataille, D., and Epstein, A. L. (1995) Herpes simplex virus type 1 replication and recombination. Biochemie, 77, 787-795.

Blümel, J., & Matz, B. (1995) Thermo-sensitive UL9 gene function is required for early stages of herpes simplex virus type 1 DNA synthesis. Journal of General Virology, 76, 3119-24.

Broach, J. R., & Volkert F. C. (1991) Circular DNA plasmids of yeast. In: The Molecular and Cellular Biology of the Yeast Saccharomyces (eds J. R. Broach, JR Pringle, E. W. Jones) pp.297-331. New York: Cold Spring Harbor Laboratory Press.

Butler, D. K., Yasuda, L. E., & Yao, M. C. (1996) Induction of large DNA palindrome formation in yeast: implications for gene amplification and genome stability in eukaryotes. Cell, 87, 1115-1122.

Cowell J. K. (1982) Double minutes and homogeneously staining regions: gene amplification in mammalian cells. Annual Review of Genetics, 16, 21-59.

Debatisse, M., & Malfor, B. (2005) In Nigg., E. A. (ed), Genome Instability in Cancer Development. Springer, Netherlands, pp343-361.

Devonshire, A. L., & Field, L. M. (1991) Gene amplification and insecticide resistance. Annual Review of Entomology, 36, 1-23.

Futcher, A. B. (1986) Copy number amplification of the 2 micron circle plasmid of Saccharomyces cerevisiae. Journal of Theoretical Biology 119, 197-204.

Galagan, J. E., & Selker E. U. (2004) RIP: the evolutionary cost of genome defence. Trend in Genetics 20, 417-423.

Grossenbacher-Grunder M. A., & Thuriaux, J. (1981) Spontaneous and UV-induced recombination in radiation-sensitive mutants of Schizosaccharomyces pombe. Mutation Research, 81, 37-48.

Gusfield, D. (1997). Algorithms on Strings, Trees and Sequences: Computer Science and Computational Biology. Cambridge: Cambridge University Press.

Hammerschmidt, W., & Mankertz, J. (1991) Herpes viral DNA replication: between the known and unknown. Semin. Virology. 2, 257-296.

Hudspeth ME, Shumard DS, Bradford CJ, & Grossman LI. (1983) Organization of Achlya mtDNA: a population with two orientations and a large inverted repeat containing the rRNA genes. Proceeding of National Academy of Science USA, 80, 142-146.

Hyrien, O., Debatisse, M, Buttin G., & de Saint Vincent B. R.(1988) The multi-copy appearance of a large inverted duplica-tion and the sequence at the inversion joint suggest a new model for gene amplification. EMBO Journal. 7, 407-17.

Jackson, S. A., & DeLuca N. A. (2003) Relationship of herpes simplex virus genome configuration to productive and per-sis-tent infections. Proceeding of National Academy of Science USA, 100, 7871–7876.

Jayaram, M., & Broach, J. R. (1983) Yeast plasmid 2-micron circle promotes recombination within bacterial transposon Tn5. Proceeding of National Academy of Science USA, 80, 7264-7268.

Jenkins, F. J., & Roizman, B. (1986) Herpes simplex virus 1 recombinants with noninverting genomes frozen in different isomeric arrangements are capable of independent replication. Journal of Virology, 59, 494-9.

Kobayashi, T & Horiuchi, T. (1996) A yeast gene product, Fob1 protein, required for both replication fork blocking and recombinational hotspot activities. Genes to Cells, 1, 465-74

Kobayashi, T., Heck, J. D., Nomura, M., & Horiuchi, T. (1998) Expansion and contraction of ribosomal DNA repeats in Saccharomyces cerevisiae: requirement of replication fork blocking (Fob1) protein and the role of RNA polymerase I. Genes and Development, 12, 3821-3830.

Kobayashi, T., Horiuchi, T., Tongaonlar, T., Vu, L., & Nomura, M. (2004) SIR2 regulates recombination between different rDNA repeats, but not recombination within individual rDNA genes in Yeast. Cell, 77, 441-453.

Kobayashi, T., Nomura, M., & Horiuchi, T. (2001) Identification of DNA cis-elements essential for expansion of ribosomal DNA repeats in Saccharomyces cerevisiae. Molecular and Cellular Biology, 21, 136-147.

Kolodner R, & Tewari K. K., (1979) Inverted repeats in chloroplast DNA from higher plants. Proceeding of National Academy of Science USA, 76, 41-5.

Kraus, E., Leung, W. Y., & Haber J. E. (2001) Break-induced replication: a review and an example in budding yeast. Proceeding of National Academy of Science USA, 17, 8255-62.

Lehman and Boehmer (1999) Replication of Herpes Simplex Virus DNA. Journal of Biological Chemistry, 274, 28059-28062

Ma, C., Martin, S., Trask, B., & Hamlin, J. L. (1993) Sister chromatid fusion initiates amplification of the dihydrofolate reductase gene in Chinese hamster cells. Genes and Development, 7, 605-20

McClintock, B. (1941) The stability of broken ends of chromosomes in Zea Mays. Genetics, 26, 234-282.

Mondello, C., Smirnova, A., & Giulotto, E. (2010) Gene amplification, radiation sensitivity and DNA double-strand breaks. Mutation Research, 704, 29-37.

Okamoto, H., Watanabe, T., & Horiuchi, T. (2011) Double rolling circle replication (DRCR) is recombinogenic. Genes to Cells, 16, 503-13.

Olmo, A., Arrebola, R., Bernier, V., González-Pacanowska, D., & Ruiz-Pérez, L. M. (1995) Co-existence of circular and multiple linear amplicons in methotrexate-resistant Leishmania. Nucleic Acid Research, 23, 2856-2864.

Palmer, J. D., (1983) Chloroplast DNA exists in two orientations. Nature, 301, 92-93.

Pipiras, E, Coquelle, A, Bieth, A, & Debatisse, M. (1998) Interstitial deletion and intra-chromosomal amplification initiated form a double –strand break targeted to a mammalian chromosome. EMBO Journal. 17, 325-333.

Poffenberger, K. L., & Roizman, B., (1985) A noninverting genome of a viable herpes simplex virus 1: presence of head-to-tail linkages in packaged genomes and requirements for circularization after infection. Journal of Virology, 53, 587-595

Poffenberger, K. L., Tabares, E., & Roizman, B., (1983) Characterization of a viable, noninverting herpes simplex virus 1 genome derived by insertion and deletion of sequences at the junction of components L and S. Proceeding of National Academy of Science USA, 80, 2690-4.

Rayko E., & Goursot, R. (1996) Amphimeric mitochondrial genomes of petite mutants of yeast. II. A model for the amplification of amphimeric mitochondrial petite DNA. Current Genetics, 30, 135-144

Roizman, B. (1979) The structure of the helps simplex virus genomes. Cell, 16, 481-494.

Roizman, B., Jacob. R. J., Knipe, D. M., Morse, L. S., & Ruyechan, W. T., (1979) On the structure, functional equivalence and replication of the four arrangements of herpes simplex virus DNA. Cold Spring Harbor Symposia on Quantitative Biology 43, 809-826.

Ruiz, J. C., & Wahl, G. M., (1988) Formation of an inverted duplication can be an initial step in gene amplification. Molecular and Cellular Biology, 8, 4302-4313.

Sauer A, Wang, J. B., Hahn, G, & McVoy, M. A., (2010) A human cytomegalovirus deleted of internal repeats replicates with near wild type efficiency but fails to undergo genome isomerization. Virology. 401, 90-5.

Schildgen, O., Gräper, S., Blümel, J., & Matz B. (2005) Genome replication and progeny virion production of herpes simplex virus type 1 mutants with temperature-sensitive lesions in the origin-binding protein. Journal of Virology, 79, 7273-7278.

Schimke, R. T. (1984) Gene amplification in cultured animal cells. Cell, 37, 705-713.

Schynts, F., McVoy, M. A., Meurens, F., Detry, B., Epstein, A. L. & Thiry, E.(2003) The structures of bovine herpesvirus 1 virion and concatemeric DNA: implications for cleavage and packaging of herpesvirus genomes. Virology. 314, 326-35.

Severini, A, C., Sevenhuysena, M., Garbutta, G. A., & Tipplesa, (2003) Structure of replicating intermediates of human herpesvirus type 6. Virology, 314, 443-450.

Severini, A, Morgan, A. R., Tovell, D. R., & Tyrrell, D. L. (1994) Study of the structure of replicative intermediates of HSV-1 DNA by pulsed-field gel electrophoresis. Virology. 200, 428-35.

Severini, A, Scraba & Tyrrell, D. L. (1996) Branch structure in the intracellular DNA of Herpes Simplex Virus Type 1, Journal of Virology, 70, 3169-3175.

Slobedman, B. & Simmons, A. (1997) Concatemeric intermediates of equine herpesvirus type 1 DNA replication contain frequent inversions of adjacent long segments of the viral genome. Virology, 229, 415-20.

Smith, K. A., Stark, M. B., Gorman, P. A. & Stark, G. R.(1992) Fusions near telomeres occur very early in the amplification of CAD genes in Syrian hamster cells. Proceeding of National Academy of Science USA, 89, 5427-31

Stark G. R. & Wahl G. M. (1984) Gene amplification. Annual Review of Biochemistry, 53, 447-491.

Stark, W. M., Boocock, M. R., & Sherratt, D. J. (1992) Catalysis by site-specific recombinases. Trends in Genetics, 8, 432-439.

Strang, B. L. & Stow, N. D. (2005) Circularization of the Herpes Simplex Virus Type 1 Genome upon Lytic Infection Journal of Virology, 79, 12487–12494.

Tanaka, H, & Yao, M.C. (2009) Palindromic gene amplification--an evolutionarily conserved role for DNA inverted repeats in the genome. Nature Review of Cancer, 9, 216-24.

Tanaka, H., Tapscott, S. J., Trask, B. J., & Yao, M. C. (2002) Short inverted duplication initiate gene amplification through the formation of a large DNA palindrome in mammalian cells. Proceeding of National Academy of Science USA, 99, 8772-8777.

Umene, K. (1999) Mechanism and application of genetic recombination in Herpesviruses. Review of Medical Virology, 9, 171-182.

Volkert, F. C. & Broach, J. R. (1986) Site specific recombination promotes plasmid amplification in yeast. Cell, 46, 541-550.

Watanabe T., & Horiuchi, T. (2005) A novel gene amplification system in yeast based on double rolling-circle replication. EMBO Journal, 12, 190-8.

Watanabe, T., Tanabe, H., & Horiuchi, T., (2011) Gene amplification system based on double rolling-circle replication as a model for oncogene-type amplification. Nucleic Acid Research, 39, e106.

Weller, S. K., & Coen, D. M. (2012) Herpes Simplex Viruses: Mechanisms of DNA replication. Cold Spring Harbor Perspective Biology, 4(9): a013011.

Wilkinson, D. E., & Weller, S. K. (2003) The role of DNA recombination in Herpes Simplex Virus DNA replication. IUBMB Life, 55, 451-458.

Zhang, X., Efstathiou, S., & Simmons, A. (1994) Identification of novel Herpes Simplex Virus replicative intermediates by Field Inversion gel electrophoresis: Implication for Viral DNA amplification strategies. Virology, 202, 530-539.

West Nile Virus Transmission by Ticks: An Oddity or Unexplored Reality?

María Armesto Álvarez
Department of Oncology
Biodonostia Research Institute, San Sebastián, Spain

Charles H. Lawrie
Department of Oncology
Biodonostia Research Institute, San Sebastián, Spain

IKERBASQUE
Basque Foundation for Science, Bilbao, Spain

Nuffield Department of Clinical Laboratory Sciences
University of Oxford, United Kingdom

1 Introduction

West Nile virus (WNV) was first identified in 1937 in Uganda in eastern Africa (Smithburn, *et al.*, 1940), and subsequently associated with major outbreaks of the disease in Africa, Eurasia, Australia and the Middle East. In the 1990s outbreaks began to be reported in both Southern and Northern Europe often associated with more severe disease than seen previously including viral encephalitis and neurological symptoms (Hubalek, *et al.*, 1999). The first report of an outbreak within the Western hemisphere occurred in 1999 in New York City and resulted in human, equine and avian mortalities (Lanciotti, *et al.*, 1999). Since this time WNV outbreaks have been reported in all the states of the US, as well as Canada, Central and South America, and parts of the Caribbean (Aiken, 2003; 2002a; Kramer, *et al.*, 2008). The latest statistics on US WNV infections can be found at the dedicated Center for Disease Control website: (http://www.cdc.gov/ncidod/dvbid/westnile/index.htm).

WNV is a member of the genus *Flavivirus* that contains over seventy identified viruses, most of which are vectored by mosquitoes or ticks, although a few have no known vectors (Monath, *et al.*, 1996). The virus has been isolated from 60 species of mosquito in the US (Centers for Disease Control and Prevention, 2002b; Hayes, *et al.*, 2005), *Culex pipiens* being the most important (Campbell, *et al.*, 2002; Donaldson, 1966). However, WNV has also been repeatedly isolated from hard (ixodid) and soft (argasid) tick species in endemic regions of Europe, Africa and Asia (Hoogstraal, 1972; Hoogstraal, *et al.*, 1976; Iakimenko, *et al.*, 1991; L'Vov, et al., 2002; Lvov, *et al.*, 1975; Mathiot, *et al.*, 1990; Platonov, 2001). Ticks rank second only to mosquitoes in their importance as vectors of human pathogens and transmit a greater variety of infectious agents than any other arthropod group (Sonenshine, 1991). Current strategies to control WNV in the US are largely based upon measures to avoid exposure and to control vector species, but at present only mosquito species are targeted by government surveillance and preventative control programmes (http://www.cdc.gov/ncidod/dvbid/westnile/index.htm).

The epidemiology of arthropod-borne diseases is a function of both ecological and physiological parameters, of which vector competency is arguably the most important (Sonenshine, *et al.*, 1994). Vector competency, the ability of biting arthropods to acquire, maintain and transmit infectious agents from reservoir hosts to susceptible hosts, is determined by extrinsic and intrinsic factors including fundamentally, the physiological ability of vector tissue to become infected and to maintain a particular infectious agent (Lane, 1994).

We therefore set out to test whether or not ticks were competent vectors for WNV firstly by testing the physiological ability of tick tissue to become infected with WNV and to maintain the virus. The susceptibility of a cell line derived from a particular arthropod vector to infection by a specific infectious agent can provide information about the determinants of virus transmission and viral persistence in the natural environment (Mussgay, *et al.*, 1975). We undertook a comparative study of the susceptibility of mammalian Vero cells, a clonal mosquito cell line (C6/36) and cell lines derived from the ticks *Ixodes ricinus* (L.) (IRE/CTVM18), *I. scapularis* (Say) (ISE6), *Rhipicephalus appendiculatus* (Neumann) (RAE/CTVM1) and *Amblyomma variegatum* (Fabricius) (AVL/CTVM17) to infection with twelve flaviviruses, including WNV, using immunofluorescence microscopy and plaque assay techniques.

Secondly we assessed the ability of both ixodid (*I. ricinus*) and argasid tick species (*Ornithodoros moubata*) ticks to acquire WNV through feeding, maintain the virus through molting (transtadial transmission) and egg production (transovarial transmission), and finally the ability to infect hosts and other ticks.

In this chapter we describe the results of these experiments and discuss some of the consequential experimental data that has arisen since, within the context of assessing whether or not ticks *really* are important vectors of WNV. The following experimental details were taken in part from previously published research (Lawrie, *et al.*, 2004a; Lawrie, *et al.*, 2004b).

2   Materials and Methods

2.1   Viruses, Cell Lines and Infection Procedures

Twelve flaviviruses (Table 1) were used to assess the susceptibility of mammalian (Vero), mosquito (C6/36) and tick cells (IRE/CTVM18; ISE6; RAE/CTVM1; AVL/CTVM17) to infection and measure persistence of infection. The origin of these viruses, and of the cell lines used in these experiments are described in detail in reference (Lawrie, *et al.*, 2004a). In particular, WNV (tick strain), was isolated from ticks feeding on an unidentified bird in the Astrakhan region of the former Soviet Union and had undergone four passes in newborn mouse brain (Lvov, *et al.*, 1975), and Dr Robert Shope of the University of Texas kindly provided WNV (NY99 strain), that had undergone three passes in newborn mouse brain (Lanciotti, *et al.*, 1999). High titer mouse brain suspension stocks of WNV (NY99 strain) (2.9×10^7 pfu ml^{-1}) were diluted in PBS (pH 7.2) to a concentration of 10^5 pfu ml^{-1} before use in animal transmission studies.

Vector	Virus	Vero	C6/36	RAE/CTVM1	ISE6	IRE/CTVM18	AVL/CTVM17
Mosquito	Yellow fever virus	+	+	-	-	-	-
	Dengue-2	+	+	-	-	-	-
	St. Louis encephalitis virus	+	+	-	-	-	ND
	West Nile Virus (NY99 strain)	+	+	+[a]	+[a]	+[a]	+[a]
	West Nile Virus (tick strain)	+	+	+[a]	+[a]	+[a]	+[a]
Tick	Tick-borne encephalitis virus	+	-	+[a]	+[a]	+[a]	+[a]
	Powassan virus	+	-	+[a]	+	+	+
	Louping-ill virus (Inverness strain)	+	-	+[a]	+	+	+
	Louping-ill virus (Loch strain)	+	-	+[a]	+	ND	ND
	Negishi virus	+	-	+	+	+	ND
No known vector	Apoi virus	+	-	-	-	-	ND
	Modoc virus	+	-	-	-	-	ND

[a]Viruses were subcultured three times. ND, not done.

Table 1: Susceptibility of Vero, C6/36 (mosquito) and the tick cell lines RAE/CTVM1, ISE6, IRE/CTVM18 and AVL/CTVM17 to flavivirus infection as measured by immunofluorescence assay (IFA). Viruses were subcultured at least once in the appropriate cell line before IFA unless indicated.

Cell line	Subculture 1	Subculture 2	Subculture 3
C6/36	7.1×10^4	8.2×10^4	1.4×10^5
RAE/CTVM1	2.4×10^4	3.0×10^4	6.0×10^4

Table 2: Titration of WNV viruses by plaque assay in PS cells after culture in C6/36 or RAE/CTVM1 cells. Titers are expressed as the mean (n=3) pfu ml^{-1} of recovered media (4 ml total).

All cells were grown in L-15 (Leibovitz) medium supplemented with fetal calf serum. Vero cells and AVL/CTVM17 cells were grown at 37°C; IRE/CTVM18, RAE/CTVM1 and C6/36 cell lines were grown at 28°C; and the ISE6 cell line was grown at 30°C. Approximately 4×10^5 cells were infected with 10^4 pfu (MOI of 0.03) of a particular virus or 100 μl of harvested infectious cell-free culture supernatant. For transmission studies, samples of tick (or mouse brain) homogenate (100 μl) were used to infect 2×10^6 C6/36 cells. The cultures were incubated at the appropriate temperature for 3 days, after which coverslips were removed and fixed in cold acetone before being examined by immunofluorescence microscopy (IFA).

2.2 Ticks

We tested a hard tick species, *I. ricinus* and a soft tick species, *O. moubata* for their vector competence with WNV (NY99 strain). These species are not native to the US and were chosen mainly for their availability. *O. moubata* ticks were considered potential vectors for the Eg101 strain of WNV in a study by Whitman and Aitken in 1960 (Whitman, *et al.*, 1960). *I. ricinus* ticks are the primary vectors of *Borrelia burgdorferi*, the aetiological agent of Lyme disease in Europe and important vectors of the flaviviruses *Tick-borne encephalitis virus* (TBEV) and *Louping-ill virus* (LIV) (Sonenshine, *et al.*, 1994).

Ticks were taken from colonies reared and maintained for many generations at CEH Oxford according to standard methods (Jones, *et al.*, 1988). Colony ticks were WNV negative by RT-PCR testing (15 individuals tested of each species).

2.3 Tick Infection and Co-feeding Transmission Experiments

Seven groups of six BALB/c mice (female, 4-6 weeks old) were inoculated by sub-cutaneous injection with 10^4 pfu of WNV. Three of the mice were bled daily from the tail to follow the course of viremia by plaque assay. Two groups of mice were infested with *I. ricinus* nymphs (twenty per mouse); one group was infested three days prior to inoculation, the other four days after inoculation (Swallow, 1985). The other five groups of mice were infested with 2nd instar *O. moubata* ticks (ten per mouse) on either the same day (day 0), or 1, 2, 3, or 4 days after inoculation (Table 3). After the initial experiment, and in order to increase the number of positive ticks available for experimentation, a further twelve mice were infested with *O. moubata* two days after inoculation with WNV.

Ticks housed in gauze-covered neoprene feeding chambers on mice (Jones, *et al.*, 1988) were removed when fully engorged; 24 hours after infestation in the case of *O. moubata* ticks and six days after infestation in the case of *I. ricinus* nymphs. The engorged ticks were then stored at 20°C in KCl saturated desiccators until testing for the presence of WNV or until ready for a further bloodmeal (duration of storage indicated in Table 3). After storage, the ticks (pools and individuals) were homogenised in 500 μl of PBS using plastic homogenisers under sterile conditions. The homogenates were frozen and stored

Species	Developmental stage	Days from inoculation to infestation	Days after engorgement[a]	IFA[b] (+/-)	RT-PCR[c] (no. positive/no. tested)
O. moubata		0	1, 2,7	- (8)	ND
	2nd instar	1	1,2,3,4,5,6,7	- (5)	ND
1st bloodmeal (infected mice)		2	1,2,3,4,5,6,7,14	+ (5)	+ (5)
		3	1,2,3,4,5,6,7,14	+ (5)	+ (5)
		4	1, 3,7	- (5)	ND
	3rd instar	2	22	+ (5)	ND
		3	22	+ (5)	ND
		2	132	+ (5)	7/14
2nd bloodmeal (uninfected mice)	3rd instar	2	60 (3)	+ (5)	+ (5)
		2	64 (7)	+ (5)	+ (5)
	4th instar	2	75 (25)	+ (5)	+ (5)
Uninfected co-fed	2nd instar	N/A	5	ND	15/66
O. moubata ticks	3rd instar	N/A	45	ND	4/15
I. ricinus	Nymph	4	2	ND	0/12
1st bloodmeal (infected mice)		-3[d]	2	ND	2/12
		-3[d]	30	ND	0/25
BALB/c mice[e]	N/A	N/A	N/A	- (1)	1/17

[a] Number of days after the ticks had completed feeding on inoculated mice at which the ticks were tested for virus infection. Where indicated brackets depict those ticks that had fed a 2nd time and the number of days after which the ticks were tested.

[b] Tick homogenate samples were scored positive if >10% of inoculated C6/36 cells showed specific fluorescence with both 813 and 546 monoclonal antibodies. Numbers of ticks in each pool are shown in parenthesis.

[c] Where indicated by +, pools of ticks were tested; numbers of ticks in each pool are shown in parenthesis. ND, not done.

[d] I. ricinus ticks depicted -3 were attached to hosts 3 days prior to inoculation with WNV.

[e] Mice were infested with infected O. moubata ticks and after 14 days were sacrificed and the brain homogenates tested by IFA and RT-PCR. N/A, not applicable.

Table 3: Results of immunofluorescence assay (IFA) and/or nested RT-PCR from O. moubata and I. ricinus ticks fed either on WNV inoculated BALB/c mice or non-infected mice (co-fed ticks).

at -70°C until analysed. Tick homogenates were assayed for infectious virus antigen (by immunofluorescence assay) and/or viral RNA (by RT-PCR).

Co-feeding transmission experiments were carried out by infesting clean BALB/c mice (n=7 (Harlan, UK)) with ten 3rd instar O. moubata ticks 57 days after they had taken an infectious bloodmeal, and ten uninfected ticks (2nd instar) in separate feeding chambers. The two feeding chambers were separated by at least 1 cm. Co-feeding experiments lasted 15 days.

To investigate tick to host transmission ten BALB/c mice were infested with cohorts of five, ten, fifteen or twenty 3rd instar O. moubata ticks 57 days after an infectious bloodmeal. Fifteen days after infestation, the mice (including those used for co-feeding) were euthanised and the brains removed. The brains were homogenised in 1 ml of sterile PBS and stored at -70°C until they were tested for WNV.

2.4   Immunofluorescence Assays (IFA)

Indirect immunofluorescence assays (IFA) were carried out on fixed cells as described previously (E. A. Gould, *et al.*, 1985a). Cells were treated with a monoclonal antibody (mAb813) that is specific for the E-protein of flaviviruses and is broadly cross-reactive (E. A. Gould, *et al.*, 1985a). WNV infected cells were additionally probed with WNV-specific monoclonal antibody (mAb 546) (E.A. Gould, *et al.*, 1990). Goat anti-mouse polyvalent antiserum conjugated with fluorescein-isothiocyanate (Sigma) was used as a secondary antibody. Incubation times for each antibody were 1 hr at 37°C. Washes (x3) were carried out in PBS at room temperature. Infected cells were visualized using an Olympus epifluorescence microscope and photographs taken using a Nikon epifluorescence microscope and camera. Uninfected cultures of each cell line were used as negative controls and appropriately infected Vero cells were used as positive controls. Examples of typically infected cells are shown in Figure 1. Cell cultures were designated infected if more than 5% of cells showed specific fluorescence (Table 1). Unless indicated, IFA were carried out on cells from the second sub-culture. Tick samples were deemed positive when more than 10% of the cells showed specific fluorescence with both monoclonal antibodies (Table 3).

2.5   Virus Titration by Plaque Assay

The porcine kidney cell line PS was grown in Eagles Minimal Essential Medium containing 7% fetal calf serum and plaque assays were carried out in 24-well plates using a 1.5% CMC overlay as described previously (E.A. Gould, *et al.*, 1985b). Cells were incubated at 37°C (+5% CO_2) for 4 days and the plates were then stained with naphthalene black.

2.6   Nested RT-PCR Assay

RNA was extracted from homogenised samples (100 µl) using RNAgents total RNA extraction kit in accordance with the manufacturer's instructions (Promega). cDNA synthesis was carried out with Superscript II reverse transcriptase (Invitrogen) and 3'(1) primer (primer sequences can be found at (Lawrie, *et al.*, 2004a)) for 50 minutes at 42°C, in a total volume of 20 µl. PCR was carried out on the cDNA (1µl) using 5'(1) and 3'(1) primers. Nested PCR was carried out on 1 µl of the first-round PCR product using the nested primers 5'(2) and 3'(2). All PCR reactions were carried out in a 50 µl volume with REDTaq DNA polymerase (Sigma). A Hybaid Touchdown thermal cycler was used with the following programme: 94.5 °C for 1min, thirty cycles of 94 °C for 40s, 56°C for 1 min and 72°C for 1 min followed by a final extension step of 72°C for 10 mins. Viral stock, RNA extracted from uninfected ticks and PBS only containing samples were used as control reactions. Positive samples gave a PCR product of about 1.2 kbp. This method could detect RNA from a viral stock equivalent of 9 pfu (data not shown).

To confirm the identity of RT-PCR products, PCR products were gel purified using QIAquick (Qiagen) columns in accordance with manufacturer's instructions. The purified DNA was sequenced with an ABI automatic sequencer and the nested primers 5'(2) and 3'(1), and a primer based upon the internal sequence of the E gene of WNV (not shown).

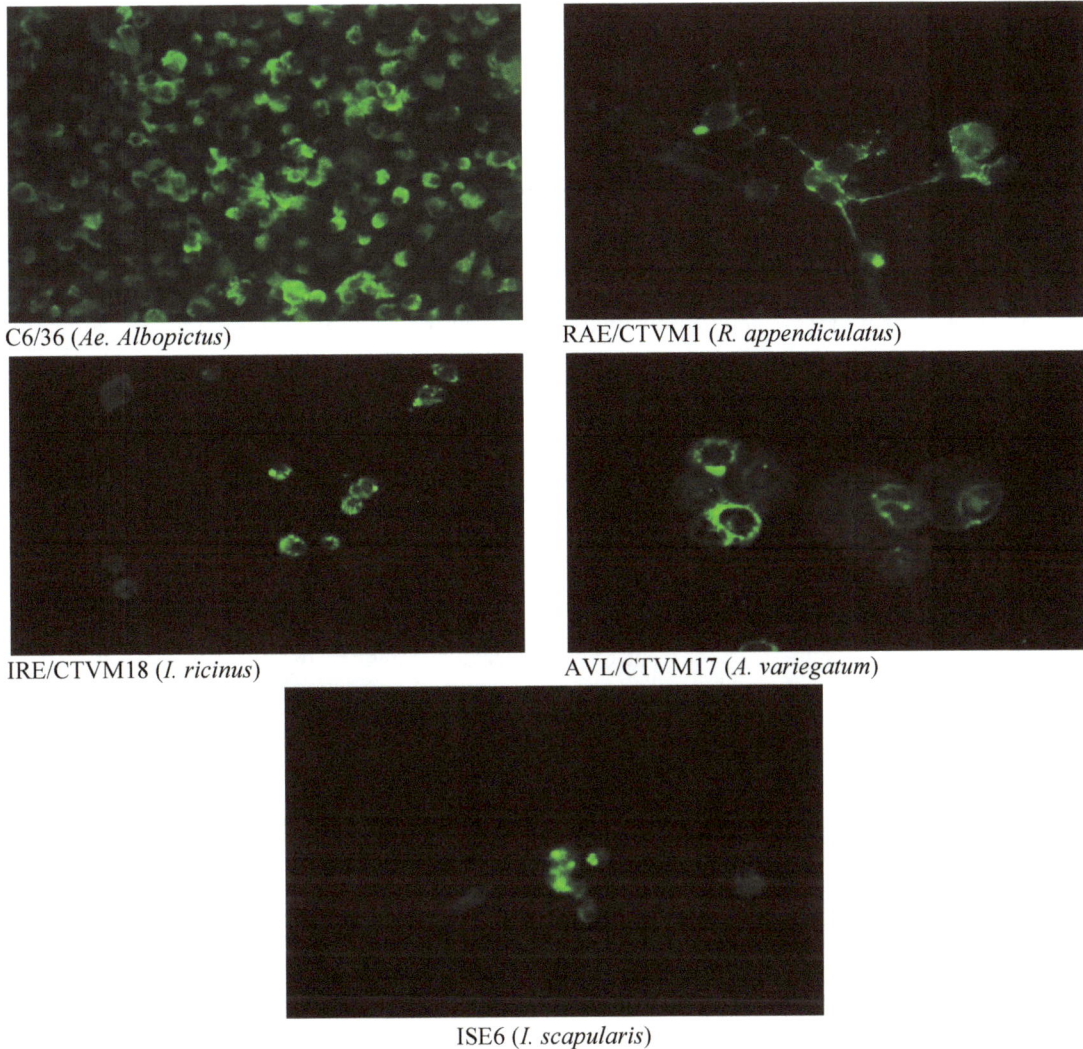

C6/36 (*Ae. Albopictus*)

RAE/CTVM1 (*R. appendiculatus*)

IRE/CTVM18 (*I. ricinus*)

AVL/CTVM17 (*A. variegatum*)

ISE6 (*I. scapularis*)

Figure 1: Examples of mosquito and tick cells infected with WNV (NY-99 strain). Cells were visualized using a Nikon epifluorescence microscope with FITC filter. Magnification 20x. *Reproduced from Lawrie et al (2004) Med. Vet. Entomol., 18*(3), 268-274.

3   Results

3.1   Physiological Competence of Tick Cells for WNV infection

The mosquito cell line C6/36 showed no signs of infection by the tick-borne viruses tested, or by *Apoi virus* or *Modoc virus,* that have no known vector. By contrast, C6/36 cells were positive for viral antigen after infection with the mosquito-borne flaviviruses (Table 1). The tick cell lines RAE/CTVM1, IRE/CTVM18, AVL/CTVM17 and ISE6 were tested for their susceptibility to infection with the viruses indicated in Table 1. All the different tick cell lines tested were susceptible to infection by the same viruses. Moreover, there was no appreciable difference in the cytoplasmic distribution of viral antigen in infected cells between either individual cell lines or the different viruses tested (Figure 1).

All tick cell lines were susceptible to infection by the tick-borne flaviviruses but not the mosquito-borne flaviviruses, with the exception of WNV (both strains). The mean titer of recovered WNV (NY99) sub-cultured three times in RAE/CTVM1 cells was 4.1 x 10^4 pfu ml-1 (Table 2). Examples of RAE/CTVM1, IRE/CTVM18, AVL/CTVM17 and ISE6 cells infected with WNV (NY99) and immunoprobed with mAb813 are shown in Figure 1.

3.2 Host to Tick Transmission

BALB/c mice inoculated with WNV were weakly viremic, two and three days after injection, with mean titers of $6x10^3$ and $3x10^3$ pfu ml^{-1} blood respectively. After four days, viremia was no longer detectable by plaque assay although the mice developed severe neurological symptoms after five or six days and were humanely killed. *O. moubata* ticks that had fed on mice on days corresponding to the viremic period (i.e. days 2 and 3 after inoculation), but not those fed outside this period, contained viral antigen as measured by IFA (Table 3). Two days after engorgement, 17% (n=12) *I. ricinus* ticks that started to feed on hosts three days prior to WNV inoculation, but not those that had started to feed four days after inoculation, were positive for WNV RNA. When the former group of ticks was tested 28 days later no evidence of infection was found. Infected *O. moubata* ticks in contrast maintained the virus after having molted into the next instar (i.e. 3rd instar), following a second non-infectious bloodmeal and after having molted for a second time into 4th instars. Fifty percent of the individual ticks (n=14) tested by RT-PCR were positive for WNV RNA when examined 132 days after the initial infectious bloodmeal.

3.3 Co-feeding Transmission

Five days post-engorgement, 23% (n=66) of uninfected 2nd instar *O. moubata* ticks that had co-fed with infected cohorts of 3rd instar ticks on non-infected mice were positive for WNV RNA (Table 3). The remaining unfed ticks (n=15) were tested after they had molted into 3rd instars, 45-days after co-feeding. Four of these ticks (27%) were positive for WNV RNA. The identities of the PCR products obtained from three positive samples were confirmed by sequence analysis.

3.4 Tick to Host Transmission

Infected cohorts of *O. moubata* ticks (3rd instar) were fed on uninfected mice in order to investigate tick to host transmission. Of the seventeen uninfected mice used (including mice used in co-feeding experiments), none showed clinical signs of infection. One of the brains tested, from a mouse infested with an infected cohort of 20 ticks, was positive by RT-PCR but negative when tested by IFA (Table 3). The PCR product was sequenced to confirm the identity of WNV.

4 Discussion

The distinction between mosquito-borne and tick-borne flaviviruses was initially based upon immunological and ecological relationships (Gould *et al.*, 1985; Gould *et al.*, 1990). More recently, phylogenetic analysis has confirmed this classification and revealed the existence of mosquito-borne, tick-borne and NKV clades within the Flavivirus genus (Gaunt *et al.*, 2001). Arthropod primary cell and tissue cultures, and subsequently continuous cell lines have proven to be valuable tools in the study of arboviruses (Mussgay *et al.*, 1975; Pudney, 1987; Singh, 1972). However, relatively little is known of the susceptibility of tick cell lines to arbovirus infection as until recently few tick cell lines were available. This study and others show that in general the ability of a particular flavivirus to infect either mosquito or tick cells, or in the case of NKV viruses neither cell types, reflects this classification. Nevertheless, despite the evolutionary distance between the mosquito-borne and tick-borne virus lineages, it is clear that some flaviviruses such as WNV can infect and replicate in both mosquito and tick cell lines.

Although WNV is phylogenetically and serologically defined as a mosquito-borne flavivirus (Gaunt *et al.*, 2001), our results demonstrated that WNV can infect and maintain infection in tick-derived cell lines. These results are consistent with previous studies of *R. appendiculatus*, *Boophilus microplus* (Canestrini) and *D. parumapertus* (Neumann) cell lines (Pudney, 1987; Varma, *et al.*, 1975), although a *Haemaphysalis spinigera* (Neumann) derived cell line tested by Banerjee *et al* was not susceptible to WNV infection (Banerjee, *et al.*, 1977). So in other words it appears that unlike other mosquito-borne flaviviruses, there is no intrinsic cellular barrier to infection of tick-derived tissue by WNV.

Next we tested the transmission ability of ticks as vectors for WNV. Our study demonstrated that both *I. ricinus* and *O. moubata* ticks become infected with WNV (NY99 strain) through feeding upon virus-inoculated rodent hosts, but only when these hosts were viremic (i.e. systemic transmission). Thirty days after engorgement, however, we no longer found any evidence of WNV infection in the *I. ricinus* ticks. This suggests that this tick species does not support replication of the virus, and therefore is not a competent vector of WNV. Consequent research has shown similar results with other ixodid species. *I. scapularis* (the main US Lyme disease vector), *A. americanum (L.)*, *Dermacentor andersoni*, and *D. variabilis* ticks were demonstrated to acquire WNV, and retain the virus transstadially, but were not able to transmit WNV back to the host (J.F. Anderson, *et al.*, 2003b). More recently *I. pacificus* ticks fed on viremic song sparrows were also able to acquire WNV but unable to effectively transmit the virus to either birds or western fence lizards, the natural host species of this tick (Reisen, *et al.*, 2007). *Hyalomma marginatum* ticks were fed on rabbits infected with WNV and all three developmental stages were found to acquire the virus, and to maintain it transstadially but not trans-ovarially (Formosinho, *et al.*, 2006).

In contrast to *I. ricinus* ticks, we found that infected *O. moubata* ticks maintained infectious virus for at least 132 days (length of experiment) and WNV persisted transtadially through at least two developmental stages. Evidence for tick to host transmission of WNV was found in our study, although the level of infection observed was low (i.e. sub-clinical). Again these data are consistent with previous transmission studies carried out with soft tick species. Whitman & Aitken observed much higher levels of transmission from WNV-infected *O. moubata* ticks to day-old chicks than in our study, but only when very high feeding densities were used (49 ticks per chick) (Whitman, *et al.*, 1960). *O. maritimus* and *O. erraticus* infected ticks were shown to transmit WNV to uninfected mice (Vermeil, *et al.*, 1959, 1960), although *O. savignyi* and *O. erraticus* ticks did not (Hurlbut, 1956; Taylor, *et al.*, 1956). An artificial membrane system was used to infect *A. arboreus* ticks, which were then able to transmit the virus to uninfected hosts (Abbassy, *et al.*, 1994), and more recently *Carios capensis* ticks were shown to acquire and effectively transmit WNV to pekin ducklings (*Anas domesticus*) (Hutcheson, *et al.*, 2005).

The transmission of flaviviruses such as *Tick-borne encephalitis virus* (TBEV) and *Louping-ill virus* (LIV) from infected to non-infected ixodid ticks through co-feeding on non-viraemic hosts (non-systemic transmission) is a well-established phenomenon (Randolph, *et al.*, 1996). Indeed this mode of transmission is believed to play a significant role in the epidemiology of these diseases (Randolph, *et al.*, 1999). Therefore we tested for co-feeding transmission of WNV between infected and uninfected *O. moubata* ticks. Over 22% of the uninfected ticks were positive for WNV RNA five days after co-feeding. A similar percentage of ticks were positive forty days later, after having molted to the next developmental stage. As co-fed ticks were in contact with the mice for less than 24 hours, this strongly suggests that WNV was non-systemically transmitted between infected and uninfected ticks, as there was insufficient time for viremia to develop. Consistent with these findings consequent research by Higgs *et al* demonstrated that the primary vector of WNV, *C. pipiens* could also become infected through co-feeding on non-viremic hosts (Higgs, *et al.*, 2005).

In summary, these data suggest that argasid (soft) but not ixodid (hard) tick species can mechanically acquire, maintain and transmit WNV. These data are however somewhat at odds with field collected records that describe the frequent isolation of WNV not only from soft ticks (Hoogstraal, 1972; Hoogstraal, *et al.*, 1976; Lvov, *et al.*, 1975), but also hard ticks including *I. ricinus, I. lividus, R. turanicus, A. variegatum, H. marginatum, D. marginatus* species (reviewed by Anderson *et al.*, (J. F. Anderson, *et al.*, 2003a). This discrepancy suggests that ixodid ticks are dead-end vectors for WNV transmission but can acquire infection naturally, most likely due to exposure to viremic hosts, although given the results of the experiments mentioned above it would be tempting to believe that co-feeding between ticks and vector-competent mosquito species might also occur.

So what about argasid (soft) ticks, are they likely to be important vectors of WNV? Like other arboviruses, WNV is naturally maintained by an enzootic cycle, consisting of *C. pipiens,* the major vector species and passerine birds as the major amplifying hosts (Komar, *et al.*, 2003). Although WNV infects a number of non-avian vertebrates, most mammals, including humans, appear to be dead-end hosts as they routinely fail to develop sufficient viraemia in order to re-infect a vector and hence continue the transmission cycle. Even though argasid ticks appear to have the ability to be physiologically competent vectors for WNV, in reality the low level of virus infection acquired by these ticks coupled with the fact that tick-to-host transmission appears to be very inefficient when compared to mosquito transmission (Hurlbut, 1956), suggests that ticks are unlikely to be important vectors of WNV. Furthermore, the relative scarcity of WNV isolation from field collected ticks suggest that whilst natural infections can occur, the frequency is insufficient to play a significant role in the natural transmission cycle of WNV. Additionally, in any case it is important to realise that argasid ticks are highly unlikely to represent a danger to the public in the current US epidemic, as although these ticks are common in Northern America, unlike hard ticks, soft ticks only very rarely parasitize land animals or humans (Sonenshine, 1991).

Acknowledgements

This study was supported by funding from the Starmer-Smith memorial lymphoma fund, Leukaemia and Lymphoma Research and Ikerbasque, the Basque Foundation for Science.

References

Abbassy, M.M., Stein, K.J., & Osman, M. (1994). New artificial feeding technique for experimental infection of Argas ticks (Acari: Argasidae). J Med Entomol, 31(2), 202-205.

Aiken, L. (2003). Health Canada "nearly blindsided" by West Nile virus incidence. Can. Med. Assoc. J., 168(6), 756.

Anderson, J.F., Main, A.J., Andreadis, T.G., Wikel, S.K., & Vossbrinck, C.R. (2003a). Transstadial transfer of West Nile virus by three species of ixodid ticks (Acari: Ixodidae). J Med Entomol, 40(4), 528-533.

Anderson, J.F., Main, A.J., Andreadis, T.G., Wikel, S.K., & Vossbrinck, C.R. (2003b). Transstadial transfer of West Nile virus by three species of ixodid ticks (Acari: Ixodidae). J. Med. Entomol., 40(4), 528-533.

Banerjee, K., Guru, P.Y., & Dhanda, V. (1977). Growth of arboviruses in cell cultures derived from the tick Haemaphysalis spinigera. Indian J. Med. Res., 66(4), 530-536.

Campbell, G.L., Marfin, A.A., Lanciotti, R.S., & Gubler, D.J. (2002). West Nile virus. Lancet Infectious Diseases, 2, 519-529.

Centers for Disease Control and Prevention. (2002a). Provisional surveillance summary of the West Nile virus epidemic-United States, January-November 2002. MMWR. Morb. Mortal. Wkly. Rep., 51(50), 1129-1133.

Centers for Disease Control and Prevention. (2002b). West Nile virus- Entomology, from http://www.cdc.gov/ncidod/dvbid/westnile/mosquitoSpecies.htm

Donaldson, J.M. (1966). An assessment of Culex pipiens quinquefasciatus say as a vector of viruses in the Witwatersrand region of the Transvaal. I. West Nile virus. S Afr J Med Sci, 31(1), 1-10.

Formosinho, P., & Santos-Silva, M.M. (2006). Experimental infection of Hyalomma marginatum ticks with West Nile virus. Acta Virol, 50(3), 175-180.

Gould, E.A., Buckley, A., Cammack, N., Barrett, A.D.T., Clegg, J.C.S., Ishak, R., & Varma, M.G.R. (1985a). Examination of the immunological relationships between flaviviruses using yellow fever virus monoclonal antibodies. J. Gen. Virol., 66(7), 1369-1382.

Gould, E.A., Buckley, A., Higgs, S., & Gaidamovich, S.Y. (1990). Antigenicity of flaviviruses. Arch Virol, Sup. 1, 137-152.

Gould, E.A., & Clegg, J.C.S. (1985b). Growth, titration and purification of alphaviruses and flaviviruses. In B. W. J. Mahy (Ed.), Virology- A practical approach (pp. 43-78). Oxford: IRL.

Hayes, E.B., Komar, N., Nasci, R.S., Montgomery, S.P., O'Leary, D.R., & Campbell, G.L. (2005). Epidemiology and transmission dynamics of West Nile virus disease. Emerg Infect Dis, 11(8), 1167-1173.

Higgs, S., Schneider, B.S., Vanlandingham, D.L., Klingler, K.A., & Gould, E.A. (2005). Nonviremic transmission of West Nile virus. Proc Natl Acad Sci U S A, 102(25), 8871-8874. doi: 0503835102 [pii] 10.1073/pnas.0503835102

Hoogstraal, H. (1972). Birds as tick hosts and as reservoirs and disseminators of tickborne infectious agents. Wiad. Parazytol., 18(4), 703-706.

Hoogstraal, H., Clifford, C.M., Keirans, J.E., Kaiser, M.N., & Evans, D.E. (1976). The Ornithodoros (Alectorobius) capensis group (Acarina: Ixodoidea: Argasidae) of the palearctic and oriental regions. O. (A.) maritimus: identity, marine bird hosts, virus infections, and distribution in western Europe and northwestern Africa. J. Parasitol., 62(5), 799-810.

Hubalek, Z., & Halouzka, J. (1999). West Nile fever--a reemerging mosquito-borne viral disease in Europe. Emerg Infect Dis, 5(5), 643-650.

Hurlbut, H.S. (1956). West Nile virus infection in arthropods. Am J Trop Med Hyg, 5, 76-85.

Hutcheson, H.J., Gorham, C.H., Machain-Williams, C., Lorono-Pino, M.A., James, A.M., Marlenee, N.L., Winn, B., Beaty, B.J., & Blair, C.D. (2005). Experimental transmission of West Nile virus (Flaviviridae: Flavivirus) by Carios capensis ticks from North America. Vector Borne Zoonotic Dis, 5(3), 293-295. doi: 10.1089/vbz.2005.5.293

Iakimenko, V.V., Bogdanov, II, Tagil'tsev, A.A., Drokin, D.A., & Kalmin, O.B. (1991). The characteristics of the relationships of arthropods of the refuge complex with the causative agents of transmissible viral infections in bird rookeries. Parazitologiia, 25(2), 156-162.

Jones, L.D., Davies, C.R., Steele, G.M., & Nuttall, P.A. (1988). The rearing and maintenance of ixodid and argasid ticks in the laboratory. Animal Technology, 39(2), 99-106.

Komar, N., Langevin, S., Hinten, S., Nemeth, N., Edwards, E., Hettler, D., Davis, B., Bowen, R., & Bunning, M. (2003). Experimental infection of north american birds with the new york 1999 strain of west nile virus. Emerg Infect Dis, 9(3), 311-322.

Kramer, L.D., Styer, L.M., & Ebel, G.D. (2008). *A global perspective on the epidemiology of West Nile virus. Annu Rev Entomol, 53, 61-81. doi: 10.1146/annurev.ento.53.103106.093258*

L'Vov, D.K., Dzharkenov, A.F., L'Vov D, N., Aristova, V.A., Kovtunov, A.I., Gromashevskii, V.L., Vyshemirskii, O.I., Galkina, I.V., Al'khovskii, S.V., Samokhvalov, E.I., Prilipov, A.G., Deriabin, P.G., Odolevskii, E.I., & Ibragimov, R.M. (2002). *Isolation of the West Nile fever virus from the great cormorant Phalacrocorax carbo, the crow Corvus corone, and Hyalomma marginatum ticks associated with them in natural and synanthroic biocenosis in the Volga delta (Astrakhan region, 2001). Vopr Virusol, 47(5), 7-12.*

Lanciotti, R.S., Roehrig, J.T., Deubel, V., Smith, J., Parker, M., Steele, K., Crise, B., Volpe, K.E., Crabtree, M.B., Schrret, J.H., Hall, R.A., MacKenzie, J.S., Cropp, C.B., Panigrahy, B., Ostlund, E., Schmitt, B., Malkinson, M., Banet, C., Weissman, J., Komar, N., Savage, H.M., Stone, W., McNamara, T., & Gubler, D.J. (1999). *Origin of the West Nile virus responsible for an outbreak of encephalitis in the northeastern United States. Science, 286, 2333-2337.*

Lane, R.S. (1994). *Competence of ticks as vectors of microbial agents with an emphasis on Borrelia burgdorferi. In D. E. Sonenshine & T. N. Mather (Eds.), Ecological dynamics of tick-borne zoonoses (pp. 45-67). Oxford: Oxford University Press.*

Lawrie, C.H., Uzcategui, N.Y., Armesto, M., Bell-Sakyi, L., & Gould, E.A. (2004a). *Susceptibility of mosquito and tick cell lines to infection with various flaviviruses. Med Vet Entomol, 18(3), 268-274.*

Lawrie, C.H., Uzcategui, N.Y., Gould, E.A., & Nuttall, P.A. (2004b). *Ixodid and argasid tick species and west nile virus. Emerg. Infect. Dis., 10(4), 653-657.*

Lvov, D.K., Timopheeva, A.A., Smirnov, V.A., Gromashevsky, V.L., Sidorova, G.A., Nikiforov, L.P., Sazonov, A.A., Andreev, A.P., Skvortzova, T.M., Beresina, L.K., & Aristova, V.A. (1975). *Ecology of tick-borne viruses in colonies of birds in the USSR. Med. Biol., 53(5), 325-330.*

Mathiot, C.C., Georges, A.J., & Deubel, V. (1990). *Comparative analysis of West Nile virus strains isolated from human and animal hosts using monoclonal antibodies and cDNA restriction digest profiles. Res. Virol., 141(5), 533-543.*

Monath, T.P., & Heinz, F.X. (1996). *Flaviviruses. In B. N. Fields, D. M. Knipe & P. M. Howley (Eds.), Fields Virology (3 ed., Vol. 1, pp. 961-1034). New York: Lippincott-Raven.*

Mussgay, M., Enzmann, P.-J., Horzinek, M.C., & Weiland, E. (1975). *Growth cycle of arboviruses in vertebrate and arthropod cells. Prog. Med. Virol., 19, 257-323.*

Platonov, A.E. (2001). *West Nile encephalitis in Russia 1999-2001: Were we ready? Are we ready? Ann N Y Acad Sci, 951, 102-116.*

Pudney, M. (1987). *Tick cell lines for the isolation and assay of arboviruses. In Yunker (Ed.), Arboviruses in arthropod cells in vitro. Boca Raton: CRC Press.*

Randolph, S.E., Gern, L., & Nuttall, P.A. (1996). *Co-feeding ticks: Epidemiological significance for tick-borne pathogen transmission. Parasitology Today, 12(12), 472-479.*

Randolph, S.E., Miklisova, D., Lysy, J., Rogers, D.J., & Labuda, M. (1999). *Incidence from coincidence: patterns of tick infestations on rodents facilitate transmission of tick-borne encephalitis virus. Parasitology, 118(Pt 2), 177-186.*

Reisen, W.K., Brault, A.C., Martinez, V.M., Fang, Y., Simmons, K., Garcia, S., Omi-Olsen, E., & Lane, R.S. (2007). *Ability of transstadially infected Ixodes pacificus (Acari: Ixodidae) to transmit West Nile virus to song sparrows or western fence lizards. J Med Entomol, 44(2), 320-327.*

Smithburn, K.C., Hughes, T.P., Burke, A.W., & Paul, J.H. (1940). *A Neurotropic Virus Isolated from the Blood of a Native of Uganda. American Journal of Tropical Medicine 20, 471-472.*

Sonenshine, D.E. (1991). *Biology of ticks (Vol. 1). Oxford: Oxford University Press.*

Sonenshine, D.E., & Mather, T.N. (1994). *Ecological dynamics of tick-borne zoonoses. Oxford: Oxford University Press.*

Swallow, W.H. (1985). *Group testing for estimating infection rates and probabilities of disease transmission. Phytopathology, 75, 882-889.*

Taylor, R.M., Work, T.H., Hurlbut, H.S., & Rizk, F. (1956). A study of the ecology of West Nile virus in Egypt. Am J Trop Med Hyg, 5, 579-620.

Varma, M.G., Pudney, M., & Leake, C.J. (1975). The establishment of three cell lines from the tick Rhipicephalus appendiculatus (Acari: Ixodidae) and their infection with some arboviruses. J. Med. Entomol., 11(6), 698-706.

Vermeil, C., Lavillaureix, J., & Reeb, E. (1959). Infection et transmission experimentales du virus West Nile par Ornithodorus coniceps (Canestrini) de souche Tunisienne. Bull. Soc. Pathol. Exot., 51, 489-495.

Vermeil, C., Lavillaureix, J., & Reeb, E. (1960). Sur la conservation et la transmission du virus West Nile par quelques arthropodes. Bull Soc Path Exot, 53, 273-279.

Whitman, L., & Aitken, T.H.G. (1960). Potentiality of Ornithodorus moubata Murray (Acarina, Argasidae) as a reservoir-vector of West Nile virus. Ann. Trop. Med. Parasitol., 54, 192-204.

The Risk of Introducing Tick-Borne Encephalitis and Crimean-Congo Hemorrhagic Fever into Southwestern Europe (Iberian Peninsula)

Ana M. Palomar, Aránzazu Portillo
Department of Infectious Diseases
Hospital San Pedro-Centre of Biomedical Research of La Rioja, Spain

José M. Eiros
Department of Pathological Anatomy, Microbiology, Preventive Medicine and Public Health
University of Valladolid, Spain

José A. Oteo
Department of Infectious Diseases
Hospital San Pedro-Centre of Biomedical Research of La Rioja, Spain

1   Introduction

Arboviral infections are world-wide distributed viral infections transmitted by arthropods, such as insects and ticks.

Ticks are arthropods (Arachnida belonging to Acari), ectoparasites and blood-sucking of vertebrates (mammals, birds and reptiles). They may act as vectors, intermediate hosts and reservoirs of a wide variety of infectious agents.

There are three families of ticks: Nutalliellidae, Argasidae (soft ticks) and Ixodidae (hard ticks). This last one is the most diverse, with at least 692 described species in the world (Nava *et al.*, 2009), and with great importance in human and animal (veterinary) health (Jongejan & Uilenberg, 2004). The life cycle of a tick comprises three growth stages: larva, nymph and adult (male and female) (Figure 1). In this cycle, animals (wildlife, livestock and/or companion animals) can act as reservoirs or amplifier hosts and humans are accidental hosts. In favourable conditions, it takes from months (i.e. *Rhipicephalus* spp.) to 1-3 years (i.e. *Ixodes ricinus*) for the tick to hatch from the egg, go through all three stages, reproduce, and then die. Ticks normally feed on more than one host. This fact gives them a high potential for pathogens transmission such as bacteria, protozoa or viruses.

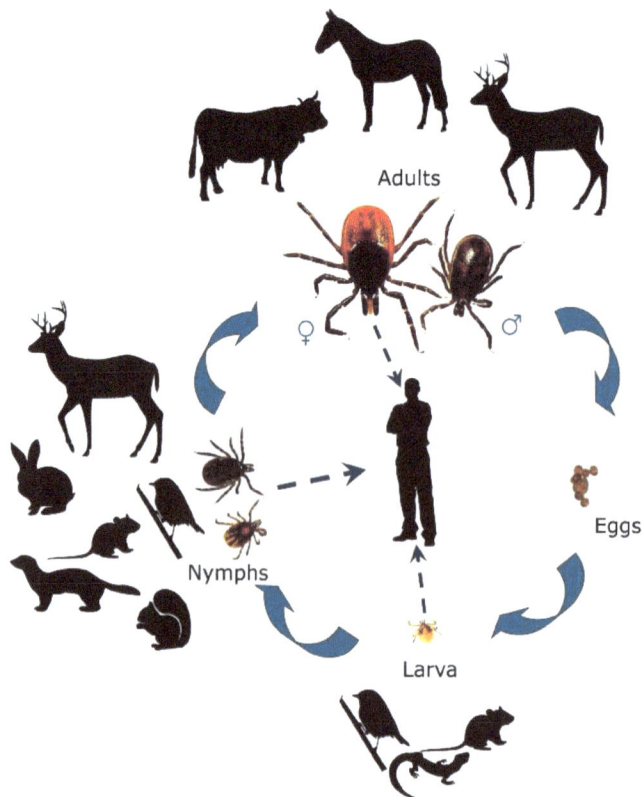

Figure 1. Life cycle of the hard tick *Ixodes ricinus* (courtesy of the authors).

Tick-bites may cause diseases by different pathogenic mechanisms. They may cause anaemia in animals they parasite (in some cases there are hundreds of ticks feeding on a unique animal), preventing them to get fatter and causing important economic losses. Ticks may also cause paralysis by inoculation of neurotoxins, allergic reactions and local injury with subsequent risk of super-infection by skin bacteria. Nevertheless, the most important mechanism of disease transmission is through the inoculation of pathogenic microorganisms.

Among factors for a tick-borne disease to be present in a certain area, we should consider: (1) The presence of the tick vector (each tick species is associated to particular microorganisms); (2) the presence of the reservoir (an organism able to maintain and amplify the pathogen without developing disease, and that in some cases may be the tick); (3) the susceptibility of each individual to the inoculated agent.

The Iberian Peninsula has different geographic and climatic zones with great contrasts, from wetlands up to desert areas. This fact coupled with the diversity of the fauna, favours the presence of many species of hard ticks and a broad spectrum of associated diseases (Table 1).

Tick (Vector of disease)	Pathogen	Disease	Presence of human TBD in the Iberian Peninsula	Reference of human TBD in the Iberian Peninsula
Ixodes ricinus	*B. burgdorferi* s.l.	Lyme borreliosis	Yes	Oteo *et al.*, 2000a
	A. phagocytophilum	Human anaplasmosis	Yes	Oteo *et al.*, 2000b
	R. monacensis	Rickettsiosis	Yes	Jado *et al.*, 2007
	Babesia spp.	Babesiosis	Yes	Miguelez *et al.*, 1996
	Louping ill virus	TBE-Like	No[1]	
Dermacentor marginatus	*R. slovaca*	DEBONEL/TIBOLA	Yes	Oteo *et al.*, 2004
	Candidatus R. rioja	DEBONEL/TIBOLA	Yes	Portillo *et al.*, 2009
Hyalomma spp.	CCHFV	CCHF	NC	Filipe *et al.*, 1985
	Dhori virus	Innominated	NC	Filipe *et al.*, 1985
Rhipicephalus sanguineus group	*R. conorii*	MSF	Yes	Bacellar *et al.*, 1999
	R. massiliae	Rickettsiosis	Yes[2]	García-García *et al.*, 2010
	Thogoto virus	Innominated	NC	Filipe *et al.*, 1985
Haemaphysalis punctata	Bhanja virus (Palma virus)	Innominated	NC	Filipe *et al.*, 1985

TBD: Tick-borne disease; *B.*: *Borrelia*; s.l.: sensu lato; *A.*: *Anaplasma*; *R.*: *Rickettsia*; TBE: Tick-Borne Encephalitis; DEBONEL: *Dermacentor*-borne necrosis erythema lymphadenopathy; TIBOLA: Tick-borne lymphadenopathy; CCHFV: Crimean-Congo Hemorrhagic Fever Virus; CCHF: Crimean-Congo Hemorrhagic Fever; NC: not confirmed (only serological evidence in humans); MSF: Mediterranean spotted fever.

[1] Only detected in sheep and goats (Gonzalez *et al.*, 1987; Balseiro *et al.*, 2012).

[2] Confirmed in a patient returning to Spain from Argentina.

Table 1. Species of hard ticks with medical importance present in the Iberian Peninsula as well as the main pathogens they transmit and the associated human tick-borne diseases.

The list of tick-borne diseases (TBD) has grown in the last years. There are recent reviews of TBD caused by bacteria (Parola *et al.*, 2005; Stanek *et al.*, 2011; Oteo & Portillo, 2012; Portillo & Oteo; 2012). However, other TBD can be under-diagnosed or misdiagnosed in our environment due to the lack of clinical or diagnostic tools, or because they have not been previously present. This could be the case of human infection with *Candidatus* Neoehrlichia mikurensis. Only five cases of this bacterial infection have been reported in Europe (Welinder-Olsson *et al.*, 2010; von Loewenich *et al.*, 2010; Fehr *et al.*, 2010; Pekova *et al.*, 2011). Nevertheless, the identification of the causative agent in European *I. ricinus* ticks suggests that the incidence of this TBD could be higher.

At present, prevalence and geographic distribution of infections caused by tick-borne arboviruses (the arboviruses with greatest importance in human health, after dengue virus) also appear to increase (Ergonul, 2006; Mansfield *et al.*, 2009; Ergonul, 2012; Hubálek & Rudolf, 2012). This may be due to better diagnostic tools and greater knowledge and surveillance on ticks (Donoso Mantke *et al.*, 2011) but there are other factors that may influence this increase. Thus, climate change may favour the increase in populations of vectors and hosts in some regions (Parola *et al.*, 2008; Estrada-Peña *et al.*, 2012a). Cultural, social and economic changes that favour the conservation of natural areas and their enjoyment are associated to an increase in tick populations and greater exposure of humans to tick-bites (Figure 2). Migrations of the hosts favour the circulation of their ectoparasites and consequently of their infectious agents (Waldenström *et al.*, 2007; Palomar *et al.*, 2012). Furthermore, the import of livestock (Chisholm *et al.*, 2012), hunting species or pets such as exotic reptiles that may be parasitized by infected ticks, should also be considered (Pietzsch *et al.*, 2006; Nowak, 2010a; Nowak, 2010b; Rataj *et al.*, 2011).

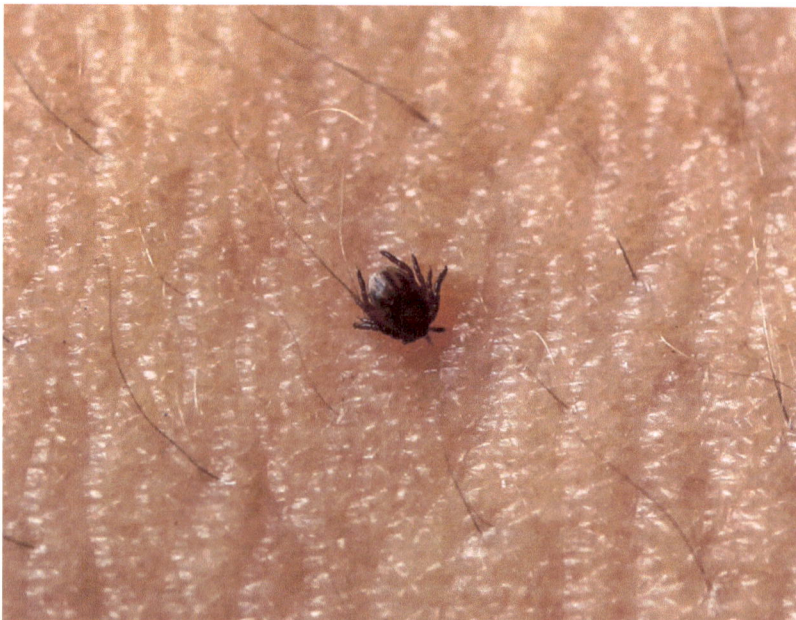

Figure 2. *Ixodes ricinus* nymph attached to a patient (courtesy of the authors)

At least, 27 tick-borne viruses have been described in Europe (Hubálek & Rudolf, 2012). Some of them cause serious diseases (i.e. Tick-Borne Encephalitis Virus, TBEV), while others (i.e. Eyach virus) are less pathogenic or seem to be associated (serological data) with infrequently reported human infections in Western Europe (Málková *et al.*, 1980; Herpe *et al.*, 2007). In this chapter, we will focus on TBEV and Crimean-Congo Hemorrhagic Fever Virus (CCHFV) because of their severity and distribution.

2   Tick-Borne Encephalitis Virus (TBEV)

TBEV is a single-stranded RNA virus that belongs to the *Flavivirus* genus, family Flaviviridae. Virions are of small size (40-60 nm), with lipid envelope and spherical structure (Figure 3). TBEV has three main subtypes: European, Siberian, and Far Eastern (Mansfield *et al.*, 2009). Some authors also include Louping ill virus in the TBE complex (Grard *et al.*, 2007).

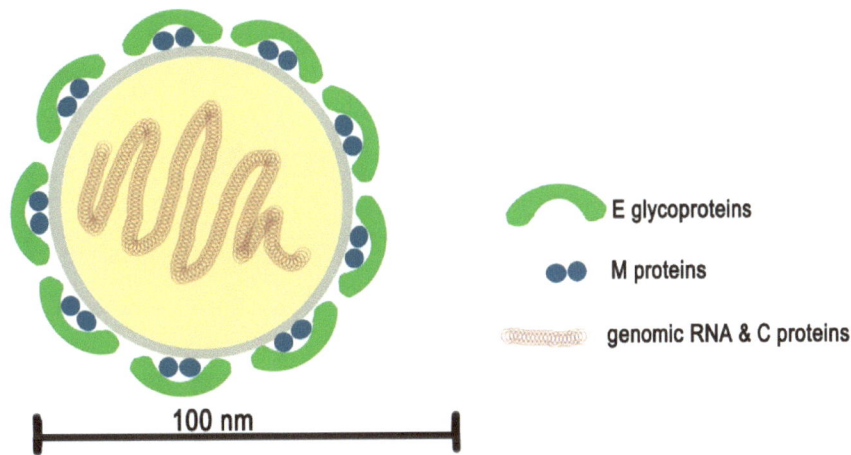

E glycoproteins

M proteins

genomic RNA & C proteins

100 nm

Figure 3: Structure of the mature phase of Tick-Borne Encephalitis virus (courtesy of the authors).

TBEV has been identified in several species of ticks and *I. ricinus* (European subtype), *Ixodes persulcatus* (Siberian and Far-Eastern subtypes) and *Ixodes ovatus* (Far-Eastern subtype in some areas of Japan) are recognized vectors (Figure 4). The virus has transovarial and transestadial transmission in ticks. Thus, the arthropod acts as vector and reservoir. Nevertheless, some authors defend the necessity of the co-feeding (transmission of pathogens between two ticks that feed very near on a host at the same time) for the viral infection to persist (Randolph, 2011). In addition to ticks, small mammals such as rodents of the genera *Apodemus* and *Myodes* (bank vole) (Süss, 2011) may act as amplifiers of the infection and, probably, as reservoirs (if the microorganism may persist in the rodent for a long time). Transmission of the infection occurs mainly by tick-bites, but cases of infection by the ingestion of contaminated, not pasteurized milk have been also reported (Süss, 2011).

TBE is the main viral disease transmitted by ticks in Eurasia, where cases of the disease have been reported in at least 32 countries (Süss, 2011). The disease is distributed in endemic foci in middle latitudes from Japan to France, and it has been also reported in South of the Scandinavian countries, North of Greece, Anatolia and Central and Northern China (Figure 5) (Petri *et al.*, 2010; Süss, 2011; Ergunay, 2011). The incidence of infection is increasing, even reaching 400% increase in countries without vaccination programme (Süss, 2008).

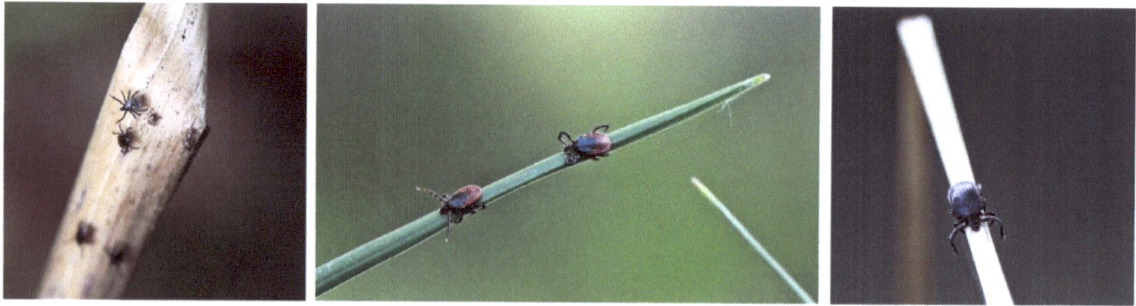

Figure 4: *Ixodes ricinus* specimens waiting for hosts over vegetation. Left to right: Larvae and nymphs; two females; a male (courtesy of the authors).

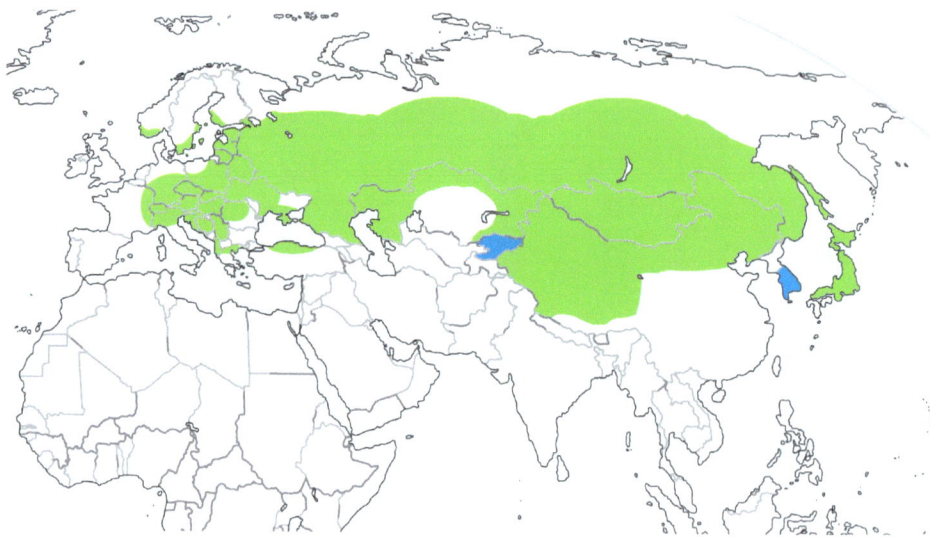

Figure 5: Known distribution of cases of Tick-Borne Encephalitis Virus (modified from Süss, 2011 and Dobler *et al.*, 2012). Countries with autochthonous cases of the disease are shown in green. Countries without reported cases of illness but where the virus has been amplified from ticks and/or from cattle are shown in blue.

TBE is the main viral disease transmitted by ticks in Eurasia, where cases of the disease have been reported in at least 32 countries (Süss, 2011). The disease is distributed in endemic foci in middle latitudes from Japan to France, and it has been also reported in South of the Scandinavian countries, North of Greece, Anatolia and Central and Northern China (Figure 5) (Petri *et al.*, 2010; Süss, 2011; Ergunay, 2011). The incidence of infection is increasing, even reaching 400% increase in countries without vaccination programme (Süss, 2008).

Up to date, the presence of TBEV has not been detected in the Iberian Peninsula, although conditions are ideal for the circulation of the virus: Vectors (*I. ricinus* is the tick species that more frequently bites humans in the North of the Iberian Peninsula) as well as reservoirs are part of the faunal diversity. In addition, the presence of the Louping ill virus (closely related to TBEV) has been confirmed in countries such as Spain (González *et al.*, 1987; Balseiro *et al.*, 2012). Furthermore, the possibility of co-feeding of larval and nymphal *I. ricinus* in Spain has been reported (Barandika *et al.*, 2010), and we have observed co-feeding in birds from La Rioja (northern Spain) (Figure 6).

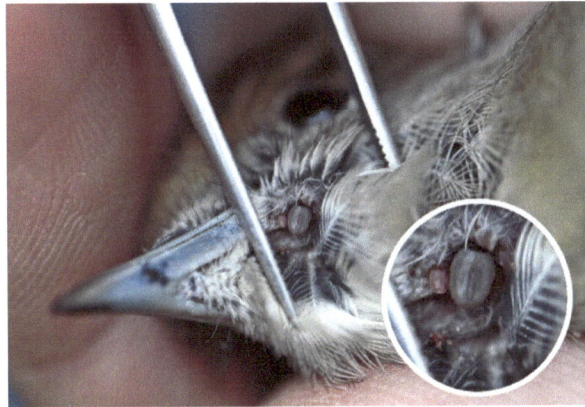

Figure 6. *Ixodes ricinus* nymph and larva feeding on a Eurasian Blackcap (*Sylvia atricapilla*) captured in Spain (courtesy of the authors).

The disease has a biphasic febrile clinical course. After an incubation period ranging from 7 to 14 days, appears the initial phase or viremia that lasts from 2 to 4 days. In this phase the symptoms are not very specific (fever, anorexia, headache, nausea, myalgia and arthralgia). After around 8 days of remission, a second phase that affects the central nervous system, causing meningitis and/or encephalitis and/or radiculitis may appear. The mortality rate is 0-3%, and patients may have important neurological sequelae (Mansfield *et al.*, 2009). In some cases, TBE may co-exist with Lyme borreliosis since both diseases share ecological niche and vector. Clinical laboratory findings are nonspecific and may include leukopenia, thrombocytopenia, discrete elevation of transaminases at a first stage and later, elevation of leukocytes (Figure 7).

In the first phase, the virus can be detected by reverse transcription polymerase chain reaction (RT-PCR) techniques or by culture from patient specimens (cerebrospinal fluid, serum and/or heparinized plasma). This last procedure requires a Biosafety Level 3-Laboratory. In the following stages diagnosis is based on the detection of IgG and IgM antibodies using enzyme-linked immunosorbent assay (ELISA). This technique has cross reactions with other flaviviruses antibodies, and it is not useful if the patient has been previously vaccinated (Mansfield *et al.*, 2009).

Prevention measures of TBE are to avoid tick-bites and the ingestion of unpasteurized milk. There are vaccines for primary prophylaxis of the infection that have showed to be very effective in endemic areas.

3   Crimean-Congo Hemorrhagic Fever Virus (CCHFV)

CCHFV, which is the causal agent of the CCHF, belongs to the *Nairovirus* genus, family Bunyaviridae. Virions are spherical, approximately 90-100nm in diameter, with lipid envelope and three genomic segments (S, M and L) of single-stranded RNA and negative polarity (Figure 8). Up to 8 different genotypes are known (Ergonul & Whitehouse, 2007).

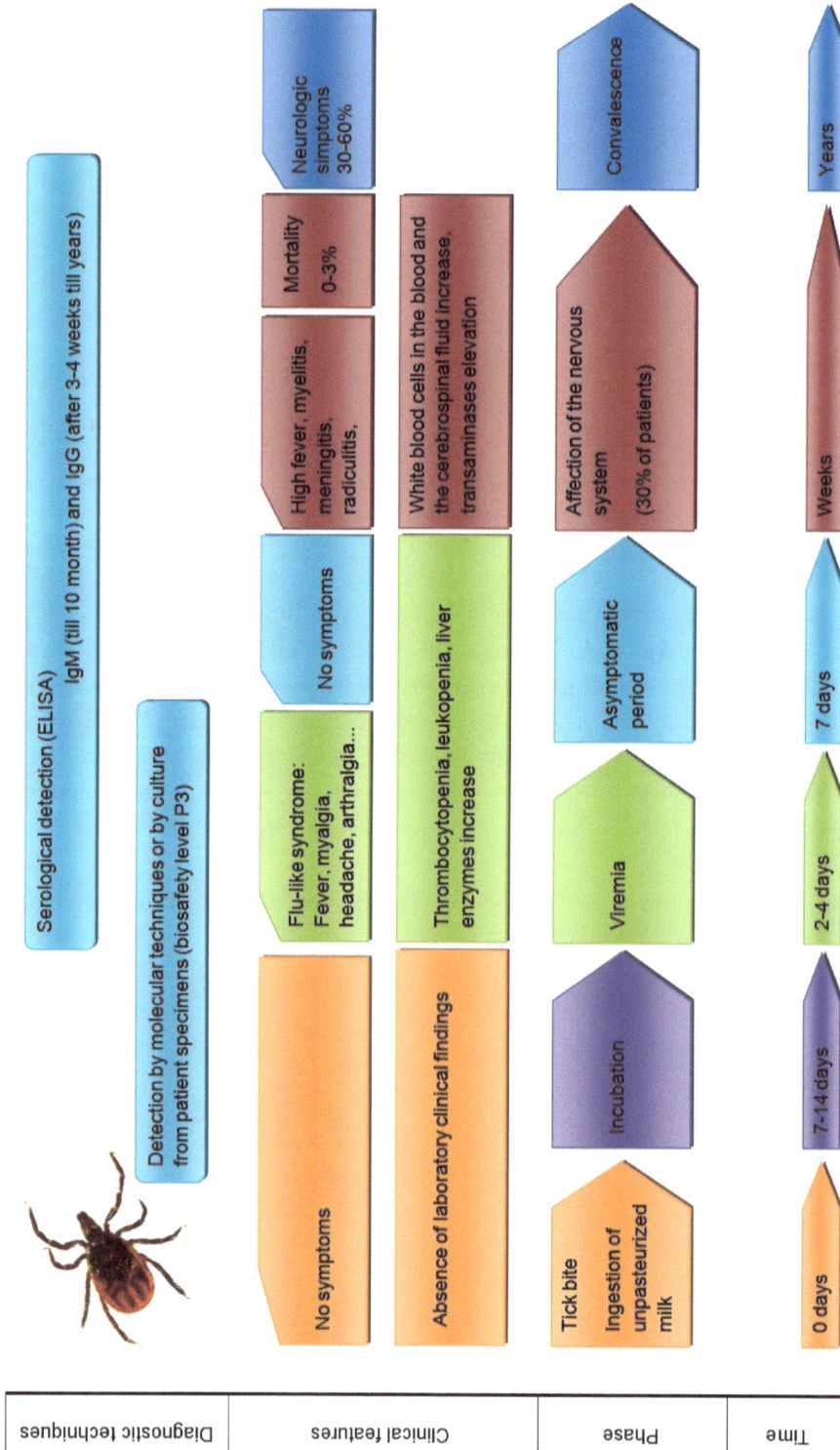

'**Figure 7.** Clinical and laboratory course of Tick-Borne Encephalitis Virus (courtesy of the authors).

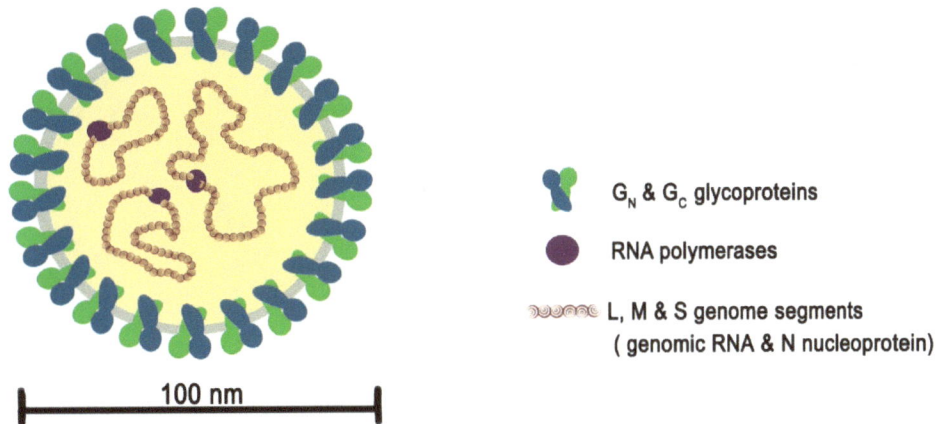

Figure 8. Structure of the mature phase of Crimean-Congo Hemorrhagic Fever Virus (courtesy of the authors).

CCHF is, after dengue, the arboviral disease with the greatest importance in human health due to its wide geographic distribution (Africa, Asia and South-Eastern Europe), the risk of acquisition, and its potential high percentage of mortality (up to 30%, and even >60% in outbreaks) (Khan *et al*., 1997; Ergonul, 2006; Ergonul, 2012).

The virus circulates in a cycle of enzootic tick-vertebrate-tick in which there is no evidence that cause disease in animals. Humans become infected through tick bites, by crushing infected ticks, after contact with a patient with CCHF during the acute phase of infection, or by contact with blood or tissues from infected livestock.

CCHFV has been isolated from at least 33 tick species belonging to the genera: *Hyalomma, Amblyomma, Rhipicephalus, Boophilus, Ixodes, Dermacentor, Haemaphysalis, Argas* and *Ornithodoros*, but most of them are not competent vectors. *Hyalomma marginatum* is considered the most important vector of the disease (Figure 9) (Turell, 2007). This tick species acts as reservoir since CCHFV is transmitted transovarial and transestadially. Small mammals (rodents) are also major reservoirs. Larger mammals and some birds such as ostriches seem to be important for the epidemiology of the virus (Ergonoul & Whitehouse, 2007). Birds harboring infected ticks suggest the dispersion of the virus during migrations, as it has been published by our group (Palomar *et al*., 2013), among others (Lindeborg *et al*, 2012). Although recent studies report low environmental suitability for the survival of foreign immature *H. marginatum* ticks introduced in Spain by migratory birds (EFSA, 2010; Bosch *et al*., 2012), the average temperatures recorded in spring in northern Spain during 2011 would have allowed ticks to molt.

Since the first documented and confirmed cases of CCHF in Crimea (1944) and Democratic Republic of the Congo (1956), outbreaks have been reported in the Balkans (Albania, ex-Yugoslavia), Bulgaria, Turkey, Iran, Iraq, United Arab Emirates, Saudi Arabia, Kuwait, Oman, Pakistan, Afghanistan, Former USSR, China, Uganda, Namibia, South Africa, Tanzania, Senegal, Kenya, Mauritania and Burkina Faso (Ergonul, 2006). More recently, cases of infection have been also described in Sudan, Greece, Georgia and India (Papa *et al*., 2008; Zakhashvili *et al*., 2010; Aradaib *et al*., 2011; Patel *et al*., 2011; Ergonul, 2012) (Figure 10). In addition, seroepidemiological studies in healthy population have evidenced the circulation of the virus in countries such as Turkmekistan, Nigeria, Egypt, Madagascar, Hungary, France, Portugal, Benin, Zimbabwe, Guinea, Cameroon, Congo and Romania (David-West *et al*.,

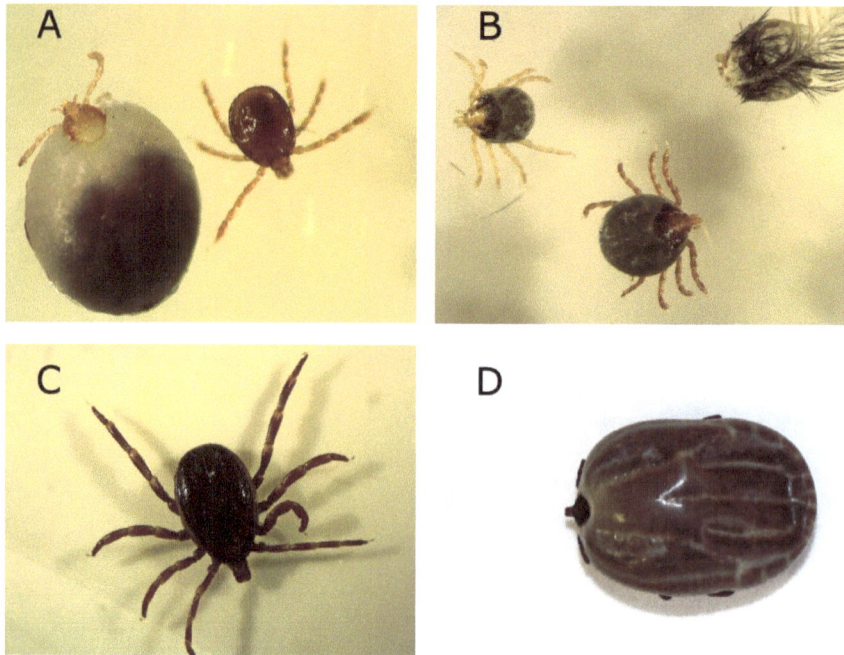

Figure 9. *Hyalomma marginatum* specimens. A: Larvae (unfed and engorged); B: Nymphs; C: Male; D: Engorged female (courtesy of the authors).

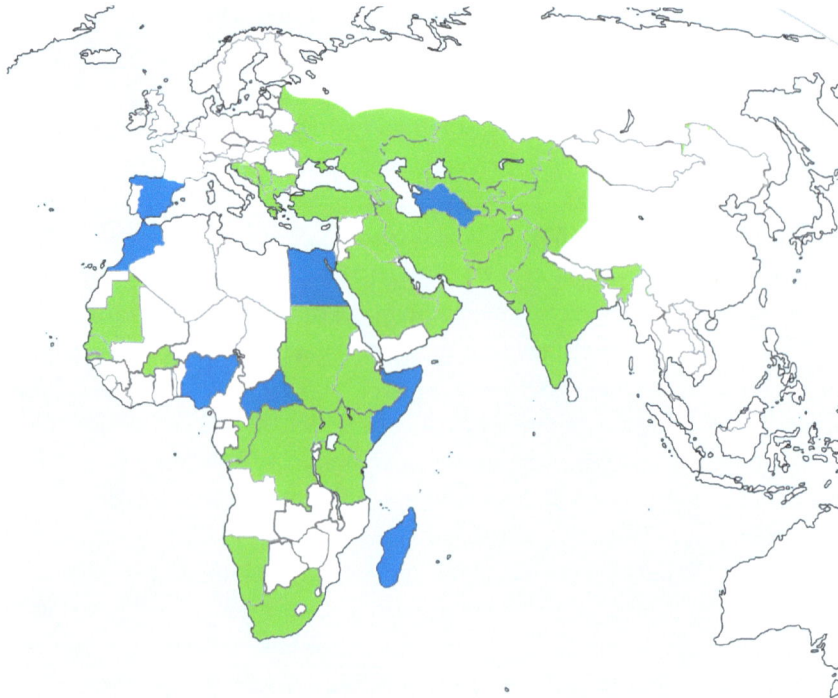

Figure 10. Known distribution of cases of Crimean-Congo Hemorrhagic Fever Virus, year 2012. Countries with autochthonous cases of the disease are shown in green. Countries without autochthonous cases of illness but where the virus has been amplified from ticks and/or from cattle are shown in blue.

1974; Smirnova *et al.*, 1978; Blackburn *et al.*, 1982, Gonzalez *et al.*, 1989; Andriamandimby *et al.*, 2011; Ergonul, 2012; Ceianu *et al.*, 2012). Furthermore, imported cases of CCHF have been diagnosed in other European countries such as England, Germany and France (Jauréguiberry *et al.*, 2005; ECDC 2008; Tall *et al.*, 2009).

Generally, the CCHF infection courses in four phases. The incubation period varies between 3 and 7 days after the acquisition of the virus. Fever (39-41°C), headache, myalgia and dizziness may appear for about 3 days during the prehemorrhagic period. In the hemorrhagic period (2-3 days following the onset of the disease), ecchymosis and petechiae of the skin and mucous membranes, as well as gastrointestinal bleeding are common. This phase may cause the death of the patient. During the period of convalescence (about 10 days), breathing difficulties, tachycardia, loss of hair, hearing or memory may be present in survivors (Ergonul, 2006; Ergonul, 2012). Thrombocytopenia, leukopenia and increased levels of lactate dehydrogenase, some aminotransferases and creatinine phosphokinase (CPK) are the typical clinical laboratory findings. Alterations in coagulation may be observed (Figure 11).

Cell cultures (only sensitive in the first five days of infection and carried out in a Biosafety Level 4-Laboratory) as well as RT-PCR assays from blood samples (sensitive in the first 9 days of infection) and the detection of IgG antibodies by ELISA (from the first week and up to 5 years) are used for diagnosis of CCHF.

There is no commercial vaccine or demonstrably effective treatment. Nevertheless, the use of ribavirin for the treatment is recommended (Ergonul, 2012).

4   Situation in the Iberian Peninsula (Southwestern Europe)

The climatic and geographic heterogeneity of Southwestern Europe, located between two very contrasting areas such as Eurasia and Africa, is responsible for the high diversity of habitats and their biological richness, with abundant and diverse tick populations, and accordingly, their associated diseases. The changes of the environmental conditions (climatic and anthropological changes) could favor the establishment of new populations of ticks and their tick-borne pathogens (Estrada *et al.*, 2012a). In this context, we will focus on the Iberian Peninsula, which is located in Southwestern Europe and has environmental and climatic conditions that favor the presence of several tick species (up to 29 species of hard ticks have been identified) and reservoirs, and where numerous tick-borne diseases have been reported. Some of them, such as Lyme borreliosis, Mediterranean spotted fever and *Dermacentor*-borne, necrosis, erythema and lymphadenopahy (DEBONEL) are endemic or very prevalent in our environment (Oteo *et al.*, 2000a; Oteo & Portillo, 2012).

The presence of CCHFV and TBEV in European areas with climate conditions, vegetation and fauna similar to those in the Iberian Peninsula (Hubálek & Rudolf, 2012), along with the presence of tick populations recognized as main vectors of these viruses (*I. ricinus* and *H. marginatum*), the increasing number of human tick-bites from these tick species observed in our area (Figure 12), the previous detection of Louping ill virus (closely related to TBEV) in ticks and livestock (González *et al.*, 1987; Balseiro *et al.*, 2012), the import of livestock and pets, and the existence of febrile syndromes and encephalitis cases of unknown etiology after tick-bites have made necessary monitoring the presence of these viruses in our country. Moreover, the Iberian Peninsula is a stopover or breeding site in the migratory routes of several bird species (Hoyo *et al.*, 2004), and migratory birds have been demonstrated to be carriers of infected ticks (Palomar *et al.*, 2013). The existence of the co-feeding has been also suggested (Barandika *et al.*, 2010), and this phenomenon has been observed by our group (Figure 6).

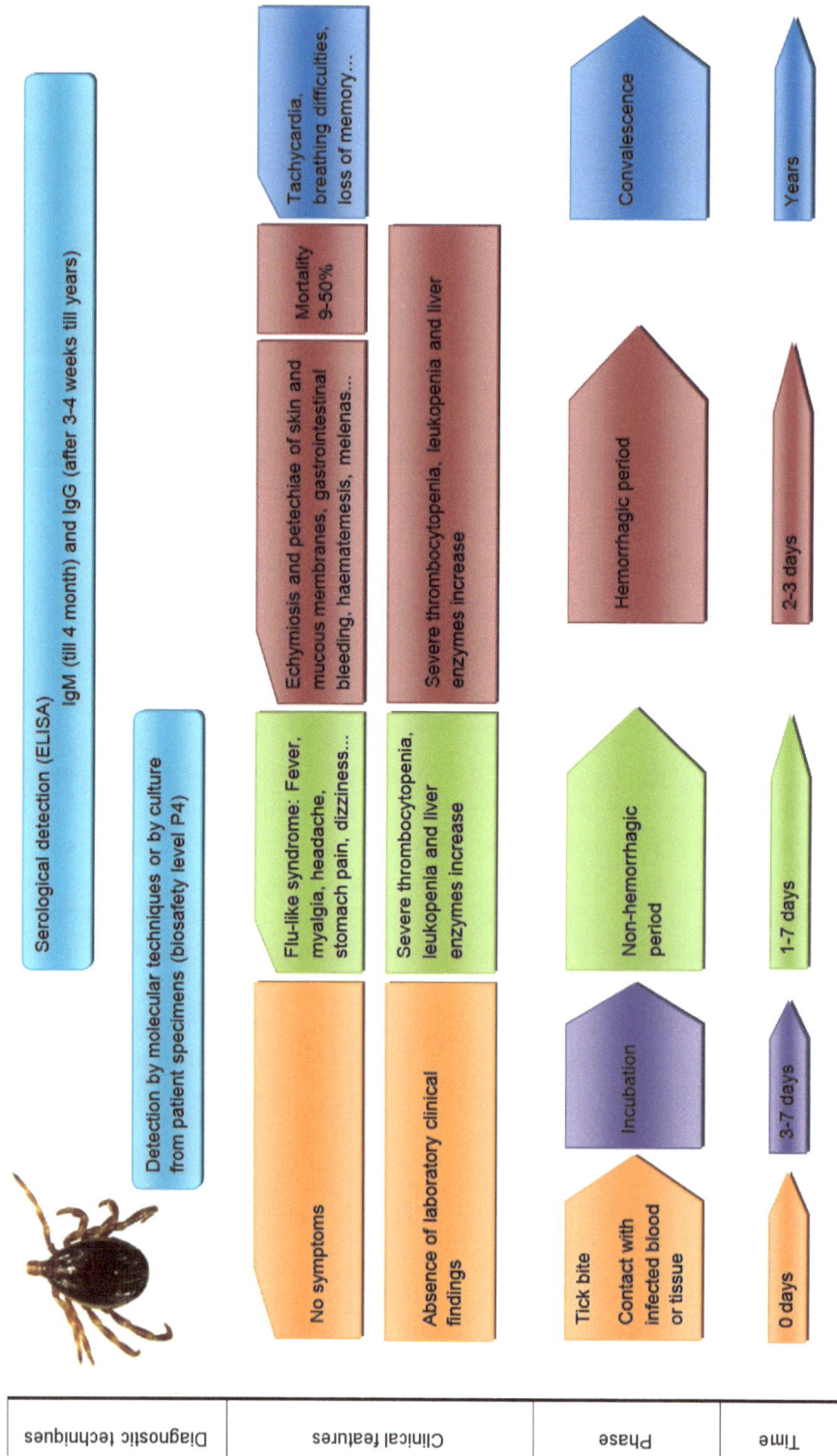

Figure 11. Clinical and laboratory course of Crimean–Congo Hemorrhagic Fever (courtesy of the authors).

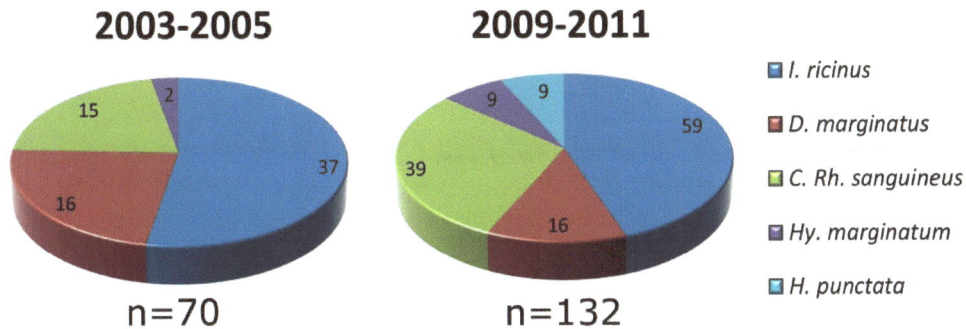

Figure 12. Number of ticks removed from patients at the Hospital of La Rioja (North of Spain; 320,000 inhabitants in the province). Years, **A**: 2003-2005; **B**: 2009-2011. *I.*: *Ixodes*; *D.*: *Dermacentor*; C: Complex; *Rh.*: *Rhipicephalus*; *Hy.*: *Hyalomma*; *H*: *Haemaphysalis*.

The reasons for the absence of these viral diseases in Southwestern Europe are unknown, and even febrile syndromes and encephalitis cases may have been misdiagnosed. Thus, an investigation aimed to detect TBEV and CCHFV in ixodid ticks from La Rioja (North of Spain) and other Spanish provinces is being performed at the Centre of Rickettsiosis and Arthropod-Borne Diseases, Area of Infectious Diseases, Hospital San Pedro-Centre of Biomedical Research from La Rioja (CIBIR), Logroño, Spain. This project was funded by the "Fondo de Investigación Sanitaria", Ministry of Science and Innovation (PS09/02492), Spain. The following sections detail the methodology and results obtained from January 2010 to June 2012. Other study about the risk of TBEV infection was carried out in the same area (Barandika *et al.*, 2010).

4.1 TBEV in Spain

Ticks belonging to *I. ricinus* species were captured from vegetation (blanket dragging technique) and mammals (cows and deer) during years 2010 and 2011. Collected specimens, except larvae (n=1,055), were processed for the study of the presence of TBEV in La Rioja. A total of 1,000 nymphs and 1,020 adults were grouped in pools of 10 or 5 individuals, respectively. Samples were homogenized and RNA was extracted using RNeasy Mini Kit (Qiagen, Hilden, Germany) according to the manufacturer's recommendations. Reverse transcription to cDNA was performed using Omniscript RT (Qiagen, Hilden, Germany). The presence of TBEV was tested using qPCR for the detection of a fragment of the noncoding 3' region (Schwaiger & Cassinotti, 2003).

TBEV was not found in any samples. Our results agree with those obtained in a previous study carried out in ticks from the North of Spain (Basque Country and La Rioja) (Barandika *et al.*, 2010). Nevertheless, these data support but do not confirm the absence of the virus in Spain (Stefanoff *et al.*, 2012).

Disease surveillance plans should be followed. As previously stated, in Spain there are established tick populations of the TBEV vector (*I. ricinus*) and reservoirs (small mammals), the phenomenon of co-feeding occurs (our observation; Figure 6), as previously suggested (Barandika *et al.*, 2010), and the circulation of a subtype of the virus (Louping ill) transmitted by the same tick species has been demonstrated in our environment (González *et al.*, 1987; Balseiro *et al.*, 2012). Furthermore, in Europe, TBE and

Lyme borreliosis have similar distribution (epidemiology), and Lyme borreliosis is endemic in the North of Spain (Oteo *et al.*, 2000a).

4.2   CCHFV in Spain

From the end of 2009 to mid-2012, removal of *H. marginatum* specimens from cattle and poultry was carried out in La Rioja. In addition, *Hyalomma lusitanicum* specimens were collected over deer in the province of Cáceres (Southwestern Spain) in November 2010. A total of 473 *H. marginatum* ticks (12 larvae, 21 nymphs and 440 adult ticks), and 117 *H. lusitanicum* adult specimens were processed. Specimens were grouped in pools of 10 specimens or individually if immature, homogenized and RNA was extracted using RNeasy Mini Kit (Qiagen, Hilden, Germany) according to the recommendations of the manufacturer. Reverse transcription to cDNA was performed using Omniscript RT (Qiagen, Hilden, Germany). Conventional PCR and qPCR assays for the amplification of different fragments of the S segment of CCHFV were performed (Midilli *et al.*, 2007; 2009; Burt & Swanepoel, 2005; Atkinson *et al.*, 2012).

CCHFV was not detected in *H. marginatum*, but it was found in *H. lusitanicum*. Two out of 12 analyzed pools were positive using a fragment of the S segment (211 bp) as PCR target (Midilli *et al.*, 2009). Only one sequence could be obtained. When compared with those deposited in GenBank, it showed 98% identity with CCHFV strains from Sudan and Mauritania (Estrada-Peña *et al.*, 2012b). These results were confirmed by the National Centre for Microbiology (Instituto de Salud Carlos III, Madrid, Spain).

This is the first detection of CCHFV in Southwestern Europe (Figure 10). The genetic identity with African strains (and not European), allowed us to hypothesize about the presence of the virus in Spain and the arrival of CCHFV-infected ticks through migratory birds (Estrada-Peña *et al.*, 2012b). Furthermore, in April 2011 bird ringings were carried out in Zoula (Morocco), which is on the route of birds that migrate from central and southern Africa to Europe in spring. Ticks parasitizing these birds were collected for the investigation of CCHFV. A total of 52 *H. marginatum* specimens (all immature stages) were studied. RNA was extracted using AllPrep DNA/RNA Mini Kit (Qiagen, Hilden, Germany). Reverse transcription to cDNA was performed using Omniscript RT (Qiagen, Hilden, Germany). A total of 6 pools were tested by PCR as previously described (Midilli *et al.*, 2009) and four pools yielded positive results, showing a minimum infection rate of 7.7%. Sequences (n=3) obtained from the S fragment (211 bp) were identical each other, and homologous (100% identity) to Sudan AB1-2009 and Mauritania ArD39554 strains, showing almost 99% identity with those previously detected in ticks from Cáceres (Palomar *et al.*, 2013). These PCR-positive pools contained ticks removed from long-distance migratory bird species that nest and/or make stopover in the Iberian Peninsula. This is the first detection of CCHFV in Morocco (Figure 10). The study confirms the role of birds as dispersal of infected ticks, and supports the theory of the entry of the virus in the Iberian Peninsula through migratory birds coming from Africa (Palomar *et al.*, 2013) (Figure 13).

The data presented herein confirm the need to establish a CCHFV surveillance plan for European countries with risk of receiving bird populations from Africa, such as Spain or Portugal. Furthermore, healthcare workers should be informed about the CCHF and the clinical picture in the potential "endemic" areas. Moreover, potential risk groups (healthcare workers, hunters, farmers…), and potential reservoirs (livestock) should be further investigated.

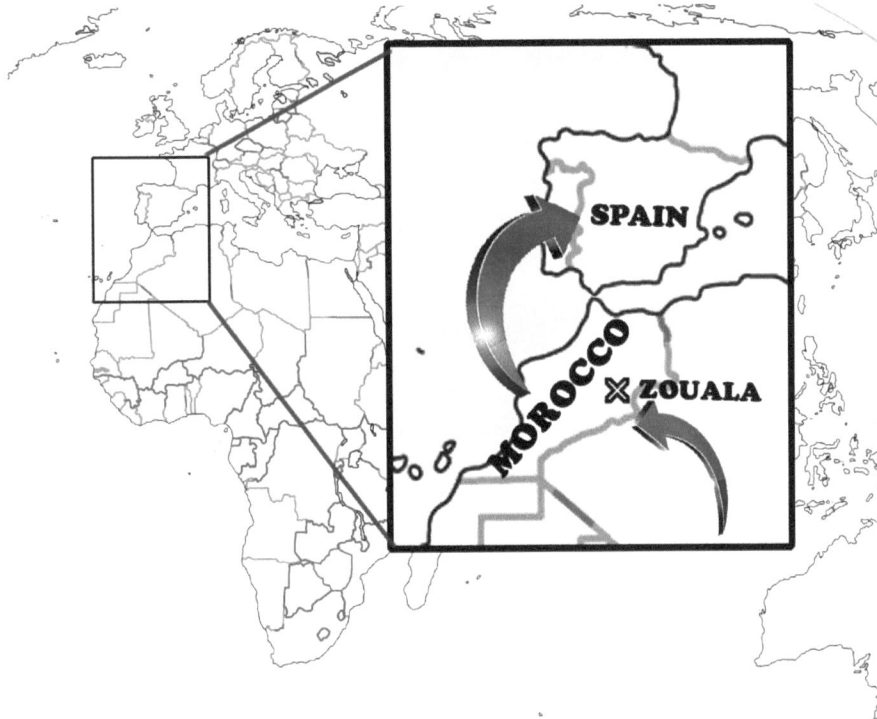

Figure 13. Map showing some of the migratory routes of birds from Central and South of Africa to Zouala (Morocco), and from there to Southwestern Europe.

In summary, these data suggest that the TBEV could establish in the Iberian Peninsula although, to our knowledge, it has not been detected in our area. In addition, the circulation of the CCHFV has been demonstrated and the risk of acquiring CCHF exists in Southwestern Europe. To raise awareness of healthcare workers is crucial in risk areas, and TBEV and CCHFV surveillance systems are required.

Acknowledgement

This study was partly supported by grants from Fondo de Investigación Sanitaria, Ministerio de Ciencia e Innovación, Spain (PS09/02492 and PI12/02579).

References

Andriamandimby, S.F., Marianneau, P., Rafisandratantsoa, J.T., Rollin, P.E., Heraud, J.M., Tordo, N., Reynes, J.M. (2011). Crimean-Congo hemorrhagic fever serosurvey in at-risk professionals, Madagascar, 2008 and 2009. Journal of Clinical Virology, 52, 370-372.

Aradaib, I.E., Erickson, B.R., Karsany, M.S., Khristova, M.L., Elageb, R.M., Mohamed, M.E., & Nichol, S.T. (2011). Multiple Crimean-Congo hemorrhagic fever virus strains are associated with disease outbreaks in Sudan, 2008-2009. PLOS Neglected Tropical Diseases, 5, e1159.

Atkinson, B., Chamberlain, J., Logue, C.H., Cook, N., Bruce, C., Dowall, S.D. & Hewson, R. (2012). Development of a real-time RT-PCR assay for the detection of Crimean-Congo hemorrhagic fever virus. Vector-Borne and Zoonotic Diseases, 12, 786-793.

Bacellar, F., Beati, L., França, A., Poças, J, & Regnery, R., & Filipe, A. (1999). Israeli Spotted Fever Rickettsia (Rickettsia conorii complex) associated with human disease in Portugal. Emerging Infectious Diseases 5, 835-836.

Balseiro, A., Royo, L.J., Martínez, C.P., Fernández de Mera, I.G., Höfle, Ú., Polledo, L., Marreros, N., Casais, R., & Marín, J.F. (2012). Louping ill in goats, Spain, 2011. Emerging Infectious Diseases, 18, 976-978.

Barandika, J.F., Hurtado, A., Juste, R.A., & García-Pérez, A.L. (2010). Seasonal dynamics of Ixodes ricinus in a 3-year period in northern Spain: first survey on the presence of tick-borne encephalitis virus. Vector-Borne and Zoonotic Diseases, 10, 1027-1035.

Blackburn, N.K., Searle, L., Taylor, P. (1982). Viral haemorrhagic fever antibodies in Zimbabwe schoolchildren. Transactions of the Royal Society of Tropical Medicine and Hygiene, 76, 803-805.

Bosch, J., Muñoz, M.J., Martínez, M., de la Torre, A., & Estrada-Peña, A. (2012). Vector-borne pathogen spread through ticks on migratory birds: A probabilistic spatial risk model for South-Western Europe. Transboundary and Emerging Diseases, (In press).

Burt, F.J. & Swanepoel, R. (2005). Molecular epidemiology of African and Asian Crimean-Congo haemorrhagic fever isolates. Epidemiology & Infection, 133, 659-666.

Ceianu, C.S., Panculescu-Gatej, R.I., Coudrier D., Bouloy, M. (2012). First serologic evidence for the circulation of crimean-congo hemorrhagic Fever virus in romania. Vector-Borne and Zoonotic Diseases, 12, 718-721.

Chisholm, K., Dueger, E., Fahmy, N.T., Samaha, H.A., Zayed, A., Abdel-Dayem, M., Villinski, J.T. (2012). Crimean-congo hemorrhagic fever virus in ticks from imported livestock, Egypt. Emerging Infectious Diseases, 18, 181-182.

David-West, T.S., Cooke, A.R., David-West, A.S. (1974). Seroepidemiology of Congo virus (related to the virus of Crimean haemorrhagic fever) in Nigeria. Bulletin of the World Health Organization, 51, 543-546.

Dobler, G., Gniel, D., Petermann, R., & Pfeffer, M. (2012). Epidemiology and distribution of tick-borne encephalitis. Wiener medizinische Wochenschrift, 162, 230-238.

Donoso Mantke, O., Escadafal, C., Niedrig, M., Pfeffer, M., Working Group For Tick-Borne Encephalitis Virus C. (2011). Tick-borne encephalitis in Europe, 2007 to 2009.Euro Surveillance, 29, 16. pii: 19976.

ECDC. (2008). Consultation on Crimean-Congo haemorragic fever prevention and control. Stockholm, September 2008

European Food Safety Authority Panel on Animal Health and Welfare (EFSA). (2010). Scientific opinion on the role of tick vectors in the epidemiology of Crimean-Congo hemorrhagic fever and African swine fever in Eurasia. EFSA Journal, 8, 1703.

Ergonul, O. (2012). Crimean-Congo hemorrhagic fever virus: new outbreaks, new discoveries. Current Opinion in Virology, 2, 215-220.

Ergonul, O. (2006). Crimean-Congo haemorrhagic fever. The Lancet Infectious Diseases, 6, 203-214.

Ergonul, O. & Whitehouse, C.A. (2007). Crimean-Congo hemorrhagic fever: A global perspective, Dordrecht, The Netherlands: Springer.

Ergunay, K., Whitehouse, C.A., & Ozkul, A. (2011). Current status of human arboviral diseases in Turkey. Vector-Borne and Zoonotic Diseases, 11, 731-741.

Estrada-Peña, A., Ayllón, N., & de la Fuente, J. (2012a). Impact of climate trends on tick-borne pathogen transmission. Frontiers in Physiology, 3, 64.

Estrada-Peña, A., Palomar, A.M., Santibáñez, P., Sánchez, N., Habela, M.A., Portillo, A., Romero, L., & Oteo, J.A. (2012b). Crimean-Congo hemorrhagic fever virus in ticks, Southwestern Europe, 2010. Emerging Infectious Diseases, 18, 179-180.

Fehr, J.S., Bloemberg, G.V., Ritter, C., Hombach, M., Lüscher, T.F., Weber, R., & Keller, P.M. (2010). Septicemia caused by tick-borne bacterial pathogen Candidatus Neoehrlichia mikurensis. Emerging Infectious Diseases, 16, 1127-1129.

Filipe, A.R., Calisher, C.H., & Lazuick, J. (1985). Antibodies to Congo-Crimean haemorrhagic fever, Dhori, Thogoto and Bhanja viruses in southern Portugal. Acta Virologica, 29, 324-328.

García-García, J.C., Portillo, A., Núñez, M.J., Santibáñez, S., Castro, B., & Oteo, J.A. (2010). A patient from Argentina infected with Rickettsia massiliae. American Journal of Tropical Medicine and Hygiene, 82, 691-692.

González, L., Reid, H.W., Pow, I., & Gilmour, J.S. (1987). A disease resembling louping-ill in sheep in the Basque region of Spain. Veterinary Record, 121, 12-13.

Gonzalez, J.P., Josse, R., Johnson, E.D., Merlin, M., Georges, A.J., Abandja, J., Danyod, M., Delaporte, E., Dupont, A., Ghogomu, A., et al. (1989). Antibody prevalence against haemorrhagic fever viruses in randomized representative Central African populations. Research in Virology, 140, 319-331.

Grard, G., Moureau, G., Charrel, R.N., Lemasson, J.J., Gonzalez, J.P., Gallian, P., Gritsun, T.S., Holmes, E.C., Gould, E.A., & de Lamballerie, X. (2007). Genetic characterization of tick-borne flaviviruses: new insights into evolution, pathogenetic determinants and taxonomy. Virology, 361, 80-92.

Herpe, B., Schuffenecker, I., Pillot, J., Malvy, D., Clouzeau, B., Bui, N., Vargas, F., Gruson, D., Zeller, H., Lafon, M.E., Fleury, H, & Hilbert G. (2007). Tickborne encephalitis, southwestern France. Emerging Infectious Diseases, 13, 1114-1116.

Hoyo, J., Elliot, A., Christie, D.A. (2004). Handbook of the birds of the world. Volumes 10-11. Barcelona: Lynx Edicions.

Hubálek, Z. & Rudolf, I. (2012). Tick-borne viruses in Europe. Parasitology Research, 111, 9-36.

Jado, I., Oteo, J.A., Aldámiz, M., Gil, H., Escudero, R., Ibarra, V., Portu, J., Portillo, A., Lezaun, M.J., García-Amil, C., Rodríguez-Moreno, I., & Anda, P. (2007). Rickettsia monacensis and human disease, Spain. Emerging Infectious Diseases, 13, 1405-1407.

Jauréguiberry, S., Tattevin, P., Tarantola, A., Legay, F., Tall, A., Nabeth, P., Zeller, H., Michelet, C. (2005). Imported Crimean-Congo hemorrhagic Fever. Journal of Clinical Microbiology, 43, 4905-4907.

Jongejan, F., & Uilenberg, G. (2004). The global importance of ticks. Parasitology, 129, Suppl. S3-14.

Khan, A.S., Maupin, G.O., Rollin, P.E., Noor, A.M., Shurie, H.H., Shalabi, A.G., Wasef, S., Haddad, Y.M., Sadek, R., Ijaz, K., Peters, C.J., & Ksiazek, T.G. (1997). An outbreak of Crimean-Congo hemorrhagic fever in the United Arab Emirates, 1994-1995. American Journal of Tropical Medicine and Hygiene, 57, 519-525.

Lindeborg, M., Barboutis, C., Ehrenborg, C., Fransson, T., Jaenson, T.G.T., Lindgren, P-E, Lundkvist, A., Nyström, F., Salaneck, E., Waldenström, J., & Olsen, B. (2012). Migratory birds, ticks, and Crimean-Congo hemorrhagic fever virus. Emerging Infectious Diseases, 18, 2095-2097.

Málková, D., Holubová, J., Kolman, J.M., Marhoul, Z., Hanzal, F., Kulková, H., Markvart, K., & Simková, L. (1980). Antibodies against some arboviruses in persons with various neuropathies. Acta Virologica, 24, 298.

Mansfield, K.L., Johnson, N., Phipps, L.P., Stephenson, J.R., Fooks, A.R., & Solomon, T. (2009). Tick-borne encephalitis virus - a review of an emerging zoonosis. Journal of General Virology, 90, 1781-1794.

Midilli, K., Gargili, A., Ergonul, O., Elevli, M., Ergin, S., Turan, N., Sengöz, G., Ozturk, R., & Bakar, M. (2009). The first clinical case due to AP92 like strain of Crimean-Congo hemorrhagic fever virus and a field survey. BMC Infectious Diseases, 9, 90.

Midilli, K., Gargili, A., Ergonul, O., Sengöz, G., Ozturk, R., Bakar, M., & Jongejan, F. (2007). Imported Crimean-Congo hemorrhagic fever cases in Istanbul. BMC Infectious Diseases, 7, 54.

Miguelez, M., Linares-Feria, M., Gonzalez, A., Mesa, M.C., Armas, F., & Laynez, P. (1996). Human babesiosis in a patient after splenectomy. Medicina Clinica (Barcelona), 106, 427-429.

Nava, S., Guglielmone, A.A., Mangold, A.J. (2009). An overview of systematics and evolution of ticks. Frontiers in Bioscience, 14, 2857-2877.

Nowak M. (2010a). Parasitisation and localisation of ticks (Acari: Ixodida) on exotic reptiles imported into Poland. Annals of Agricultural and Environmental Medicine, 17, 237-242.

Nowak M. (2010b). The international trade in reptiles (Reptilia)--the cause of the transfer of exotic ticks (Acari: Ixodida) to Poland. Veterinary Parasitology, 11, 169, 373-381

Oteo, J. A., Blanco, J. R., Martínez de Artola, V., Grandival, R., Ibarra, V., Dopereiro, R. (2000a). Erythema migrans (Lyme borreliosis). Clinicoepidemiological characteristics of 50 patients. Revista Clínica Española, 200, 60-63.

Oteo, J.A., Blanco, J.R., Martínez de Artola, V., & Ibarra, V. (2000b). First report of human granulocytic ehrlichiosis from southern Europe (Spain). Emerging Infectious Diseases, 6, 430-432.

Oteo, J.A., Ibarra, V., Blanco, J.R., Martínez de Artola, V., Márquez, F.J., Portillo, A., Raoult, D., & Anda, P. (2004). Dermacentor-borne necrosis erythema and lymphadenopathy: clinical and epidemiological features of a new tick-borne disease. Clinical Microbiology and Infection, 10, 327-331.

Oteo, J.A. & Portillo, A. (2012). Tick-borne rickettsioses in Europe. Ticks and Tick-Borne Diseases, 3, 271-278.

Palomar, A.M., Santibáñez, P., Mazuelas, D., Roncero, L., Santibáñez, S., Portillo, A., & Oteo, J.A. (2012). Role of birds in dispersal of etiologic agents of tick-borne zoonoses, Spain, 2009. Emerging Infectious Diseases, 18, 1188-1191.

Palomar, A.M., Portillo, A., Santibáñez, P., Mazuelas, D., Arizaga, J., Crespo, A., Gutiérrez, O., Cuadrado, J.F., & Oteo J.A. (2013). Crimean-Congo Hemorrhagic Fever Virus, ticks, migratory birds, Morocco, Spain, Europe. Emerging Infectious Diseases, 19, 260-263.

Patel, A.K., Patel, K.K., Mehta, M., Parikh, T.M., Toshniwal, H., Patel, K. J. (2011). First Crimean-Congo hemorrhagic fever outbreak in India. Association of Physicians of India, 59,585-589.

Papa A., Maltezou H.C., Tsiodras S., Dalla V.G., Papadimitriou T., Pierroutsakos I., Kartalis, G.N., Antoniadis, A. (2008). A case of Crimean-Congo haemorrhagic fever in Greece, June 2008. Euro Surveillance, 13, 18952.

Parola, P., Socolovschi, C., Jeanjean, L., Bitam, I., Fournier, P.E., Sotto, A., Labauge, P., Raoult, D. (2008). Warmer weather linked to tick attack and emergence of severe rickettsioses. PLOS Neglected Tropical Diseases, 2, e338.

Parola, P., Paddock, C.D., Raoult, D. (2005). Tick-borne rickettsioses around the world: emerging diseases challenging old concepts. Clinical Microbiology Reviews, 18, 719-756.

Pekova, S., Vydra, J., Kabickova, H., Frankova, S., Haugvicova, R., Mazal, O., Cmejla, R., Hardekopf, D.W., Jancuskova, T., & Kozak, T. (2011). Candidatus Neoehrlichia mikurensis infection identified in 2 hematooncologic patients: benefit of molecular techniques for rare pathogen detection. Diagnostic Microbiology and Infectious Diseases, 69, 266-270.

Petri, E., Gniel, D., Zent, O. (2010). Tick-borne encephalitis (TBE) trends in epidemiology and current and future management. Travel medicine and infectious disease, 8, 233-245.

Pietzsch, M., Quest, R., Hillyard, P.D., Medlock, J.M., & Leach, S. (2006). Importation of exotic ticks into the United Kingdom via the international trade in reptiles. Experimental and Applied Acarology, 38, 59-65.

Portillo, A., Ibarra, V., Santibáñez, S., Pérez-Martínez, L., Blanco, J.R., & Oteo, J.A. (2009). Genetic characterisation of ompA, ompB and gltA genes from Candidatus Rickettsia rioja. Clinical Microbiology and Infection, 15 Suppl 2, 307-308.

Portillo, A. & Oteo, J.A. (2012). Rickettsiosis as threat for the traveller. Current Topics in Tropical Medicine. Dr. Alfonso Rodriguez-Morales (Ed.), ISBN: 978-953-51-0274-8, InTech, Available from: http://www.intechopen.com/books/current-topics-in-tropical-medicine/rickettsiosis-as-threat-for-the-traveller

Randolph, S.E. (2011). Transmission of tick-borne pathogens between co-feeding ticks: Milan Labuda's enduring paradigm. Ticks and Tick-Borne Diseases, 2, 179-182.

Rataj, A.V., Lindtner-Knific, R., Vlahović, K., Mavri, U., & Dovč, A. (2011). Parasites in pet reptiles. Acta Veterinaria Scandinavica, 53, 33.

Schwaiger, M. & Cassinotti, P. (2003). Development of a quantitative real-time RT-PCR assay with internal control for the laboratory detection of tick borne encephalitis virus (TBEV) RNA. Journal of Clinical Virology, 27, 136-145.

Smirnova, S.E., Mamaev, V.I., Nepesova, N.M., Filipenko, P.I., Kalieva, V.I. (1978). [Study of the circulation of Crimean hemorrhagic fever virus in Turkmenistan]. Zh Mikrobiol Epidemiol Immunobiol. 1, 92-97. Russian.

Stanek, G., Reiter, M. (2011). The expanding Lyme Borrelia complex--clinical significance of genomic species? Clinical Microbiology and Infection, 17, 487-493.

Stefanoff, P., Pfeffer, M., Hellebrand, W., Rogalska, J., Rúhe, F., Makowka, A., Michalik, J., Wodecka, B., Rymasszewska, A., Kiewra, D., Baumann-Popczyk, A., & Dobler, G. (2012). Virus detection in questing ticks is not a sensitive indicator for risk assessment of tick-borne encephalitis in humans. Zoonosis and Public Health (In press)

Süss J. (2008). Tick-borne encephalitis in Europe and beyond—the epidemiological situation as of 2007. Euro Surveillance 13.

Süss J. (2011). Tick-borne encephalitis 2010: epidemiology, risk areas, and virus strains in Europe and Asia-an overview. Ticks and Tick-Borne Diseases, 2, 2-15.

Tall, A., Sall, A.A., Faye, O., Diatta, B., Sylla, R., Faye, J., Faye, P.C., Faye, O., Ly, A.B., Sarr, F.D., Diab, H., Diallo, M. (2009) [Two cases of Crimean-Congo haemorrhagic fever (CCHF) in two tourists in Senegal in 2004]. [Article in French] Bull Societe de Pathologie Exotique, 102, 159-161.

Turell, M.J. (2007). Role of ticks in the transmission of Crimean-Congo hemorrhagic fever virus. In: Ergonul, O, Whitehouse, CA, eds. Crimean-Congo hemorrhagic fever: A global perspective. Springer, 143-154.

von Loewenich, F.D., Geissdorfer, W., Disque, C., Matten, J., Schett, G., & Sakka, S.G. (2010). Detection of "Candidatus Neoehrlichia mikurensis" in two patients with severe febrile illnesses: evidence for a European sequence variant. Journal of Clinical Microbiology, 48, 2630-2635.

Waldenström, J., Lundkvist, A., Falk, K., Garpmo, U, Bergström, S., Lindegren, G., Sjöstedt, A., Mejlon, H., Fransson, T., Haemig, P.D., & Olsen, B. (2007). Migrating birds and tick-borne encephalitis virus. Emerging Infectious Diseases, 13, 1215–1218.

Welinder-Olsson C, Kjellin E, Vaht K, Jacobsson S, & Wenneras C. (2010). First case of human "Candidatus Neoehrlichia mikurensis" infection in a febrile patient with chronic lymphocytic leukemia. Journal of Clinical Microbiology, 48, 1956-1959.

Zakhashvili, K., Tsertsvadze, N., Chikviladze, T., Jghenti, E., Bekaia, M., Kuchuloria, T., Hepburn, M.J., Imnadze, P., & Nanuashvili, A. (2010). Crimean-Congo hemorrhagic fever in man, Republic of Georgia, 2009. Emerging Infectious Diseases, 16, 1326-1328.

microRNAs: New Actors in Retinoic Acid Signaling in the Differentiation of Neuroblastoma Cells

Salvador Meseguer
Instituto de Biomedicina de Valencia
Consejo Superior de Investigaciones Científicas, Valencia, Spain

Juan-Manuel Escamilla
Instituto de Biomedicina de Valencia
Consejo Superior de Investigaciones Científicas, Valencia, Spain

Domingo Barettino
Instituto de Biomedicina de Valencia
Consejo Superior de Investigaciones Científicas, Valencia, Spain

1   Introduction

The discovery of microRNAs (miRNAs, miRs) led to a profound change on our vision about the regulation of gene expression in eukaryotes. MicroRNAs are an emerging class of small non-coding endogenous RNAs that participate on the fine tuning of gene expression at the post-transcriptional level. First discovered at the early 90s in the nematode *C. elegans* (Lee *et al.*, 1993), microRNAs have been involved in multiple important biological processes both in animal as in plant cells. These regulatory RNAs are transcribed as primary longer transcripts, which are then processed into 19-23-nt mature miRNAs. One strand of the mature miRNA is then incorporated into the RNA-induced silencing complex (RISC) to regulate gene expression by targeting the 3'-untranslated region (3'UTR) of mRNAs with consequent translational repression and/or target mRNA degradation. This mode of action demonstrates the great regulatory potential of miRNAs, since a unique mRNA can be targeted by diverse miRNAs and conversely each miRNA may have hundreds of different target mRNAs. In recent years miRNAs have been established as important regulators of tumor development, progression and metastasis, and have demonstrated to be useful for tumor diagnosis and classification. Moreover, miRNA regulation might represent a new avenue for cancer treatment in a near future.

Neuroblastoma is the most common extracranial solid tumor in childhood and the most common tumor in infants, which originates from aberrant development of primordial neural crest cells. Several lines of evidence support the idea that microRNA deregulation could contribute to neuroblastoma pathogenesis and progression (Chen & Stallings, 2007; Welch *et al.*, 2007), and the usefulness of miRNA profiles for neuroblastoma diagnostics, classification and prognosis has been recently reported (De Preter *et al.*, 2011). Neuroblastoma cell lines can be induced to differentiate *in vitro* by several agents, including Retinoic Acid (RA) (Sidell, 1982; Pahlman *et al.*, 1984), the biologically active form of vitamin A. RA treatments lead to proliferative arrest and neuronal differentiation (Sidell, 1982; Thiele *et al.*, 1985) and to a reduction of the biological aggressiveness of neuroblastoma cells, by reducing their migratory and invasive abilities (Voigt & Zintl, 2003; Joshi *et al.*, 2006; Escamilla *et al.*, 2012). As a consequence of this, RA and its derivatives have been introduced into therapeutic protocols for neuroblastoma patients (Matthay *et al.*, 1999; Matthay & Reynolds, 2000; Matthay *et al.*, 2009).

In this article we want to review recent evidences supporting the contribution of miRNA regulation to RA-induced differentiation of neuroblastoma cells. We will show that miRNA contribute to the gene-expression changes associated with neuroblastoma cell differentiation and that specific RA-induced miRNAs target the expression of relevant genes in the context of neural differentiation. In addition RA-regulated miRNAs contribute to the reduction in the biological aggressiveness elicited by RA *in vitro*. We put forward the idea that miRNA regulation is part of the RA signaling pathway, and that miRNAs are essential mediators of the actions of RA in neuroblastoma cells.

2   The Basics of miRNA Actions

2.1   Biogenesis of miRNAs

miRNAs use complementary base pairing and the RNA induced silencing complex (RISC) to bind and either block translation and/or promote degradation of their target mRNAs. miRNAs are 19-22 nt-long RNA molecules transcribed mainly from non- coding regions of the genome, although some are embedded within genes, primarily as part of intronic sequences (Zhu *et al.*, 2009). In addition, clusters of miR-

NAs were also found in the genome (Rodriguez *et al.*, 2004). miRNAs are transcribed as larger hairpin-containing molecules, called pri-miRNA, that are cleaved in the nucleus by the microprocessor complex, involving Drosha and Pasha/DGCR8 proteins (Lee *et al.*, 2002; Lee *et al.*, 2003). The result of this cleavage is a shorter precursor hairpin (approx. 70 nt), called pre-miRNA. Pre-miRNAs are exported through exportin-5 to the cytoplasm (Yi *et al.*, 2003) where undergo further cleavage by Dicer to yield a transient intermediate imperfect duplex of approx 19-22 bp miRNA (Hutvagner *et al.*, 2001). Subsequently, the duplex is loaded into RISC complex together with proteins of the Argonaute (Ago) family, and unwinds (Meister *et al.*, 2004). The miRNA strand in RISC acts as a guide strand to find the complementary site in mRNA, and thereby suppressing the translational activity of the target mRNA (Figure 1). The complementary strand (known as miRNA* or as passenger strand) is degraded when the duplex is unwound, although recent evidences show that in some cases miRNA* accumulated at physiological levels and support the idea of a role for miRNA* on gene regulation (Mah *et al.*, 2010).

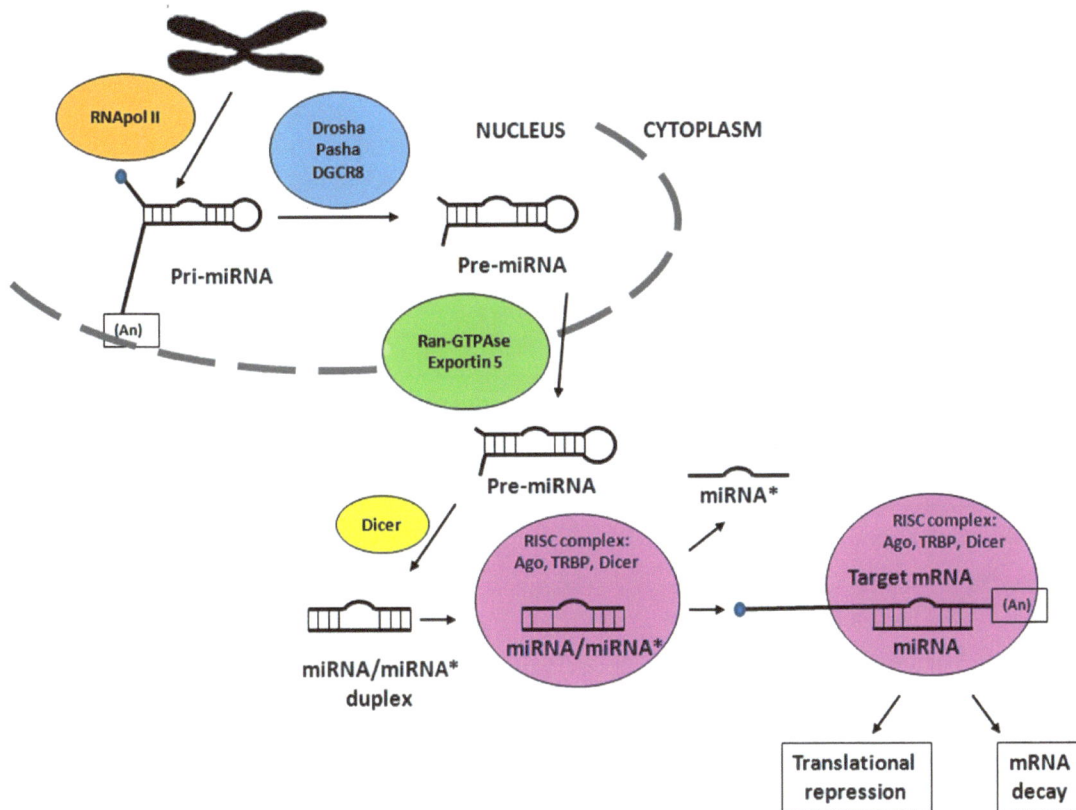

Figure 1: miRNA Biogenesis. The scheme depicts the different steps in the biogenesis of miR-NAs, the enzymes involved and the intermediate miRNA forms.

2.2   miRNA Target Binding

miRNAs interact primarily with the 3'-untranslated (3'UTR) region of their target mRNAs, although recent evidences show that miRNAs can also associate with sites located within the coding region of their target genes (Forman & Coller, 2010). In fact, complex arrays of multiple binding sites for either the same or different miRNAs located both in the 3'UTR as well as in the coding region of the target genes have been reported (Annibali *et al.*, 2012) . The base pairing of miRNA and mRNA in vertebrates requires only partial homology, with a preference for contiguous pairing occurring only at the "seed" region, located at nucleotides 2-7 of the guide strand. The lack of stringency results in a many-to-many relationship between miRNAs and mRNA targets, with the consequence that a high percentage of the genome may be regulated post-transcriptionally by a comparatively small set of miRNAs. A consequence of that is also that bioinformatic prediction of miRNA target mRNAs becomes relatively inaccurate. The guide strand binds to its complementary region in the 3'UTR of its target mRNA through Watson–Crick base pairing of the seed residues. Several alternative seed binding arrangements have been observed that involved different number of residues and therefore could have different binding affinity (Bartel, 2009).

2.3   Suppression of mRNA Translation and/or mRNA Degradation Mediated by miRNAs

The binding of miRNA-RISC complex to its cognate mRNA target leads to mRNA silencing through suppression of mRNA translation and/or mRNA decay. (reviewed in Fabian *et al.*, 2010) Several mechanisms involving different protein complexes have been proposed. mRNA translation could be blocked at initiation step as well as post-initiation stages. The miRNA-RISC complex inhibits translation initiation by interfering with eIF4F-cap recognition and 40S small ribosomal subunit recruitment or by antagonizing 60S subunit joining and preventing 80S ribosomal complex formation. The interaction of the GW182 protein with the poly(A)-binding protein (PABP) might interfere with the closed-loop formation mediated by the eIF4G-PABP interaction and thus contribute to the repression of translation initiation. The miRNA-RISC might inhibit also translation at postinitiation steps by inhibiting ribosome elongation, inducing ribosome drop-off, or promoting proteolysis of nascent polypeptides. To promote mRNA degradation, the miRNA-RISC complex interacts with the CCR4-NOT1 deadenylase complex to facilitate deadenylation of the mRNA poly(A) tail. Deadenylation requires the direct interaction of the GW182 protein with the PABP. Following deadenylation, the 5'-terminal cap (m^7G) is removed by the DCP1-DCP2 decapping complex. Although miRNA-mediated deadenylation followed by mRNA degradation appear to be widespread events, not all miRNA-targeted mRNAs are destabilized. miRNA-targeted translationally repressed mRNAs can accumulate in discrete cytoplasmic foci, such as P or GW bodies, or stress granules. A fraction of GW bodies co-localizes with multivesicular bodies (MVBs), membrane structures that play a role in miRNA-mediated repression. Compelling evidences support a role for miRNAs at the nucleus, acting on transcriptional regulation via chromatin remodeling and epigenetic mechanisms (Huang & Li, 2012).

3   Profiling miRNA Expression During Retinoic-Acid-Induced Neuroblastoma Cell Differentiation

3.1   Profiling miRNA Expression during Retinoic-Acid Induced Neuroblastoma Cell Differentiation

Several studies have addressed the changes in the expression of miRNAs upon RA-dependent induction of differentiation of neuroblastoma cells, with somewhat different results depending on the cell line, treatment duration, analysis platform used, etc. (Chen & Stallings, 2007; Beveridge *et al.*, 2009; Chen *et al.*, 2010; Foley *et al.*, 2011; Meseguer *et al.*, 2011). To analyze the contribution of microRNA regulation to RA-induced differentiation of neuroblastoma cells, we have studied the changes in the pattern of expression of 667 different human miRNAs upon RA treatment of SH-SY5Y neuroblastoma cells. We used miRNA profiling with TaqMan RT-PCR Low Density Arrays, and we found that 452 miRNAs were expressed above detection level. From them, 42 specific miRNAs change significatively their expression levels (26 upregulated and 16 downregulated) during RA-induced differentiation. This suggests miRNAs as an additional post-transcriptional regulatory layer under RA control (Meseguer *et al.*, 2011). (Figure 2)

3.2   A Role for miRNAs-10a and -10b in RA-dependent Regulation of Neuroblastoma Differentiation

We have focused our study on the closely related miR-10a and -10b, that showed the most prominent expression changes in SH-SY5Y cell line. Similar results have been reported for other neuroblastoma cell lines, like LA-N-1, LAN5 and SK-N-BE (Foley *et al.*, 2011; Meseguer *et al.*, 2011).

Loss of function experiments with anti-sense anti-miRs antagonists could show that miR-10a and -10b contribute to the regulation of RA-induced differentiation. RA-induced neurite outgrowth was impaired in cells with experimentally reduced levels of miR-10a or -10b, and the expression of several neural differentiation markers like Tyrosine Kinase receptors *NTRK2* (*trkB*) and *RET, GAP43,* Neuron-specific Enolase (*ENO2*), medium-size neurofilament protein NEFM and the enzyme Tyrosine Hydroxylase (TH) was abrogated or severely impaired after suppression of miR-10a or -10b (Figure 3). Conversely, the downregulation of the members of the ID gene family, *ID1, ID2* and *ID3* was abolished in RA-treated cells transfected with anti-miR-10a and anti-miR-10b. However, miR-10a and -10b did not appear to play a relevant role in RA-induced proliferation arrest, because the strong reduction of the incorporation of ^{3}H-Thymidine (to approximately 30% of the control values) and the decrease in the percentage of cells in S- phase (to 50% of the control) induced by RA treatment, was equivalent in neuroblastoma cells transfected with anti-miR-10a and anti-miR-10b (Meseguer *et al.*, 2011). However, a reduction in the cell growth in SK-N-BE neuroblastoma cells when transfected with pre-miR-10a and -10b has been reported (Foley *et al.*, 2011). Overexpression of miR-10 and -10b by transfecting synthetic precursor pre-miRs could not trigger full differentiation itself and although the mRNA levels of *RET, NTRK2, GAP43* and *ENO2* or the protein levels of NEFM and TH were slightly enhanced by transfection of pre-miR-10a and -10b, the attained expression levels for all the markers analyzed were far below those obtained by RA treatment. Similarly, ectopic expression of miR-10a and -10b led to certain increase in neurite outgrowth, but lower to that obtained for RA treatment (Meseguer *et al.*, 2011). Therefore, miR-10a and-10b appeared to be necessary but not sufficient for full neural differentiation, and consequently additional actions of RA must contribute to differentiation.

3.3   miRNAs-10a and -10b Contribute to the Reduction on the Biological Aggressiveness of Neuroblastoma Cells Induced by RA

It has been reported that RA treatment of neuroblastoma cells results in a reduction in their biological aggressiveness, by decreasing their migratory and invasive abilities (Voigt & Zintl, 2003; Joshi *et al.*, 2006; Escamilla *et al.*, 2012). We wanted to analyze whether RA-induced expression of miR-10a and -10b could be related to the reduction in migratory and invasive potential of neuroblastoma cells. To test the migratory potential of SH-SY-5Y cells we used a modified, light-opaque Boyden chamber assay (Falcon HTS FluoroBlok, 8 µm pore size). Cells were transfected with anti-miR-10a or -10b or the corre-

(A)

(B)

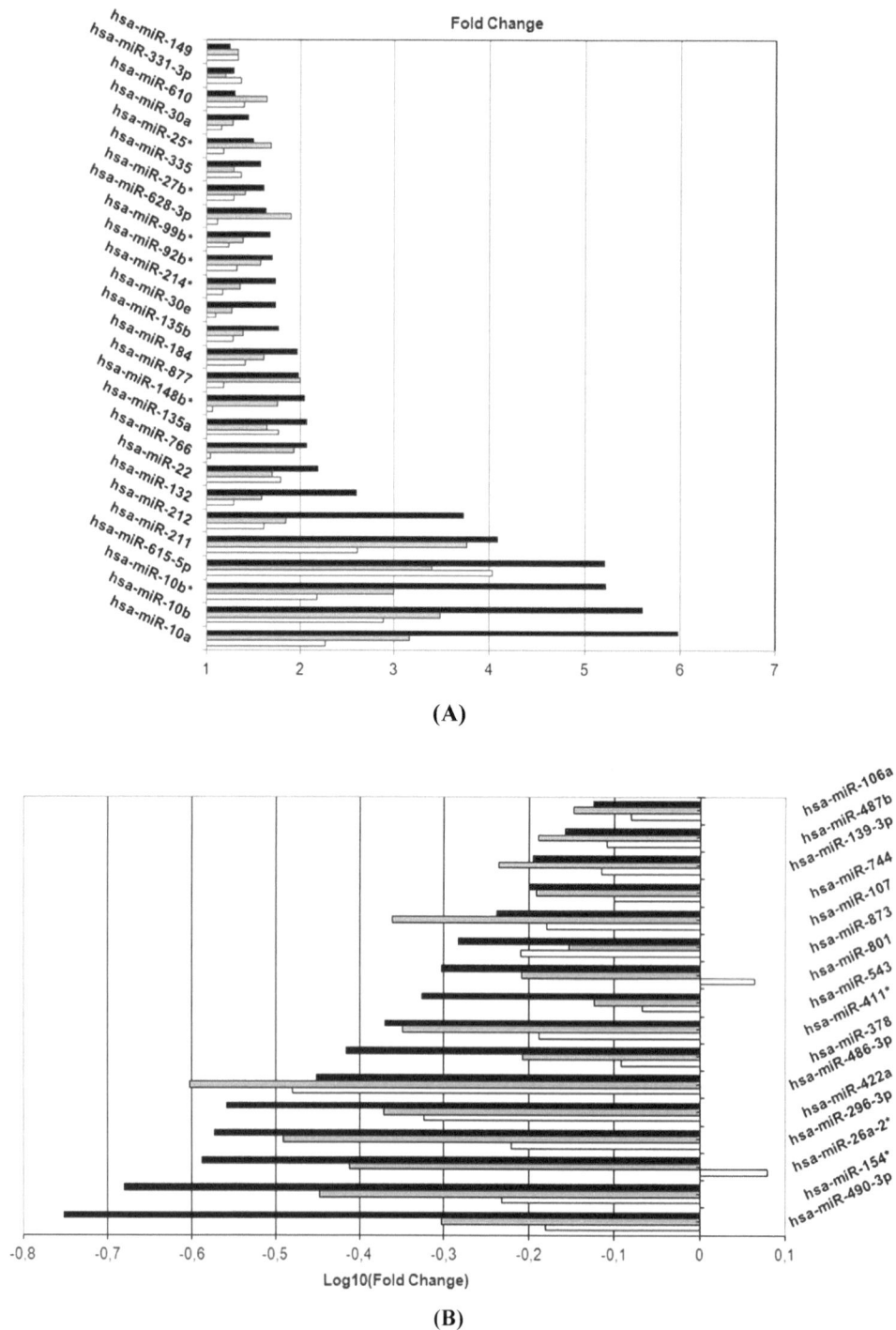

Figure 2: miRNA expression profiling in differentiating SH-SY5Y cells. Relative expression values detected in TaqMan microRNA Low Density Arrays for microRNAs with FDR<0.05 at least in two of the three treated versus non-treated comparisons, for upregulated **(A)** and downregulated miRNAs **(B)**. The values for 24 (empty bars), 48 (grey bars) and 96 (black bars) h of RA treatment are represented.

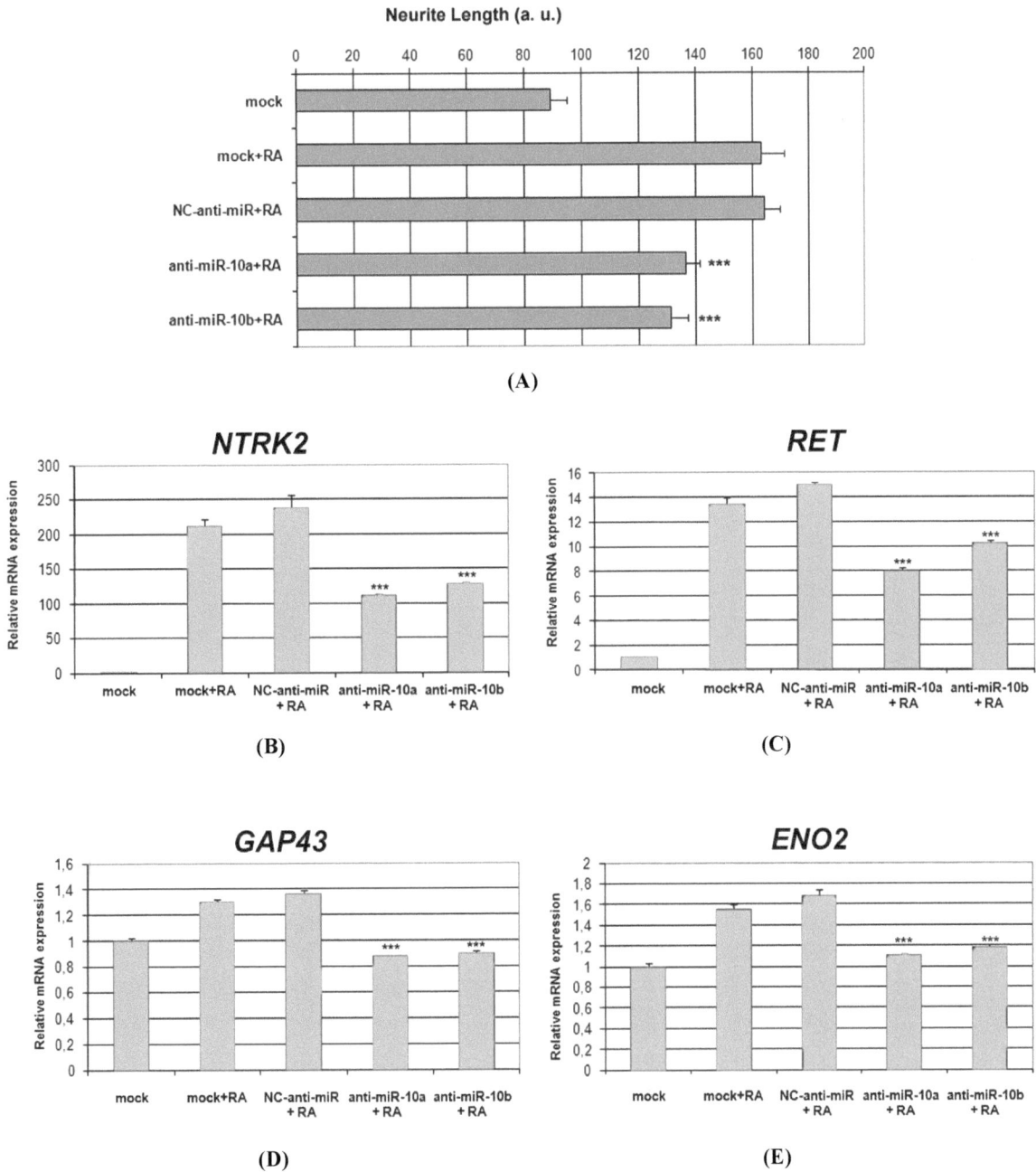

Figure 3: Knock-down of miR-10a and -10b impaired RA-induced differentiation. Blocking the action of miR-10a and -10b by transfection of their cognate anti-miRs diminished neurite outgrowth (A) and reduced the expression of neuronal differentiation markers *NTRK2* (B), *RET* (C), *GAP43* (D) and *ENO2* (E), as shown by quantitative RT-PCR. (Statistical signification in the Figures: *: p<0.05; **: p<0.01; ***: p<0,001; ns: non significative)

sponding Negative Control anti-miR, treated with 1 μM RA or vehicle in culture medium during 96 h, and labeled in the plate with Calcein AM. Labeled cells were counted and added to the upper chamber of the boyden chamber, and allow to migrate towards de lower chamber, filled with medium containing 10% FBS as chemoattractant. The results show that indeed RA-treatment reduced the migration of neuro-blastoama cells. However suppressing miR-10a or -10b expression not only abolished that reduction but increased migration over basal levels, supporting a contribution of RA-induced miR-10a and 10b to the reduction of migratory activity produced by RA (Meseguer *et al.*, 2011) (Figure 4A).

For invasion assays we used a similar assay, with the difference that the porous membrane separating the upper and lower cahambers of the Boyden chamber was covered with BD *Matrigel* matrix (5 μg/cm^2 in serum-free medium). The lower chamber contained 10% FBS as chemoattractant to promote cell invasion. In this case RA treatment results in increased invasive potential, whereas in cells transfected with anti-miR-10a or 10b the same treatment the increase in invasion induced by RA treatment is even larger, supporting the idea that the expression of miR-10a and -10b contributes to a reduction in the invasive potential (Meseguer *et al.*, 2011) (Figure 4B).

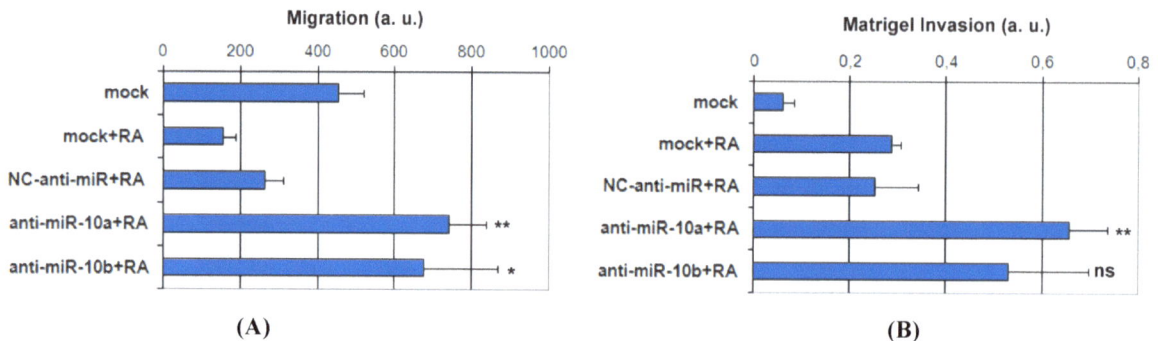

(A)   **(B)**

Figure 4: Involvement of miR-10a and -10b on the effects of RA in migratory and invasive potential of neuroblastoma cells. Mock-transfected cells and cells transfected with Negative Control (NC) anti-miR, anti-miR-10a or anti-miR-10b were treated with 1 μM RA or vehicle for 96 h and used in migration **(A)** or matrigel invasion **(B)** transwell assays. The graph shows a representative experiment performed in triplicate (mean ± SD). Statistical significance was analyzed by comparing samples transfected with anti-miR-10a and -10b with those transfected with NC-anti-miR.

To analyze the effects of RA treatment on the metastatic potential of neuroblastoma cells we used the chicken embryo chorioallantoic membrane assays (also known as CAM assay; (Zijlstra *et al.*, 2002). This assay is useful to study intravasation and metastasis *in vivo*, since it recapitulates all the steps of the metastatic process. In the CAM assay the cells to be tested are inoculated on the chorioallantoic membrane of 10-day-old chicken embryos. After a week, the egg is opened, the embryo is obtained and secondary organs like liver or lungs were dissected. The presence of human cells in the chicken organs is evaluated and quantified after obtaining their genomic DNA, by detecting the presence of human-specific *Alu*-sequences by Real-Time PCR. As this is a complex technique that requires a higher number of replicate experiments we have simplified the study to analyze only the effects of miR-10a suppression. Neuroblastoma cells could be detected in the chicken lungs after 7 days incubation. Suppresion of miR-10a expression with its cognate anti-miR resulted in an increase of the metastatic cells. As expected, RA treatment led to a reduction of the number of neuroblastoma cells reaching the lungs. However this inhibitory effect of RA was abolished in cells having a reduced amount of miR-10a by transfecting the corresponding anti-miR-10a (Meseguer *et al.*, 2011) (Figure 5).

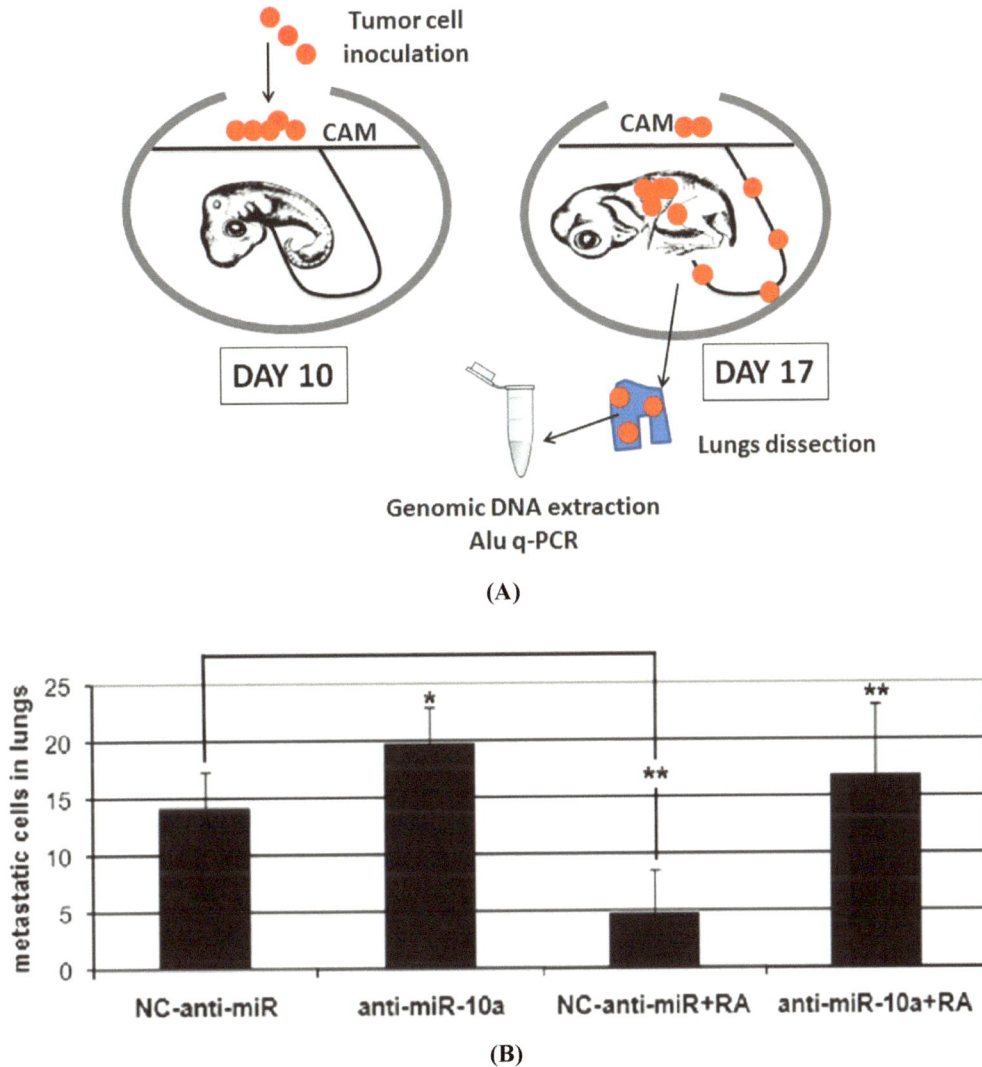

(A)

(B)

Figure 5: Chorioallantoic Membrane Metastasis Assay. (A) Schematic representation of the experiment. Cells from the different treatment groups were transferred to the upper chorioallantoic membrane of 10-day-old chicken embryos and the number of metastatized cells into the lungs evaluated 7 days later. (B) Cells transfected with Negative Control (NC) anti-miR or anti-miR-10a were treated with 1 μM RA or vehicle for 96 h as indicated in the figure. The graph represents the values obtained from six parallel assays (mean $\pm$ SD). Statistical significance was analyzed by comparing samples transfected with anti-miR-10a with those transfected with NC-anti-miR. In addition samples transfected with NC-anti-miR treated with vehicle were compared to those treated with RA.

In good agreement with our results, it has been reported that miR-10a and -10b reduces the ability of neuroblastoma cells to form colonies in soft agar (Foley *et al.*, 2011), a phenotype that is characteristic of malignant cells. All these results support the idea that miR-10a and -10b expression contribute to to reduction of migratory, invasive and metastatic activities induced by RA. In a recent report it has been shown that a protein involved in cell migration, Tiam1, is targeted by miR-10b in mammary tumor cells. Overexpression of miR-10b suppresses the ability of breast carcinoma cells to migrate and invade (Moriarty *et al.*, 2010). Consistent to that, it has been reported an association between lower miR-10a expression and lower overall survival for a subclass of neuroblastoma tumors (11q- tumor cohort) (Foley *et al.*, 2011). However other reports seem to involve the members of the miR-10 family as promoters of migration and metastasis in different tumors (Ma *et al.*, 2007; Sasayama *et al.*, 2009; Veerla *et al.*, 2009; Weiss *et al.*, 2009; Ma *et al.*, 2010; Nakata *et al.*, 2011; Liu *et al.*, 2012; Lu *et al.*, 2012). This apparent controversy may suggest that the role of the microRNAs from the miR-10 family in tumorigenesis and metastasis would depend on their molecular targets and therefore would depend on the cellular context.

4   Molecular Targets of miR-10a and -10b in the Differentiation of Neuroblastoma Cells

4.1   The Search for the Molecular Targets for miRNAs

The identification of molecular targets for miRNAs is a crucial step towards the understanding of miRNA function. Because an ever growing number of experimentally validated targets for miRNAs are being reported, a simple way to identify miRNA targets is to search for validated targets in the literature or in databases as TarBase (Vergoulis *et al.*, 2012). A validated target for miR-10b in breast cancer cells is the homeobox gene *HOXD10* (Ma *et al.*, 2007; Ma & Weinberg, 2008). However, we could not find regulation of *HOXD10* in SH-SY5Y neuroblastoma cells, when treated with RA or when the levels of miR-10a and -10b were experimentally altered (Meseguer *et al.*, 2011).

A lot of effort has been made to generate computational miRNA target prediction tools (reviewed in Maziere & Enright, 2007), mainly based on the search for complementary sequences in the genome. However, that is not an easy task, because short sequences are problematic for the algorithms usually developed for complementarity analysis. As indicated in 2.2, the base pairing of miRNA and mRNA in vertebrates requires only partial homology, with a preference for contiguous pairing occurring only at the "seed" region, located at nucleotides 2-7 of the guide strand, and this makes even more difficult to find the right target sequence in the genome. Several authors have approached this problem from different startpoints, using mainly complementarity analysis of the complete miRNA sequence, complementarity analysis of the seed sequence, or adding thermodynamic stability analysis of duplex sequences or 3'UTR sequence conservation to the complementarity analysis. Nowadays a set of miRNA target prediction resources are available, mainly as web-based tools. However it becomes striking to the new users of these tools how different results can be obtained when using the same sequence with different prediction tools. In addition, prediction tools generate lists of hundreds of genes for each of the miRNAs, and the fact of having sequence diversity at the 3'UTR by alternative polyadenylation sites could also complicate the analysis (for discussion see Clancy *et al.*, 2011).

To find relevant targets for miR-10a and-10b in neuroblastoma cells we choose to combine bioinformatic prediction tools together with experimental analysis. We created a list of potential miR-10a and -

10b targets by including the common predicted genes using three different prediction resources: miRbase targets (John *et al.*, 2004), TargetScan (Lewis *et al.*, 2003) and PicTar (Krek *et al.*, 2005). Only mRNAs that contained evolutionarily conserved miRNA binding sequences on their 3'UTR were considered. This list was crossed with the dataset of an Affymetrix microarray experiment containing the genes downregulated after 48 h RA treatment. In the resulting list, two members of the Arginin/serine-rich splicing factors, *SFRS1* (SF2/ASF) and *SFRS10* (TRA2B), as well as the nuclear receptor co-repressor *NCOR2* (SMRT) were on top (Meseguer *et al.*, 2011).

4.2   Regulation of *SFRS1* (SF2/ASF) by miR-10a and -10b

The regulation of *SFRS1* (SF2/ASF) by miR-10a and-10b was experimentally validated at mRNA and protein levels in HeLa and SH-SY5Y cells (Figure 6). In addition regulation by miR-10a and -10b was shown in transfection experiments with reporter plasmids containing *SFRS1* 3'UTR sequences linked to the Luciferase gene. miR-10a and -10b are new players in the complex regulation of *SFRS1* protein through a mechanism involving enhanced mRNA cleavage. In addition, we showed how changes in miR-10a and -10b expression levels may influence some molecular activities in which the product of *SFRS1* is involved, such as translation enhancement of certain mRNAs and alternative splicing, that could have importance in the neural differentiation process (Meseguer *et al.*, 2011) (Figure 7). We have reported that the activation of signaling pathways by RA treatment results in rapid changes in the phosphorylation pattern of SR proteins, including SFRS1 and subsequently, changes in alternative splicing selection and an increase of the translation of mRNAs containing SFRS1 binding sites take place (Laserna *et al.*, 2009). In this context, the reduction in *SFRS1* levels trough miR-10a and -10b regulation could be interpreted as the closing of the feedback regulatory loop of RA on the activities of *SFRS1*.

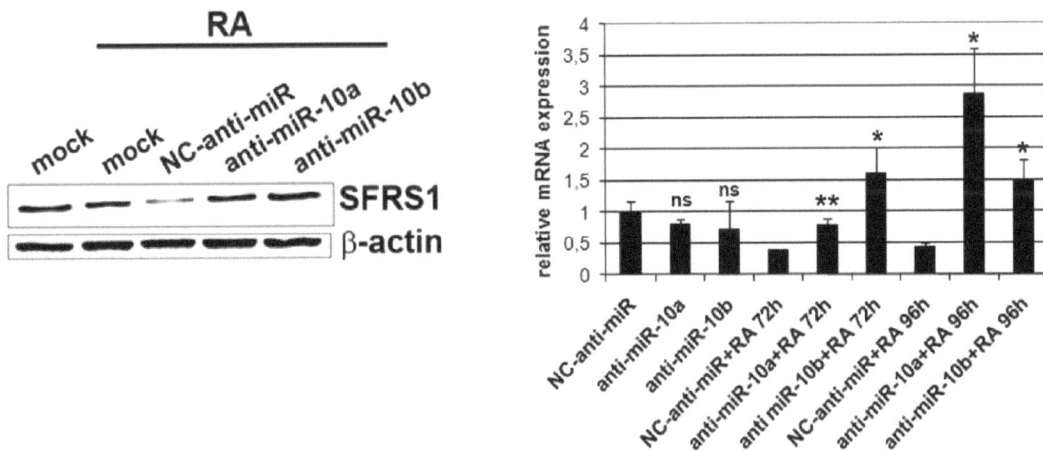

Figure 6: miR-10a/-10b knockdown leads to increased SFRS1 protein and mRNA levels in HeLa and SH-SY5Y cells. (left panel) Western blot of SFRS1 protein expression after anti-miR-10a, -10b and negative control NC-anti-miR transfection of SH-SY5Y cells followed by 1μM RA treatment. The blot was reprobed with actin beta antibodies as loading control. **(right panel)** RT-qPCR analysis of SFRS1 mRNA levels in same conditions. The graph shows expression levels relative to that of RA untreated, NC-anti-miR transfected cells (mean ± SD of a triplicate experiment). Statistical analysis for right panel was made by comparing the values from cells transfected with anti-miR-10a or -10b to those from cells transfected with NC-anti-miR.

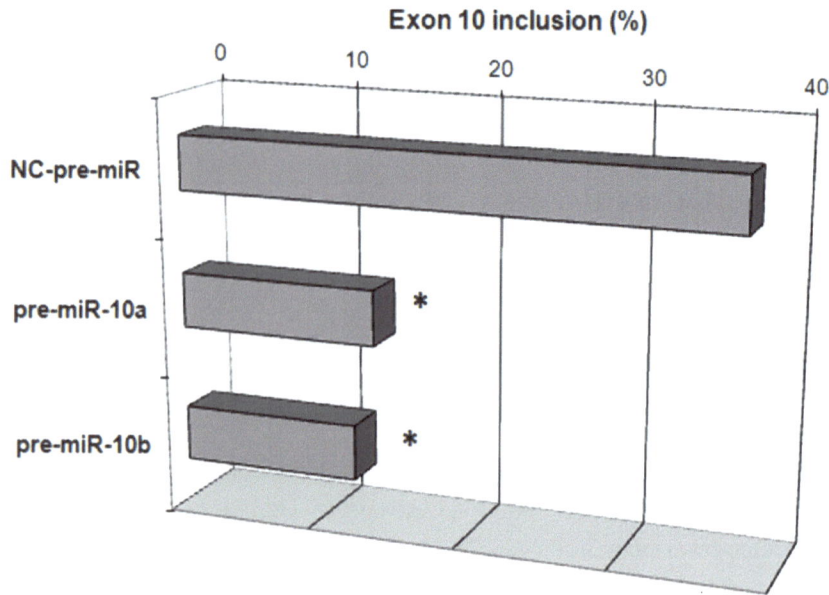

Figure 7: Experimental alteration of miR-10a and -10b levels resulted in an impairment of SFRS1 functions in the regulation of alternative splicing . Alternative splicing of *tau* protein exon 10 is altered by transfection of anti-miR-10a and -10b. RT-PCR was performed on RNA extracted from anti-miR-10a, -10b or negative control (NC) anti-miR transfected SH-SY5Y cells. *tau* Exon 10 flanking primers were used in RT-PCR reaction according to (Kondo *et al.*, 2004). Quantification of the percentage of exon 10 inclusion. The graph shows the average from 3 independent experiments. Statistical analysis was made by comparing the values from cells transfected with pre-miR-10a or -10b to those from cells transfected with NC-pre-miR.

4.2   Regulation of *NCOR2* (SMRT) by miR-10a and -10b

The regulation of *NCOR2* by miR-10a and-10b was experimentally validated at mRNA and protein levels in SK-N-BE neuroblastoma cells. Moreover, a luciferase reporter construct containing the *NCOR2* 3'UTR showed a significant decrease in luciferase activity when co-transfected with mature miR-10a, -10b or 10a/10b mimics in SK-N-BE cells. This decrease in luciferase activity was completely abolished when the putative miR-10a and -10b target site was mutated in its seed sequence. Knock-down of *NCOR2* expression through transfection of siRNAs to SK-N-BE cells recapitulates most of the changes induced by RA, like neurite outgrowth, proliferative arrest, expression of neural markers, downregulation of MYCN and expression of miR-10a (Foley *et al.*, 2011). *NCOR2* acts as co-repressor in the regulation of many genes, especially as co-regulator of nuclear receptor-regulated genes. Bound to the unliganded receptor, *NCOR2* maintains the promoters of nuclear receptor-regulated genes in a repressed state, and its release from the complex with the receptor upon ligand binding allows transcriptional activation (Xu *et al.*, 1999). It has been reported that *NCOR2* represses expression of the jumonji-domain containing gene *JMJD3*, a direct retinoic-acid-receptor target that functions as a histone H3 trimethyl K27 demethylase and which is capable of activating specific components of the neurogenic program (Jepsen *et al.*, 2007). Therefore, downregulation of *NCOR2* by miR-10a and -10b would potentiate the actions of RA through

RARs and RXRs and could contribute to some of the changes in gene expression associated with neural differentiation.

5   Other miRNA-based Regulatory Networks under the Control of Retinoic Acid in the Differentiation of Neuroblastoma Cells

5.1   Targeting of the differentiation inhibitor ID2 by miR-9 and miR-103

The HLH transcription factor *ID2* is a repressor of cell differentiation and has been involved in neuroblastoma pathogenesis (Lasorella *et al.*, 2002). RA treatments downregulate the expression of *ID2*, as well as other ID genes as *ID1* and *ID3* (Jogi *et al.*, 2002; Lopez-Carballo *et al.*, 2002). Repression of ID genes appears to be a pre-requisite for neuroblastoma differentiation (Iavarone & Lasorella, 2006). It has been recently reported that *ID2* mRNA is targeted by two RA-induced miRNAs, miR-9 and miR-103 (Annibali *et al.*, 2012). Binding of miR-9 occurs within the coding sequence of *ID2* mRNA, whereas miR-103 target site is located in the 3'-UTR as usual. Forced expression of miR-9 and miR-103 results in reduced cell proliferation, expression of differentiation markers and morphological differentiation, a similar result to that obtained by expressing an engineered HLH domain blocking ID2 protein action (Ciarapica *et al.*, 2009). Consistent to all this, a non-targetable version of *ID2* mRNA could restore proliferation and N-Myc expression to RA-induced differentiating cells (Annibali *et al.*, 2012). Therefore the miR-9/miR-103/*ID2* module could represent a new regulatory network under the control of RA involved in neuroblastoma differentiation.

5.2   Changes in DNA Methylation Induced by RA and Mediated by miRNAs

RA has been reported to induce a global change in the methylation pattern of gene promoters during differentiation of neuroblastoma cell lines (Das *et al.*, 2010; Stallings *et al.*, 2011) . Genome-wide changes in the methylation patterns could be associated to a downregulation of DNA methylases *DNMT1* and *DNMT3b*. The expression of those two DNA methylases could be under the control of RA-induced miRNAs. *DNMT1* was targeted by miR-152 and *DNMT3b* is a potential target for miR-26a/b and miR-125a/b. These miRNAs are under repressive control by *MYCN*, an important gene in neuroblastoma proliferation and pathogenesis (Westermark *et al.*, 2011), whose expression is downregulated by RA treatments (Thiele *et al.*, 1985). DNA de-methylation affects to a significative number of promoter regions, and results in the re-expression of several differentiation associated-genes as is the case of *NOS1*, a gene that has been involved in neurite outgrowth and neuroblastoma differentiation (Ciani *et al.*, 2004). Using an novel integrated approach for analyzing DNA methylation coupled with miRNA and mRNA expression data sets Stallings and co-workers (Das *et al.*, 2012) identified 67 epigenetically regulated miRNAs in neuroblastoma, many of them were underexpressed in tumors and could be associated to poor patient survival. This set of methylation-repressed miRNAs regulated the expression of a large set of genes that were consistently overexpressed in highly malignant tumors. Ectopic expression of some of these epigenetically silenced miRNAs in neuroblastoma cell lines resulted in a reduction of cell viability, stressing the role of those miRNAs on neuroblastoma pathogenesis. In particular ectopic expression of miR-340 led to apoptotic cell death or differentiation depending on the cell context. miR-340 levels are increased during RA-induced differentiation through de-methylation of an upstream promoter region. miR-340 targeted the transcription factor *SOX2*, providing a mechanism for the repression of *SOX2* mediated by

RA in neuroblastoma cells. *SOX2* has been involved in the maintenance of the undifferentiated phenotype in neural stem cells (Wegner & Stolt, 2005). However downregulation of *SOX2* does not appear to be required for RA-induced neuroblastoma cell differentiation, because neurite outgrowth and proliferative arrest occurred even in cells overexpressing *SOX2*. Thus, the interplay between miRNA regulation and gene activation mediated by DNA de-methylation appears to have an important role in the complex process of neuroblastoma cell differentiation triggered by RA.

6   Concluding Remarks

MicroRNAs are essential players in the process on neural differentiation of neuroblastoma cells, and contribute to the transduction of Retinoic Acid signaling. In addition miRNAs have been reported to participate in the pathogenesis and progression of human neuroblastoma tumors (Chen & Stallings, 2007; Welch *et al.*, 2007), and miRNA profiles have been recently proven to be useful for classification and prognosis (De Preter *et al.*, 2011). Finally miRNAs open new avenues for the treatment of neuroblastoma cells, and proof of concept experiments showing a therapeutic action of miRNA-based treatments in animal models of neuroblastoma tumors have been reported (Tivnan *et al.*, 2010; Tivnan *et al.*, 2011; Tivnan *et al.*, 2012). Therefore, we have to expect an increased interest of the neuroblastoma researchers community in the study of microRNAs for the next years.

Acknowledgements

The authors' research work described in this article was financed through grants of the Spanish National Plan for Research, Development and Innovation (SAF2007-60780, SAF2010-15032 and SAF2011-23869), Generalitat Valenciana (ACOMP 09/212) and Genoma España to D. Barettino. S. Meseguer was the recipient of an EACR training and travel fellowship award and a CSIC I3P predoctoral fellowship/contract.

References

Annibali, D., Gioia, U., Savino, M., Laneve, P., Caffarelli, E. & Nasi, S. (2012). A new module in neural differentiation control: two microRNAs upregulated by retinoic acid, miR-9 and -103, target the differentiation inhibitor ID2. PLoS One, 7, e40269.

Bartel, D. P. (2009). MicroRNAs: target recognition and regulatory functions. Cell, 136, 215-233.

Beveridge, N. J., Tooney, P. A., Carroll, A. P., Tran, N. & Cairns, M. J. (2009). Down-regulation of miR-17 family expression in response to retinoic acid induced neuronal differentiation. Cell Signal, 21, 1837-1845.

Ciani, E., Severi, S., Contestabile, A. & Bartesaghi, R. (2004). Nitric oxide negatively regulates proliferation and promotes neuronal differentiation through N-Myc downregulation. J Cell Sci, 117, 4727-4737.

Ciarapica, R., Annibali, D., Raimondi, L., Savino, M., Nasi, S. & Rota, R. (2009). Targeting Id protein interactions by an engineered HLH domain induces human neuroblastoma cell differentiation. Oncogene, 28, 1881-1891.

Clancy, J. L., Wei, G. H., Echner, N., Humphreys, D. T., Beilharz, T. H. & Preiss, T. (2011). mRNA isoform diversity can obscure detection of miRNA-mediated control of translation. Rna, 17, 1025-1031.

Chen, H., Shalom-Feuerstein, R., Riley, J., Zhang, S. D., Tucci, P., Agostini, M., Aberdam, D., Knight, R. A., Genchi, G., Nicotera, P., Melino, G. & Vasa-Nicotera, M. (2010). miR-7 and miR-214 are specifically expressed during neuroblastoma differentiation, cortical development and embryonic stem cells differentiation, and control neurite outgrowth in vitro. Biochem Biophys Res Commun, 394, 921-927.

Chen, Y. & Stallings, R. L. (2007). Differential patterns of microRNA expression in neuroblastoma are correlated with prognosis, differentiation, and apoptosis. Cancer Res, 67, 976-983.

Das, S., Bryan, K., Buckley, P. G., Piskareva, O., Bray, I. M., Foley, N., Ryan, J., Lynch, J., Creevey, L., Fay, J., Prenter, S., Koster, J., van Sluis, P., Versteeg, R., Eggert, A., Schulte, J. H., Schramm, A., Mestdagh, P., Vandesompele, J., Speleman, F. & Stallings, R. L. (2012). Modulation of neuroblastoma disease pathogenesis by an extensive network of epigenetically regulated microRNAs. Oncogene.

Das, S., Foley, N., Bryan, K., Watters, K. M., Bray, I., Murphy, D. M., Buckley, P. G. & Stallings, R. L. (2010). MicroRNA mediates DNA demethylation events triggered by retinoic acid during neuroblastoma cell differentiation. Cancer Res, 70, 7874-7881.

De Preter, K., Mestdagh, P., Vermeulen, J., Zeka, F., Naranjo, A., Bray, I., Castel, V., Chen, C., Drozynska, E., Eggert, A., Hogarty, M. D., Izycka-Swieszewska, E., London, W. B., Noguera, R., Piqueras, M., Bryan, K., Schowe, B., van Sluis, P., Molenaar, J. J., Schramm, A., Schulte, J. H., Stallings, R. L., Versteeg, R., Laureys, G., Van Roy, N., Speleman, F. & Vandesompele, J. (2011). miRNA expression profiling enables risk stratification in archived and fresh neuroblastoma tumor samples. Clin Cancer Res, 17, 7684-7692.

Escamilla, J. M., Bäuerl, C., López, C. M. R., Pekkala, S. P., Navarro, S. & Barettino, D. (2012). Retinoic-Acid-Induced Downregulation of the 67 KDa Laminin Receptor Correlates with Reduced Biological Aggressiveness of Human Neuroblastoma Cells. Neuroblastoma-Present and Future. H. Shimada. Rijeka, InTech, 217-232.

Fabian, M. R., Sonenberg, N. & Filipowicz, W. (2010). Regulation of mRNA translation and stability by microRNAs. Annu Rev Biochem, 79, 351-379.

Foley, N. H., Bray, I., Watters, K. M., Das, S., Bryan, K., Bernas, T., Prehn, J. H. & Stallings, R. L. (2011). MicroRNAs 10a and 10b are potent inducers of neuroblastoma cell differentiation through targeting of nuclear receptor corepressor 2. Cell Death Differ, 18, 1089-1098.

Forman, J. J. & Coller, H. A. (2010). The code within the code: microRNAs target coding regions. Cell Cycle, 9, 1533-1541.

Huang, V. & Li, L. C. (2012). miRNA goes nuclear. RNA Biol, 9, 269-273.

Hutvagner, G., McLachlan, J., Pasquinelli, A. E., Balint, E., Tuschl, T. & Zamore, P. D. (2001). A cellular function for the RNA-interference enzyme Dicer in the maturation of the let-7 small temporal RNA. Science, 293, 834-838.

Iavarone, A. & Lasorella, A. (2006). ID proteins as targets in cancer and tools in neurobiology. Trends Mol Med, 12, 588-594.

Jepsen, K., Solum, D., Zhou, T., McEvilly, R. J., Kim, H. J., Glass, C. K., Hermanson, O. & Rosenfeld, M. G. (2007). SMRT-mediated repression of an H3K27 demethylase in progression from neural stem cell to neuron. Nature, 450, 415-419.

Jogi, A., Persson, P., Grynfeld, A., Pahlman, S. & Axelson, H. (2002). Modulation of basic helix-loop-helix transcription complex formation by Id proteins during neuronal differentiation. J Biol Chem, 277, 9118-9126.

John, B., Enright, A. J., Aravin, A., Tuschl, T., Sander, C. & Marks, D. S. (2004). Human MicroRNA targets. PLoS Biol, 2, e363.

Joshi, S., Guleria, R., Pan, J., DiPette, D. & Singh, U. S. (2006). Retinoic acid receptors and tissue-transglutaminase mediate short-term effect of retinoic acid on migration and invasion of neuroblastoma SH-SY5Y cells. Oncogene, 25, 240-247.

Kondo, S., Yamamoto, N., Murakami, T., Okumura, M., Mayeda, A. & Imaizumi, K. (2004). Tra2 beta, SF2/ASF and SRp30c modulate the function of an exonic splicing enhancer in exon 10 of tau pre-mRNA. Genes Cells, 9, 121-130.

Krek, A., Grun, D., Poy, M. N., Wolf, R., Rosenberg, L., Epstein, E. J., MacMenamin, P., da Piedade, I., Gunsalus, K. C., Stoffel, M. & Rajewsky, N. (2005). Combinatorial microRNA target predictions. Nat Genet, 37, 495-500.

Laserna, E. J., Valero, M. L., Sanz, L., del Pino, M. M., Calvete, J. J. & Barettino, D. (2009). Proteomic analysis of phosphorylated nuclear proteins underscores novel roles for rapid actions of retinoic acid in the regulation of mRNA splicing and translation. Mol Endocrinol, 23, 1799-1814.

Lasorella, A., Boldrini, R., Dominici, C., Donfrancesco, A., Yokota, Y., Inserra, A. & Iavarone, A. (2002). Id2 is critical for cellular proliferation and is the oncogenic effector of N-myc in human neuroblastoma. Cancer Res, 62, 301-306.

Lee, R. C., Feinbaum, R. L. & Ambros, V. (1993). The C. elegans heterochronic gene lin-4 encodes small RNAs with antisense complementarity to lin-14. Cell, 75, 843-854.

Lee, Y., Ahn, C., Han, J., Choi, H., Kim, J., Yim, J., Lee, J., Provost, P., Radmark, O., Kim, S. & Kim, V. N. (2003). The nuclear RNase III Drosha initiates microRNA processing. Nature, 425, 415-419.

Lee, Y., Jeon, K., Lee, J. T., Kim, S. & Kim, V. N. (2002). MicroRNA maturation: stepwise processing and subcellular localization. Embo J, 21, 4663-4670.

Lewis, B. P., Shih, I. H., Jones-Rhoades, M. W., Bartel, D. P. & Burge, C. B. (2003). Prediction of mammalian microRNA targets. Cell, 115, 787-798.

Liu, Z., Zhu, J., Cao, H., Ren, H. & Fang, X. (2012). miR-10b promotes cell invasion through RhoC-AKT signaling pathway by targeting HOXD10 in gastric cancer. Int J Oncol, 40, 1553-1560.

Lopez-Carballo, G., Moreno, L., Masia, S., Perez, P. & Barettino, D. (2002). Activation of the phosphatidylinositol 3-kinase/Akt signaling pathway by retinoic acid is required for neural differentiation of SH-SY5Y human neuroblastoma cells. J Biol Chem, 277, 25297-25304.

Lu, Y. C., Chen, Y. J., Wang, H. M., Tsai, C. Y., Chen, W. H., Huang, Y. C., Fan, K. H., Tsai, C. N., Huang, S. F., Kang, C. J., Chang, J. T. & Cheng, A. J. (2012). Oncogenic function and early detection potential of miRNA-10b in oral cancer as identified by microRNA profiling. Cancer Prev Res (Phila), 5, 665-674.

Ma, L., Reinhardt, F., Pan, E., Soutschek, J., Bhat, B., Marcusson, E. G., Teruya-Feldstein, J., Bell, G. W. & Weinberg, R. A. (2010). Therapeutic silencing of miR-10b inhibits metastasis in a mouse mammary tumor model. Nat Biotechnol, 28, 341-347.

Ma, L., Teruya-Feldstein, J. & Weinberg, R. A. (2007). Tumour invasion and metastasis initiated by microRNA-10b in breast cancer. Nature, 449, 682-688.

Ma, L. & Weinberg, R. A. (2008). Micromanagers of malignancy: role of microRNAs in regulating metastasis. Trends Genet, 24, 448-456.

Mah, S. M., Buske, C., Humphries, R. K. & Kuchenbauer, F. (2010). miRNA*: a passenger stranded in RNA-induced silencing complex? Crit Rev Eukaryot Gene Expr, 20, 141-148.

Matthay, K. & Reynolds, C. (2000). Is there a role for retinoids to treat minimal residual disease in neuroblastoma? Br J Cancer, 83, 1121-1123.

Matthay, K. K., Reynolds, C. P., Seeger, R. C., Shimada, H., Adkins, E. S., Haas-Kogan, D., Gerbing, R. B., London, W. B. & Villablanca, J. G. (2009). Long-term results for children with high-risk neuroblastoma treated on a randomized trial of myeloablative therapy followed by 13-cis-retinoic acid: a children's oncology group study. J Clin Oncol, 27, 1007-1013.

Matthay, K. K., Villablanca, J. G., Seeger, R. C., Stram, D. O., Harris, R. E., Ramsay, N. K., Swift, P., Shimada, H., Black, C. T., Brodeur, G. M., Gerbing, R. B. & Reynolds, C. P. (1999). Treatment of high-risk neuroblastoma with intensive chemotherapy, radiotherapy, autologous bone marrow transplantation, and 13-cis- retinoic acid. Children's Cancer Group. N Engl J Med, 341, 1165-1173.

Maziere, P. & Enright, A. J. (2007). Prediction of microRNA targets. Drug Discov Today, 12, 452-458.

Meister, G., Landthaler, M., Patkaniowska, A., Dorsett, Y., Teng, G. & Tuschl, T. (2004). Human Argonaute2 mediates RNA cleavage targeted by miRNAs and siRNAs. Mol Cell, 15, 185-197.

Meseguer, S., Mudduluru, G., Escamilla, J. M., Allgayer, H. & Barettino, D. (2011). MicroRNAs-10a and -10b Contribute to Retinoic Acid-induced Differentiation of Neuroblastoma Cells and Target the Alternative Splicing Regulatory Factor SFRS1 (SF2/ASF). J Biol Chem, 286, 4150-4164.

Moriarty, C. H., Pursell, B. & Mercurio, A. M. (2010). miR-10b targets Tiam1: implications for Rac activation and carcinoma migration. J Biol Chem, 285, 20541-20546.

Nakata, K., Ohuchida, K., Mizumoto, K., Kayashima, T., Ikenaga, N., Sakai, H., Lin, C., Fujita, H., Otsuka, T., Aishima, S., Nagai, E., Oda, Y. & Tanaka, M. (2011). MicroRNA-10b is overexpressed in pancreatic cancer, promotes its invasiveness, and correlates with a poor prognosis. Surgery, 150, 916-922.

Pahlman, S., Ruusala, A. I., Abrahamsson, L., Mattsson, M. E. & Esscher, T. (1984). Retinoic acid-induced differentiation of cultured human neuroblastoma cells: a comparison with phorbolester-induced differentiation. Cell Differ, 14, 135-144.

Rodriguez, A., Griffiths-Jones, S., Ashurst, J. L. & Bradley, A. (2004). Identification of mammalian microRNA host genes and transcription units. Genome Res, 14, 1902-1910.

Sasayama, T., Nishihara, M., Kondoh, T., Hosoda, K. & Kohmura, E. (2009). MicroRNA-10b is overexpressed in malignant glioma and associated with tumor invasive factors, uPAR and RhoC. Int J Cancer, 125, 1407-1413.

Sidell, N. (1982). Retinoic acid-induced growth inhibition and morphologic differentiation of human neuroblastoma cells in vitro. J Natl Cancer Inst, 68, 589-596.

Stallings, R. L., Foley, N. H., Bray, I. M., Das, S. & Buckley, P. G. (2011). MicroRNA and DNA methylation alterations mediating retinoic acid induced neuroblastoma cell differentiation. Semin Cancer Biol, 21, 283-290.

Thiele, C. J., Reynolds, C. P. & Israel, M. A. (1985). Decreased expression of N-myc precedes retinoic acid-induced morphological differentiation of human neuroblastoma. Nature, 313, 404-406.

Tivnan, A., Foley, N. H., Tracey, L., Davidoff, A. M. & Stallings, R. L. (2010). MicroRNA-184-mediated inhibition of tumour growth in an orthotopic murine model of neuroblastoma. Anticancer Res, 30, 4391-4395.

Tivnan, A., Orr, W. S., Gubala, V., Nooney, R., Williams, D. E., McDonagh, C., Prenter, S., Harvey, H., Domingo-Fernandez, R., Bray, I. M., Piskareva, O., Ng, C. Y., Lode, H. N., Davidoff, A. M. & Stallings, R. L. (2012). Inhibition of neuroblastoma tumor growth by targeted delivery of microRNA-34a using anti-disialoganglioside GD2 coated nanoparticles. PLoS One, 7, e38129.

Tivnan, A., Tracey, L., Buckley, P. G., Alcock, L. C., Davidoff, A. M. & Stallings, R. L. (2011). MicroRNA-34a is a potent tumor suppressor molecule in vivo in neuroblastoma. BMC Cancer, 11, 33.

Veerla, S., Lindgren, D., Kvist, A., Frigyesi, A., Staaf, J., Persson, H., Liedberg, F., Chebil, G., Gudjonsson, S., Borg, A., Mansson, W., Rovira, C. & Hoglund, M. (2009). MiRNA expression in urothelial carcinomas: important roles of miR-10a, miR-222, miR-125b, miR-7 and miR-452 for tumor stage and metastasis, and frequent homozygous losses of miR-31. Int J Cancer, 124, 2236-2242.

Vergoulis, T., Vlachos, I. S., Alexiou, P., Georgakilas, G., Maragkakis, M., Reczko, M., Gerangelos, S., Koziris, N., Dalamagas, T. & Hatzigeorgiou, A. G. (2012). TarBase 6.0: capturing the exponential growth of miRNA targets with experimental support. Nucleic Acids Res, 40, D222-229.

Voigt, A. & Zintl, F. (2003). Effects of retinoic acid on proliferation, apoptosis, cytotoxicity, migration, and invasion of neuroblastoma cells. Med Pediatr Oncol, 40, 205-213.

Wegner, M. & Stolt, C. C. (2005). From stem cells to neurons and glia: a Soxist's view of neural development. Trends Neurosci, 28, 583-588.

Weiss, F. U., Marques, I. J., Woltering, J. M., Vlecken, D. H., Aghdassi, A., Partecke, L. I., Heidecke, C. D., Lerch, M. M. & Bagowski, C. P. (2009). Retinoic acid receptor antagonists inhibit miR-10a expression and block metastatic behavior of pancreatic cancer. Gastroenterology, 137, 2136-2145 e2131-2137.

Welch, C., Chen, Y. & Stallings, R. L. (2007). MicroRNA-34a functions as a potential tumor suppressor by inducing apoptosis in neuroblastoma cells. Oncogene, 26, 5017-5022.

Westermark, U. K., Wilhelm, M., Frenzel, A. & Henriksson, M. A. (2011). The MYCN oncogene and differentiation in neuroblastoma. Semin Cancer Biol, 21, 256-266.

Xu, L., Glass, C. K. & Rosenfeld, M. G. (1999). Coactivator and corepressor complexes in nuclear receptor function. Curr Opin Genet Dev, 9, 140-147.

Yi, R., Qin, Y., Macara, I. G. & Cullen, B. R. (2003). Exportin-5 mediates the nuclear export of pre-microRNAs and short hairpin RNAs. Genes Dev, 17, 3011-3016.

Zhu, Y., Kalbfleisch, T., Brennan, M. D. & Li, Y. (2009). A MicroRNA gene is hosted in an intron of a schizophrenia-susceptibility gene. Schizophr Res, 109, 86-89.

Zijlstra, A., Mellor, R., Panzarella, G., Aimes, R. T., Hooper, J. D., Marchenko, N. D. & Quigley, J. P. (2002). A quantitative analysis of rate-limiting steps in the metastatic cascade using human-specific real-time polymerase chain reaction. Cancer Res, 62, 7083-7092.

Geminiviral Co-option of Post-Translational Modification Pathways

Rosa Lozano-Durán
Departamento de Biología celular, Genética y Fisiología
University of Málaga
Instituto de Hortofruticultura Subtropical y Mediterránea' La Mayora'
Consejo Superior de Investigaciones Científicas (IHSM-UMA-CSIC), Spain

Eduardo R Bejarano
Departamento de Biología celular, Genética y Fisiología
University of Málaga
Instituto de Hortofruticultura Subtropical y Mediterránea' La Mayora'
Consejo Superior de Investigaciones Científicas (IHSM-UMA-CSIC), Spain

1   Geminiviruses, Plant DNA Viruses with Devastating Effects in Agriculture

Geminiviruses are insect-transmitted plant viruses with circular, single-stranded (ss) DNA genomes that cause some of the most economically important diseases in vegetable and field crops worldwide (Mansoor *et al.*, 2003; Rojas *et al.*, 2005; Briddon and Stanley, 2009). Members of the Geminivirus family posses one of the smallest known genomes for an independently replicating virus (Rojas *et al.*, 2005), comprised of one (monopartite) or two (bipartite) components, each of which is ~2.5 – 3.0 Kb in size. For efficient coding of proteins, geminiviruses utilize bidirectional and overlapping genes, with the regulatory sequences, both promoters and origin of replication, localized within the intergenic region (IR) (Figure 1) (reviewed in Rojas *et al.*, 2005; Briddon and Stanley, 2009; Jeske, 2009).

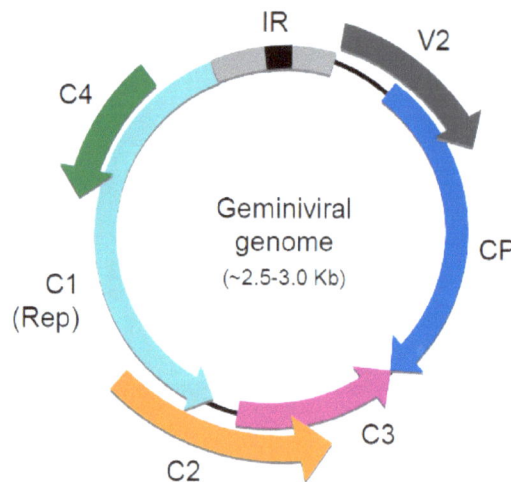

Figure 1: Genome organization of a monopartite geminivirus (modified from Rojas *et al.*, 2005).

Based on genome organization, insect vector and host range, the family *Geminiviridae* is classified into four genera: *Begomovirus*, *Curtovirus*, *Topocuvirus* and *Mastrevirus* (Table 1) (Fauquet *et al.*, 2008). The genomes of curtoviruses, topocuviruses and monopartite begomoviruses have similar features and genome organization: members of these genera encode 6 proteins in the one DNA molecule that constitutes their genome; based on their functions and their position on the viral genome, their proteins have been named V2 (also known as pre-coat protein), CP (also known as V1), C3 (also known as L3 or REn – for replication enhancer-), C2 (also known as L2 or TrAP –for transcriptional activating protein-), replication-associated protein (Rep, also known as C1 or L1) and C4 (also known as L4) (Figure 1). Bipartite begomoviruses have a genome comprising two molecules, named DNA-A and DNA-B. The DNA-A is equivalent to the genome of monopartite geminiviruses, and contains the same genes described above. In addition to these, bipartite begomoviruses encode two additional proteins in the DNA-B component, named movement protein (MP) and nuclear shuttle protein (NSP).

Genus	Type member	Host range	Insect vector	Genome
Mastrevirus	*Maize streak virus* (MSV)	Monocots (and a few dicots)	Leafhoppers (fam. *Cicadellidae*)	Monopartite
Curtovirus	*Beet curly top virus* (BCTV)	Dicots	Leafhoppers (fam. *Cicadellidae*)	Monopartite
Begomovirus	*Bean golden mosaic virus* (BGMV)	Dicots	Whiteflies (*Bemisia tabaci*)	Monopartite or bipartite
Topocuvirus	*Tomato pseudo-curly top virus* (TPCTV)	Dicots	Treehoppers (fam. *Membracidae*)	Monopartite

Table 1: Currently recognized genera of the Geminiviridae family, their type members and properties (host range, insect vector, and genome organization) (modified from Rojas *et al.,* 2005).

Geminiviruses have proliferated worldwide in the past few decades, resulting in extensive yield losses in food and fibre crops, such as tomato, bean, cotton or cassava (Moffat, 1999; Briddon and Stanley, 2009; Jeske, 2009; Moriones and Navas-Castillo, 2010), posing a major threat to sustainable agriculture and food security at a global scale. The study of the mechanisms underlying the pathogenicity and spread of these viruses constitutes an essential step in the fight of the devastating plant diseases they cause.

2   The Limited Weaponry of Geminiviruses

The establishment of a successful infection is a complicated and delicate task that involves a succession of superimposed challenges for the viral pathogen. On one hand, geminiviruses have to replicate their genomes, a process that entails getting to the nucleus and subverting the cellular DNA replication machinery: geminiviruses do not encode their own DNA polymerase, so they broadly rely on the host biosynthetic machinery for viral DNA replication (Hanley-Bowdoin *et al*., 2000). Moreover, geminiviruses usually infect terminally differentiated, non-dividing cells, in which the DNA replication machinery is no longer available; the virus is then forced to reprogram the host cell, gaining control over the cell cycle (Hanley-Bowdoin *et al*., 2000). On the other hand, viruses must have the capacity to move between cells, as well as spread systemically throughout the plant. For this purpose, some mechanism for trafficking through plasmodesmata is probably essential, also opening the door for long-distance transport in the phloem stream. Another vital requisite for the establishment of an infection is the ability to suppress or evade the wide range of host defence responses, overcoming the lethal impediments these responses pose. And last but not least, geminiviruses need to be acquired by their insect vectors and subsequently transmitted to naïve plants to initiate new infections and continue their spread.

The size limitation of the geminiviral genome imposes an efficient, space-effective bidirectional and overlapping protein coding. The resulting proteins are small in size (ranging approximately from 80 to 360 amino acids) and multifunctional; at the same time, different proteins encoded by the same viral genome may target the same or very similar processes, if these are crucial for the infection. For example, geminiviruses encode at least four different gene silencing suppressor proteins not related to each other that may have complementary functions (Nawaz-ul-Rehman and Fauquet, 2009). These data reinforce the idea that geminiviruses posses an important evolutionary potential and are in a constant exploratory mode for survival, a scenario similar to that presented in the proposed evolutionary 'arms race' between host and pathogen (de Wit, 2007). Obviously, the competency of geminiviruses to manipulate the plant cell is the result of a prolonged co-evolution between parasite and host, and is constricted by this process; in other words, the capability of the virus to modulate the cellular homeostasis for its own benefit is evolutionary-shaped. This evolutionary dependency implies that the geminiviral exploitation of the host cell is not static, but rather the outcome of the dynamic interplay between a virus and a plant across evolution.

3   Postranslational Modifications in Plants

Plants are sessile organisms forced to endure all kind of environmental changes, including continuous attacks by potential pathogens. In order to mount fast, effective, reversible responses to both biotic and abiotic stresses, plants extensively rely on proteomic plasticity, since it allows for rapid, dynamic changes in the proteome to adapt to varying environmental cues with minimal energetic cost. The reversible addition of small molecules to target proteins, a process known as post-translational protein modification (PTM), plays a central role in the achievement of the aforementioned proteomic plasticity. This may be particularly relevant in the plant kingdom, where PTMs are proposed to rival transcription as the dominant regulatory mechanism (Dreher & Callis, 2007; Smalle & Vierstra, 2004).

PTMs result in changes in the properties of the modified target protein, namely stability, molecular interactions, activity or localization, ultimately leading to functional changes. A diverse array of molecules have been found to be chemically added to target proteins as post-translational modifications, including biochemically functional groups such as phosphate, acetate, lipids and carbohydrates, and also small peptides such as ubiquitin or ubiquitin-like modifiers (e.g. SUMO or RUB1).

4   Geminiviruses and Ubiquitination

Ubiquitination is a well-characterized PTM in which the 76-amino-acid protein ubiquitin is covalently attached to a target protein through an enzymatic catalytic cascade. Ubiquitination confers one of several possible fates depending on the number of ubiquitin molecules attached and the location of their attachment. The most general destiny of ubiquitinated proteins is their breakdown by the 26S proteasome, a proteolytic protein complex; other possible, less common consequences of ubiquitination include regulation of the activity or localization of the target protein (Mukhopadhyay & Riezman, 2007).

The ubiquitin-26S proteasome system (UPS) is essential in eukaryotes, and it plays a central regulatory role in plants (Vierstra, 2009). The UPS begins with the sequential actions of three enzyme families, E1 ubiquitin-activating enzyme (UBA), E2 ubiquitin-conjugating enzyme, and E3 ubiquitin ligase, which in turn covalently attach one or more ubiquitin molecules to a specific target protein. Given that the final step in the ubiquitination cascade serves as the primary substrate recognition event, E3 enzymes are the key factors determining substrate specificity of the process. Ubiquitination is a reversible modification: the ubiquitin conjugate can be disassembled from the targeted protein by deubiquitinating enzymes (DUBs).

The importance and complexity of the UPS in plants can be foreseen by phylogenetic analysis: over 1,600 loci, expressing nearly 6% of the proteome, have been identified in *Arabidopsis thaliana* to encode core components of the UPS. Moreover, the hierarchical importance of each component is clearly illustrated by its diversity: Arabidopsis, for example, expresses two E1s, at least 37 E2s, and potentially over 1,400 different E3s (Vierstra, 2009).

Four main classes of E3s are described in plants, classified by their mechanisms of action and sub-unit composition: HECT, RING, U-box and cullin-RING ligases (CRLs), the latter being multisubunit E3s. All CRLs contain a small RING domain-containing protein, a cullin protein, and one or several additional cullin-specific subunit(s) with substrate recognition or adaptor functions (Hotton and Callis, 2008; Vierstra, 2009).

To date, three cullins have been described to form CRLs in plants, CULLIN1, CULLIN3 and CULLIN4, defining the three classes of CRL complexes. Gene families encode substrate recognition subunits for each class of CRL; classes are named typically after their common motif. For CULLIN 1 (CUL1)-based CRLs, the substrate-binding subunit is an F-box protein. The extensive number of potential substrate recognition subunits in the proteome of plants, together with the combinatorial assembly of CRLs, suggests that this class of E3 ligases must have complex and highly diverse roles. Of note, one of the largest gene families in *A. thaliana* encodes the F-box subunits of SCF complexes (Gagne *et al.,* 2002), with nearly 700 members.

During the past few years, a growing body of reports has unveiled ubiquitination as an important player in plant-virus interactions (Alcaide-Loridan and Jupin, 2012). Components of the ubiquitination pathway have been shown to change their expression level in response to viral infection (Takizawa *et al.,* 2005; Ascencio-Ibanez *et al.,* 2008; Alfenas-Zerbini *et al.,* 2009; Lai *et al.,* 2009), and ubiquitination of viral proteins has been detected in some cases (Hazelwood and Zaitlin, 1990; Barajas *et al.,* 2009; Barajas and Nagy, 2010). Moreover, the list of direct interactions between viral proteins and components of the ubiquitination pathway is growing every year.

An increasing number of reports have made it clear that geminiviruses interact with the ubiquitination pathway, probably at multiple levels, to promote their virulence.

Infection by the geminivirus *Cabbage leaf curl virus* (CaLCuV) triggered changes in the transcription of a wide array of genes encoding components of the UPS in Arabidopsis: 32 genes encoding subunits of the 26S proteasome complex were up-regulated, as were the two genes encoding E1 ubiquitin-activating enzymes, eight out of 37 E2 ubiquitin-conjugating enzymes, and 149 out of 1,570 E3 ubiquitin ligases, whereas only 23 genes encoding E3 ligases were down-regulated (Ascencio-Ibanez *et al.,* 2008).

Transgenic expression of individual geminiviral proteins also leads to altered expression of UPS elements (Lai *et al.,* 2009; Lozano-Duran *et al.,* 2011b). One particularly interesting case is that of C4 from *Beet severe curly top virus* (BSCTV), which promotes expression of the RING E3 ligase *RKP* (for Related to KPC1); since RKP controls cell cycle progression through degradation of the cell cycle inhibitors ICK/KRPs (Ren *et al.,* 2008; Lai *et al.,* 2009), C4-mediated up-regulation of *RKP* could result in the re-entry of cell cycle, a requirement for geminivirus replication. In agreement with this idea, the protein level of ICK/KRP1 was decreased upon BSCTV infection, and overexpression of *ICK1/KRP1* in Arabidopsis reduced the susceptibility to BSCTV (Lai *et al.,* 2009).

The physical association between geminiviral proteins and components of the UPS has also been reported (Table 2). One example is the interaction between the βC1 protein (which is encoded in a satellite βDNA) from *Cotton leaf curl Multan virus* (CLCuMV) and the tomato ubiquitin E2 enzyme SlUBC3 (Eini *et al.,* 2009). Transgenic expression of *βC1* in tobacco led to a reduction in the level of polyubiquitinated proteins, suggesting that βC1 is interfering with ubiquitination in a general, non-specific manner, probably through its interaction with the SlUBC3 homologue.

Geminiviral protein	Geminivirus species	Plant interactor (species)	Reference
Rep	*African cassava mosaic virus* (ACMV)	SUMO conjugating enzyme E1 (*Nicotiana benthamiana*)	Castillo *et al.*, 2004
Rep	*Tomato golden mosaic virus* (TGMV)	SUMO conjugating enzyme E1 (*Nicotiana benthamiana*)	Castillo *et al.*, 2004; Sanchez-Durán *et al.*, 2011
Rep	*Tomato yellow leaf curl Sardinia virus* (TYLCSV)	SUMO conjugating enzyme E1 (*Nicotiana benthamiana*)	Castillo *et al.*, 2004
C2	*Tomato golden mosaic virus* (TGMV)	ADK (Arabidopsis)	Wang *et al.*, 2003
C2	*Tomato golden mosaic virus* (TGMV)	SNF1 (Arabidopsis)	Hao *et al.*, 2003
C2	*Beet curly top virus* (BCTV)	ADK (Arabidopsis)	Wang *et al.*, 2003
C2	*Beet curly top virus* (BCTV)	CSN5 (Arabidopsis, tomato)	Lozano-Duran *et al.*, 2011b
C2	*Beet curly top virus* (BCTV)	SNF1 (Arabidopsis)	Hao *et al.*, 2003
C2	*Tomato yellow leaf curl virus* (TYLCV)	CSN5 (Arabidopsis, tomato)	Lozano-Duran *et al.*, 2011b
C2	*Tomato yellow leaf curl Sardinia virus* (TYLCSV)	UBA1 (tomato)	Hericourt *et al.*, in preparation
C2	*Tomato yellow leaf curl Sardinia virus* (TYLCSV)	CSN5 (Arabidopsis, tomato)	Lozano-Duran *et al.*, 2011b
C4	*Tomato golden mosaic virus* (TGMV)	AtSKeta (Ararbidopsis)	Piroux *et al.*, 2007
C4	*Tomato golden mosaic virus* (TGMV)	AtSKzeta (Arabidopsis)	Piroux *et al.*, 2007
C4	*Beet curly top virus* (BCTV)	AtSKeta (Ararbidopsis)	Piroux *et al.*, 2007
C4	*Beet curly top virus* (BCTV)	AtSKzeta (Arabidopsis)	Piroux *et al.*, 2007
C4	*Tomato yellow leaf curl virus-Australia* (ToLCV)	SlSK (tomato)	Dogra *et al.*, 2009
C4	*Tomato yellow leaf curl Sardinia virus* (TYLCSV)	BAM1 (Arabidopsis)	Hericourt *et al.*, in preparation
C4	*Tomato yellow leaf curl Sardinia virus* (TYLCSV)	AtSKkappa (Arabidopsis)	Hericourt *et al.*, in preparation
NSP	*Cabbage leaf curl virus* (CaLCuV)	NsAK (Arabidopsis)	Florentino *et al.*, 2006
NSP	*Tomato crinkle leaf yellow virus* (TCrLYV)	NIK1-3 (Arabidopsis)	Fontes *et al.*, 2006
NSP	*Tomato golden mosaic virus* (TGMV)	NIK1-3 (Arabidopsis)	Fontes *et al.*, 2006
βC1	*Cotton leaf curl Multan virus* (CLCuMV)	SlUBC3 (tomato)	Eini *et al.*, 2009
βC1	*Tomato yellow leaf curl China virus* (TYLCCNV)	SlSnRK1 (tomato)	Shen *et al.*, 2011

Table 2: Geminiviral proteins found to interact with host proteins involved in post-translational modification pathways.

The results obtained with CLCuMV indicate that ubiquitination could be globally detrimental for the infection by geminiviruses, and therefore a preferred target for viral effectors. In agreement with this hypothesis, it has been recently shown that silencing of the ubiquitin-activating enzyme UBA1 in *Nicotiana benthamiana* results in enhanced *Tomato yellow leaf curl Sardinia virus* (TYLCSV) infection (Lozano-Duran *et al.*, 2011a). Interestingly, the tomato UBA1 has been found to interact with TYLCSV

C2 in yeast (Hericourt *et al.,* in preparation) (Table 2), which raises the idea that C2 could be inhibiting UBA1 during the viral infection as a virulence strategy.

Along the same lines, a negative impact of geminiviral C2 on ubiquitination has been described, at least for TYLCSV, *Tomato yellow leaf curl virus* (TYLCV) and *Beet curly top virus* (BCTV). These three C2 proteins interact with CSN5, catalytic subunit of the CSN complex (see section 'Geminiviruses and rubylation'; Table 2), and their transgenic expression in Arabidopsis seemed to result in the altered regulation of CULLIN1-based SCF complexes (Lozano-Duran *et al.,* 2011b). Consistently, an array of SCF-regulated pathways, such as the response to the plant hormones jasmonates, auxins, gibberellins and ethylene, was affected in these transgenic lines. Again, given the relevance of SCF complex-mediated regulation for a plethora of physiological processes in plants (Hua and Vierstra, 2011), the geminiviruses' ability to globally interfere with this machinery in the host cell could mean a very potent virulence strategy.

A very tantalizing model suggests that a finer mechanism could act superimposed to the C2-mediated general inhibition of SCF complexes. This idea is based on the finding that overexpression of a given F-box protein can overcome the C2-mediated inhibition of SCF complexes (Lozano-Duran and Bejarano, 2011a); therefore, it is enticing to speculate that geminiviruses may not only impair, but rather redirect the activity of the SCF complex by inducing the expression of selected F-box proteins, and in this way co-opt the SCF-mediated ubiquitination pathway to benefit viral functions.

5   Geminiviruses and Rubylation

The activity of the CRLs (see section 'Geminiviruses and ubiquitination') is essential in eukaryotes and highly diverse, controlling multiple cellular processes. Since there is a plethora of substrate-binding subunits for each CRL, the molecular composition of the complexes in the cell must be tightly regulated according to developmental or environmental cues. On the other hand, the activity of specific CRLs must be modulated as well to ensure a prompt response to the said stimuli. CRLs are subject to regulation by another protein modification pathway, the related-to-ubiquitin (RUB1) pathway: all three *Arabidopsis* CULLINs are regulated by a cycle of covalent attachment and removal of the ubiquitin-like protein RUB1 (known as Nedd8 in fission yeast and animals) (Dreher and Callis, 2007). The RUB1 pathway has an analogous enzymatic cascade to that of ubiquitination, with E1, E2 and E3 enzymes, and ends with the covalent attachment of RUB1 to the target protein. Like ubiquitination, rubylation is essential in eukaryotes.

As in other post-translational protein modifications, rubylation is reversible: RUB1 can be detached from CULLINs by the CSN (COP9 signalosome) complex. The CSN is a multiprotein complex, conserved in eukaryotes, which possesses isopeptidase activity (Wei *et al.,* 2008). This complex comprises eight subunits, named CSN1 to CSN8, where CSN5 functions as the catalytic centre (Wei *et al.,* 2008); the derubylating activity, however, requires an intact CSN holocomplex, and all eight subunits are essential for the integrity and subsequent functionality of the complex (Wei *et al.,* 2008).

RUB1/Nedd8 conjugation seems to stimulate CRL activity *in vitro* (Read *et al.,* 2000; Wu *et al.,* 2000). Surprisingly, derubylation also appears to be needed for *in vivo* robust CRL activity (Osterlund *et al.,* 2000; Lyapina *et al.,* 2001; Schwechheimer *et al.,* 2001; Cope and Deshaies, 2003): loss-of-function mutations in either rubylation or derubylation pathways in *Arabidopsis* result in shared phenotypes, with CRL substrate accumulation in both cases (Hotton and Callis, 2008). These apparently contradictory results have led to a model in which a dynamic cycling of RUB1 modification and removal is required for proper CRL activity (Lyapina *et al.*, 2001). A possible explanation for this paradox comes from the observation that rubylation leads to auto-ubiquitination and destabilization of CRL components, which would result in reduced CRL activity (Denti *et al.*, 2006; Wu *et al.*, 2006; Schmidt *et al.*, 2009; Stuttmann *et al.*, 2009). On the other hand, it has been proposed that CULLIN rubylation and derubylation might act coupled with a functional cycle, coordinating a CRL activity-promoting event such as the assembly/disassembly of the complex. This assembly/disassembly event would be essential for switching the substrate-binding subunit of the complex, allowing the ubiquitination of new substrates in response to developmental or environmental stimuli (Wu *et al.*, 2006; Schmidt *et al.*, 2009; Stuttmann *et al.*, 2009).

The rubylation status of CULLIN1 has been shown to be specifically affected by C2 from the geminiviruses TYLCSV, TYLCV and BCTV. These three C2 proteins interact with CSN5 (Table 2) and their transgenic expression in Arabidopsis results in the hyperaccumulation of CULLIN1 in its rubylated state, suggesting that C2 could be interfering with the CSN de-rubylating activity over CULLIN1 (Lozano-Duran *et al.*, 2011b). As described in the previous section, this in turn seems to be coupled with the malfunction of multiple SCF complexes and the concomitant altered physiological responses.

Because infection by BCTV seems to be hindered in an Arabidopsis *csn5a* knock-down line (Lozano-Duran and Bejarano, 2011b), it could be hypothesized that geminiviruses may be redirecting the activity of the CSN complex to efficiently co-opt the SCF-mediated ubiquitination, rather than generally suppressing this process. This idea is supported by the finding that silencing of *CSN3* in *N. benthamiana*, which is expected to result in loss of the entire CSN complex (Wei *et al.*, 2008), has a negative impact on the infection by TYLCSV (Lozano-Duran *et al.*, 2011a).

Since SCF complexes control a plethora of cell functions, by aiming at the regulation of the SCF complexes, geminiviruses could be tampering with multiple cellular processes at once with minimal costs. In agreement with this idea, CSN5 has been recently described as a cellular hub convergently targeted by independently evolved virulence effectors from different pathogens (Mukhtar *et al.*, 2011).

6   Geminiviruses and Sumoylation

Sumoylation is a PTM in which peptides belonging to the family of small ubiquititin-like modifier (SUMO) are covalently attached to a target protein. SUMOs and ubiquitin are highly similar structurally, despite being diverse in sequence, and the enzymatic cascade leading to SUMO conjugation also resembles that of ubiquitination. Like for others PTMs, sumoylation is essential in eukaryotes, reversible, and seems to regulate an abundance of cell processes such as cell cycle, transcription or subcellular trafficking (Ulrich, 2009; Castro *et al.*, 2012). Unlike ubiquitination, SUMO attachment does not mostly result in protein degradation, and instead a major consequence of sumoylation is thought to be the modificacion of protein-protein interactions through alteration of interacting surfaces. Since both SUMO and ubiquitin are linked to Lys residues, these peptides have been shown to compete for target proteins, indicating that SUMO can also modulate protein stability and subcellular localization (Ulrich, 2009).

The importance of sumoylation in geminivirus-plant interactions is illustrated by the finding that the essential Rep proteins from *Tomato golden mosaic virus* (TGMV), *African cassava mosaic virus* (ACMV) and TYLCSV physically interact with the host SUMO-conjugating enzyme E1 (Castillo *et al.*, 2004) (Table 2). Viral replication was strongly reduced by altered expression of SUMO, either positively or negatively (Castillo *et al.*, 2004), suggesting that the accumulation of this peptide needs to be carefully fine-tuned for successful geminiviral replication, therefore highlighting its importance in this process. This idea is further supported by the fact that silencing of SUMO-conjugating enzyme in *N. benthamiana* results in suppression of TYLCSV infection (Castillo *et al.*, 2007).

The interaction between geminivirus Rep and the host SUMO E1 has been proven required for viral replication and infectivity (Sanchez-Duran *et al.*, 2011). Interestingly enough, overexpression of Rep does not dramatically alter the general pattern of sumoylation in the plant, but seems to trigger changes in specific proteins, resulting in increased or *de novo* sumoylation (Sanchez-Duran *et al.*, 2011). Therefore, it has been proposed that the Rep-mediated modulation of sumoylation in the infected cell may be limited to certain target host proteins; these targets, however, remain to be identified (Sanchez-Duran *et al.*, 2011).

7 Geminiviruses and Myristoylation

Myristoylation is a post-translational (or co-translational) modification consisting in the covalent attachment of a myristoyl group via an amide bond to the alpha-amino group of an N-terminal glycine of a popyleptide. Myristoylation is catalyzed by the enzyme N-myristoyltransferase (NMT). Unlike other PTMs, myristoylation is essentially irreversible, and it plays a pivotal role in directing and anchoring proteins to membranes, although it can also affect protein-protein interactions (Martin *et al.*, 2011). As a result, the addition of the myristate moiety is involved in signal transduction and regulation of different cell processes.

The βC1 protein from CLCuMV (see section 'Geminiviruses and ubiquitination') needs to undergo myristoylation in order to interact with the tomato SlUBC3 (Eini *et al.*, 2009), and mutation of the myristoylated motif of βC1 results in its inability to induce the typical DNA-β-specific symptoms (Eini *et al.*, 2009). Even though βC1 is localized in the cell periphery and the nucleus and impairing myristoylation could disrupt its plasma membrane localization, it seems to also affect the interaction with SlUBC3 specifically, since the loss of interaction can be detected using the yeast two-hybrid system, in which both bait and pray proteins are artificially targeted to the nucleus.

Interestingly, the C4 protein from begomoviruses, curtoviruses and topocuviruses harbours a conserved myristoylation motif, which has been shown to be required for membrane localization and symptom production in the begomovirus *East African cassava mosaic Cameroon virus* (EACMCV) and the curtovirus BCTV (Fondong *et al.*, 2007; Piroux *et al.*, 2007). C4 is a pathogenicity determinant, and has been shown to function as a suppressor of gene silencing in several geminiviral species (Fondong *et al.*, 2007; Gopal *et al.*, 2007; Dogra *et al.*, 2009; Amin *et al.*, 2011; Luna *et al.*, 2012); why membrane targeting is relevant for the biological role of C4, and whether disruption of membrane localization affects all or only a subset of the activities exerted by this potentially multifunctional pathogenicity factor, remains to be elucidated.

8 Geminiviruses and Phosphorylation

Protein phosphorylation is a PTM consisting in the covalent addition of a phosphate group to a serine, threonine or tyrosine residue. Phosphorylation is reversible and constitutes one of the most common mechanisms of regulation of protein function; proteins can switch between a phosphorylated and an unphosphorylated form, displaying a differential activity in each state. The enzymes that phosphorylate proteins are protein kinases, and those in charge of the removal of the phosphate group are called phosphatases.

The sequential phosphorylation of proteins, or phosphorelay, in a given signalling pathway provides the basis for complex signalling and regulatory networks in response to multiple cues. Interestingly, the Arabidopsis genome contains more than 1,000 predicted protein kinases (Lukowitz *et al.*, 2000), almost twice as many as the human genome (Manning *et al.*, 2002), suggesting that phosphorylation plays a crucial role in the regulation of plant responses. Using mass spectrometry, the phosphoproteome of Arabidopsis and rice have been shown to comprise more than 1,400 (Reiland *et al.*, 2009) and almost 3,400 phosphorylated proteins, respectively (Nakagami *et al.*, 2010); current efforts are being aimed at identifying dynamic changes in plant phosphoproteomes in response to specific signals, such as abiotic stresses or pathogen attack.

Several geminiviral proteins, such as the MP from *Abutilon mosaic virus* (Kleinow *et al.*, 2009), are known to be phosphorylated in the plant cell; in a few examples, the interacting plant kinase responsible for this modification has been identified (Table 2). That is the case of the βC1 from *Tomato yellow leaf curl China* β-satellite, which is phosphorylated upon interaction with the tomato SlSnRK (Shen *et al.*, 2011), or that of the NSP from CaLCuV, TGMV and *Tomato crinkle leaf yellow virus* (TCrLYV), all three interacting with an Arabidopsis PERK-like receptor named NsAK (for NSP-associated kinase) (Florentino *et al.*, 2006). However, the impact of phosphorylation of these viral proteins on viral infectivity seems to differ in the previous two examples. Phosphorylation of βC1 by SlSnRK is most likely detrimental for the virus, as indicated by infection experiments of plants overexpressing or silenced for this kinase or infections with *βC1* mutants harbouring phospho-mimetic or phospho-dead residues at the phosphorylation sites (Shen *et al.*, 2011). On the contrary, loss of NsAK function reduces the efficiency of CaLCuV infection and attenuates symptom development, indicating that NsAK is most likely a positive regulator of geminiviral infection, possibly contributing to NSP function (Florentino *et al.*, 2006).

Interestingly, two plant kinases, BAM1 and SK4-1 (Shaggy-related kinase kappa), both of which interact with TYLCSV C4 in yeast (Héricourt *et al.*, in preparation), have been suggested to be required for geminiviral infection, since their silencing results in the delay or suppression of TYLCSV infection (Lozano-Duran *et al.*, 2011a). Shaggy-like protein kinases also interact with other geminiviral C4 proteins, namely those of BCTV, TGMV and *Tomato leaf curl virus-Australia*, and this interaction is required to trigger disease symptoms and for C4 function as suppressor of gene silencing (Piroux *et al.*, 2007; Dogra *et al.*, 2009). At least one of these shaggy-like proteins, AtSKeta, phosphorylates C4 from BCTV and, to a lesser extent, C4 from TGMV *in vitro* (Piroux *et al.*, 2007), raising the idea that this family of plant kinases may be co-opted by C4 to promote its own phosphorylation and enhance its virulence function.

Some geminiviral effectors interact with plant kinases not as substrates, but rather as inhibitors, as part of their virulence function. L2 from BCTV and AL2 from TGMV, for example, interact with and inactivate Adenosine kinase (ADK) and SNF1 (Hao *et al.*, 2003; Wang *et al.*, 2003), which contributes to pathogenicity. The NSP from TGMV and TCrLYV binds three leucine-rich repeat receptor-like kinases (LRR-RLK) in Arabidopsis, named NIK1 to NIK3, and inhibit their kinase activity; the positive correlation between infection rate and loss of NIK1 and NIK3 function suggests the involvement of these NIKs in antiviral defence responses (Fontes *et al.*, 2004).

9 Conclusions

A growing body of reports generated during the past few years highlights the importance of post-translational modifications in host-virus interactions. In plants, post-translational modifications play a prevalent role in the regulation of physiological processes and responses to stimuli, what makes them a very attractive target for viruses.

Works by different researchers have unveiled that geminiviruses interact with a wide array of post-translational modification pathways, including ubiquitination, sumoylation, rubylation, myristoylation and phosphorylation, and in some cases have determined how these interactions ultimately impact pathogenicity. It is noteworthy that geminiviruses have an extremely limited coding capacity due to size constrictions; in this scenario, aiming at hub regulators of the host cell biology, such as post-translational modifications, would probably mean a very cost-effective, powerful virulence strategy. Current efforts by laboratories in different parts of the world will hopefully help gain insight into the intricate interactions between geminiviruses and post-translational modification pathways in the near future.

References

Alcaide-Loridan, C., and Jupin, I. (2012). Ubiquitin and Plant Viruses, Let's Play Together! Plant Physiol 160, 72-82.

Alfenas-Zerbini, P., Maia, I.G., Favaro, R.D., Cascardo, J.C., Brommonschenkel, S.H., and Zerbini, F.M. (2009). Genome-wide analysis of differentially expressed genes during the early stages of tomato infection by a potyvirus. Mol Plant Microbe Interact 22, 352-361.

Amin, I., Hussain, K., Akbergenov, R., Yadav, J.S., Qazi, J., Mansoor, S., Hohn, T., Fauquet, C.M., and Briddon, R.W. (2011). Suppressors of RNA silencing encoded by the components of the cotton leaf curl begomovirus-betasatellite complex. Mol Plant Microbe Interact 24, 973-983.

Ascencio-Ibanez, J.T., Sozzani, R., Lee, T.J., Chu, T.M., Wolfinger, R.D., Cella, R., and Hanley-Bowdoin, L. (2008). Global analysis of Arabidopsis gene expression uncovers a complex array of changes impacting pathogen response and cell cycle during geminivirus infection. Plant Physiol 148, 436-454.

Barajas, D., and Nagy, P.D. (2010). Ubiquitination of tombusvirus p33 replication protein plays a role in virus replication and binding to the host Vps23p ESCRT protein. Virology 397, 358-368.

Barajas, D., Li, Z., and Nagy, P.D. (2009). The Nedd4-type Rsp5p ubiquitin ligase inhibits tombusvirus replication by regulating degradation of the p92 replication protein and decreasing the activity of the tombusvirus replicase. J Virol 83, 11751-11764.

Briddon, R.W., and Stanley, J. (2009). Geminiviridae. eLS.

Castillo, A.G., Kong, L.J., Hanley-Bowdoin, L., and Bejarano, E.R. (2004). Interaction between a geminivirus replication protein and the plant sumoylation system. J Virol 78, 2758-2769.

Castillo, A.G., Morilla, G., Lozano, R., Collinet, D., Perez-Luna, A., Kashoggi, A., and Bejarano, E.R. (2007). Identification of Plant Genes Involved in TYLCV Replication. In Tomato Yellow Leaf Curl Virus Disease. Management, Molecular Biology, Breeding for Resistance., H. Czosnek, ed (Springer).

Castro, P.H., Tavares, R.M., Bejarano, E.R., and Azevedo, H. (2012). SUMO, a heavyweight player in plant abiotic stress responses. Cell Mol Life Sci 69, 3269-3283.

Cope, G.A., and Deshaies, R.J. (2003). COP9 signalosome: a multifunctional regulator of SCF and other cullin-based ubiquitin ligases. Cell 114, 663-671.

de Wit, P. (2007). How plants recognize pathogens and defend themselves. Cell Mol Life Sci. 64, 2726-2732.

Denti, S., Fernandez-Sanchez, M.E., Rogge, L., and Bianchi, E. (2006). The COP9 signalosome regulates Skp2 levels and proliferation of human cells. J Biol Chem 281, 32188-32196.

Dogra, S.C., Eini, O., Rezaian, M.A., and Randles, J.W. (2009). A novel shaggy-like kinase interacts with the Tomato leaf curl virus pathogenicity determinant C4 protein. Plant Mol Biol 71, 25-38.

Dreher, K., and Callis, J. (2007). Ubiquitin, hormones and biotic stress in plants. Ann Bot 99, 787-822.

Eini, O., Behjatnia, S.A., Dogra, S., Dry, I.B., Randles, J.W., and Rezaian, M.A. (2009). Identification of sequence elements regulating promoter activity and replication of a monopartite begomovirus-associated DNA beta satellite. J Gen Virol 90, 253-260.

Fauquet, C.M., Briddon, R.W., Brown, J.K., Moriones, E., Stanley, J., Zerbini, M., and Zhou, X. (2008). Geminivirus strain demarcation and nomenclature. Arch Virol 153, 783-821.

Florentino, L.H., Santos, A.A., Fontenelle, M.R., Pinheiro, G.L., Zerbini, F.M., Baracat-Pereira, M.C., and Fontes, E.P. (2006). A PERK-like receptor kinase interacts with the geminivirus nuclear shuttle protein and potentiates viral infection. J Virol 80, 6648-6656.

Fondong, V.N., Reddy, R.V., Lu, C., Hankoua, B., Felton, C., Czymmek, K., and Achenjang, F. (2007). The consensus N-myristoylation motif of a geminivirus AC4 protein is required for membrane binding and pathogenicity. Mol Plant Microbe Interact 20, 380-391.

Fontes, E.P., Santos, A.A., Luz, D.F., Waclawovsky, A.J., and Chory, J. (2004). The geminivirus nuclear shuttle protein is a virulence factor that suppresses transmembrane receptor kinase activity. Genes Dev 18, 2545-2556.

Gopal, P., Pravin Kumar, P., Sinilal, B., Jose, J., Kasin Yadunandam, A., and Usha, R. (2007). Differential roles of C4 and betaC1 in mediating suppression of post-transcriptional gene silencing: evidence for transactivation by the C2 of Bhendi yellow vein mosaic virus, a monopartite begomovirus. Virus Res 123, 9-18.

Hanley-Bowdoin, L., Settlage, S.B., and Robertson, D. (2004). Reprogramming plant gene expression: a prerequisite to geminivirus DNA replication. Mol. Plant Pathol. 5.

Hanley-Bowdoin, L., Settlage, S.B., Orozco, B.M., Nagar, S., and Robertson, D. (2000). Geminiviruses: models for plant DNA replication, transcription, and cell cycle regulation. Crit Rev Biochem Mol Biol 35, 105-140.

Hao, L., Wang, H., Sunter, G., and Bisaro, D.M. (2003). Geminivirus AL2 and L2 proteins interact with and inactivate SNF1 kinase. Plant Cell 15, 1034-1048.

Hazelwood, D., and Zaitlin, M. (1990). Ubiquitinated conjugates are found in preparations of several plant viruses. Virology 177, 352-356.

Hotton, S.K., and Callis, J. (2008). Regulation of cullin RING ligases. Annu Rev Plant Biol 59, 467-489.

Hua, Z., and Vierstra, R.D. (2011). The cullin-RING ubiquitin-protein ligases. Annu Rev Plant Biol 62, 299-334.

Jeske, H. (2009). Geminiviruses. Curr Top Microbiol Immunol 331, 185-226.

Kleinow, T., Tanwir, F., Kocher, C., Krenz, B., Wege, C., and Jeske, H. (2009). Expression dynamics and ultrastructural localization of epitope-tagged Abutilon mosaic virus nuclear shuttle and movement proteins in Nicotiana benthamiana cells. Virology 391, 212-220.

Lai, J., Chen, H., Teng, K., Zhao, Q., Zhang, Z., Li, Y., Liang, L., Xia, R., Wu, Y., Guo, H., and Xie, Q. (2009). RKP, a RING finger E3 ligase induced by BSCTV C4 protein, affects geminivirus infection by regulation of the plant cell cycle. Plant J 57, 905-917.

Lozano-Duran, R., and Bejarano, E.R. (2011a). Geminivirus C2 protein might be the key player for geminiviral co-option of SCF-mediated ubiquitination. Plant Signal Behav 6.

Lozano-Duran, R., and Bejarano, E.R. (2011b). Mutation in Arabidopsis CSN5A partially complements the lack of Beet curly top virus pathogenicity factor L2. Journal of Plant Pathology & Microbiology 2:108. doi:10.4172/2157-7471.1000108.

Lozano-Duran, R., Rosas-Diaz, T., Luna, A.P., and Bejarano, E.R. (2011a). Identification of host genes involved in geminivirus infection using a reverse genetics approach. PLoS One 6, e22383.

Lozano-Duran, R., Rosas-Diaz, T., Gusmaroli, G., Luna, A.P., Taconnat, L., Deng, X.W., and Bejarano, E.R. (2011b). Geminiviruses subvert ubiquitination by altering CSN-mediated derubylation of SCF E3 ligase complexes and inhibit jasmonate signaling in Arabidopsis thaliana. Plant Cell 23, 1014-1032.

Lukowitz, W., Gillmor, C.S., and Scheible, W.R. (2000). Positional cloning in Arabidopsis. Why it feels good to have a genome initiative working for you. Plant Physiol 123, 795-805.

Luna, A.P., Morilla, G., Voinnet, O., and Bejarano, E.R. (2012). Functional analysis of gene-silencing suppressors from tomato yellow leaf curl disease viruses. Mol Plant Microbe Interact 25, 1294-1306.

Lyapina, S., Cope, G., Shevchenko, A., Serino, G., Tsuge, T., Zhou, C., Wolf, D.A., Wei, N., and Deshaies, R.J. (2001). Promotion of NEDD-CUL1 conjugate cleavage by COP9 signalosome. Science 292, 1382-1385.

Manning, G., Whyte, D.B., Martinez, R., Hunter, T., and Sudarsanam, S. (2002). The protein kinase complement of the human genome. Science 298, 1912-1934.

Mansoor, S., Briddon, R.W., Zafar, Y., and Stanley, J. (2003). Geminivirus disease complexes: an emerging threat. Trends Plant Sci 8, 128-134.

Martin, D.D., Beauchamp, E., and Berthiaume, L.G. (2011). Post-translational myristoylation: Fat matters in cellular life and death. Biochimie 93, 18-31.

Moffat, A. (1999). Geminiviruses emerge as serious crop threat. Science, 1835.

Moriones, E., and Navas-Castillo, J. (2010). Tomato Yellow Leaf Curl Disease Epidemics. In Bemisia: Bionomics and magements of a global pest, P.A. Stansly and S.E. Naranjo, eds (Springer Netherlands).

Mukhopadhyay, D., and Riezman, H. (2007). Proteasome-independent functions of ubiquitin in endocytosis and signaling. Science 315, 201-205.

Mukhtar, M.S., Carvunis, A.R., Dreze, M., Epple, P., Steinbrenner, J., Moore, J., Tasan, M., Galli, M., Hao, T., Nishimura, M.T., Pevzner, S.J., Donovan, S.E., Ghamsari, L., Santhanam, B., Romero, V., Poulin, M.M., Gebreab, F., Gutierrez, B.J., Tam, S., Monachello, D., Boxem, M., Harbort, C.J., McDonald, N., Gai, L., Chen, H., He, Y., Vandenhaute, J., Roth, F.P., Hill, D.E., Ecker, J.R., Vidal, M., Beynon, J., Braun, P., and Dangl, J.L. (2011). Independently evolved virulence effectors converge onto hubs in a plant immune system network. Science 333, 596-601.

Nakagami, H., Sugiyama, N., Mochida, K., Daudi, A., Yoshida, Y., Toyoda, T., Tomita, M., Ishihama, Y., and Shirasu, K. (2010). Large-scale comparative phosphoproteomics identifies conserved phosphorylation sites in plants. Plant Physiol 153, 1161-1174.

Nawaz-ul-Rehman, M.S., and Fauquet, C.M. (2009). Evolution of geminiviruses and their satellites. FEBS Lett 583, 1825-1832.

Osterlund, M.T., Wei, N., and Deng, X.W. (2000). The roles of photoreceptor systems and the COP1-targeted destabilization of HY5 in light control of Arabidopsis seedling development. Plant Physiol 124, 1520-1524.

Piroux, N., Saunders, K., Page, A., and Stanley, J. (2007). Geminivirus pathogenicity protein C4 interacts with Arabidopsis thaliana shaggy-related protein kinase AtSKeta, a component of the brassinosteroid signalling pathway. Virology 362, 428-440.

Read, M.A., Brownell, J.E., Gladysheva, T.B., Hottelet, M., Parent, L.A., Coggins, M.B., Pierce, J.W., Podust, V.N., Luo, R.S., Chau, V., and Palombella, V.J. (2000). Nedd8 modification of cul-1 activates SCF(beta(TrCP))-dependent ubiquitination of IkappaBalpha. Mol Cell Biol 20, 2326-2333.

Reiland, S., Messerli, G., Baerenfaller, K., Gerrits, B., Endler, A., Grossmann, J., Gruissem, W., and Baginsky, S. (2009). Large-scale Arabidopsis phosphoproteome profiling reveals novel chloroplast kinase substrates and phosphorylation networks. Plant Physiol 150, 889-903.

Ren, H., Santner, A., del Pozo, J.C., Murray, J.A., and Estelle, M. (2008). Degradation of the cyclin-dependent kinase inhibitor KRP1 is regulated by two different ubiquitin E3 ligases. Plant J 53, 705-716.

Rojas, M.R., Hagen, C., Lucas, W.J., and Gilbertson, R.L. (2005). Exploiting chinks in the plant's armor: evolution and emergence of geminiviruses. Annu Rev Phytopathol 43, 361-394.

Sanchez-Duran, M.A., Dallas, M.B., Ascencio-Ibanez, J.T., Reyes, M.I., Arroyo-Mateos, M., Ruiz-Albert, J., Hanley-Bowdoin, L., and Bejarano, E.R. (2011). Interaction between geminivirus replication protein and the SUMO-conjugating enzyme is required for viral infection. J Virol 85, 9789-9800.

Schmidt, M.W., McQuary, P.R., Wee, S., Hofmann, K., and Wolf, D.A. (2009). F-box-directed CRL complex assembly and regulation by the CSN and CAND1. Mol Cell 35, 586-597.

Schwechheimer, C., Serino, G., Callis, J., Crosby, W.L., Lyapina, S., Deshaies, R.J., Gray, W.M., Estelle, M., and Deng, X.W. (2001). Interactions of the COP9 signalosome with the E3 ubiquitin ligase SCFTIRI in mediating auxin response. Science 292, 1379-1382.

Shen, Q., Liu, Z., Song, F., Xie, Q., Hanley-Bowdoin, L., and Zhou, X. (2011). Tomato SlSnRK1 protein interacts with and phosphorylates betaC1, a pathogenesis protein encoded by a geminivirus beta-satellite. Plant Physiol 157, 1394-1406.

Smalle, J., and Vierstra, R.D. (2004). The ubiquitin 26S proteasome proteolytic pathway. Annu Rev Plant Biol 55, 555-590.

Stuttmann, J., Lechner, E., Guerois, R., Parker, J.E., Nussaume, L., Genschik, P., and Noel, L.D. (2009). COP9 signalosome- and 26S proteasome-dependent regulation of SCFTIRI accumulation in Arabidopsis. J Biol Chem 284, 7920-7930.

Takizawa, M., Goto, A., and Watanabe, Y. (2005). The tobacco ubiquitin-activating enzymes NtE1A and NtE1B are induced by tobacco mosaic virus, wounding and stress hormones. Mol Cells 19, 228-231.

Ulrich, H.D. (2009). The SUMO system: an overview. Methods Mol Biol 497, 3-16.

Vierstra, R.D. (2009). The ubiquitin-26S proteasome system at the nexus of plant biology. Nat Rev Mol Cell Biol 10, 385-397.

Wang, H., Hao, L., Shung, C.Y., Sunter, G., and Bisaro, D.M. (2003). Adenosine kinase is inactivated by geminivirus AL2 and L2 proteins. Plant Cell 15, 3020-3032.

Wei, N., Serino, G., and Deng, X.W. (2008). The COP9 signalosome: more than a protease. Trends Biochem Sci 33, 592-600.

Wu, J.T., Chan, Y.R., and Chien, C.T. (2006). Protection of cullin-RING E3 ligases by CSN-UBP12. Trends Cell Biol 16, 362-369.

Wu, K., Chen, A., and Pan, Z.Q. (2000). Conjugation of Nedd8 to CUL1 enhances the ability of the ROC1-CUL1 complex to promote ubiquitin polymerization. J Biol Chem 275, 32317-32324.

The Role of Measles Virus Receptor CD150 in Measles Immunopathogenesis

Olga Romanets

CIRI, International Center for Infectiology Research, IbIV team, Inserm, U1111, CNRS UMR5308, Université Lyon 1, Ecole Normale Supérieure de Lyon, Lyon, France
R.E. Kavetsky Institute of Experimental Pathology, Oncology and Radiobiology
The National Academy of Sciences of Ukraine, Kyiv, Ukraine

Svetlana Sidorenko

R.E. Kavetsky Institute of Experimental Pathology, Oncology and Radiobiology
The National Academy of Sciences of Ukraine, Kyiv, Ukraine

Branka Horvat

CIRI, International Center for Infectiology Research, IbIV team, Inserm, U1111, CNRS, UMR5308, Université Lyon 1, Ecole Normale Supérieure de Lyon, Lyon, France

1 Introduction

Measles virus (MV) is one of the most contagious pathogens for humans. Despite the existence of an efficient vaccine, measles outbreaks still occur all around the world. Three different cell surface receptors have been identified to serve for MV entry. The major viral receptor CD150 that is mainly expressed on hematopoietic cells, mediates viral entry in respiratory tract and systemic propagation in lymphoid tissues. Recently identified MV receptor poliovirus receptor-related 4 (PVRL4) or nectin-4 is expressed on the basal side of the respiratory epithelium and facilitates virus release from the airways. The third MV receptor, CD46, though expressed on all nucleated human cells, serves as the entry receptor for only laboratory adapted MV strains. Binding to cell receptors is achieved via viral envelope protein hemagglutinin. Interaction between measles virus and CD150 could play a significant role in the modulation of the immune response, seen during measles. The immediate effect of this interaction results with virus-cell fusion, cytolytic viral replication and consequent elimination of CD150-positive immunocompetent cells. Among them are T and B lymphocytes, dendritic cells, activated monocytes and macrophages. This instant effect along with the MV-induced modulation of immunocompetent cell functions leads to the development of profound immunosuppression. Since CD150 is a potent immunosignaling receptor and its ligation on cell surface can change the cytokine profile and functions of dendritic cells, T cells and macrophages, it is thus likely that its interaction with MV hemagglutinin could be also implicated in measles immunopathogenesis. CD150 is linked to signal transduction pathways that are involved in regulation of immune response and cell differentiation: Akt/PKB, ERK1/2, p38 MAPK, and JNK1/2. Understanding the signaling events upon CD150 ligation with measles virus hemagglutinin may answer the multiple questions concerning the molecular mechanism of measles virus mediated immunosuppression.

2 Measles Virus

Measles is a highly infectious and potentially fatal disease. The causative agent for this infection is measles virus (MV), a member of the family *Paramyxoviridae*, genus *Morbillivirus*. *Morbillivirus*es also include rinderpest virus (RPV), canine distemper virus (CDV), peste des petits ruminants virus (PPRV), phocine distemper virus, cetacean morbillivirus and seal distemper virus (Lamb & Parks, 2007). MV is one of the most highly contagious infectious agents and outbreaks can occur in populations in which less than 10% of individuals are susceptible to infection. Live attenuated and effective vaccines were developed more than 40 years ago to limit this severe and fatal disease. After a global campaign for vaccination, estimated global measles mortality decreased by 74% from 535,300 deaths in 2000 to 139,300 in 2010. Measles mortality was reduced by more than three-quarters in all WHO regions except the WHO Southeast Asia region. India accounted for 47% of estimated measles mortality in 2010, and the WHO African region accounted for 36% (Simons *et al.*, 2012). Despite all efforts to eradicate measles, it has still not been achieved because of the limitation of the licensed vaccines, including their instability at room temperature, the requirement of two-dose application and necessity of vaccine coverage of greater than 95% to prevent further outbreaks. In addition, the vaccination cannot be provided in early infancy as maternal antibodies reduce its efficiency and to immunocompromised persons as it could potentially be dangerous. All the factors mentioned above together with anti-vaccine opposition on religious or philosophical grounds in some communities limit the possibility of global measles elimination. Measles virus is a close relative of and shares a lot of biological properties with another member of the genus *Morbilli-*

virus, RPV. As in 2011 the Food and Agriculture Organization officially announced rinderpest to be eradicated from the globe. This experience may help in the future eradication of measles (OIE, 25 May 2011).

Clinically apparent measles begins with a prodrome characterized by fever, cough, coryza (runny nose) and conjunctivitis and ends with the characteristic erythematous and maculopapular rash. Though pneumonia appears to be the most common fatal complication of measles, complications have been described in almost every organ system including the central nervous system (CNS). The CNS involvement accounts for acute postinfectious measles encephalomyelitis with either infectious or autoimmune etiology, measles inclusion body encephalitis (MIBE) and subacute sclerosing panencephalitis (SSPE) (Schneider-Schaulies *et al.*, 2003).

MV is a spherical enveloped virus with a single stranded RNA genome of negative polarity that contains 6 genes encoding eight proteins. V and C proteins are encoded by the P gene in addition to phosphoprotein (P) via RNA editing process and use of alternative translational frame respectively. Of the six structural proteins, P, large protein (L) and nucleoprotein (N) form the nucleocapsid that encloses the viral RNA. The hemagglutinin protein (H), fusion protein (F) and matrix protein (M), together with lipids from the host cell membrane, form the viral envelope (Griffin, 2007; Figure 1). Unlike some other members of the *Paramyxoviridae*, which utilize sialic acid moieties on glycoproteins and glycolipids to enter cells, *Morbilliviruses* use specific cellular receptors. In case of MV they are: CD46 for laboratory MV strains (Dorig *et al.*, 1993; Naniche *et al.*, 1993), CD150, for both, wild-type and laboratory MV strains (Tatsuo *et al.*, 2000; de Vries, Lemon *et al.*, 2010), and recently discovered PVRL4 (nectin-4), allowing viral egress from the respiratory tract (Muhlebach *et al.*, 2011; Noyce *et al.*, 2011; Figure 2A).

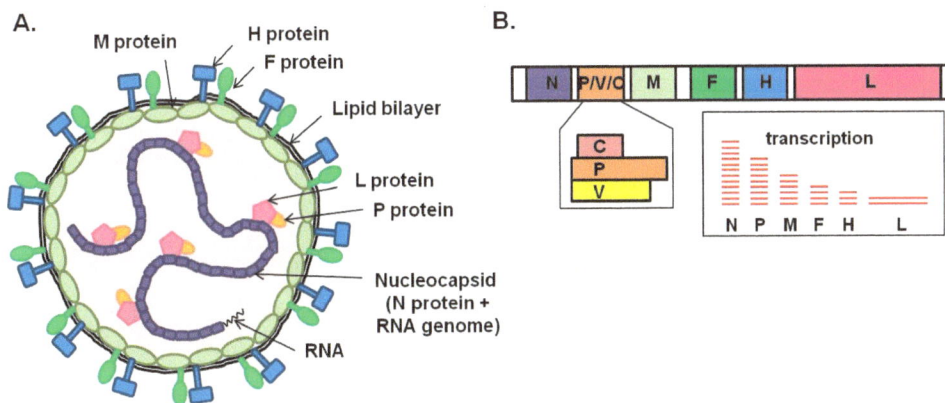

Figure 1: Measles virus particle and genome. A. The structure of measles virus particle. B. Schematic representation of measles virus genome.

Although they do not serve as entry receptors, the C-type lectins, DC-SIGN (CD209) and Langerin (CD207) facilitate MV attachment to the myeloid dendritic cells (de Witte *et al.*, 2008) and Langerhans cells (van der Vlist *et al.*, 2011) respectively (Figure 2B). CD150 and PVRL4 account for the lymphotropic and epitheliotropic properties of natural MV. MV is also endotheliotropic and neurotropic, however the entry receptors for MV on the surface of these types of cells have not yet been identified.

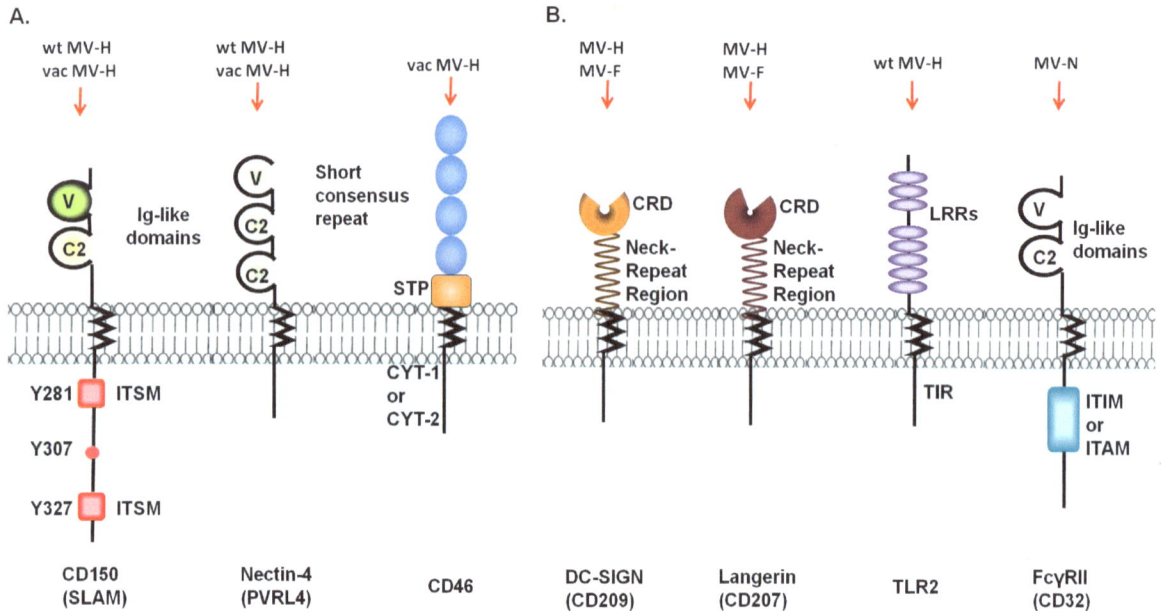

Figure 2: Schematic presentation of structure of measles virus receptors. **A.** Three entry MV receptors, able to interact with MV hemagglutinin have been identified: CD46 for laboratory MV strains, CD150 for both, wild type and laboratory MV strains in lymphoid cells, and nectin-4, for both MV strains again, but in epithelial cells. **CD46** consists of four short consensus repeats (SCR) on N-terminus, followed by alternatively spliced serine, threonine and proline-rich region (STP), transmembrane domain and one of two cytoplasmic tails (CYT-1 or CYT-2). **CD150** comprises two immunoglobuline(Ig)-like domains (V and C2) on N-terminus, transmembrane region and cytoplasmic tail containing three tyrosine residues which could be phosphorylated, two of which form the core of immunoreceptor tyrosine-based switch motif (ITSM). The structure of **PVRL4** (nectin-4) is defined by three extracellular Ig-like domains (V and two C2-type domains), a single transmembrane helix, and an intracellular domain. **B.** Cell membrane molecules interacting with MV, but not allowing virus fusion. Four other surface molecules have been found to interact with MV proteins: DC-SIGN, Langerin, TLR2 and FcγRII. **DC-SIGN** (CD209) consists of carbohydrate recognition domain (CRD) and neck-repeat region in the extracellular region, after that transmembrane and cytoplasmic domains. It interacts with both MV membrane glycoproteins: H and F. **Langerin** (CD207) and DC-SIGN are highly homologous, share some ligands, but are expressed by different cell types. While DC-SIGN represents a trimer, Langerin is present as tetramer on cell surface. Langerin also has an additional carbohydrate-binding Ca^{2+}-independent site in its CRD domain. **TLR2** is composed of extracellular multiple leucine-rich repeats (LRRs), transmembrane domain and cytoplasmic region with Toll/IL-1R (TIR) domain and interacts only with wt MV-H. **FcγRII** (CD32) has two Ig-like domains on N-terminus, followed by transmembrane and cytoplasmic regions. FcγRII receptors represent two subfamilies: activatory FcγRII with immunoreceptor tyrosine-based activation motif (ITAM) in their cytoplasmic tail, and inhibitory FcγRII containing immunoreceptor tyrosine-based inhibitory motif (ITIM) instead of ITAM. In contrast to other described receptors, FcγRII binds measles virus N protein.

3   CD150 receptor

3.1   CD150 Structure and Expression

The CD150 cell surface receptor was first described as 'IPO-3 antigen' (Pinchouk *et al.*, 1988; Pinchouk *et al.*, 1986; Sidorenko & Clark, 1993) on activated human lymphocytes. Its preferential expression on cells of hematopoietic tissues, biochemical and functional features has been characterized (Sidorenko & Clark, 1993). In 1995 the cDNA for this receptor was cloned under the name signaling lymphocyte activation molecule (SLAM) (Cocks *et al.*, 1995). The monoclonal antibody IPO-3 was submitted for the international collaborative studies in the frame of 5-7 workshops on Human Leukocyte Differentiation Antigens (HLDA). In 1996 on the 6th workshop on HLDA (Kobe, Japan) the IPO-3 antigen received international nomenclature CDw150 (Sidorenko, 1997) that was transformed into CD150 at the 7th HLDA workshop (Harrogate, Great Britain, 2000) (Sidorenko, 2002).

CD150 (IPO-3/SLAM F1) is a member of SLAM family within the immunoglobulin superfamily of surface receptors. According to the nomenclature accepted by 9th international Workshop on Human Leukocyte Differentiation Antigens (Barcelona, 2010) SLAM family includes nine members: SLAMF1 (CD150 or IPO-3, SLAM), SLAMF2 (CD48 or BCM1, Blast-1, OX-45), SLAMF3 (CD229 or Ly9), SLAMF4 (CD244 or 2B4, NAIL), SLAMF5 (CD84 or Ly9B), SLAMF6(CD352 or NTB-A, SF2000, Ly108), SLAMF7 (CD319 or CRACC, CS1, 19A24), SLAMF8 (CD353 or BLAME) and SLAMF9 (SF2001 or CD84-H1). The characteristic signature of CD150 family is within the extracellular region: an N-terminal variable (V) Immunoglobulin (Ig) domain lacking disulfide bonds is followed by a truncated Ig constant 2 (C2) domain with two intradomain disulfide bonds (Figure 2A). The genes of the SLAM family are clustered close together on the long arm of chromosome 1 at bands 1q21-24 (Sidorenko & Clark, 2003). The gene structure for all CD150/SLAM family receptors is similar with the signal peptides and each of the Ig domains encoded by separate exons. All these receptors are type I transmembrane proteins with the exception of CD48 (Cannons *et al.*, 2011).

CD150 is a single chain transmembrane phosphoglycoprotein of 75-95 kDa in size with a 42 kDa protein core. It is heavily N-glycosylated with terminal sialic acid residues on oligosaccharide chains. Moreover, it was shown that this receptor is associated with tyrosine (Y) and serine/threonine (S/T) kinases and is phosphorylated at tyrosine and serine residues (Sidorenko & Clark, 1993).

In addition to transmembrane form of CD150 (mCD150), activated T and B lymphocytes, CD40 ligand-activated dendritic cells and also lymphoblastoid and Hodgkin's lymphoma cell lines express mRNA encoding secreted form of CD150 (sCD150) that lacks 30 amino acids – the entire transmembrane region (TM), mRNAs for cytoplasmic form (cCD150) lacking the leader sequence, and a variant membrane CD150 (vmCD150) with truncated cytoplasmic tail (CY). However, expression of vmCD150 (tCD150) isoform was not confirmed at the protein level (Bleharski *et al.*, 2001; Cocks *et al.*, 1995; Punnonen *et al.*, 1997; Sidorenko & Clark, 2003; Yurchenko *et al.*, 2005).

CD150 receptor is mainly expressed within hematopoietic cell lineage. Its expression was detected on immature thymocytes, activated and memory T cells, $CD4^+$ T cells with much higher expression level on Th1 cells, $CD4^+CD25^+$ regulatory and follicular helper T cells, peripheral blood and tonsillar B cells, mature dendritic cells and macrophages. The level of CD150 expression on subpopulations of tonsillar B cells differs with its maximum levels on plasma cells. The activation of T and B cells leads to the rapid upregulation of CD150 expression. Low level of CD150 expression was also found on NKT cells, platelets and eosinophiles. The expression of CD150 on peripheral blood monocytes could be induced by mitogen and cytokines stimulation, and also by measles virus particles (Browning *et al.*, 2004; Cocks *et al.*,

1995; Kruse *et al.*, 2001; Minagawa*et al.*, 2001; Sidorenko & Clark, 1993, 2003; Veillette *et al.*, 2007; Yurchenko *et al.*, 2010). CD150 expression is a distinguishing feature of hematopoetic stem cells (HSC) in mice (Hock, 2010). CD150 was also found on malignant cells of leukemias and lymphomas mainly with an activated cell phenotype (Mikhalap *et al.*, 2004).

3.2 CD150 Ligands

With the exception of CD48 and CD244/2B4 (receptor-ligand pair), all SLAM family receptors are self-ligands. Intriguingly, there is a marked variation in the apparent affinity of these self-associations (Kd=0.5–200 µM), suggesting that the various members of the CD150 family may modulate immune cell functions to a different extent. Crystallographic determination of the structures of SLAM family members homodimers indicated that self-association is mediated by the N-terminal variable (V)-type Ig-like (IgV) domain, which enables head-to-head contact between two monomers (Mavaddat *et al.*, 2000; Sintes & Engel, 2011; Veillette *et al.*, 2007). CD150 binds to itself with low affinity (Kd=>200µM). Although the affinity of this receptor is low, the binding avidity increases due to the redistribution or clustering of molecules after cell activation. It is probable that the binding is affected by other receptor–ligand interactions that help to bring the membranes into proximity and induce changes in the lateral mobility of receptors (Engel *et al.*, 2003; Mavaddat *et al.*, 2000).

CD150 was found to be the major receptor for several *Morbilliviruses* (Tatsuo & Yanagi, 2002). In case of MV the role of attachment protein is played by hemagglutinin (MV-H), which directly binds the cellular receptors of the virus (CD150, CD46 and nectin-4), mediating virus entry into the cell (Fig. 2A). Human CD150 (hCD150) was reported as a cellular receptor for wild type (wt) measles virus (Tatsuo *et al.*, 2000). The hCD150 V domain is necessary and sufficient for its function as a MV receptor; however, the other regions of hCD150, including the C2 domain, TM, and CY are not required for this function (Ono *et al.*, 2001). Histidine (H) at position 61 appears to be critical for CD150 to act as a receptor for MV. Isoleucine (I) at position 60, Valine (V) 63, lysine (K) at position 58 and S59 also appear to contribute to receptor function of hCD150 (Ohno *et al.*, 2003; Xu *et al.*, 2006). The mutagenesis of the H protein based on its ability to induce SLAM-dependent cell–cell fusion has revealed that residues important for interaction with SLAM are I194, D505, D507, D530, R533, F552 and P554 (Masse *et al.*, 2004; Navaratnarajah *et al.*, 2008; Vongpunsawad *et al.*, 2004).

CD150 receptors from human, mouse, dog, cow and marmoset have about 60–70% identity at the amino acid level, except human and marmoset CD150, which have 86% identity. The sequences at positions 58–67 are well conserved among these species, especially I60 and H61 which are conserved in human, marmoset, dog and cow CD150 (Ohno *et al.*, 2003). Mouse CD150 has functional and structural similarity to human CD150 (60% identity at the amino acid level), but it cannot act as a receptor for MV, partly explaining why mice are not susceptible to MV. It has been proposed that amino acid substitutions at the positions 60, 61, 63 to human-type residues may make mouse CD150 act as an MV receptor, as introduction of changes at these positions compromises the receptor function of human CD150., while introduction of changes at these positions compromises the receptor function of human CD150 (Yanagi *et al.*, 2009). CDV and RPV use dog and bovine CD150 respectively as cellular receptors. Furthermore, it was found that MV, CDV and RPV can use CD150 of non-host species as receptors but with lower efficiency (Yanagi *et al.*, 2009).

CD150 is not only a self ligand and a receptor for Morbilliviruses, but also a bacterial sensor that regulates intracellular enzyme activities involved in the removal of Gram-negative bacteria (Berger *et al.*, 2010; Sintes & Engel, 2011).

3.3   CD150-mediated Signaling

Engagement of CD150 on cell membrane results in numerous intracellular signaling events. CD150-mediated signals can be divided into receptor-proximal, including immediate binding partners (Figure 3A), and distal – signal transduction pathways (Figure 3B). CD150 receptor interacts with intracellular partners through its cytoplasmic tail (CD150ct), specifically via three key tyrosine residues which could be phosphorylated: Y281, Y307 and Y327 (Y288, Y315 and Y335 in mice respectively). The first and the last tyrosine residues form the core for the unique immunoreceptor tyrosine-based switch motifs (ITSMs) (Shlapatska *et al.*, 2001; Figure 2A). Six members of SLAM family receptors contain 1 to 4 ITSMs. The cytoplasmic tail of CD150 has 2 ITSMs. Upon the tyrosine phosphorylation by Src family kinases ITSMs bind key SH2-containing components of signal transduction pathways, including the adaptor proteins SH2D1A, SH2D1B (EAT-2) and SH2D1C (ERT) (Shlapatska *et al.*, 2001; Sidorenko & Clark, 2003).

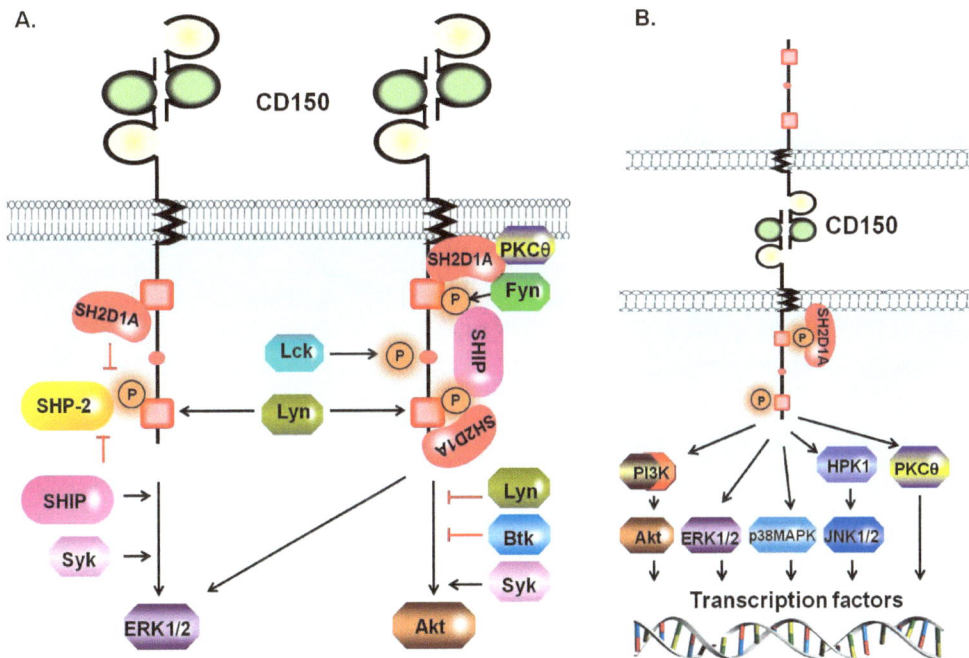

Figure 3: CD150-mediated signaling. A. Receptor-proximal signaling events triggered by CD150 ligation could be divided on those which are dependent on CD150-SH2D1A interaction and those which are not. Upon ligation, three tyrosine residues in cytoplasmic tail could be phosphorylated. Lck, Lyn and Fyn kinases were shown to be able to do it. Afterward several SH2- and SH3-containing molecules were shown to be able to bind to these tyrosines either via SH2D1A (Fyn, SHIP, PKCθ) or not (SHP-2). CD150 ligation mediates the activation of Akt signaling pathway (requires Syk and SH2D1A and is negatively regulated by Lyn and Btk) and ERK signaling pathway (requires SHIP and Syk, but not SH2D1A). B. Receptor-distal signaling events after CD150 ligation: activation of Akt, ERK1/2, JNK1/2, p38MAPK signaling pathways that lead to the activation of transcription factors, e.g. FoxO1, c-Jun and NF-κB.

Upon antigen receptor cross-linking the cytoplasmic tail of CD150 becomes phosphorylated, while after CD150 ligation with the IPO-3 antibodies – the opposite effect is observed (Mikhalap *et al.*, 1999). It was suggested that A12 antibody is antagonistic, while the outcome of IPO-3 cross-linking is similar to the effect of hemophilic stimulation with CD150 recombinant protein (Punnonen *et al.*, 1997; Veillette, 2004). Several Src-family kinases, namely Lck phosphorylates Y307, Lyn – Y327 and Fyn – Y281, were found to be able to phosphorylate key tyrosine residues of CD150 (Howie *et al.*, 2002; Mikhalap *et al.*, 2004; Figure 3A).

The signaling events downstream of CD150 could be divided on those that are dependent on CD150-SH2D1A interaction and those which are not. SH2D1A binds Y281 of CD150 cytoplasmic tail independently of phosphorylation, does not bind Y307, and binds Y327 only after phosphorylation (Howie *et al.*, 2002). The SH2D1A interaction with Y281 of SLAM is mediated via R32 of SH2D1A (Sayos *et al.*, 1998).

The coupling of CD150 to signal transduction pathways is provided by two SH2D1A functions: recruitment of enzymes or, alternatively, blocking binding of SH2-containing proteins. SH2D1A SH2 domain binds to the SH3 domain of FynT and indirectly couples FynT to CD150. The crystal structure of a ternary CD150-SH2D1A-Fyn-SH3 complex reveals that SH2D1A SH2 domain binds the FynT SH3 domain through a R78-based motif which does not involve canonical SH3 or SH2 binding interactions (Chan *et al.*, 2003; Latour *et al.*, 2001; Latour *et al.*, 2003). The observed mode of binding to the Fyn-SH3 domain is expected to preclude the auto-inhibited conformation of Fyn, thereby promoting activation of the kinase after recruitment (Chan *et al.*, 2003). SHIP also is recruited in CD150-SH2D1A signaling complex via binding of its SH2 domain to phosphorylated Y315 and/or Y335 of mouse CD150 and appeares to be the intermediate molecule that links CD150-SH2D1A to Dok-related adaptors and RasGAP (Latour *et al.*, 2001). This signaling cascade is dependent on the generation of a ternary CD150-SH2D1A-Fyn complex for CD150 phosphorylation. The presence of SH2D1A facilitates binding of SHIP to CD150 (Latour *et al.*, 2001; Shlapatska *et al.*, 2001). Although SHIP possesses only one SH2 domain, both Y281 and Y327 in CD150 are important for its association with SHIP (Shlapatska *et al.*, 2001).

R78 residue of SH2D1A is also critical for its constitutive association with PKCθ in T cells. This SH2D1A-PKCθ interaction is Fyn independent. Moreover, CD150 engagement increases TCR-induced PKCθ recruitment to the site of T cell stimulation (Cannons *et al.*, 2010). As PKCθ could be detected as part of the CD150-SH2D1A complex following TCR ligation, CD150 engagement can facilitate PKCθ recruitment, nuclear p50 NF-κB levels, and IL-4 production via a ternary CD150-SH2D1A–PKCθ complex (Cannons *et al.*, 2004; Cannons *et al.*, 2010).

SH2D1A is capable of not only bridging the interaction of FynT, PKCθ or SHIP with CD150 but also inhibiting the binding of SHP-2 to phosphorylated CD150 (Sayos *et al.*, 1998; Shlapatska *et al.*, 2001). SH2 domains of SHIP and SHP-2 bind to the same sites in the receptors of SLAM family as does SH2D1A strongly suggesting that these three proteins are competing binding partners. Apparently, displacement of SHP-2 by SH2D1A makes Y281 and Y327 available for binding by SHIP, which also requires Y281 and Y327 (Li *et al.*, 2003; Shlapatska *et al.*, 2001).

CD150 also associates with CD45 in human B lymphoblastoid cell lines MP-1 and CESS that express SH2D1A, however it is not clear whether CD150-CD45 association is direct, or is mediated via SH2D1A (Mikhalap *et al.*, 1999). It should be noted that in SH2D1A negative B cell lines CD150 is strongly associated with SHP-2 that binds only tyrosine phosphorylated ITSMs (Shlapatska *et al.*, 2001). Since BCR engagement induces CD150 tyrosine phosphorylation (Mikhalap *et al.*, 1999) it could be that activation of B cells is required for SHP-2 binding to CD150. In B cells CD150 is associated with Src-family kinases Fgr and Lyn (Mikhalap *et al.*, 1999), however only Lyn is able to phosphorylate CD150 *in vitro* (Mikhalap *et al.*, 2004).

CD150-binding partners link it to several signal transduction pathways, among them are MAPK and Akt/PKB signaling networks (Figure 3B). In T and B cells CD150 crosslinking alone results in an increase in serine phosphorylation of Akt/PKB on S473, which is the hallmark of kinase activation state (Mikhalap *et al.*, 1999; Howie *et al.*, 2002). CD150-mediated Akt phosphorylation requires Syk and SH2D1A, is negatively regulated by Lyn and Btk, but is SHIP independent as was shown in the model of DT40 chicken knockout cell sublines transfected with SH2D1A and/or CD150 (Mikhalap *et al.* 2004). In B cells CD150-induced ERK phosphorylation requires SHIP and Syk but not SH2D1A. Lyn, Btk, and SHP-2 appear to be involved in the regulation of constitutive levels of ERK1/2-phosphorylation. These data allow proposing of the hypothesis that CD150 and SH2D1A are co-expressed during a narrow window of B-cell maturation and SH2D1A may be involved in regulation of B-cell differentiation via switching the CD150-mediated signaling pathways (Mikhalap *et al.*, 2004; Figure 3A).

It was also shown that Akt kinase could be phosphorylated via CD150 both in naïve and activated primary tonsillar B cells. CD150-mediated activation of Akt kinase depends on CD150-SH2D1A interaction followed by phosphorylation of CD150ct and attraction of p85α regulatory subunit of phosphatidylinositol-3-kinase (PI3K). As was demonstrated by surface plasmon resonance, p85α subunit of PI3K via its N terminal SH2 domain could directly bind CD150ct, and this interaction takes place in normal tonsillar B cells and lymphoblastoid cell line MP-1. One of the downstream targets of Akt kinase in B cells is transcription factor FoxO1. Despite the high basal level of pFoxO1, CD150 mediates FoxO1 phosphorylation in normal tonsillar B cells and MP-1 cell line (Yurchenko *et al.*, 2011).

In primary tonsillar B cells and Hodgkin's lymphoma cell lines CD150 signaling not only induces the activation of ERK1/2 kinases but also regulates the activation of two other families of MAPK kinases – p38 MAPK and JNK1/2. CD150 mediates the activation of JNK1/2 p54 and JNK2-γ isoforms in all tested human B cells. Furthermore, the CD150-mediated JNK activation is significantly enhanced after HPK1 overexpression and HPK1 is co-precipitated with CD150, suggesting that HPK1 is downstream of CD150 in this signaling pathway (Yurchenko *et al.*, 2010).

All these facts demonstrate that signaling properties of CD150 depend on the cell type and availability of other components of signal transduction networks. However, it is clear that downstream of CD150-mediated signaling pathways are transcription factors that regulate cell biology and could modulate immune response.

3.4   CD150 Functions

Several models were used to study CD150 functions: ligation of CD150 with monoclonal antibodies or CD150 recombinant protein in human and murine *in vitro* system and CD150 knockout mice, where the expression of murine CD150 was genetically deleted. These experimental approaches revealed numerous roles of CD150 in the functions of different immune cell subsets.

3.4.1   CD150 Functions in Lymphocytes

CD150 is involved in the regulation of interferon-gamma (IFN-γ) response. Initial studies showed that the engagement of human CD150 with mAb A12 enhances the antigen-specific proliferation, cytokine production by CD4[+] T cells, particularly IFN-γ, and direct the proliferating cells to a T0/Th1 phenotype (Aversa *et al.*, 1997; Cocks *et al.*, 1995). Similarly, antibodies against mouse CD150 also enhanced IFN-γ production (Howie *et al.*, 2002; Castro *et al.*, 1999). However, it seems that some anti-CD150 antibodies, including A12 mAb, are antagonistic, since CD150 ligation on T cells inhibits IFN-γ production rather than stimulate it. It was shown that expression of full-length CD150 and SH2D1A in BI-141 T cell transfectants, activated with anti-CD3, abolished the production of IFN-γ (Latour *et al.*, 2001). In addition, homophilic CD150-CD150 interactions between T cells and artificial CD150 expressing APC (antigen-presenting cell) line reduced IFN-γ expression (Cannons *et al.*, 2004, Figure 4). It was also shown that SH2D1A deficient T cells produce more IFN-γ in response to CD3 triggering (Cannons *et al.*, 2004; Howie *et al.*, 2002).

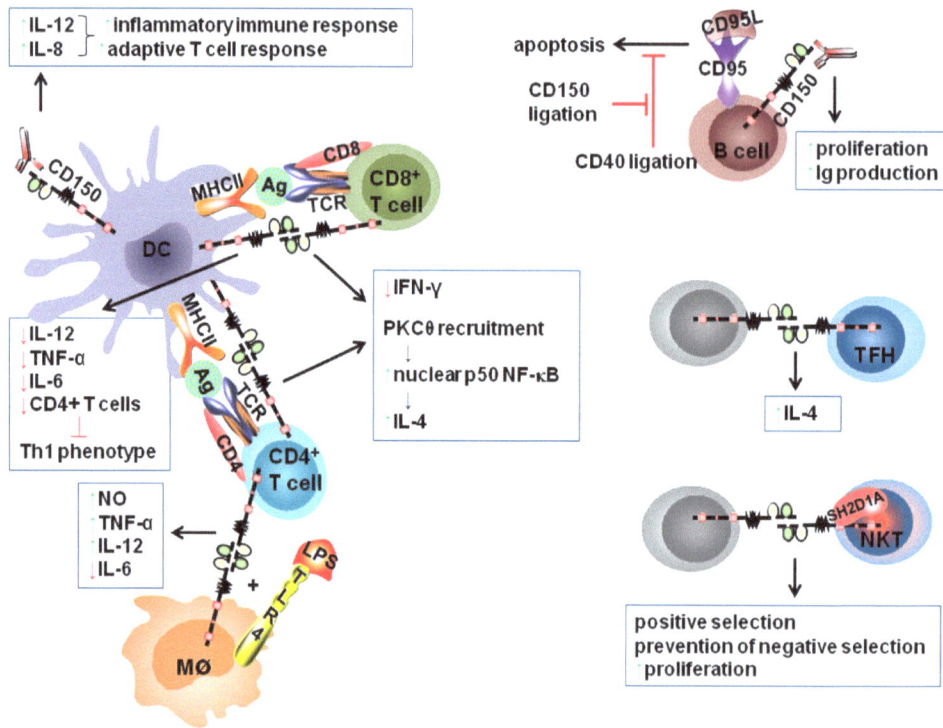

Figure 4: CD150 functions. CD150 is expressed on several cell populations in immune system: T and B lymphocytes, dendritic cells, macrophages, follicular helper T cells and NKT lymphocytes. It has been shown that CD150 ligation mediates the functional changes in these cell types. In **CD4+ and CD8+ T cells** CD150 engagement mediates the inhibition of IFN-γ, but activation of IL-4 production via increase of nuclear p50 NF-κB levels in PKCθ-dependent manner. In **DCs**, CD150 ligation with different ligands had (exerted) the opposite effects. Stimulation with anti-CD150 antibodies resulted in activation of inflammatory and adaptive T cell responses due to the increase of IL-12 and IL-18 production, while CD150 self-ligation mediated inhibition of IL-12, TNF-α and IL-6 production by DCs, leading to the inhibition of naïve CD4+ T cell differentiation towards Th1 phenotype. In **macrophages** CD150 acts as a co-receptor that regulates signals transduced by the major LPS receptor TLR4, controlling the production of TNF-α, NO, IL-12 and IL-6. CD150 ligation blocks the rescue of **B cells** by CD40 ligation from CD95-mediated apoptosis. Besides, it augments B cell proliferation and enhances Ig production by CD40-activated B cells. In **follicular helper T cells (TFH)** CD150 engagement leads to upregulation of IL-4 production, and finally in **NKT cells** it promotes positive selection and enhances their proliferation. *Ag* - antigen; *Mø* - macrophage; *MHCII* – major histocompatibility complex class II; *TCR* – T cell receptor.

Studies of CD150-knockout mice revealed an important role for CD150 in regulation of Th2 development. In CD150-deficient CD4$^+$ T cells a significant decrease in TCR-mediated IL-4 production and slight upregulation in IFN-γ secretion was observed (Wang *et al.*, 2004). Moreover, CD150 receptor positively regulates TCR-induced IL-4 production by naive and activated CD4$^+$ T cells, but negatively regulates IFN-γ secretion by CD8$^+$ and to a lesser extent by CD4$^+$ cells (Wang *et al.*, 2004). SH2D1A expression may be a limiting factor coordinating the TCR and CD150-mediated signaling pathways contributing to IL-4 regulation, as overexpression of SH2D1A potentiates the effects of CD150 on IL-4 production (Cannons *et al.*, 2010).

CD150 is also specifically required for IL-4 production by germinal center (GC) T follicular helper (TFH) cells, CD4$^+$ T cells, specialized in B cell help. On the model of CD150 knockout mice it was shown, that for optimal help to B cells TFH cells require CD150 signaling to produce IL-4 (Yusuf *et al.*, 2010; Figure 4).

Studies with knockout mice revealed that CD150-SH2D1A mediated signaling may contribute to some functions of innate-like lymphocytes (Griewank *et al.*, 2007; Jordan *et al.*, 2007; Nichols *et al.*, 2005; Veillette *et al.*, 2007). Innate-like lymphocytes are subsets of lymphocytes which, when activated, exhibit faster and more robust effector functions. The prototypical innate-like lymphocytes are the NKT cells (Godfrey & Berzins, 2007; Veillette *et al.*, 2007). It was demonstrated that SH2D1A-driven signals may be necessary for the positive selection, proliferation, and/or prevention of negative selection of immature NKT cells. One possibility is that SH2D1A-mediated signals are triggered by homotypic interactions between SLAM family receptors expressed on double-positive thymocytes. CD150 and Ly108 seem to be the predominant SLAM family receptors triggering the function of SH2D1A during NKT cell development (Griewank *et al.*, 2007). Another indication of CD150 role in NKT differentiation comes from the characterization of the *Nkt1* locus on mouse chromosome 1. The differential expression of *Slamf1* and *Slamf6* genes mediates the control of NKT cell numbers attributed to the *Nkt1* gene (Jordan *et al.*, 2007; Figure 4).

CD150 is also involved in the regulation of cell proliferation and survival. Ligation of CD150 with monoclonal antibody IPO-3, signaling properties of which are opposite to A12 mAb, as well as homotypic CD150-CD150 interactions augment proliferation of resting human B lymphocytes, induced by BCR or CD40 ligation, mitogens or cytokines, especially IL-4. Ligation of CD150 also enhances immunoglobulin production by CD40-activated B cells (Punnonen *et al.*, 1997; Sidorenko & Clark, 1993). CD150-induced signals can both synergize with and augment CD95-mediated apoptosis in human B cells and T cells (Mikhalap *et al.*, 1999). In human B cell lines MP-1, RPMI-1788, and Raji, signaling via CD40 rescues cells from CD95-mediated apoptosis, but ligation of CD150 can block CD40-mediated protection. Conversely, CD40 ligation cancels out the synergistic effect of CD95 and CD150 (Mikhalap *et al.*, 1999; Figure 4). Besides, CD150 could inhibit cell proliferation of Hodgkin's lymphoma cell lines and induce apoptosis in one of them (Yurchenko *et al.*, 2010).

3.4.2 CD150 Functions in Antigen-Presenting Cells

CD150 also plays an important role in immune responses of macrophages. CD150 acts as a co-receptor that regulates signals transduced by Toll-like receptor (TLR) 4, the major lipopolysaccharide (LPS) receptor on the surface of mouse macrophages (Wang *et al.*, 2004). In CD150$^{-/-}$ macrophages LPS-induced IL-12 and TNF secretion is impaired, while IL-6 is overproduced even in the absence of any extraneous stimuli. Moreover, CD150$^{-/-}$macrophages produce reduced amounts of nitric oxide (NO) upon stimulation with LPS (Figure 4). However, CD150 does not regulate phagocytosis or responses to peptidoglycan or

CpG (Wang *et al.*, 2004). In SLAM-deficient (Slamf1$^{-/-}$) mice macrophages also exhibit impaired LPS-induced production of TNF-α and nitric oxide. These experiments allow to conclude that CD150 acts as a vital regulator in the innate immune defense against Gram-negative bacteria in macrophages controlling two main independent bactericidal processes: phagosome maturation and the production of free radical species by the NOX2 complex (Berger *et al.*, 2010).

Macrophages of CD150$^{-/-}$ C57Bl/6 mice are defective at clearing the parasite *Leishmania major* (Wang *et al.*, 2004). The activation of CD150 may also promote the cell-mediated immune response mediated by IFN-γ to intracellular bacterial pathogens, namely to *Mycobacterium leprae* (Garcia *et al.*, 2001). Finally, CD150 is required for the replication of *Trypanosoma cruzi* (*T.cruzi*) in macrophages and DCs (Calderon *et al.*, 2012). *T. cruzi*, the protozoan parasite responsible for Chagas' disease, causes severe myocarditis. In the absence of CD150, macrophages and DCs are less susceptible to *T. cruzi* infection and produce less myeloid cell specific factors that are keys in influencing the host response to parasite and the outcome of the infection. Consequently, CD150 deficient mice are resistant to *T. cruzi* infection.

These findings clearly define CD150 as a novel bacterial sensor (Sintes & Engel, 2011) and suggest its role in the regulation of some parasite infections.

CD150 is highly expressed on mature dendritic cells (DCs) but only at a low level on immature DCs (Polacino *et al.*, 1996). CD150 surface expression is strongly up-regulated by IL-1β that leads to an increased DC-induced T cell response (Kruse *et al.*, 2001). CD150 expression is rapidly increased on DCs during the maturation process (Bleharski *et al.*, 2001; Polacino *et al.*, 1996). CD150 could be upregulated on DCs with CD40L, poly(I:C) (polyinosinic polycytidylic acid) or LPS. mRNA encoding both membrane-bound and soluble secreted isoforms of CD150 was detected in CD40 ligand-activated DCs. The functional outcome of CD150 ligation on DCs surface depends on the nature of its ligands. Particularly, engagement of CD150 with anti-CD150 mAbs IPO-3 enhances production of IL-12 and IL-8 by DC, but has no effect on the production of IL-10 (Bleharski *et al.*, 2001). At the same time, another group of scientists has obtained the opposite results with the stimulation of CD150 on the surface of DCs with its self-ligand, CD150, expressed on transfected cells (Rethi *et al.*, 2006). This may suggest that the differential functional outcome of CD150 signaling in DCs depends on the receptor region, engaged by its ligand. CD150/CD150 interactions did not interfere with sCD40L induced DC maturation. CD150/CD150 associations inhibited IL-12, TNF-α, and IL-6 secretion by CD40L-activated DCs. CD150 signaling also modulated the function of CD40L-activated DCs by reducing their ability to promote naïve T-cell differentiation toward IFN-γ–producing effector cells (Figure 4). CD150 inhibited the differentiation of CD4$^+$ naive T cells into Th1-type effector cells without promoting their differentiation into Th2 cells which was shown by the lack of IL-4 production and the low levels of IL-13 in the presence of high concentration of IFN-γ (Rethi *et al.*, 2006).

Thus, CD150 isoforms are expressed on a wide range of lymphoid cell types. With its extracellular part, CD150 binds to several types of ligands, including CD150 by itself, glycoproteins of *Morbilliviruses* and bacterial antigens, while its cytoplasmic tail may interact with key signaling molecules that connect CD150 to several intracellular signal transduction pathways. This allows CD150 to be involved in the regulation of cell transcription programs and gene expression and therefore control cell proliferation, differentiation and survival. In the context of all these findings CD150 has attracted a lot of interest in terms of its involvement in the measles virus induced immunosuppression. As the major measles virus receptor and a dual-function signaling lymphocyte receptor, CD150 may play an important role in mediating the inhibition of immune response by measles virus and its proteins.

4   Measles Immunopathogenesis

4.1   Measles Virus Major Cell Targets and Spreading in the Host

Measles represents a typical childhood disease, which is contracted only once in the lifetime of an individual because the anti-viral immune responses are efficiently induced and persist (Avota *et al.*, 2010). But paradoxically measles virus infection induces both an efficient MV-specific immune response and a transient but profound immunosuppression. This depression of host immune response leads to an increased susceptibility to secondary infections following measles, which are responsible for its high mortality rate.

It is currently postulated that the primary cell targets for MV are CD150-positive alveolar macrophages, dendritic cells and lymphocytes in the respiratory tract. This concept is also supported with the fact that almost all CD14[+] monocytes in human tonsils express CD150. DC infection has been observed in experimentally infected cotton rats (Niewiesk *et al.*, 1997), transgenic mice (Shingai *et al.*, 2005; Ferreira *et al.*, 2010), and macaques (de Swart *et al.*, 2007; Lemon *et al.*, 2011). Both cultured CD1a[+] DCs and epidermal Langerhans cells can be infected *in vitro* by both vaccine and wild type strains of MV. Both vaccine and wild-type strains of MV undergo a complete replication cycle in DCs (Grosjean *et al.*, 1997).

In peripheral tissues DCs are found in immature state but in response to danger signals they undergo maturation and upregulate co-stimulatory molecules as well as MHC class I and II. MV replication induces maturation of immature DCs, causing down-regulation of CD1a, CD11c, and CD32 expression; up-regulation of MHCI, MHCII, CD80, and CD40 expression; and induction of CD25, CD69, CD71, CD86, and CD83 expression, alteration in the expression of chemokines, chemokine receptors, and chemotaxis (Abt *et al.*, 2009; Schnorr *et al.*, 1997; Servet-Delprat *et al.*, 2000; Zilliox *et al.*, 2006). Such dramatic changes allow DCs to increase their migratory potential and effectively realize their function – antigen presentation and activation of effector cells. All these events are also supported with the production of respective cytokines by DCs. Infection of DCs results in rapid induction of IFN-β mRNA and protein and multiple IFN-α mRNAs, as well as upregulation of IL-10 and IL-12 secretion and acquisition of MIP-3β responsiveness, which provides the migratory capacity to DCs (Dubois *et al.*, 2001; Zilliox *et al.*, 2006). DC infection with vaccine strains of MV also induces their functional maturation (Schnorr *et al.*, 1997).

Infection spreads in DC cultures, but release of infectious virus is minimal unless cells are activated (Fugier-Vivier *et al.*, 1997; Grosjean *et al.*, 1997). Immature DCs do not express CD150 receptor at a high level. However, DC maturation is followed by the upregulation of CD150 expression level on their surface which could be used for viral spreading. Immature DCs form a network within all epithelia and mucosa, including the respiratory tract (Servet-Delprat *et al.*, 2003). MV may exploit the DC network to travel to secondary lymphoid organs by infecting immature DCs, inducing their maturation and migration to these organs (Hahm *et al.*, 2004). Moreover, the virus could be transported attached to DC-SIGN molecule on the surface of uninfected dendritic cells. DCs expressing either CD150 or DC-SIGN can transmit MV to co-cultured T cells (de Witte *et al.*, 2008). The interaction of lymphocytes with MV-infected DCs results in lymphocyte infection, DC activation, and enhanced MV replication, leading to DC death (Fugier-Vivier *et al.*, 1997; Murabayashi *et al.*, 2002; Servet-Delprat *et al.*, 2000). Thus, some of dendritic cells get infected but some carry the virus to the lymph nodes where MV meets its main lymphoid targets – B and T cells (Condack *et al.*, 2007; de Swart *et al.*, 2007). However, MV transmission to T cells occurs most efficiently from cis-infected DCs, and this involves the formation of polyconjugates and an organized virological synapse (Koethe *et al.*, 2012).

4.2   Induction of Innate and Adaptive Immune Response by Measles Virus

MV infection activates the innate immunity with the induction of a type I interferon (IFN) response *in vitro* and *in vivo* (Devaux *et al.*, 2008; Gerlier & Valentin, 2009; Herschke *et al.*, 2007; Plumet *et al.*, 2007). Type I interferons (IFN-α/β) are an important part of innate immunity to viral infections because they induce an antiviral response and limit viral replication until the adaptive response clears the infection. Type I IFNs are induced upon pathogen recognition by the pattern recognition receptors which include TLRs, RIG-I like receptors (RLRs) and Nod-like receptors (NLRs). RLRs are RNA helicases, expressed by all nucleated cells, that recognize RNA molecules, which are absent in cell cytoplasm in normal conditions. Three types of RLRs, namely RIG-I, MDA5 and LGP2, could be distinguished depending on their ligands. MDA5 recognizes long double-stranded RNAs, RIG-I detects short double-stranded RNAs with a 5'-triphosphate residue, while LGP2 has greater affinity for dsRNA and regulates function of RIG-I and MDA5. This RNA detection induces IFN-β gene transcription and activation of the transcription factors: IFN regulatory factor 3 (IRF3) and nuclear factor-κB (NF-κB) (Griffin, 2010; Figure 5).

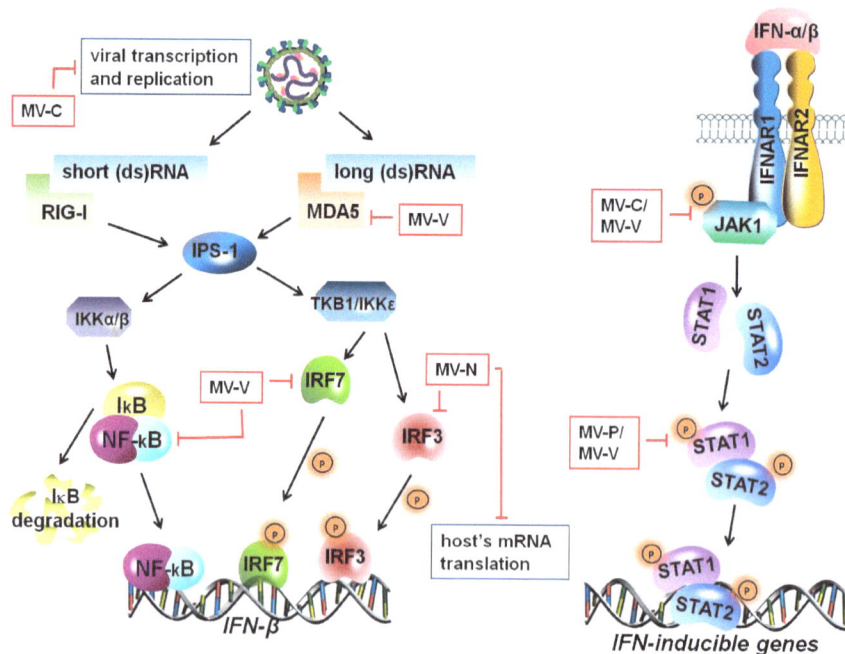

Figure 5: Innate anti-measles immune response and viral escape from its detection. MV leader RNA interacts with and activates RIG-I and to a lesser extent MDA5. Both pathways lead to the induction of signal transduction pathways with the activation of several transcription factors that regulate the expression of IFN genes. MV has developed several strategies to escape the induction of IFN response, some of which do not depend on viral replication but only the presence of viral proteins and their interaction with host cell proteins.

During MV replication MV RNA interacts with RIG-I and less with MDA5 and thus stimulates IFN-β transcription in responsive cells. Moreover, measles N protein can interact with and activate IRF3 by itself (Herschke *et al.*, 2007; Plumet *et al.*, 2007; Figure 5). However, MV infection usually suppresses type I IFN production in PBMCs (Naniche *et al.*, 2000), CD4[+] T cells (Sato *et al.*, 2008; Figure 5) and has a variable effect in plasmacytoid DCs (Druelle *et al.*, 2008; Schlender *et al.*, 2005). In addition wild type MV is less able to induce IFN, than MV vaccine strains most of the time (Naniche *et al.*, 2000).

Besides of RNA helicases, measles viral components or replication intermediates could also be recognized by pattern-recognizing host machinery of TLRs. Pattern recognition by antigen-presenting cells via TLRs is an important element of innate immunity (Beutler, 2004). TLR2 was found to interact with the hemagglutinin of wild-type measles virus (Figure 2B). This effect of MV-H could be abolished by mutation of a single amino acid, asparagine at position 481 to tyrosine, which is found in attenuated strains and is important for interaction with CD46. TLR2 activation by MV wild-type H protein induces surface CD150 expression in human monocytes and stimulates IL-6 production (Bieback *et al.*, 2002).

The induction of adaptive immune response during measles infection coincides with the appearance of its clinical manifestations, including skin rash. At the time of the rash, both MV-specific antibody and activated T cells are detectable in circulation, however in few days after its appearance the virus is cleared from peripheral blood cells. The central role in viral clearance belongs to CD8$^+$ T cells that is supported by studies in infected macaques (Permar *et al.*, 2003; de Vries, Yuksel *et al.*, 2010). In early immune response, CD4$^+$ T cells produce type 1 cytokines, including IFN-γ and IL-2, while after clearance of infectious virus they switch to the production of type 2 cytokines, like IL-4, IL-10, and IL-13 (Moss *et al.*, 2002; Figure 6). Th2 cytokine skewing after acute measles infection facilitates the development of humoral responses important for lifelong memory protection against any new measles infection, but depresses the induction of type 1 responses that is necessary for fighting new pathogens. However, recent studies on macaque model showed that humoral responses could also be abrogated upon MV infection. MV efficiently replicates in B lymphocytes, resulting in follicular exhaustion and disorganization of the germinal centers, which are essential in actively ongoing humoral immune responses (de Vries *et al.*, 2012; Figure 6).

4.3   Measles Virus Strategies for Suppression of Immune Response

The immunosuppressive effects of measles were first recognized and quantified by von Pirquet in the 19th century, in his study of delayed type hypersensitivity (DTH) skin test responses during a measles outbreak in a tuberculosis sanitarium (Von Pirquet, 1908). In addition to depressed immune responses to recall antigens (such as tuberculin), the cellular immune responses and antibody production to new antigens are impaired during and after the acute measles (Moss *et al.*, 2004). The fact that just a small proportion of peripheral blood cells are infected during measles allows us to speculate about alternative mechanisms of immunosuppression that do not involve direct viral infection of lymphoid cells. During several weeks after resolution of the rash and visible recovery, infectious virus is no longer detectable, but viral RNA continues to be present in PBMCs, as well as in respiratory secretions and urine (Permar *et al.*, 2001; Riddell *et al.*, 2007). A number of different potential mechanisms for MV-induced immunosuppression have been proposed, including lymphopenia, prolonged cytokine imbalance, leading to inhibition of cellular immunity, suppression of lymphocyte proliferation and compromised DC functions (Avota *et al.*, 2010; Griffin, 2010). The interaction of measles viral proteins with cellular receptors and other intracellular elements involved in the induction of immune response may play an important role in MV-induced immunosuppression.

4.3.1   The Role of Viral Glycoproteins in Measles Immunosuppression

Measles virus glycoproteins are highlyimplicated in the suppression of lymphocyte proliferation during and after measles acute infection even in the absence of MV replication. In cotton rat model transiently transfected cells expressing the viral glycoproteins (hemagglutinin and fusion protein) inhibit lymphocyte proliferation after intraperitoneal inoculation (Niewiesk *et al.*, 1997). This is not connected to cell fusion or unresponsiveness to IL-2, but rather to the retardation of the cell cycle that correlates with inhibition of proliferation. This inhibitory signal prevents entry of T cells into S phase and results in the reduction of cyclin-dependent kinase complexes and delayed degradation of p27Kip leading to cell cycle retardation and accumulation of cells in the G0/G1 phase (Engelking *et al.*, 1999; Niewiesk *et al.*, 1999; Schnorr *et al.*, 1997). Similarly, the complex of both MV glycoproteins, F and H, is critical in triggering MV-induced suppression of mitogen-dependent proliferation of human PBLs *in vitro* (Dubois *et al.*, 2001; Schlender *et al.*, 1996). It is also supported by the data that human DCs expressing MV glycoproteins *in vitro* fail to deliver a stimulation signal for proliferation to T cells, despite the presence of co-stimulatory molecules on their surface (Klagge *et al.*, 2000). However, the nature of the receptor responsible for mediating MV glycoprotein-induced immunosuppression has not been identified so far.

Some immunosuppressive effects of measles virus were shown to be caused by direct interaction of its glycoproteins with CD46 receptor. Thus, upon the intraperitoneal injection of UV-inactivated MV in hapten-sensitized CD46-transgenic mice a significant decrease in dendritic cell IL-12 production from draining lymph nodes was observed, providing *in vivo* evidence of the systemic modulation of IL-12 production by MV proteins (Marie *et al.*, 2001). Down-regulation of IL-12 production in primary human monocytes, could be induced in the absence of viral replication by cross-linking of CD46 with an antibody or with the complement activation product C3b (Karp *et al.*, 1996). Moreover, the engagement of distinct CD46 isoforms (CD46-1 and CD46-2) induces different effects in immune response. CD46-2 induces increased generation of specific CD8$^+$ T cells and decreases proliferation of CD4$^+$ T cells, which is associated with strongly suppressed IL-10 secretion. In contrast, CD46-1 engagement decreases the inflammatory response as well as the generation of specific CD8$^+$ T cells. Moreover, it markedly increases the proliferation of CD4$^+$ T cells which are capable of producing the anti-inflammatory cytokine IL-10 (Marie *et al.*, 2002).

CD46 downregulation can be rapidly induced in uninfected cells after surface contact with MV particles or MV-infected cells. Contact-mediated CD46 modulation can lead to complement-mediated lysis of uninfected cells that also may cause lymphopenia (Schneider-Schaulies *et al.*, 1996; Schnorr *et al.*, 1995). Recent discovery of Notch ligand Jagged1, as a natural ligand for CD46, which induces Th1 differentiation (Le Friec *et al.*, 2012), opens new possibilities to explain the importance of CD46-pathogen interaction in the modulation of the immune response. However, CD46 is most probably involved in the pathogenesis of only vaccine strains of measles virus, while most of wild type MV strains do not use this receptor.

4.3.2   The Impact of Measles Non-Structural Proteins on Antiviral Immune Response

MV non-structural proteins can block the induction of IFN response using multiple strategies. The MV V protein interacts with RNA helicase MDA5 and inhibits the IFN response (Andrejeva *et al.*, 2004; Childs *et al.*, 2007; Figure 5). Moreover, in plasmacytoid dendritic cells MV V can be a substrate for IKKα, which results in competition between MV-V and IRF7 for the phosphorylation by IKKα. In addition MV V can bind to IRF7 and inhibit its transcriptional activity. Binding to both IKKα and IRF7 requires the 68-amino-acid unique C-terminal domain of V (Pfaller & Conzelmann, 2008; Figure 5). Both P and V proteins can inhibit the phosphorylation of STAT1 and the signal cascade downstream from the IFNAR (Caignard *et al.*, 2007; Devaux *et al.*, 2007). In MV-infected cells, C and V proteins of measles virus form a complex containing IFNAR1, RACK1, and STAT1 and inhibit the Jak1 phosphorylation (Yokota *et al.*, 2003). Moreover, MV V protein could act as an inhibitor of cell death by preventing the activation of the apoptosis regulator PUMA (Cruz *et al.*, 2006). The nonstructural C protein inhibits type I IFN induction and signaling, in part by decreasing viral RNA synthesis, and has been implicated in prevention of cell death (Escoffier *et al.*, 1999; Reutter *et al.*, 2001; Shaffer *et al.*, 2003; Figure 5). Recombinant MV lacking the C protein grows poorly in cells possessing the intact IFN pathway and this growth defect is associated with reduced viral translation and genome replication. The translational inhibition correlates with phosphorylation of the alpha subunit of eukaryotic translation initiation factor 2 (eIF2α) (Nakatsu *et al.*, 2006). In addition, the protein kinase PKR plays an important role as an enhancer of IFN-β induction during measles virus infection via activation of mitogen-activated protein kinase and NF-κB (McAllister *et al.*, 2010). Besides the anti-IFN-α/β properties of V and C proteins *in vivo*, both C and V proteins are required for MV to strongly inhibit the inflammatory response in the peripheral blood monocytic cells of infected monkeys. In the absence of V or C protein, virus-induced TNF-α downregulation is alleviated and IL-6 is upregulated (Devaux *et al.*, 2008).

In addition, MV P efficiently stabilizes the expression and prevents the ubiquitination of the human p53-induced-RING-H2 (PIRH2), an ubiquitin E3 ligase belonging to the RING-like family. PIRH2 is involved in the ubiquitination of p53 and the ε-subunit of the coatmer complex, ε–COP, which is part of the COP-I secretion complex. As such, PIRH2 can regulate cell proliferation and the secretion machinery (Chen *et al.*, 2005).

4.3.3   The Effect of MV Nucleoprotein in the Regulation of Immune Response

Measles virus nucleoprotein (N) interacts with FcγR receptor on dendritic cells via its C-terminal part (Laine *et al.*, 2003; Ravanel *et al.*, 1997; Figure 2B). This interaction is critical for MV-induced immunosuppression of inflammatory responses *in vivo* that was shown by the inhibition of hypersensitivity responses in CD46-transgenic mice. MV N protein impairs the APC function affecting the priming of naïve CD8$^+$ lymphocytes during sensitization as well as the development of the effector phase following secondary antigen contact (Marie *et al.*, 2001). It has been difficult to understand how this cytosolic viral protein could leave an infected cell and then perturb the immune response. Finally it was shown that intracellularly synthesized nucleoprotein enters the late endocytic compartment, where it recruits its cellular ligand, the FcγR. Nucleoprotein is then expressed at the surfaces of infected leukocytes associated with the FcγR and is secreted into the extracellular compartment, allowing its interaction with uninfected cells. Cell-derived nucleoprotein inhibits the secretion of IL-12 and the generation of the inflammatory reaction, both shown to be impaired during measles (Marie *et al.*, 2004). MV N was also shown to induce an anti-inflammatory regulatory immune response and its repetitive administration into apolipoprotein E-deficient mice resulted in the reduction of atherosclerotic lesions (Ait-Oufella *et al.*, 2007). Finally, the immunosuppressive properties of MV N seem to be shared with the other members of *Morbilliviruses*, since both PPRV and CDV nucleoproteins bind FcγR and suppress delayed hypersensitivity responses (Kerdiles *et al.*, 2006).

Interestingly, N protein also binds to the eukaryotic initiation factor 3 (eIF3-p40). The interaction between MV-N and eIF3-p40 *in vitro* inhibits the translation of a reporter mRNAs (Sato *et al.*, 2007). This is the first observation indicating that MV can repress the translation in host cells. Therefore, viral mRNAs may selectively escape requirement for eIF3-p40 initiation factor for translation of viral proteins (Gerlier & Valentin, 2009).

4.3.4   The Effect of Measles Virus Infection on Host Pathophysiology

MV infection is associated with lymphopenia with decreased numbers of T cells and B cells in circulation during the rash. Increased surface expression of CD95 (Fas) and Annexin V staining on both $CD4^+$ and $CD8^+$ T cells during acute measles suggests that apoptosis of uninfected lymphocytes may account for some of the lymphopenia. While B cell numbers may remain low for weeks, T cell counts return to normal within few days (Ryon et al., 2002). MV-induced lymphopenia could be due to loss of precursors, albeit MV interaction with $CD34^+$ human hematopoetic stem cells (HSCs) or thymocytes did not affect viability and/or differentiation in vitro (Avota et al., 2010).

Recent studies on macaque model proposed the alternative explanation for MV-induced lymphopenia and its relation to immunosuppression. It showed that MV preferentially infects $CD45RA^-$ memory T lymphocytes and follicular B lymphocytes, resulting in high infection levels in these populations, which causes temporary immunological amnesia thus explaining the short duration of measles lymphopenia yet long duration of immune suppression. Therefore, MV infection wipes immunological memory, resulting in increased susceptibility to opportunistic infections (de Vries et al., 2012).

The influence of measles virus infection on gene expression by human peripheral blood mononuclear cells (PBMCs) was examined with cDNA microarrays. MV infection up-regulated the NF-κB p52 subunit and B cell lymphoma protein-3 (Bcl-3). This finding suggests the modulation of the activity of NF-κB, transcription factor that regulates the expression of a wide range of genes involved in inducing and controlling immune responses (Bolt et al., 2002). MV also upregulated the activating transcription factor 4 (ATF-4) and the pro-apoptotic and growth arrest-inducing CHOP/GADD153 genes indicated that MV infection induces the endoplasmic reticulum (ER) stress response in PBMCs. It is possible that the ER stress response is involved in the MV-induced reduction of lymphocyte proliferation through the induction of CHOP/GADD153 (Bolt et al., 2002).

It was shown that MV infection induces downregulation of human receptor CD150 (hCD150) in transgenic mice, inhibits cell division and proliferation of $hCD150^+$ but not $hCD150^-$ T cells, and makes them unresponsive to mitogenic stimulation. The role of CD150 in this process was studied on the transgenic mice expressing hCD150 under the control of the lck proximal promoter. The use of the lck proximal promoter in producing transgenic mice results in specific expression of CD150 protein on immature and mature T lymphocytes in blood, spleen, and thymus that partially mimics the CD150 expression in human T cells (Hahm et al., 2003).

Activation of the PI3K/Akt kinase pathway is an important target for MV interference in T cells. Shortly after MV exposure in vivo and in vitro this pathway was shown to be efficiently inhibited after IL-2R or CD3/CD28 ligation in T cells (Avota et al., 2001; Avota et al., 2004). In the absence of MV replication, MV H/F can inhibit T cell proliferation in vitro and the intracellular pathway involves the impairment of the Akt kinase activation (Avota et al., 2001). Downstream effectors of Akt kinase include molecules essentially involved in S-phase entry such as subunits of cyclin-dependent kinases, and consequently, these were found deregulated in T-cell cultures exposed to MV (Engelking et al., 1999; Figure 6). Active Akt kinase largely abolished MV-induced proliferation arrest (Avota et al., 2001). The regulatory subunit of the PI3K, p85, which acts upstream Akt kinase activation, was tyrosine phosphorylated shortly after TCR ligation in MV-exposed T cells, yet failed to redistribute to cholesterol-rich detergent-resistant membranes (DRMs) and this correlated with a lack of TCR-stimulated degradation of Cbl-b protein (Avota et al., 2004). This signal also impairs actin cytoskeletal remodeling in T cells, which lose their ability to adhere to and promote microvilli formation (Muller et al., 2006). The role of Akt pathway in the MV infection may be cell dependent, as its specific inhibitor strongly reduces the replication of several *Paramyxoviruses*, including MV (Sun *et al.*, 2008). In this study Akt signaling was shown to support the viral replication either directly or by promoting host cell survival and cell cycle entry in non-lymphoid cell types.

Another measles strategy to influence the intracellular signaling in immunocompetent cells is to cause ceramide accumulation in human T cells in a neutral (NSM) and acid (ASM) sphingomyelinase–dependent manner (Avota *et al.*, 2011; Figure 6). Ceramides promote formation of membrane microdomains and are essential for clustering of receptors and signaling platforms in the plasma membrane. They also act as signaling modulators, namely by regulating relay of PI3K signaling. In T cells ceramides, induced by MV, downmodulate chemokine-induced T cell motility on fibronectin that is mimicks extracellular matrix interaction (Avota *et al.*, 2011; Gassert *et al.*, 2009). In human DCs SMase activation and subsequent ceramide accumulation are directly linked to c-Raf-1 and ERK activation in response to DC-SIGN ligation. DC-SIGN signaling in turn may weaken TLR4 signaling, thereby downregulating inflammatory responses. SMase activation also promotes surface translocation and compartmentalization of CD150 receptor, promoting MV fusion (Avota *et al.*, 2011).

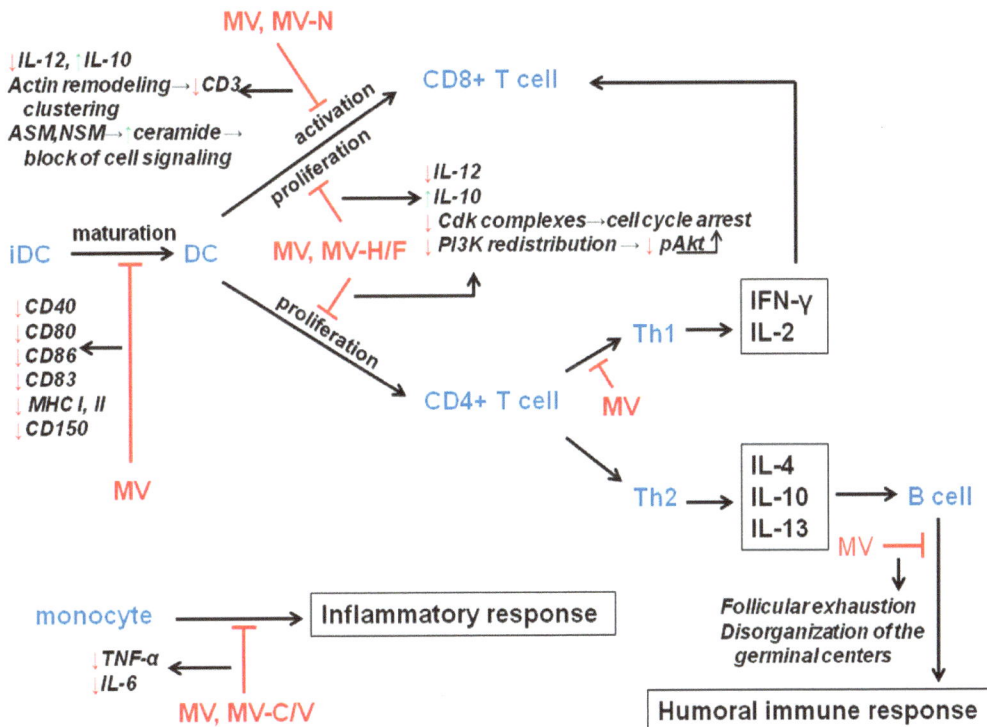

Figure 6: MV evasion strategies to avoid host adaptive immune response. Dendritic cells lay in the center of regulation of antiviral immune responses. By abrogation of DC maturation via down-regulation of surface markers like CD40, CD80, CD86, CD83, MHCI/II, CD150, and deregulation of cytokine production (IL-12 and IL-10), MV influences different stages of DC life cycle, and inhibits not only DC function, but also other immune cell responses. The mechanisms of such action include the disruption of cell signaling (PI3K/Akt pathway), cytoskeletal remodeling that crashes the stable immunological synapses, ceramide accumulation, etc.

MV exposure also results in an almost complete collapse of membrane protrusions associated with reduced phosphorylation levels of cofilin and ezrin/radixin/moesin (ERM) proteins. The signal elicited by MV prevents efficient clustering and redistribution of CD3 to the central region of the immunological synapse in T cells. Thus, by inducing microvillar collapse and interfering with cytoskeletal actin remodeling, MV signaling disturbs the ability of T cells to adhere, spread, and cluster receptors essential for sustained T-cell activation (Muller *et al.*, 2006). Together, these findings highlight an as yet unrecognized concept of pathogenesis where a virus causes membrane ceramide accumulation or cytosceletal remodeling to reorganize the immunological synapses and to target essential processes in T cell activation.

Different murine models have been generated to analyze the effect of MV infection *in vivo*. Suckling mice ubiquitously expressing CD150 were highly susceptible to the intranasal MV infection (Sellin *et al.*, 2006) and generated FoxP3$^+$ T regulatory cells. After being crossed to IFN-I deficient background, adult mice developed generalized immunosuppression with strong reduction of hypersensitivity responses (Sellin *et al.*, 2009). In double transgenic mice, expressing both CD150 and CD46 in the IFN-I deficient background, wild-type MV induced infection of DCs, but functional immunological defect was not further analyzed (Shingai *et al.*, 2005). Finally, the transgenic murine model, capable of reproducing several aspects of measles-induced immunosuppression was made by introducing the V domain of human CD150 to mouse CD150 that allows MV infection in mice. The infected mice developed lymphopenia, impaired T cell proliferation and cytokine imbalance (Koga *et al.*, 2010) illustrating potential *in vivo* role of CD150 in measles immunopathogenesis, although the effect on MV replication and its interaction with CD150 on the modulation of immune responses was not clearly dissociated in any of these transgenic models.

4.3.5   MV Interference with the Function of Dendritic Cells

The initiation of adaptive immune responses to viruses and bacterial infections relies on the activation of T and B cells by professional antigen-presenting cells, dendritic cells (Trifilo *et al.*, 2006). Maturation of DCs includes the up-regulation of co-stimulatory molecules and expression of proinflammatory cytokines, shown to be impaired during measles infection (Trifilo *et al.*, 2006). At initial stages of infection, MV replication induces maturation of immature DCs. However, CD40-dependent maturation of DCs is inhibited by MV replication, which is demonstrated by repressed induction of co-stimulatory membrane molecules (CD40, CD80, CD86) and a lack of activation (CD25, CD69, CD71) and maturation (CD83) marker expressions (Figure 6). The inhibition of CD80 and CD86 expression could be related to the impairment of CD40 signaling, which is demonstrated by inhibition of tyrosine-phosphorylation in MV-infected CD40-activated DCs (Servet-Delprat *et al.*, 2000). The same effect of MV infection was observed in transgenic mice expressing hCD150 on dendritic cells under the *CD11c* promoter. After infection with wt MV, murine splenic hCD150$^+$ DCs decreased the expression level of B7-1 (CD80), B7-2 (CD86), CD40, MHC class I, and MHC class II molecules and increased the rate of apoptosis (Figure 6). Furthermore, MV-infected DCs failed to stimulate allogeneic T cells. Analysis of CD8$^+$ T cells showed that they were poorly or even not activated, as judged by their low expression levels of CD44, CD25, and CD69 molecules and by their inability to proliferate (Hahm *et al.*, 2004).

After the first contact with pathogen antigens DCs undergo morphological changes and increase migratory capacities. Upon measles virus infection antigen-presenting function of DCs is partly damaged. Antigen uptake, as measured by mannose receptor-mediated endocytosis, is not affected (Grosjean *et al.*, 1997). However, the ability of MV-infected DCs to stimulate proliferation of heterologous CD4$^+$ T cells is affected that was shown in mixed leukocyte reaction (MLR) (Dubois *et al.*, 2001; Fugier-Vivier *et al.*, 1997; Grosjean *et al.*, 1997; Schnorr *et al.*, 1997). MV infection of DCs alsoprevents CD40L-dependent

CD8$^+$ T cell proliferation (Servet-Delprat *et al.*, 2000). The full T-cell activation does not occur probably because T-cell conjugation with DCs is unstable and short (Shishkova *et al.*, 2007). MV-exposed T cells are recruited into conjugates with DCs *in vitro* but have impaired clustering of receptors needed for sustained T-cell activation, in part due to accumulation of ceramide and preventing stimulated actin cytoskeletal dynamics and recruitment of surface receptors and membrane-proximal signaling complexes (Gassert *et al.*, 2009).

Measles virus attached to DC-SIGN (de Witte *et al.*, 2008) or Langerin (Van der Vlist *et al.*, 2011) probably uses DCs as the vehicle to the secondary lymphoid organs. However DCs are not found in efferent lymphatic vessels as they probably undergo apoptosis in the lymph nodes. MV-infected DCs develop increased sensitivity to CD95L and undergo CD95-mediated apoptosis when co-cultured with activated T cells. Moreover, CD95-dependent DC apoptosis participates in MV release (Servet-Delprat *et al.*, 2000). IFN-α/β production induced by MV in human DCs, triggers the synthesis of functional TRAIL (tumor necrosis factor (TNF)-related apoptosis-inducing ligand) on their surface. TRAIL belongs to TNF family receptors and was shown to be involved in apoptosis of several tumor cell lines. Moreover, MV was found to induce functional TRAIL expression also in monocytes after activation of IFN-α/β expression (Vidalain *et al.*, 2000). Thus, IFN-α/β-activated DCs and monocytes may exert an innate TRAIL-mediated cytotoxic activity towards surrounding MV-infected cells (Servet-Delprat *et al.*, 2003).

Prolonged suppression of IL-12 production has been observed in children with measles that is critical for the orchestration of cellular immunity (Atabani *et al.*, 2001). CD40-induced cytokine pattern in DCs is also modified *in vitro* by MV replication: IL-12 and IL-1α/β mRNA are decreased, whereas IL-10 mRNA is induced (Fugier-Vivier *et al.*, 1997; Servet-Delprat *et al.*, 2000; Figure 6).

When infected with MV, transgenic mice, which express human CD150 receptor on DCs are defective in the selective synthesis of IL-12 in response to stimulation of TLR4 signaling, but not to engagements of TLR2, 3, 7 or 9. MV suppressed the TLR4-mediated IL-12 induction in DCs even in the presence of co-stimulation with other ligands for TLR2, 3, 7 or 9. MV V and C proteins are not responsible for IL-12 suppression mediated TLR4 signaling, while the interaction of MV-H with human CD150 facilitates this suppression. IL-12 is a key cytokine inducing cellular immune responses to protect host from the pathogenic infections. It is possible that expressed on MV-infected cells MV-H , interacts with CD150 receptor on uninfected cells to cause the inhibition of TLR4-mediated IL-12 synthesis. Similarly, MV abrogates the function of DCs in detecting and delivering of danger signals by pathogenic components via TLRs to the host immune system (Hahm *et al.*, 2007). Modulation of TLR signaling by MV also occurs upon co-ligation of DC-SIGN, as reflected by induction of DC-SIGN-dependent Raf-1 activation, which in turn promotes IL-10 transcription in immature DCs by inducing acetylation of the NF-κB subunit p65. Measles virus induces IL-10 in the absence of LPS, because it binds to both TLR2 and DC-SIGN (Gringhuis *et al.*, 2007).

IL-10, an immunoregulatory and immunosuppressive cytokine, is also elevated for weeks in the plasma of children with measles (Moss *et al.*, 2002). It downregulates the synthesis of cytokines, suppresses macrophage activation and T cell proliferation, and inhibits delayed-type hypersensitivity responses, which could contribute to the increased susceptibility to the secondary infections), often observed during measles.

5 Conclusions

CD150 surface receptor is expressed on the main measles virus cell targets: DCs, T and B cells, activated monocytes and macrophages. Its interaction with MV hemagglutinin mediates the viral entry and therefore plays an important role in the primary steps of the infection. CD150 is described as a dual-function receptor, involved in the regulation of immune cell functions. While in B cells CD150 stimulation promotes cell activation, proliferation and Ig production, in T cells its ligation has mostly inhibitory effect (particularly, the inhibition of IFN-γ production). Moreover, by mediating the inhibition of IL-12, IL-6 and TNF-α secretion by DCs and induction of IL-4 production by NKT cells, CD150 shifts the differentiation of CD4$^+$ T cells towards Th2 phenotype, thus inhibiting the generation of IFN-γ producing Th1 cells. Engagement of CD150 was shown to regulate the activation of several signaling pathways, including MAPK and Akt/PKB. Measles virus infection is associated with dramatic suppression of cellular immune response, which is accountable for the risk of secondary infections and high mortality rate after measles infection. MV-induced immunopathogenesis is linked to the aberrant DC maturation, modulation of IL-12 production and inhibition of T cell proliferation. At the same time, MV induces virus-specific lifelong immunity, as humoral immune responses remain almost intact, presenting thus an immunological paradox associated with this infectious disease. It is possible, that measles virus uses CD150-mediated signaling machinery to inhibit cellular immune response allowing successful viral propagation. This consequence of CD150 engagement, which remains to be experimentally determined, may contribute to the establishment of the measles paradox. More complete understanding the role of CD150-measles interaction in viral immunopathogenesis may open novel avenues in the development new therapeutic approaches aiming to reduce complications of measles-induced immunosuppression and will shed new light on the immunoregulatory role of CD150.

Acknowledgments

The work was supported by INSERM, Ligue contre le Cancer and Ministère des affaires Etrangéres, Partenariat Curien franco-ukrainien "Dnipro", The State Fund for Fundamental Researches of Ukraine, National Academy of Sciences of Ukraine, FEBS Summer and Collaborative Fellowships, Bourse de Gouvernement Français and "AccueilDoc" from Region Rhone Alpes. Authors thank to A. Talekar for reading the review and English editing.

References

Abt, M., Gassert, E., & Schneider-Schaulies, S. (2009). Measles virus modulates chemokine release and chemotactic responses of dendritic cells. J Gen Virol, 90(Pt 4), 909-914.

Ait-Oufella, H., Horvat, B., Kerdiles, Y., Herbin, O., Gourdy, P., Khallou-Laschet, J., et al. (2007). Measles virus nucleoprotein induces a regulatory immune response and reduces atherosclerosis in mice. Circulation, 116(15), 1707-1713.

Andrejeva, J., Childs, K. S., Young, D. F., Carlos, T. S., Stock, N., Goodbourn, S., et al. (2004). The V proteins of paramyxoviruses bind the IFN-inducible RNA helicase, mda-5, and inhibit its activation of the IFN-beta promoter. Proc Natl Acad Sci U S A, 101(49), 17264-17269.

Atabani, S. F., Byrnes, A. A., Jaye, A., Kidd, I. M., Magnusen, A. F., Whittle, H., et al. (2001). *Natural measles causes prolonged suppression of interleukin-12 production. J Infect Dis, 184(1), 1-9.*

Aversa, G., Chang, C. C., Carballido, J. M., Cocks, B. G., & de Vries, J. E. (1997). *Engagement of the signaling lymphocytic activation molecule (SLAM) on activated T cells results in IL-2-independent, cyclosporin A-sensitive T cell proliferation and IFN-gamma production. J Immunol, 158(9), 4036-4044.*

Avota, E., Avots, A., Niewiesk, S., Kane, L. P., Bommhardt, U., ter Meulen, V., et al. (2001). *Disruption of Akt kinase activation is important for immunosuppression induced by measles virus. Nat Med, 7(6), 725-731.*

Avota, E., Gassert, E., & Schneider-Schaulies, S. (2010). *Measles virus-induced immunosuppression: from effectors to mechanisms. Med Microbiol Immunol, 199(3), 227-237.*

Avota, E., Gassert, E., & Schneider-Schaulies, S. (2011). *Cytoskeletal dynamics: concepts in measles virus replication and immunomodulation. Viruses, 3(2), 102-117.*

Avota, E., Gulbins, E., & Schneider-Schaulies, S. (2011). *DC-SIGN mediated sphingomyelinase-activation and ceramide generation is essential for enhancement of viral uptake in dendritic cells. PLoS Pathog, 7(2), e1001290.*

Avota, E., Muller, N., Klett, M., & Schneider-Schaulies, S. (2004). *Measles virus interacts with and alters signal transduction in T-cell lipid rafts. J Virol, 78(17), 9552-9559.*

Berger, S. B., Romero, X., Ma, C., Wang, G., Faubion, W. A., Liao, G., et al. (2010). *SLAM is a microbial sensor that regulates bacterial phagosome functions in macrophages. Nat Immunol, 11(10), 920-927.*

Beutler, B. (2004). *Inferences, questions and possibilities in Toll-like receptor signalling. Nature, 430(6996), 257-263.*

Bieback, K., Lien, E., Klagge, I. M., Avota, E., Schneider-Schaulies, J., Duprex, W. P., et al. (2002). *Hemagglutinin protein of wild-type measles virus activates toll-like receptor 2 signaling. J Virol, 76(17), 8729-8736.*

Bleharski, J. R., Niazi, K. R., Sieling, P. A., Cheng, G., & Modlin, R. L. (2001). *Signaling lymphocytic activation molecule is expressed on CD40 ligand-activated dendritic cells and directly augments production of inflammatory cytokines. J Immunol, 167(6), 3174-3181.*

Bolt, G., Berg, K., & Blixenkrone-Moller, M. (2002). *Measles virus-induced modulation of host-cell gene expression. J Gen Virol, 83(Pt 5), 1157-1165.*

Browning, M. B., Woodliff, J. E., Konkol, M. C., Pati, N. T., Ghosh, S., Truitt, R. L., et al. (2004). *The T cell activation marker CD150 can be used to identify alloantigen-activated CD4(+)25+ regulatory T cells. Cell Immunol, 227(2), 129-139.*

Caignard, G., Guerbois, M., Labernardiere, J. L., Jacob, Y., Jones, L. M., Wild, F., et al. (2007). *Measles virus V protein blocks Jak1-mediated phosphorylation of STAT1 to escape IFN-alpha/beta signaling. Virology, 368(2), 351-362.*

Calderon, J., Maganto-Garcia, E., Punzon, C., Carrion, J., Terhorst, C., & Fresno, M. (2012). *The receptor Slamf1 on the surface of myeloid lineage cells controls susceptibility to infection by Trypanosoma cruzi. PLoS Pathog, 8(7), e1002799.*

Cannons, J. L., Tangye, S. G., & Schwartzberg, P. L. (2011). *SLAM family receptors and SAP adaptors in immunity. Annu Rev Immunol, 29, 665-705.*

Cannons, J. L., Wu, J. Z., Gomez-Rodriguez, J., Zhang, J., Dong, B., Liu, Y., et al. (2010). *Biochemical and genetic evidence for a SAP-PKC-theta interaction contributing to IL-4 regulation. J Immunol, 185(5), 2819-2827.*

Cannons, J. L., Yu, L. J., Hill, B., Mijares, L. A., Dombroski, D., Nichols, K. E., et al. (2004). *SAP regulates T(H)2 differentiation and PKC-theta-mediated activation of NF-kappaB1. Immunity, 21(5), 693-706.*

Chan, B., Lanyi, A., Song, H. K., Griesbach, J., Simarro-Grande, M., Poy, F., et al. (2003). *SAP couples Fyn to SLAM immune receptors. Nat Cell Biol, 5(2), 155-160.*

Chen, M., Cortay, J. C., Logan, I. R., Sapountzi, V., Robson, C. N., & Gerlier, D. (2005). *Inhibition of ubiquitination and stabilization of human ubiquitin E3 ligase PIRH2 by measles virus phosphoprotein. J Virol, 79(18), 11824-11836.*

Childs, K., Stock, N., Ross, C., Andrejeva, J., Hilton, L., Skinner, M., et al. (2007). mda-5, but not RIG-I, is a common target for paramyxovirus V proteins. Virology, 359(1), 190-200.

Cocks, B. G., Chang, C. C., Carballido, J. M., Yssel, H., de Vries, J. E., & Aversa, G. (1995). A novel receptor involved in T-cell activation. Nature, 376(6537), 260-263.

Condack, C., Grivel, J. C., Devaux, P., Margolis, L., & Cattaneo, R. (2007). Measles virus vaccine attenuation: suboptimal infection of lymphatic tissue and tropism alteration. J Infect Dis, 196(4), 541-549.

Cruz, C. D., Palosaari, H., Parisien, J. P., Devaux, P., Cattaneo, R., Ouchi, T., et al. (2006). Measles virus V protein inhibits p53 family member p73. J Virol, 80(11), 5644-5650.

de Swart, R. L., Ludlow, M., de Witte, L., Yanagi, Y., van Amerongen, G., McQuaid, S., et al. (2007). Predominant infection of CD150+ lymphocytes and dendritic cells during measles virus infection of macaques. PLoS Pathog, 3(11), e178.

de Vries, R. D., Lemon, K., Ludlow, M., McQuaid, S., Yuksel, S., van Amerongen, G., et al. (2010). In vivo tropism of attenuated and pathogenic measles virus expressing green fluorescent protein in macaques. J Virol, 84(9), 4714-4724.

de Vries, R. D., Yuksel, S., Osterhaus, A. D., & de Swart, R. L. (2010). Specific CD8(+) T-lymphocytes control dissemination of measles virus. Eur J Immunol, 40(2), 388-395.

de Vries, R. D., McQuaid, S., van Amerongen, G., Yuksel, S., Verburgh, R. J., Osterhaus, A. D. M. E., et al. (2012). Measles immune suppression: lessons from the macaque model. PLOS Pathogens, 8(8), e1002885.

de Witte, L., de Vries, R. D., van der Vlist, M., Yuksel, S., Litjens, M., de Swart, R. L., et al. (2008). DC-SIGN and CD150 have distinct roles in transmission of measles virus from dendritic cells to T-lymphocytes. PLoS Pathog, 4(4), e1000049.

Devaux, P., Hodge, G., McChesney, M. B., & Cattaneo, R. (2008). Attenuation of V- or C-defective measles viruses: infection control by the inflammatory and interferon responses of rhesus monkeys. J Virol, 82(11), 5359-5367.

Devaux, P., von Messling, V., Songsungthong, W., Springfeld, C., & Cattaneo, R. (2007). Tyrosine 110 in the measles virus phosphoprotein is required to block STAT1 phosphorylation. Virology, 360(1), 72-83.

Dorig, R. E., Marcil, A., Chopra, A., & Richardson, C. D. (1993). The human CD46 molecule is a receptor for measles virus (Edmonston strain). Cell, 75(2), 295-305.

Druelle, J., Sellin, C. I., Waku-Kouomou, D., Horvat, B., & Wild, F. T. (2008). Wild type measles virus attenuation independent of type I IFN. Virol J, 5, 22.

Dubois, B., Lamy, P. J., Chemin, K., Lachaux, A., & Kaiserlian, D. (2001). Measles virus exploits dendritic cells to suppress CD4+ T-cell proliferation via expression of surface viral glycoproteins independently of T-cell trans-infection. Cell Immunol, 214(2), 173-183.

Engel, P., Eck, M. J., & Terhorst, C. (2003). The SAP and SLAM families in immune responses and X-linked lymphoproliferative disease. Nat Rev Immunol, 3(10), 813-821.

Engelking, O., Fedorov, L. M., Lilischkis, R., ter Meulen, V., & Schneider-Schaulies, S. (1999). Measles virus-induced immunosuppression in vitro is associated with deregulation of G1 cell cycle control proteins. J Gen Virol, 80 (Pt 7), 1599-1608.

Escoffier, C., Manie, S., Vincent, S., Muller, C. P., Billeter, M., & Gerlier, D. (1999). Nonstructural C protein is required for efficient measles virus replication in human peripheral blood cells. J Virol, 73(2), 1695-1698.

Ferreira, C. S., Frenzke, M., Leonard, V. H., Welstead, G. G., Richardson, C. D., & Cattaneo, R. (2010). Measles virus infection of alveolar macrophages and dendritic cells precedes spread to lymphatic organs in transgenic mice expressing human signaling lymphocytic activation molecule (SLAM, CD150). J Virol, 84(6), 3033-3042.

Fugier-Vivier, I., Servet-Delprat, C., Rivailler, P., Rissoan, M. C., Liu, Y. J., & Rabourdin-Combe, C. (1997). Measles virus suppresses cell-mediated immunity by interfering with the survival and functions of dendritic and T cells. J Exp Med, 186(6), 813-823.

Garcia, V. E., Quiroga, M. F., Ochoa, M. T., Ochoa, L., Pasquinelli, V., Fainboim, L., et al. (2001). Signaling lymphocytic activation molecule expression and regulation in human intracellular infection correlate with Th1 cytokine patterns. J Immunol, 167(10), 5719-5724.

Gassert, E., Avota, E., Harms, H., Krohne, G., Gulbins, E., & Schneider-Schaulies, S. (2009). Induction of membrane ceramides: a novel strategy to interfere with T lymphocyte cytoskeletal reorganisation in viral immunosuppression. PLoS Pathog, 5(10), e1000623.

Gerlier, D., & Valentin, H. (2009). Measles virus interaction with host cells and impact on innate immunity. Curr Top Microbiol Immunol, 329, 163-191.

Godfrey, D. I., & Berzins, S. P. (2007). Control points in NKT-cell development. Nat Rev Immunol, 7(7), 505-518.

Grabbe, S., & Schwarz, T. (1998). Immunoregulatory mechanisms involved in elicitation of allergic contact hypersensitivity. Immunol Today, 19(1), 37-44.

Griewank, K., Borowski, C., Rietdijk, S., Wang, N., Julien, A., Wei, D. G., et al. (2007). Homotypic interactions mediated by Slamf1 and Slamf6 receptors control NKT cell lineage development. Immunity, 27(5), 751-762.

Griffin, D. E. (2007). Measles virus. Field's virology. 5th edition, 2, 1551-1585.

Griffin, D. E. (2010). Measles virus-induced suppression of immune responses. Immunol Rev, 236, 176-189.

Gringhuis, S. I., den Dunnen, J., Litjens, M., van Het Hof, B., van Kooyk, Y., & Geijtenbeek, T. B. (2007). C-type lectin DC-SIGN modulates Toll-like receptor signaling via Raf-1 kinase-dependent acetylation of transcription factor NF-kappaB. Immunity, 26(5), 605-616.

Grosjean, I., Caux, C., Bella, C., Berger, I., Wild, F., Banchereau, J., et al. (1997). Measles virus infects human dendritic cells and blocks their allostimulatory properties for CD4+ T cells. J Exp Med, 186(6), 801-812.

Hahm, B., Arbour, N., Naniche, D., Homann, D., Manchester, M., & Oldstone, M. B. (2003). Measles virus infects and suppresses proliferation of T lymphocytes from transgenic mice bearing human signaling lymphocytic activation molecule. J Virol, 77(6), 3505-3515.

Hahm, B., Arbour, N., & Oldstone, M. B. (2004). Measles virus interacts with human SLAM receptor on dendritic cells to cause immunosuppression. Virology, 323(2), 292-302.

Hahm, B., Cho, J. H., & Oldstone, M. B. (2007). Measles virus-dendritic cell interaction via SLAM inhibits innate immunity: selective signaling through TLR4 but not other TLRs mediates suppression of IL-12 synthesis. Virology, 358(2), 251-257.

Herschke, F., Plumet, S., Duhen, T., Azocar, O., Druelle, J., Laine, D., et al. (2007). Cell-cell fusion induced by measles virus amplifies the type I interferon response. J Virol, 81(23), 12859-12871.

Hock, H. (2010). Some hematopoietic stem cells are more equal than others. J Exp Med, 207(6), 1127-1130.

Howie, D., Okamoto, S., Rietdijk, S., Clarke, K., Wang, N., Gullo, C., et al. (2002). The role of SAP in murine CD150 (SLAM)-mediated T-cell proliferation and interferon gamma production. Blood, 100(8), 2899-2907.

Jordan, M. A., Fletcher, J. M., Pellicci, D., & Baxter, A. G. (2007). Slamf1, the NKT cell control gene Nkt1. J Immunol, 178(3), 1618-1627.

Karp, C. L., Wysocka, M., Wahl, L. M., Ahearn, J. M., Cuomo, P. J., Sherry, B., et al. (1996). Mechanism of suppression of cell-mediated immunity by measles virus. Science, 273(5272), 228-231.

Kerdiles, Y. M., Cherif, B., Marie, J. C., Tremillon, N., Blanquier, B., Libeau, G., et al. (2006). Immunomodulatory properties of morbillivirus nucleoproteins. Viral Immunol, 19(2), 324-334.

Klagge, I. M., ter Meulen, V., & Schneider-Schaulies, S. (2000). Measles virus-induced promotion of dendritic cell maturation by soluble mediators does not overcome the immunosuppressive activity of viral glycoproteins on the cell surface. Eur J Immunol, 30(10), 2741-2750.

Koethe, S., Avota, E., & Schneider-Schaulies, S. (2012). Measles virus transmission from dendritic cells to T cells: formation of synapse-like interfaces concentrating viral and cellular components. J Virol, 86(18), 9773-9781.

Koga, R., Ohno, S., Ikegame, S., & Yanagi, Y. (2010). *Measles virus-induced immunosuppression in SLAM knock-in mice. J Virol, 84(10), 5360-5367.*

Kruse, M., Meinl, E., Henning, G., Kuhnt, C., Berchtold, S., Berger, T., et al. (2001). *Signaling lymphocytic activation molecule is expressed on mature CD83+ dendritic cells and is up-regulated by IL-1 beta. J Immunol, 167(4), 1989-1995.*

Laine, D., Trescol-Biemont, M. C., Longhi, S., Libeau, G., Marie, J. C., Vidalain, P. O., et al. (2003). *Measles virus (MV) nucleoprotein binds to a novel cell surface receptor distinct from FcgammaRII via its C-terminal domain: role in MV-induced immunosuppression. J Virol, 77(21), 11332-11346.*

Lamb, R. A., & Parks, G. D. (2007). *Paramyxoviridae: the viruses and their replication. Field's virology. 5th edition, 1, 1449-1496.*

Latour, S., Gish, G., Helgason, C. D., Humphries, R. K., Pawson, T., & Veillette, A. (2001). *Regulation of SLAM-mediated signal transduction by SAP, the X-linked lymphoproliferative gene product. Nat Immunol, 2(8), 681-690.*

Latour, S., Roncagalli, R., Chen, R., Bakinowski, M., Shi, X., Schwartzberg, P. L., et al. (2003). *Binding of SAP SH2 domain to FynT SH3 domain reveals a novel mechanism of receptor signalling in immune regulation. Nat Cell Biol, 5(2), 149-154.*

Le Friec, G., Sheppard, D., Whiteman, P., Karsten, C. M., Shamoun, S. A., Laing, A., et al. (2012). *The CD46-Jagged1 interaction is critical for human T(H)1 immunity. Nat Immunol.*

Lemon, K., de Vries, R. D., Mesman, A. W., McQuaid, S., van Amerongen, G., Yuksel, S., et al. (2011). *Early target cells of measles virus after aerosol infection of non-human primates. PLoS Pathog, 7(1), e1001263.*

Li, C., Iosef, C., Jia, C. Y., Han, V. K., & Li, S. S. (2003). *Dual functional roles for the X-linked lymphoproliferative syndrome gene product SAP/SH2D1A in signaling through the signaling lymphocyte activation molecule (SLAM) family of immune receptors. J Biol Chem, 278(6), 3852-3859.*

Marie, J. C., Astier, A. L., Rivailler, P., Rabourdin-Combe, C., Wild, T. F., & Horvat, B. (2002). *Linking innate and acquired immunity: divergent role of CD46 cytoplasmic domains in T cell induced inflammation. Nat Immunol, 3(7), 659-666.*

Marie, J. C., Kehren, J., Trescol-Biemont, M. C., Evlashev, A., Valentin, H., Walzer, T., et al. (2001). *Mechanism of measles virus-induced suppression of inflammatory immune responses. Immunity, 14(1), 69-79.*

Marie, J. C., Saltel, F., Escola, J. M., Jurdic, P., Wild, T. F., & Horvat, B. (2004). *Cell surface delivery of the measles virus nucleoprotein: a viral strategy to induce immunosuppression. J Virol, 78(21), 11952-11961.*

Masse, N., Ainouze, M., Neel, B., Wild, T. F., Buckland, R., & Langedijk, J. P. (2004). *Measles virus (MV) hemagglutinin: evidence that attachment sites for MV receptors SLAM and CD46 overlap on the globular head. J Virol, 78(17), 9051-9063.*

Mavaddat, N., Mason, D. W., Atkinson, P. D., Evans, E. J., Gilbert, R. J., Stuart, D. I., et al. (2000). *Signaling lymphocytic activation molecule (CDw150) is homophilic but self-associates with very low affinity. J Biol Chem, 275(36), 28100-28109.*

McAllister, C. S., Toth, A. M., Zhang, P., Devaux, P., Cattaneo, R., & Samuel, C. E. (2010). *Mechanisms of protein kinase PKR-mediated amplification of beta interferon induction by C protein-deficient measles virus. J Virol, 84(1), 380-386.*

Mikhalap, S. V., Shlapatska, L. M., Berdova, A. G., Law, C. L., Clark, E. A., & Sidorenko, S. P. (1999). *CDw150 associates with src-homology 2-containing inositol phosphatase and modulates CD95-mediated apoptosis. J Immunol, 162(10), 5719-5727.*

Mikhalap, S. V., Shlapatska, L. M., Yurchenko, O. V., Yurchenko, M. Y., Berdova, G. G., Nichols, K. E., et al. (2004). *The adaptor protein SH2D1A regulates signaling through CD150 (SLAM) in B cells. Blood, 104(13), 4063-4070.*

Minagawa, H., Tanaka, K., Ono, N., Tatsuo, H., & Yanagi, Y. (2001). *Induction of the measles virus receptor SLAM (CD150) on monocytes. J Gen Virol, 82(Pt 12), 2913-2917.*

Moss, W. J., & Griffin, D. E. (2006). Global measles elimination. Nat Rev Microbiol, 4(12), 900-908.

Moss, W. J., Ota, M. O., & Griffin, D. E. (2004). Measles: immune suppression and immune responses. Int J Biochem Cell Biol, 36(8), 1380-1385.

Moss, W. J., Ryon, J. J., Monze, M., & Griffin, D. E. (2002). Differential regulation of interleukin (IL)-4, IL-5, and IL-10 during measles in Zambian children. J Infect Dis, 186(7), 879-887.

Muhlebach, M. D., Mateo, M., Sinn, P. L., Prufer, S., Uhlig, K. M., Leonard, V. H., et al. (2011). Adherens junction protein nectin-4 is the epithelial receptor for measles virus. Nature, 480(7378), 530-533.

Muller, N., Avota, E., Schneider-Schaulies, J., Harms, H., Krohne, G., & Schneider-Schaulies, S. (2006). Measles virus contact with T cells impedes cytoskeletal remodeling associated with spreading, polarization, and CD3 clustering. Traffic, 7(7), 849-858.

Murabayashi, N., Kurita-Taniguchi, M., Ayata, M., Matsumoto, M., Ogura, H., & Seya, T. (2002). Susceptibility of human dendritic cells (DCs) to measles virus (MV) depends on their activation stages in conjunction with the level of CDw150: role of Toll stimulators in DC maturation and MV amplification. Microbes Infect, 4(8), 785-794.

Nakatsu, Y., Takeda, M., Ohno, S., Koga, R., & Yanagi, Y. (2006). Translational inhibition and increased interferon induction in cells infected with C protein-deficient measles virus. J Virol, 80(23), 11861-11867.

Nanda, N., Andre, P., Bao, M., Clauser, K., Deguzman, F., Howie, D., et al. (2005). Platelet aggregation induces platelet aggregate stability via SLAM family receptor signaling. Blood, 106(9), 3028-3034.

Naniche, D., Varior-Krishnan, G., Cervoni, F., Wild, T. F., Rossi, B., Rabourdin-Combe, C., et al. (1993). Human membrane cofactor protein (CD46) acts as a cellular receptor for measles virus. J Virol, 67(10), 6025-6032.

Naniche, D., Yeh, A., Eto, D., Manchester, M., Friedman, R. M., & Oldstone, M. B. (2000). Evasion of host defenses by measles virus: wild-type measles virus infection interferes with induction of Alpha/Beta interferon production. J Virol, 74(16), 7478-7484.

Navaratnarajah, C. K., Vongpunsawad, S., Oezguen, N., Stehle, T., Braun, W., Hashiguchi, T., et al. (2008). Dynamic interaction of the measles virus hemagglutinin with its receptor signaling lymphocytic activation molecule (SLAM, CD150). J Biol Chem, 283(17), 11763-11771.

Nichols, K. E., Hom, J., Gong, S. Y., Ganguly, A., Ma, C. S., Cannons, J. L., et al. (2005). Regulation of NKT cell development by SAP, the protein defective in XLP. Nat Med, 11(3), 340-345.

Niewiesk, S., Eisenhuth, I., Fooks, A., Clegg, J. C., Schnorr, J. J., Schneider-Schaulies, S., et al. (1997). Measles virus-induced immune suppression in the cotton rat (Sigmodon hispidus) model depends on viral glycoproteins. J Virol, 71(10), 7214-7219.

Niewiesk, S., Ohnimus, H., Schnorr, J. J., Gotzelmann, M., Schneider-Schaulies, S., Jassoy, C., et al. (1999). Measles virus-induced immunosuppression in cotton rats is associated with cell cycle retardation in uninfected lymphocytes. J Gen Virol, 80 (Pt 8), 2023-2029.

Noyce, R. S., Bondre, D. G., Ha, M. N., Lin, L. T., Sisson, G., Tsao, M. S., et al. (2011). Tumor cell marker PVRL4 (nectin 4) is an epithelial cell receptor for measles virus. PLoS Pathog, 7(8), e1002240.

Ohno, S., Seki, F., Ono, N., & Yanagi, Y. (2003). Histidine at position 61 and its adjacent amino acid residues are critical for the ability of SLAM (CD150) to act as a cellular receptor for measles virus. J Gen Virol, 84(Pt 9), 2381-2388.

OIE (Office international des epizooties). Organisation mondiale de la santé. No more deaths from rinderpest. OIE's recognition pathway paved way for global declaration of eradication by FAO member countries in June. 25 May 2011. http://www. oie.int/for-the-media/press-releases/detail/ article/no-more-deaths-from-rinderpest/.

Ono, N., Tatsuo, H., Tanaka, K., Minagawa, H., & Yanagi, Y. (2001). V domain of human SLAM (CDw150) is essential for its function as a measles virus receptor. J Virol, 75(4), 1594-1600.

Permar, S. R., Klumpp, S. A., Mansfield, K. G., Kim, W. K., Gorgone, D. A., Lifton, M. A., et al. (2003). Role of CD8(+) lymphocytes in control and clearance of measles virus infection of rhesus monkeys. J Virol, 77(7), 4396-4400.

Permar, S. R., Moss, W. J., Ryon, J. J., Monze, M., Cutts, F., Quinn, T. C., et al. (2001). *Prolonged measles virus shedding in human immunodeficiency virus-infected children, detected by reverse transcriptase-polymerase chain reaction. J Infect Dis, 183(4), 532-538.*

Pfaller, C. K., & Conzelmann, K. K. (2008). *Measles virus V protein is a decoy substrate for IkappaB kinase alpha and prevents Toll-like receptor 7/9-mediated interferon induction. J Virol, 82(24), 12365-12373.*

Pinchouk, V. G., Sidorenko, S. P., Gluzman, D. F., Vetrova, E. P., Berdova, A. G., & Schlapatskaya, L. N. (1988). *Monoclonal antibodies IPO-3 and IPO-10 against human B cell differentiation antigens. Anticancer Res, 8(6), 1377-1380.*

Pinchouk, V. G., Sidorenko, S. P., Vetrova, E. P., Berdova, A. G., Shlapatskaya, L. N., & Gluzman, D. F. (1986). *Monoclonal antibodies against the lymphoblastoid cell line RPMI-1788. Exp Oncol 8, 41-46.*

Plumet, S., Herschke, F., Bourhis, J. M., Valentin, H., Longhi, S., & Gerlier, D. (2007). *Cytosolic 5'-triphosphate ended viral leader transcript of measles virus as activator of the RIG I-mediated interferon response. PLoS One, 2(3), e279.*

Polacino, P. S., Pinchuk, L. M., Sidorenko, S. P., & Clark, E. A. (1996). *Immunodeficiency virus cDNA synthesis in resting T lymphocytes is regulated by T cell activation signals and dendritic cells. J Med Primatol, 25(3), 201-209.*

Punnonen, J., Cocks, B. G., Carballido, J. M., Bennett, B., Peterson, D., Aversa, G., et al. (1997). *Soluble and membrane-bound forms of signaling lymphocytic activation molecule (SLAM) induce proliferation and Ig synthesis by activated human B lymphocytes. J Exp Med, 185(6), 993-1004.*

Racaniello, V. (2011). *Virology. An exit strategy for measles virus. Science, 334(6063), 1650-1651.*

Ravanel, K., Castelle, C., Defrance, T., Wild, T. F., Charron, D., Lotteau, V., et al. (1997). *Measles virus nucleocapsid protein binds to FcgammaRII and inhibits human B cell antibody production. J Exp Med, 186(2), 269-278.*

Rethi, B., Gogolak, P., Szatmari, I., Veres, A., Erdos, E., Nagy, L., et al. (2006). *SLAM/SLAM interactions inhibit CD40-induced production of inflammatory cytokines in monocyte-derived dendritic cells. Blood, 107(7), 2821-2829.*

Reutter, G. L., Cortese-Grogan, C., Wilson, J., & Moyer, S. A. (2001). *Mutations in the measles virus C protein that up regulate viral RNA synthesis. Virology, 285(1), 100-109.*

Riddell, M. A., Moss, W. J., Hauer, D., Monze, M., & Griffin, D. E. (2007). *Slow clearance of measles virus RNA after acute infection. J Clin Virol, 39(4), 312-317.*

Ryon, J. J., Moss, W. J., Monze, M., & Griffin, D. E. (2002). *Functional and phenotypic changes in circulating lymphocytes from hospitalized zambian children with measles. Clin Diagn Lab Immunol, 9(5), 994-1003.*

Sato, H., Honma, R., Yoneda, M., Miura, R., Tsukiyama-Kohara, K., Ikeda, F., et al. (2008). *Measles virus induces cell-type specific changes in gene expression. Virology, 375(2), 321-330.*

Sato, H., Masuda, M., Kanai, M., Tsukiyama-Kohara, K., Yoneda, M., & Kai, C. (2007). *Measles virus N protein inhibits host translation by binding to eIF3-p40. J Virol, 81(21), 11569-11576.*

Sayos, J., Wu, C., Morra, M., Wang, N., Zhang, X., Allen, D., et al. (1998). *The X-linked lymphoproliferative-disease gene product SAP regulates signals induced through the co-receptor SLAM. Nature, 395(6701), 462-469.*

Schlender, J., Hornung, V., Finke, S., Gunthner-Biller, M., Marozin, S., Brzozka, K., et al. (2005). *Inhibition of toll-like receptor 7- and 9-mediated alpha/beta interferon production in human plasmacytoid dendritic cells by respiratory syncytial virus and measles virus. J Virol, 79(9), 5507-5515.*

Schlender, J., Schnorr, J. J., Spielhoffer, P., Cathomen, T., Cattaneo, R., Billeter, M. A., et al. (1996). *Interaction of measles virus glycoproteins with the surface of uninfected peripheral blood lymphocytes induces immunosuppression in vitro. Proc Natl Acad Sci U S A, 93(23), 13194-13199.*

Schneider-Schaulies, J., Meulen, V., & Schneider-Schaulies, S. (2003). *Measles infection of the central nervous system. J Neurovirol, 9(2), 247-252.*

Schneider-Schaulies, J., Schnorr, J. J., Schlender, J., Dunster, L. M., Schneider-Schaulies, S., & ter Meulen, V. (1996). *Receptor (CD46) modulation and complement-mediated lysis of uninfected cells after contact with measles virus-infected cells. J Virol, 70(1), 255-263.*

Schnorr, J. J., Dunster, L. M., Nanan, R., Schneider-Schaulies, J., Schneider-Schaulies, S., & ter Meulen, V. (1995). Measles virus-induced down-regulation of CD46 is associated with enhanced sensitivity to complement-mediated lysis of infected cells. Eur J Immunol, 25(4), 976-984.

Schnorr, J. J., Seufert, M., Schlender, J., Borst, J., Johnston, I. C., ter Meulen, V., et al. (1997). Cell cycle arrest rather than apoptosis is associated with measles virus contact-mediated immunosuppression in vitro. J Gen Virol, 78 (Pt 12), 3217-3226.

Schnorr, J. J., Xanthakos, S., Keikavoussi, P., Kampgen, E., ter Meulen, V., & Schneider-Schaulies, S. (1997). Induction of maturation of human blood dendritic cell precursors by measles virus is associated with immunosuppression. Proc Natl Acad Sci U S A, 94(10), 5326-5331.

Sellin, C. I., Davoust, N., Guillaume, V., Baas, D., Belin, M.-F., Buckland, R., et al. (2006). High Pathogenicity of Wild-Type Measles Virus Infection in CD150 (SLAM) Transgenic Mice. Journal of Virology, 80(13), 6420–6429.

Sellin, C. I., Jegou, J.-F., Renneson, J., Druelle, J., Wild, F., Marie, J. C., et al. (2009). Interplay between virus-specific effector response and Foxp3 regulatory T cells in measles virus immunopathogenesis. PLoS One, 4(3), e4948.

Servet-Delprat, C., Vidalain, P. O., Azocar, O., Le Deist, F., Fischer, A., & Rabourdin-Combe, C. (2000). Consequences of Fas-mediated human dendritic cell apoptosis induced by measles virus. J Virol, 74(9), 4387-4393.

Servet-Delprat, C., Vidalain, P. O., Bausinger, H., Manie, S., Le Deist, F., Azocar, O., et al. (2000). Measles virus induces abnormal differentiation of CD40 ligand-activated human dendritic cells. J Immunol, 164(4), 1753-1760.

Servet-Delprat, C., Vidalain, P. O., Valentin, H., & Rabourdin-Combe, C. (2003). Measles virus and dendritic cell functions: how specific response cohabits with immunosuppression. Curr Top Microbiol Immunol, 276, 103-123.

Shaffer, J. A., Bellini, W. J., & Rota, P. A. (2003). The C protein of measles virus inhibits the type I interferon response. Virology, 315(2), 389-397.

Shingai, M., Inoue, N., Okuno, T., Okabe, M., Akazawa, T., Miyamoto, Y., et al. (2005). Wild-type measles virus infection in human CD46/CD150-transgenic mice: CD11c-positive dendritic cells establish systemic viral infection. J Immunol, 175(5), 3252-3261.

Shishkova, Y., Harms, H., Krohne, G., Avota, E., & Schneider-Schaulies, S. (2007). Immune synapses formed with measles virus-infected dendritic cells are unstable and fail to sustain T cell activation. Cell Microbiol, 9(8), 1974-1986.

Shlapatska, L. M., Mikhalap, S. V., Berdova, A. G., Zelensky, O. M., Yun, T. J., Nichols, K. E., et al. (2001). CD150 association with either the SH2-containing inositol phosphatase or the SH2-containing protein tyrosine phosphatase is regulated by the adaptor protein SH2D1A. J Immunol, 166(9), 5480-5487.

Sidorenko, S. P., & Clark, E. A. (1993). Characterization of a cell surface glycoprotein IPO-3, expressed on activated human B and T lymphocytes. J Immunol, 151(9), 4614-4624.

Sidorenko, S. P. (1997). CDw150 cluster report. In: Leucocyte Typing VI Garland Publishing, Inc., p.583-584.

Sidorenko, S. P. (2002). CDl50 cluster report. In: Leucocyte Typing VII, Oxford University Press, p.104-106.

Sidorenko, S. P., & Clark, E. A. (2003). The dual-function CD150 receptor subfamily: the viral attraction. Nat Immunol, 4(1), 19-24.

Simons, E., Ferrari, M., Fricks, J., Wannemuehler, K., Anand, A., Burton, A., et al. (2012). Assessment of the 2010 global measles mortality reduction goal: results from a model of surveillance data. Lancet, 379(9832), 2173-2178.

Sintes, J., & Engel, P. (2011). SLAM (CD150) is a multitasking immunoreceptor: from cosignalling to bacterial recognition. Immunol Cell Biol, 89(2), 161-163.

Sun, M., Fuentes, S. M., Timani, K., Sun, D., Murphy, C., Lin, Y., et al. (2008). Akt plays a critical role in replication of nonsegmented negative-stranded RNA viruses. J Virol, 82(1), 105-114.

Tatsuo, H., Ono, N., Tanaka, K., & Yanagi, Y. (2000). SLAM (CDw150) is a cellular receptor for measles virus. Nature, 406(6798), 893-897.

Tatsuo, H., Ono, N., & Yanagi, Y. (2001). Morbilliviruses use signaling lymphocyte activation molecules (CD150) as cellular receptors. J Virol, 75(13), 5842-5850.

Tatsuo, H., & Yanagi, Y. (2002). The morbillivirus receptor SLAM (CD150). Microbiol Immunol, 46(3), 135-142.

Trifilo, M. J., Hahm, B., Zuniga, E. I., Edelmann, K. H., & Oldstone, M. B. (2006). Dendritic cell inhibition: memoirs from immunosuppressive viruses. J Infect Dis, 194 Suppl 1, S3-10.

van der Vlist, M., de Witte, L., de Vries, R. D., Litjens, M., de Jong, M. A., Fluitsma, D., et al. (2011). Human Langerhans cells capture measles virus through Langerin and present viral antigens to CD4(+) T cells but are incapable of cross-presentation. Eur J Immunol, 41(9), 2619-2631.

Veillette, A. (2004). SLAM Family Receptors Regulate Immunity with and without SAP-related Adaptors. J Exp Med, 199(9), 1175-1178.

Veillette, A., Dong, Z., & Latour, S. (2007). Consequence of the SLAM-SAP signaling pathway in innate-like and conventional lymphocytes. Immunity, 27(5), 698-710.

Vidalain, P. O., Azocar, O., Lamouille, B., Astier, A., Rabourdin-Combe, C., & Servet-Delprat, C. (2000). Measles virus induces functional TRAIL production by human dendritic cells. J Virol, 74(1), 556-559.

Von Pirquet, C. (1908). Das verhalten der kutanen tuberculinreaktion wa¨ hrend der ma¨ sern. Dtsch. Med. Wochenschr. 30, 1297-1300.

Vongpunsawad, S., Oezgun, N., Braun, W., & Cattaneo, R. (2004). Selectively receptor-blind measles viruses: Identification of residues necessary for SLAM- or CD46-induced fusion and their localization on a new hemagglutinin structural model. J Virol, 78(1), 302-313.

Wang, N., Satoskar, A., Faubion, W., Howie, D., Okamoto, S., Feske, S., et al. (2004). The cell surface receptor SLAM controls T cell and macrophage functions. J Exp Med, 199(9), 1255-1264.

WHO. (2011). Measles mortality reduction: a successful initiative. http://www.who.int/immunization/newsroom/measles/en/index.html.

Xu, Q., Zhang, P., Hu, C., Liu, X., Qi, Y., & Liu, Y. (2006). Identification of amino acid residues involved in the interaction between measles virus Haemagglutin (MVH) and its human cell receptor (signaling lymphocyte activation molecule, SLAM). J Biochem Mol Biol, 39(4), 406-411.

Yanagi, Y., Takeda, M., Ohno, S., & Hashiguchi, T. (2009). Measles virus receptors. Curr Top Microbiol Immunol, 329, 13-30.

Yokota, S., Saito, H., Kubota, T., Yokosawa, N., Amano, K., & Fujii, N. (2003). Measles virus suppresses interferon-alpha signaling pathway: suppression of Jak1 phosphorylation and association of viral accessory proteins, C and V, with interferon-alpha receptor complex. Virology, 306(1), 135-146.

Yurchenko, M., Shlapatska, L. M., Romanets, O. L., Ganshevskiy, D., Kashuba, E., Zamoshnikova, A., et al. (2011). CD150-mediated Akt signalling pathway in normal and malignant B cells. Exp Oncol, 33(1), 9-18.

Yurchenko, M. Y., Kashuba, E. V., Shlapatska, L. M., Sivkovich, S. A., & Sidorenko, S. P. (2005). The role of CD150-SH2D1A association in CD150 signaling in Hodgkin's lymphoma cell lines. Exp Oncol, 27(1), 24-30.

Yurchenko, M. Y., Kovalevska, L. M., Shlapatska, L. M., Berdova, G. G., Clark, E. A., & Sidorenko, S. P. (2010). CD150 regulates JNK1/2 activation in normal and Hodgkin's lymphoma B cells. Immunol Cell Biol, 88(5), 565-574.

Yusuf, I., Kageyama, R., Monticelli, L., Johnston, R. J., Ditoro, D., Hansen, K., et al. (2010). Germinal center T follicular helper cell IL-4 production is dependent on signaling lymphocytic activation molecule receptor (CD150). J Immunol, 185(1), 190-202.

Zilliox, M. J., Parmigiani, G., & Griffin, D. E. (2006). Gene expression patterns in dendritic cells infected with measles virus compared with other pathogens. Proc Natl Acad Sci U S A, 103(9), 3363-3368.

Lots of Bovine Viral Diarrhoea Virus E2 Protein: A Subunit Vaccine

Antonino S. Cavallaro, Donna Mahony, Karishma T. Mody
Timothy J. Mahonuy and Neena Mitter
Queensland Alliance for Agriculture and Food Innovation
The University of Queensland, Australia

1   Introduction

1.1   Bovine Viral Diarrhoea Virus (BVDV)

Bovine viral diarrhoea (BVD) is a prevalent cattle disease that causes serious mucosal lesions and clinical disorders such as reproductive, congenital defects and persistent infections (Houe, 1999; Nelson *et al.*, 2012). An economic analysis in 2009 has shown that yearly losses due to BVD could reach approximately US$88 per animal (Hessman *et al.*, 2009). Bovine viral diarrhoea virus (BVDV) commonly known as bovine pestivirus, is a single-stranded RNA virus which infects cattle and sheep (Gard *et al.*, 2007). BVDV isolates are classified as either BVDV-1 or BVDV-2 with BVDV-1 being the dominant species. BVDV-1 has been further divided into genotypes a to o (Yilmaz *et al.*, 2012). Both species of BVDV can exist in one of two biotypes depending on the presence or absence of cytopathic effects in culture cells referred to as cytopathic (CP) and noncytopathic (NCP) respectively (Schweizer and Peterhans, 2001). BVDV has been classified in the genus Pestivirus within family *Flaviviridae*. This genus comprises of four recognised virus species: Bovine viral diarrhoea virus 1 (BVDV-1) and BVDV-2, Border disease virus and Classical swine fever virus (Bauermann *et al.*, 2012). The viruses associated with diseases such as yellow fever, dengue, and hepatitis C also belong to the this family (Sako *et al.*, 2008b). BVDV infection in cattle is of great importance in several countries due to its clinical and economical importance. A major concern regarding pestivirus is not only limited to the substantial economic losses incurred but also to the fact that these viruses are not host specific signifying that they can easily spread amongst livestock such as sheep and pigs. It has been well established that sheep and goats can carry and be infected with BVDV and then be able to pass the virus back to cattle (Sako *et al.*, 2008a). BVDV has also been found in bison and water buffaloes (Craig *et al.*, 2008).

BVDV can cause reproductive losses, immunosuppressive effects and is associated with the disease complex, bovine respiratory disease (BRD). BRD can result from a complex interaction between stress, bacteria, viruses and the environment (Duff and Galyean, 2007) and is responsible for 60-70% of all cattle illness in Australian feedlots (Animal Health and Welfare, MLA 2006) with economic losses of AUS$40 million per year. BVDV infection is widespread throughout the world and can occur either via persistent infected (PI) or acutely infected animals. Transmission of BVDV occurs when uninfected animals come in contact with bodily fluid discharges from infected cattle. Although the prevalence of infection varies, the infection tends to be endemic in many populations, reaching a maximum level of 1–2% of the PI cattle and 60–85% of the cattle being antibody positive (Houe, 1999). The virus is mainly transmitted through PI animals as they continuously shed large amounts of virus in the environment and are an important source of virus transmission within and between herds (Houe, 1999; Corbett *et al.*, 2011).

PI animals can develop if the foetus becomes infected with the virus in the first trimester or up to the first 125 days of gestation and may lead to abortion or stillbirth resulting in reduced productivity (Divers and Peek, 2008). If an infected developing foetus survives to the end of pregnancy, the calf may be born with severe birth defects, be developmentally delayed or appear normal. Asymptomatic PI animals can act as disease reservoirs and spread BVDV to the other cattle as they constantly shed the virus throughout their life. Any secretion of body fluids may result in easy transmission of virus to susceptible animals (McGowan *et al.*, 2008). BVDV infected cattle have reduced immune responses thus making them more susceptible to other diseases like pneumonia, mastitis, BRD and diarrhoea. Immunosuppression caused by BVDV infection can lead to secondary infection, which is the major cause of death in BVDV infected cattle. Once a PI animal is detected, it is then desirable to remove and destroy the animal and search for other susceptible cattle which may have come into contact with the virus and develop management strategies to eradicate or reduce the impact of the virus on the herd (Divers and Peek, 2008).

1.2   Current Vaccines

Currently available live and inactivated BVDV vaccines are effective at preventing the majority of clinical diseases associated with acute infections however these vaccines fail to completely protect against foetal infection (Callan, 2002). To date the inactivated vaccine, Pestigard® (Pfizer) is the only BVDV vaccine approved for use in Australia. It needs to be administered as two doses, 6-8 weeks apart, with annual booster injections required thereafter; also it has a shelf-life of only one month when refrigerated. The inactivated BVDV (strain C-86) vaccine Bovilis BVD (Merck) is available in the UK. It protects the foetus against transplacental infection with BVDV and requires an annual booster dose. It has a shelf-life of 18 months at +2°C to +8°C. Once opened the vaccine shelf-life is reduced to 10 hours (Merck). BVD vaccine Arsenal® (Novartis Animal Health US), is a one-dose, modified live vaccine administered subcutaneously to weaned calves which gives protection against both BVDV Type 1 and Type 2 (Novartis, 2006).

In addition, to administering BVDV vaccines there is a strong need to develop a large-scale BVDV eradication plan. Many countries in the European Union (EU) have developed an eradication program to assist in the fight and control of the disease together with the use of vaccines (Alvarez *et al.*, 2007). The spreading of BVDV within herds can be managed by identifying and removing PI animals and by ensuring that breeding animals that are susceptible do not become infected during the eradication procedure (Niskanen and Lindberg, 2003). Current control measures for BVDV involve isolation of infected cattle, serological testing of new cattle before incorporation into a herd and vaccination.

1.3   BVDV Antigenic Determinants

The BVDV genome is a 12.3 kb single stranded RNA molecule containing a single open reading frame that is translated into a single polyprotein which is processed into individual viral proteins by viral and cellular proteases (Figure 1). The structural envelope protein E2 of BVDV is a major immunogenic determinant, and is an ideal candidate as a subunit vaccine as it evokes the production of neutralising antibodies (Bolin and Ridpath, 1996; Ciulli *et al.*, 2009; Nelson *et al.*, 2012; Patterson *et al.*, 2012; Pecora *et al.*, 2012). The neutralising antibodies produced by E2 after natural infection or vaccinations are considered as the most important protective mediator against subsequent BVDV infection (Howard *et al.*, 1989; Howard *et al.*, 1994; Ridpath *et al.*, 2003).

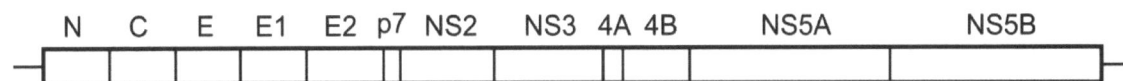

Figure 1: Schematic of the BVDV genome. Boxes represent the coding region associated with the mature viral proteins. N: N protease; C: Capsid; E: Erns; E2: glycoprotein E1; E1: glycoprotein E2; p7: non-structural protein 7; NS2: nonstructural protein 2; NS3: nonstructural protein 3; 4A: nonstructural protein 4A; 4B: nonstructural protein 4B; NS5A: nonstructural protein 5A; NS5B: nonstructural protein 5B.

The E2 protein contains 17 cysteine residues, which form intramolecular, and intermolecular disulphide bonds. These disulphide bonds lead to the *in vivo* formation of dimers of E2-E2 and E1-E2 (Branza-Nichita *et al.*, 2001). E2 dimer formation has also been observed in *E. coli* derived E2 (Cavallaro *et al.*, 2011). Expression of E2 has been documented in mammalian (Bolin and Ridpath, 1996; Donofrio *et al.*, 2006) as well as insect cell lines (Bolin and Ridpath, 1996; Pande *et al.*, 2005; Marzocca *et al.*, 2007), an insect larval system (Ferrer *et al.*, 2007) and most recently in plants (Nelson *et al.*, 2012). Friesian–Holstein bullocks immunised with BVDV E2 protein expressed on the surface of *Saccharomyces cerevisiae* exhibited both T-helper type 1 (Th1) and Th2 cell-mediated immune responses, with the production of IFN-γ, IL-4 and IL-10 (Patterson *et al.*, 2012).

We have previously detailed expression of E2 in *E. coli*, and although initially it was produced as insoluble inclusion bodies, after processing, the resultant protein was immunogenic and detectable by BVDV-E2 specific antibodies (Cavallaro *et al.*, 2011).

1.4   Protein Expression

Protein expression in *E. coli* seems ideal for expression of antigens for veterinary subunit vaccines owing to high antigen yields, ease of scale-up, and relatively low cost compared to baculovirus or mammalian expression systems (Demain and Vaishnav, 2009). However, *E. coli* protein expression also presents several disadvantages over mammalian and insect expression systems.

E. coli expressed proteins can lack post-translational modifications such as glycosylation, amidation, hydroxylation, myristoylation, palmitation or sulfation (Brondyk, 2009). Lacking these modifications may render the proteins unsuitable for use in vaccines, as they may not induce a protective immune response. We have shown that immunisation with *E. coli* derived E2 induced humoral immunity in mice (Cavallaro *et al.*, 2011). Furthermore, virus neutralising antibodies have been induced in response to immunisation with *E. coli* derived envelope protein (E) of Japanese Encephalitis Virus, also a member of the Flavivirus family (Chia *et al.*, 2001). Das *et al.* (2007) demonstrated monoclonal antibodies generated against *E. coli* expressed Ebola virus antigen recognised the glycosylated antigen expressed in mammalian cells.

A limitation of protein expression in *E. coli* is the production of insoluble proteins. These insoluble proteins form inclusion bodies (IB) within the cytosol of the bacteria (Kane and Hartley, 1988). The formation of IB has been used to an advantage as it was observed that IB contain the protein of interest in a highly pure form and can be used as a method to separate the protein of interest from endogenous proteins (Speed *et al.*, 1996; Garcia-Fruitos, 2010).

Another potential drawback of *E. coli* derived proteins is contamination with endotoxins. Endotoxins are a major component of gram negative bacterial cell walls which are released and co-purified during protein purification methods (Petsch and Anspach, 2000). Endotoxins are heat stable lipopolysaccharides with a molecular weight range from 10 to 20 kDa that form highly stable aggregates (Petsch and Anspach, 2000). Mammalian exposure to endotoxins can induce several undesirable physiological effects such as fever, leukocytosis, hypoferremia, platelet aggregation, thrombocytopenia and coagulapathies (Hurley, 1995).

The threshold human dose for endotoxin is 5 EU/kg, using this value as a starting point and, a safe endotoxin limit for a 100 μL daily dose for a 30 g mouse would be 1.5 EU/mL (Malyala and Singh, 2008). Previous studies have reported endotoxin levels of 3 EU/mL to show no deleterious effects in animal models (Fifis *et al.*, 2004; Scheerlinck *et al.*, 2006).

Techniques for removal of endotoxins from purified protein preparations include ultrafiltration, adsorption techniques, affinity chromatography and Triton X114 two-phase extraction (Adam *et al.*, 1995; Petsch and Anspach, 2000). Two-phase extraction with Triton X114 has been shown to reduce endotoxin level by 98-99% in the soluble proteins cardiac troponin I, myoglobin and creatin kinase, with a protein recovery rate of > 90% (Liu *et al.*, 1997). Aida and Pabst (Aida and Pabst, 1990) demonstrated a 1000 fold reduction of endotoxin for the soluble proteins catalase, cytochrome c, and bovine serum albumin using this method with a protein loss of 2% for cytochrome c. BVDV-E2 has been successfully purified from insoluble IB using an integrated endotoxin removal step to produce soluble, endotoxin-free protein (Cavallaro *et al.*, 2011).

1.5 Codon Optimisation

We have obtained moderate yields of E2 when expressed in *E. coil*, for immunogenic analysis in mice (Cavallaro *et al.*, 2011). However, these yields were insufficient for quantities required for vaccine production. Methods that increase heterologous gene expression include vector and strain selection, temperature optimisation, media optimisation and codon optimisation (Makrides, 1996). *E. coli* codon usuage differs from that of eukaryotic codon usage, rare codons that are used infrequently in *E. coli* may cause expression problems including reduced rate of translation (Zhou *et al.*, 2004; Chen and Texada, 2006). To overcome codon bias for heterologous genes, the intracellular tRNA pool can be modified to include plasmids expression copies of rare tRNA molecules (Makrides, 1996; Zhou *et al.*, 2004).

Heterologous genes can be modified to substitute rare codons with high frequency codons, Zhou et al. (2004) showed increased expression of the synthetic malarial protein FALVAC-1 from 36.8 mg/L to 130 mg/L when using a codon optimised construct. Although higher yields can be obtained by adjusting the codon bias, it has also been shown to impact on protein solubility; the fatty acid-binding protein 1 EgFABP1 from *Echonococcus granulosus* was insoluble when expressed in a codon optimised form (Cortazzo *et al.*, 2002; Sorensen and Mortensen, 2005). Furthermore codon optimised proteins have shown reduced enzyme activity chloramphenicol acetyltransferase shows a 20% reduction in specific activity (Komar *et al.*, 1999).

We have previously reported a successful method for BVDV-E2 expression (Cavallaro et al, 2011). In this chapter we will present our work utilising *E. coli* codon optimisation for increased yields. Furthermore we will present new immunological data supporting the viability of *E. coli* derived E2 as a subunit vaccine.

2   Materials and Methods

2.1   Cloning of E2-T1 and optiE2 into pET-SUMO Bacterial Expression Vector

The E2 gene was amplified from a plasmid containing BVDV isolate MD74 which has been identified as a type-1 isolate (Mahony *et al.*, 2005). Twenty µL of Qiagen (Venlo, The Netherlands) PCR master mix (Catalogue #201443) was used with the primers E2-T1-F and E2-T1-R (Table 1) at a final concentration of 0.5 µM. PCR cycling conditions comprised an initial incubation at 95°C for 5 minutes, followed by 35 cycles at 94°C for 30 seconds, 60°C for 30 seconds and 72°C for 90 seconds. The resultant 1040 bp product was ligated into the pET-SUMO vector (Invitrogen, Carlsbad, USA) and designated E2-T1. The ligation products were subsequently transformed into electrocompetent *E. coli* strain DH10B (Invitrogen).

An *E. coli* optimised clone of E2-T1 was synthesised by GenScript (Piscataway, USA) using their proprietary OptimumGene™ algorithm. This optimised clone was used as a PCR template following the above conditions, using corresponding primers pairs (Table 1) to produce optiE2 plus SUMO (oE2+S) and optiE2-*Nhe*I. The subsequent products were ligated into the pET-SUMO vector. Further modification of optiE2-*Nhe*I was performed by digesting with *Nhe*I, and religating.

Protein	Primers	Sequence
E2-T1	E2-T1-F	5' ATG GTG GAT CCG TGC AAG CCT 3'
	E2-T1-R	5' CTA AGA CTC GGC GAA GTA GTC CCG G 3'
optiE2-*Nhe*I	oE2-S-F	5' <u>GCT AGC</u> ATG GTG GAC CCG TGT AAA CCG 3'
(optiE2 minus SUMO precursor)	oE2-S-R	5' TCA ATG ATG ATG ATG ATG ATG GGA TTC TGC 3'
oE2+S	oE2+S-F	5' ATG GTG GAC CCG TGT AAA CCG 3'
	oE2+S-R	5' CTA GGA TTC TGC GAA ATA GTC ACG ATG 3'

Table 1: PCR primers for the production of the expression constructs E2-T1, optiE2 minus SUMO (oE2-S) and optiE2 plus SUMO (oE2+S). The *Nhe*I restriction site of oE2-S-F is underlined. The integrated 6-His tag of oE2-S-R is shaded.

Positive clones were confirmed by sequencing (AGRF, Brisbane, Australia) and transformed into *E. coli* strain BL21 (DE3, Invitrogen) cells for protein expression.

2.2   Large-Scale Expression and Purification of E2 Proteins

A single overnight culture of *E. coli* BL21 (DE3) containing the pET-SUMO-E2-T1, pET-SUMO-oE2-S or pET-SUMO-oE2+S construct was used to inoculate four 250 mL cultures of LB Miller broth (Amresco, Solon, USA) containing 50 mg/L Kanamycin-sulphate (Amresco). The cultures were grown at 37°C to an OD_{600nm} of 0.4 to 0.6, then induced with 1 mM IPTG and grown for a further 2 hours (pET-SUMO-E2-T1) or 4 hours (pET-SUMO-oE2-S, pET-SUMO-oE2+S). The bacterial pellet was collected by centrifugation at 3,800 *g*, at 4°C for 15 minutes in 4 x 250 mL centrifuge tubes. Total protein was extracted by resuspending each bacterial pellet in 50 mL *E. coli* lysis buffer (50 mM KPO_4 phosphate (pH 7.8), 400 mM NaCl, 100 mM KCl, 10% glycerol, 0.5% Triton X-100, 10 mM Imidazole), with the addition of 12.5 mg of Lysozyme (Sigma) and 750 units of Benzonase nuclease (Novagen-Merck, Darmstadt, Germany). The bacterial suspensions were incubated in lysis buffer for 20 minutes with gentle shaking. The samples were subjected to three cycles of freezing in liquid nitrogen and thawing at 42°C. The lysates were then centrifuged at 37,000 *g* for 15 minutes at 4°C.. The insoluble protein fraction (containing IB aggregates) and the supernatant (containing the soluble protein fraction) were stored at -20°C.

2.3   Purification of Soluble E2-T1

E2-T1 protein was purified from the soluble fraction by affinity chromatography using TALON (Clontech, Mountain View, USA) resin following manufacturer's instruction. Bound protein was eluted from the resin using TALON elution buffer with a step gradient of 50 mM, 80 mM, 100 mM and 150 mM imidazole, collecting ten 500 µL fractions/step. An aliquot (20 µL) of the fractions were analysed by SDS-PAGE.

2.4   Purification of Inclusion Body Aggregates of E2 Proteins

The insoluble protein fractions were recovered from the IB using BugBuster™ Master Mix (Novagen-Merck) IB pellets (equivalent to 160 mL bacterial culture) were resuspended in 2.5 mL BugBuster™ and vortexed for 2 minutes. Following the addition of 15 mL of 1:10 diluted BugBuster™ and further vortexing for 1 minute, the resuspended IB pellets were centrifuged at 5000 g at 4°C for 15 minutes. Three further washes of 25 mL 1:10 diluted BugBuster™ were performed with vortexing and centrifugation steps as above. Following the final wash step, the pellets were resuspended in 1mL 1:10 diluted BugBuster™, transferred into 1.5 mL tubes and centrifuged at 16,200 g at 4°C for 15 minutes. The supernatant was removed and the IB pellets were stored at -20°C without any detectable protein degradation.

2.5   Endotoxin Removal

All reagents were prepared in endotoxin-free water (<0.001 EU/mL, MO BIO Laboratories, Carlsbad, USA). Triton X-114 exhibits a cloud point at 22°C, above this temperature micelles aggregate forming a new phase with very low water content. Endotoxin remains in the detergent phase (Petsch and Anspach, 2000). Purified IB pellets were resuspended in 1 to 6 mL of PBS (137 mM NaCl, 2.7 mM KCl, 10 mM Phosphate buffer (pH 7.2), Amresco), and vortexed for 1 minute to disperse the insoluble protein. Dispersed protein solutions were mixed with 1% (v/v) Triton X-114 by vigorous vortexing for 1 minute. Samples were incubated on ice for 5 minutes, vortexed and subsequently incubated at 56°C for 1 minute to allow phase separation. After centrifugation at 16,200g at room temperature for 7 seconds in a microfuge the 3 phases (aqueous, oil and pellet) were recovered into separate tubes and analysed by SDS-PAGE electrophoresis. To determine the level of endotoxin in the protein samples, endotoxin assays were performed by using the Limulus Amoebocyte Lysate (LAL) assay by AMS Laboratories (Sydney, Australia).

2.6   Solubilisation of E2 Proteins

Protein pellets from the IB preparations were dissolved in 50 mM Tris (pH 6.8), 100 mM DTT, 1% SDS, 10% Glycerol, vortexed at low speed for 2 minutes and incubated at 37°C for 20 minutes. The resulting solubilised protein was dialysed at room temperature, with 3 buffer changes over 24 hours against 50 mM Tris (pH 7.0), 0.2% Igepal CA630 (Sigma-Aldrich). Following dialysis, protein integrity was determined by SDS-PAGE analysis and protein yield determined by colourimetric assay (BioRad DC Kit, Hercules, USA). Dialysis was also attempted in 1x PBS (pH 7.2).

2.7   SDS-PAGE Electrophoresis

SDS-PAGE analysis was performed using Invitrogen's XCell SureLock® Mini-Cell precast system with NuPAGE 10% BIS-Tris gels according to manufacturer instructions. Size estimations were determined against SeeBlue® Plus2 (Invitrogen) pre-stained standards. The resolved proteins were visualised by staining in 50% methanol, 10% acetic acid, 0.25% Coomassie Blue R250 for 30 minutes, followed by destaining in 30% methanol, 10% acetic acid for 10 minutes three times.

2.8   Western Hybridisation Analysis

Following SDS-PAGE electrophoresis, the resolved polypeptides were transferred to Hybond C nitrocellulose membrane (GE Healthcare, Buckinghamshire, United Kingdom) using Invitrogen XCell II™ Blot Module Kit according to manufacturer's instructions. All antibodies were diluted in BLOTTO (PBS (Amresco), 0.1% Tween 20, 1% skim milk). E2 specific monoclonal antibodies mAb-157 and mAb-348 (Deregt et al., 1998) (VMRD, Pullman, USA) were diluted to 1:100. An anti-E2 sheep sera (804) was produced in vaccinated sheep after intramuscular injection of BVDV-E2 and diluted to 1:100. Monoclonal 6xHis antibodies (Clontech) were used at 1:15,000. Sera raised against oE2-S in sheep by subcutaneous injections (Sheep # 1599) were diluted 1:10,000. Sera raised against E2-T1 in mice (M1) was diluted 1:64,000 (Cavallaro et al., 2011). Anti-mouse immunoglobulin G HRP conjugate (Chemicon, Millipore, Billerica, Massachusetts, USA) and anti sheep/goat immunoglobulin HRP conjugate (Sigma) were used at 1:2,000 and 1:10,000 respectively. Detection was carried out using an ECL detection kit (GE Healthcare). Relative purity of the expressed proteins was determined by densitometry; E2 proteins were probed with 6-His antibodies, and the resultant image was analysed using the software package ImageJ (http://rsb.info.nih.gov/ij/).

2.9   Animals

C57BL/6J mice were purchased from and housed in the Biological Resource Facility, The University of Queensland, Brisbane, Australia under specific pathogen free conditions. Female mice were housed in HEPA-filtered cages with 4 animals per cage in an environmentally controlled area with a cycle of 12 hours of light and 12 hours of darkness. Food and water were given ad libitum. All studies were conducted with 8 week old mice at the time of first injection. All procedures were approved by The University of Queensland Ethics Committee.

2.10   Immunisation of Mice with E2 Proteins

Blood samples were collected by retro-orbital bleed using heparin coated hematocrit tubes (Hirschmann Laborgeräte Heilbronn, Germany). Blood samples collected prior to the first immunisation were referred to as the preimmune samples and samples collected 2 weeks after the third immunisation were referred to as terminal bleed.

All doses of E2 were prepared in sterile conditions in a certified biological safety cabinet using sterile reagents, equipment and aseptic technique. The adjuvant QuilA (Superfor Biosector, Vedback, Denmark) was resuspended at 2 mg/mL in sterile injectable water (Pfizer, Brooklyn, USA).

Dose volumes were adjusted to 500 μL using 0.9% saline (Pfizer). 50 μg E2-T1 together with 10 μg QuilA, were administered in a final volume of 100 μL subcutaneously at the tail base using a sterile 27 gauge needle (Terumo, Tokyo, Japan). Three injections were administered at 2 week intervals and mice were sacrificed 14 days after the final immunisation. Animals were closely monitored throughout the study. All the animals remained in good health for the duration of the study with no visible deleterious health effects.

2.11   Humoral Antibody Responses

ELISA assays for the detection of E2 specific antibodies were performed by coating microtitre plates (96 well, Nunc, Maxisorb, Roskilde, Denmark) with 50 μL oE2-S antigen solution (2 ng/μL in PBS) overnight at room temperature. Antigen solution was removed from the plates which were then washed once with 1x PBS-T (1x PBS, 0.1% Tween: Sigma-Aldrich) and blocked with 200 μL per well of PBS containing 5% BSA (Sigma-Aldrich), 5% skim milk (Fonterra, Auckland, New Zealand) for 1 hour with gentle shaking at room temperature. Plates were washed three times in 200 μL 1xPBS-T as described above.

Mouse sera samples were diluted from 1:100 to 1:6400 and 50 µL of diluted sera was added to plates then incubated for 2 hours at room temperature. To detect mouse antibodies HRP conjugated poly-clonal sheep anti-mouse IgG antibodies (100 µL of 1:10000 dilution in PBS (pH 7.2), Chemicon Australia, Melbourne, Vic, Australia) was added per well and incubated for 1 hour at RT with gentle shaking. Plates were washed three times in 200 µL 1xPBS-T and 100 µL of TMB substrate (Sigma-Aldrich) was added to each well. After 15 minutes at RT 100 µL of 1N HCl was added to each well to stop the chromogenic reaction. Plates were read at 450 nm within 10 minutes.

2.12   Isolation of Murine Splenocytes and IFN-γ ELISPOT Assays

Spleens were aseptically removed following euthanasia and placed into 5 mL ice cold DMEM media supplemented with 10% foetal bovine serum (FBS), 20 mM Hepes (pH 7.3), 1 M sodium pyruvate, 1 M Glutamax, 100 units/mL penicillin G, 100 µg/mL streptomycin, 0.25 µg/mL Fungizone. Spleens were gently disrupted and passed through a 100 µm nylon mesh (Becton Dickinson, Franklin Lakes, NJ) using a syringe plunger. Cells were washed with 5 mL DMEM, centrifuged (800 g, 5 min, 4 $^{\circ}$C) and then re-suspended in 1 mL lysis buffer (0.15 M NH$_4$Cl, 10 mM KHCO$_3$, 0.1 mM Na$_2$-EDTA for 5 min at room temperature. Repeat wash steps twice with DMEM each time. Cell pellets were resuspended in 2 mL DMEM and cell numbers determined by staining with 0.2% trypan blue. Cells from each mouse spleen were seeded at 1.0 - 1.5 x 10^5 cells/well in triplicate into Polyvinylidene fluoride (PVDF) ELISPOT plates precoated with monoclonal interferon-γ (IFN-γ) (Mabtech) capture antibody. Cells were incubated in complete DMEM medium at 37 $^{\circ}$C and 5% CO$_2$ for 40 hours in the presence or absence of oE2-S protein (10 µg/mL or the polyclonal activator concavalin A (Con A, 1 µg/mL, Sigma Aldrich) as a positive control. IFN-γ ELISPOT assays were performed according to the manufacturer's specifications. The ELISPOT plates were read on an ELISPOT reader (Autoimmun Diagnostika, Strassburg, Germany).

2.13   Dynamic Light Scattering Analysis

Size, polydispersity and zeta potential data were determined by dynamic light scattering (DLS) using a Malvern Instruments Zetasizer Nano (Worcestershire, UK). E2 protein solutions (1 mL) at concentrations within the recommendations for sizing and Zeta Potential (oE2-S: 2.2 µg/µL; oE2+S 2.1 µg/µL and E2-T1 0.8 µg/µL) were placed in a clear disposable zeta cell (DTS1060C, Malvern Instruments). Size distribution and polydispersity analysis was performed using the size standard operating procedure (SOP) using the default parameters for protein analysis. Zeta potential (ZP) measurements were carried out using the zeta potential SOP with default parameters. Analysis of the data was carried out by the Malvern Zetasizer software.

2.14   Physical Properties of E2 Proteins

Physical data was obtained using ProtParam, last accessed 3 March 2011 at http://au.expasy.org/tools/protparam.html. Disulphide bond prediction was determined using the DiANNA prediction software (Ferre and Clote, 2005a; Ferre and Clote, 2005b; Ferre and Clote, 2006).

3   Results

3.1   Cloning and Expression

E2-T1 is a truncated version of the E2 gene (BVDV isolate MD74) produced by PCR using E2-T1F and E2-T1R primers (Table 1) to remove the 3' region of the ORF which encodes for the membrane binding domain (Figure 2). The resultant 1040 bp product was ligated into the pET-SUMO expression vector.

An *E. coli* optimised clone of E2-T1 was synthesised by GenScript using their proprietary algorithm. The optimised clone was used as a PCR template and with the corresponding primers pairs (Table 1); to generate optiE2+SUMO (oE2+S) which is 100% amino acid identical to E2-T1, and optiE2-*Nhe*I, a precursor for optiE2-SUMO, which also contains a second 6-His tag. The subsequent products were ligated into the pET-SUMO vector. To produce optiE2-SUMO (oE2-S), optiE2-*Nhe*I was further modified by digesting with *Nhe*I, removing 293 bp of the SUMO tag, followed by religation (Figure 2).

The physical properties of oE2+S were identical to E2-T1, whereas oE2-S generates a smaller protein with a lower calculated pI. A comparison of the physical properties of the E2 variants appears in Table 2.

	E2-T1/oE2+S	oE2-S
Nucleic Acids (bp)	1392	1116
Amino Acids	463	372
Size (kDa)	52.5	42.2
Calculated pI	6.22	7.25

Table 2: Physical properties of E2 proteins

Using the DiANNA disulphide prediction software (Ferre and Clote, 2005a; Ferre and Clote, 2005b; Ferre and Clote, 2006) the amino acid sequences of oE2-S and E2-T1/oE2+S were analysed to determine the cysteines likely to be involved in disulphide bond formation (Table 3).

oE2-S		E2-T1/oE2+S	
Position	**Cysteine residues and flanking amino acids**	**Position**	**Cysteine residues and flanking amino acids**
26 - 248	SMVDPCKPDFS – YPIGKCKLENE	124 - 288	GMVDPCKPDFS – PHRQNCVTQKT
70 - 227	TVVVWCKDGQF – GHIESCKWCGY	168 - 260	TVVVWCKDGQF – TGSVSCMLANK
81 - 203	TFMRRCAREAR – EDLYNCALGGN	179 - 301	TFMRRCAREAR – EDLYNCALGGN
128 - 279	FGLCPCDARPV – QGRVKCKIGDT	224 - 346	FEFGLCPCDAR – YPIGKCKLENE
152 - 317	AFQMVCPIGWT – VEKTACTFNYT	226 - 377	FGLCPCDARPV – QGRVKCKIGDT
162 - 190	TGSVSCMLANK – PHRQNCVTQKT	250 - 325	AFQMVCPIGWT – GHIESCKWCGY
211 - 230	GGNWTCVVGEQ – ESCKWCGYRFL	328 - 398	ESCKWCGYRFL – LGPMPCRPHDI
264 - 300	LDDTSCNRDGV – LGPMPCRPHDI	362 - 415	LDDTSCNRDGV – VEKTACTFNYT

Table 3: DiANNA disulphide bond predictions of oE2-S and E2-T1/oE2+S proteins.

```
                                                                              100
E2#    ATGGGCAGCAGCCATCATCATCATCATCACGGCAGCGGCCTGGTGCCGCGCGGCAGCGCTAGCATGTCGGACTCAGAAGTCAATCAAGAAGCTAAGCCAG
        M  G  S  S  H  H  H  H  H  H  G  S  G  L  V  P  R  G  S  A  S  M  S  D  S  E  V  N  Q  E  A  K  P

                                                                              200
E2#    AGGTCAAGCCAGAAGTCAAGCCTGAGACTCACATCAATTTAAAGGTGTCCGATGGATCTTCAGAGATCTTCTTCAAGATCAAAAAGACCACTCCTTTAAG
        E  V  K  P  E  V  K  P  E  T  H  I  N  L  K  V  S  D  G  S  S  E  I  F  F  K  I  K  K  T  T  P  L  R

                                                                              300
E2#    AAGGCTGATGGAAGCGTTCGCTAAAAGACAGGGTAAGGAAATGGACTCCTTAAGATTCTTGTACGACGGTATTAGAATTCAAGCTGATCAGACCCCTGAA
        R  L  M  E  A  F  A  K  R  Q  G  K  E  M  D  S  L  R  F  L  Y  D  G  I  R  I  Q  A  D  Q  T  P  E

                                                                              400
E2-MD74                                                       GTGGATCCGTGCAAGCCTGACTTCTCCTACGCAATCGCGA
E2-T1/74  GATTTGGACATGGAGGATAACGATATTATTGAGGCTCACAGAGAACAGATTGGTGGTATG---------------------------------------
oE2+/-S   ------------------------------------------------------------C----T--A------------------T--T--A
           D  L  D  M  E  D  N  D  I  I  E  A  H  R  E  Q  I  G  G  M  V  D  P  C  K  P  D  F  S  Y  A  I  A

                                                                              500
E2-T1/74  AGGACGAGAAGATCGGCCTACTAGGTGCTGAGAGCCTGACCACCTTCTGGAAAGACTACTCACCCGGAATGCGGTTGGAGGACGCGACGGTCGTAGTCTG
oE2+/-S   -A-----A--A---------G--G--C------ATCA-----G--G--T---------T--TAGC-----T-----TC-----A-----A--C--G--T
           K  D  E  K  I  G  L  L  G  A  E  S  L  T  T  F  W  K  D  Y  S  P  G  M  R  L  E  D  A  T  V  V  W

                                                                              600
E2-T1/74  GTGCAAGGACGGCCAGTTTACGTTCATGCGCAGGTGCGCGCGCGAGGCCCGATACCTGGCCATCTTGCACACCCGCGCCCTCCCGACCTCTGCGGTGTTC
oE2+/-S   ------A--T----------C---------TC-C--T-----T--A-----C---------T--TC----T-----T--A--G-----------T--T--T
           C  K  D  G  Q  F  T  F  M  R  R  C  A  R  E  A  R  Y  L  A  I  L  H  T  R  A  L  P  T  S  A  V  F

                                                                              700
E2-T1/74  AAAAAACTGTTTGATGGACAGAGGCAGGAGGACATCGTGGAGATGGGAGACGACTTTGAGTTCGGACTGTGCCCATGCGACGCCAGGCCCGTGATCCGCG
oE2+/-S   -----------C-----C---C--C-A--A----T-----A-----C--T-------A-----T-------G--T--T-AC-T--G--T------
           K  K  L  F  D  G  Q  R  Q  E  D  I  V  E  M  G  D  D  F  E  F  G  L  C  P  C  D  A  R  P  V  I  R

                                                                              800
E2-T1/74  GGAAGTTCAACACCACGCTGCTAAACGGGCCAGCCTTCCAGATGGTGTGCCCCATCGGATGGACGGGGTCTGTCAGCTGCATGCTGGCTAACAAAGACAT
oE2+/-S   -T--A--T--------------C----T--C--G-----C--------------C-----G--T--C-----C--T-----GTC---T--------G-----T-
           G  K  F  N  T  T  L  L  N  G  P  A  F  Q  M  V  C  P  I  G  W  T  G  S  V  S  C  M  L  A  N  K  D  I

                                                                              900
E2-T1/74  CCTGGACACCACTACGGTGCAGACCTACAGGAGGGCCAAGCCATTCCCTCACCGCCAGAACTGCGTCACCCAGAAAACTGTGGGGGAAGACCTCTACAAC
oE2+/-S   ------------G--C----------TC-TC--C-----A--G--T--G-----T-----T------G--G--A-----C--T--T----T--G--T--
           L  D  T  T  T  V  Q  T  Y  R  R  A  K  P  F  P  H  R  Q  N  C  V  T  Q  K  T  V  G  E  D  L  Y  N

                                                                              1000
E2-T1/74  TGCGCCCTGGGAGGAAACTGGACATGCGTAGTGGGGGAGCAGCTACAATACACGGGGGGCCACATCGAGTCATGCAAGTGGTGCGGTTACAGGTTCCTCA
oE2+/-S   -----G-----C--T--T-----G--T--G--T--C--A-----G--------C--C--T--T--T--T--A-------A-----T-----TC-C-----G-
           C  A  L  G  G  N  W  T  C  V  V  G  E  Q  L  Q  Y  T  G  G  H  I  E  S  C  K  W  C  G  Y  R  F  L

                                                                              1100
E2-T1/74  AGGGTGAGGGATTGCCACATTACCCGATTGGCAAGTGCAAGCTAGAGAACGAGACTGGCTACAGGTTACTGGATGACACTTCTTGCAACAGGGACGGCGT
oE2+/-S   -A--C--A--TC-----G-----------C--T--A--T-A--G--A-----A--G-----C-TC-G----------C--G-----TC-T--T--T-
           K  G  E  G  L  P  H  Y  P  I  G  K  C  K  L  E  N  E  T  G  Y  R  L  L  D  D  T  S  C  N  R  D  G  V

                                                                              1200
E2-T1/74  GGCCCATAGTACCACAGGGGCGGGTGAAATGCAAAATCGGCGATACAGTCGTGCAGGTCATCGCTATGGACACCAAACTCGGGCCTATGCCTTGCCGACCA
oE2+/-S   T-----T--C--G-----T--T--T-----T-----T-----C--G--------A--------T--------G--T--G-----G-----T--G
           A  I  V  F  Q  G  R  V  K  C  K  I  G  D  T  V  V  Q  V  I  A  M  D  T  K  L  G  F  M  P  C  R  P

                                                                              1300
E2-T1/74  CACGACATCATCTCTCAAGTGAGGGGCCTGTGGGAGAAGACGGCATGCACCTTCAACTACACCAGGACGTTGAAGAACAAATACTTTGAGCCCAGAGACAGTT
oE2+/-S   --T--T--T---AGCTC---A--C--G-----A--A-----C--T-----T-----T-----T--GC-T--CC----A--T--------C--A--GC-C---TCC-
           H  D  I  I  S  S  E  G  P  V  E  K  T  A  C  T  F  N  Y  T  R  T  L  K  N  K  Y  F  E  P  R  D  S

                                                                              1400
E2-MD74  TCTTCCAGCAATACATGCTAAAAGGAGAGTACCAATACTGGTTTGACCTCGAGGTCACGGACCACCACCGGGACTACTTCGCCGAGTCTATCTTGGTGAT
E2-T1                                                                                              TAG
oE2+S    -T-----------T-----G--G--T--A--T-G------------T-G--A--T----------T--T-----T-----A--A--CTAG
          F  F  Q  Q  Y  M  L  K  G  E  Y  Q  Y  W  F  D  L  E  V  T  D  H  H  R  D  Y  F  A  E  S  I  L  V  I
oE2-S    -T-----------T-----G--G--T--A--T-G------------T-G--A--T----------T--T-----T-----A--A--CCATCATCATCA
          F  F  Q  Q  Y  M  L  K  G  E  Y  Q  Y  W  F  D  L  E  V  T  D  H  H  R  D  Y  F  A  E  S  H  H  H  H

                                                                              1480
E2-MD74  CGTGGTGGTCCTACTGGGGGGGCCGCTACGTGCTATGGTTGCTGGTCACCTACATCATCTTGTCAGAACAAAGAGCCTCGGGG
          V  V  V  L  L  G  G  R  Y  V  L  W  L  L  V  T  Y  I  I  L  S  E  Q  R  A  S  G
oE2-S    TCATCATTGA
          H  H  *
```

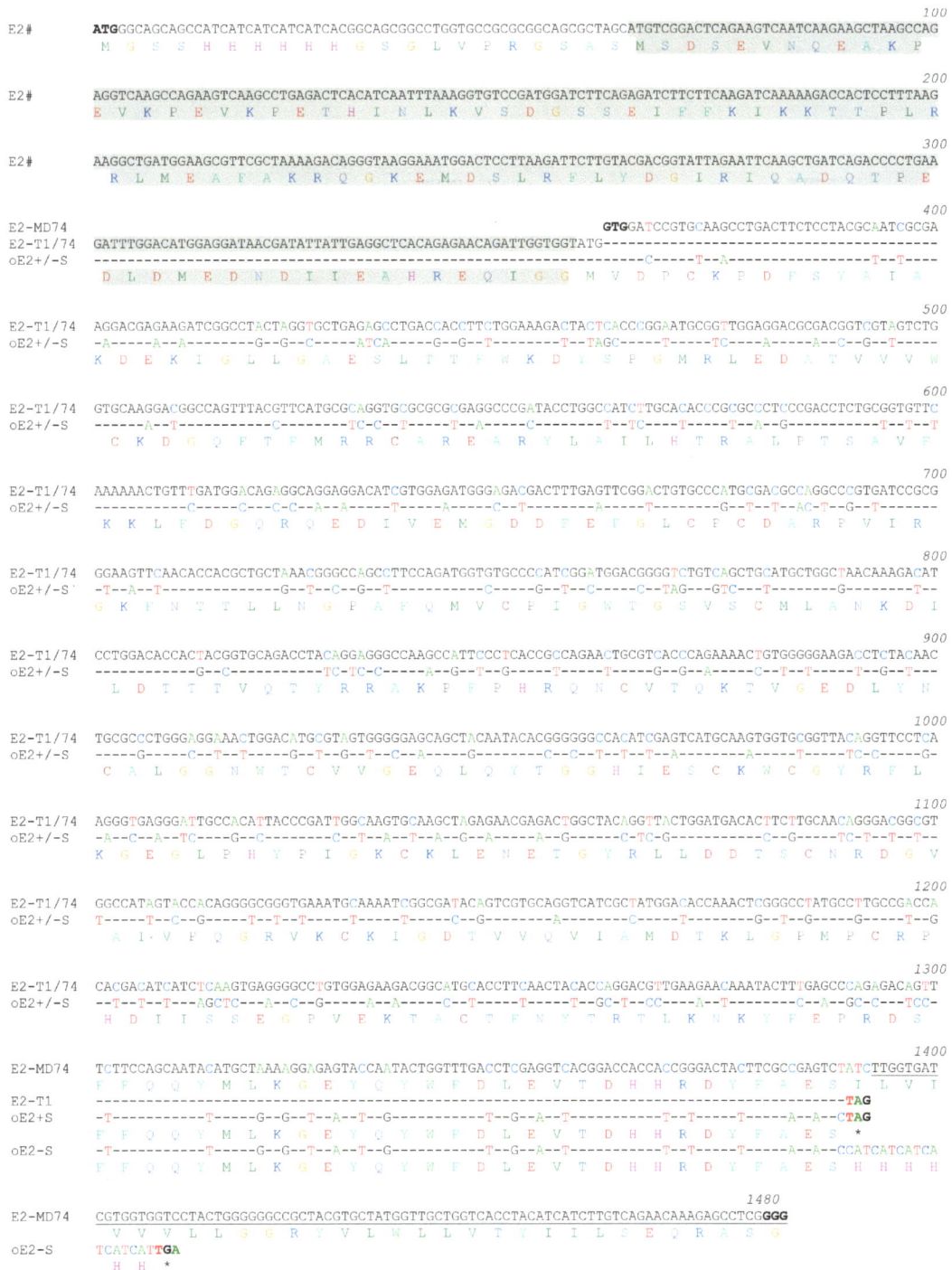

Figure 2: The nucleic acid and derived amino acid sequences of E2-MD74, E2-T1, oE2+S and oE2-S. E2-T1 and E2-MD74 are identical except for the 3' membrane binding domain which is underlined. E2-MD74 is expressed as part of the BVDV polyprotein, DNA encoding E2-MD74 commences with GTG (position 361) and concludes with GGG (position 1482) and is shown in bold. The start and stop codons of the expression constructs are in bold. The three bacterial expression constructs all contain a leader sequence; these sequences are referred to as E2# across the identical alignment, E2-T1 and oE2+S have a full length SUMO leader sequence. The *Nhe*I fragment of the SUMO leader sequence has been removed from oE2-S and is shaded. Optimised constructs are referred to as oE2+/-S across identical sequences.

Pilot expression studies carried out in BL21 (DE3) cells showed maximum protein expression (at 37°C) occurred 2 and 4 hours post induction with 1 mM IPTG for E2-T1 and oE2+S/-S respectively. The majority of the expressed proteins are contained in the insoluble fraction as inclusion bodies (Figure 3).

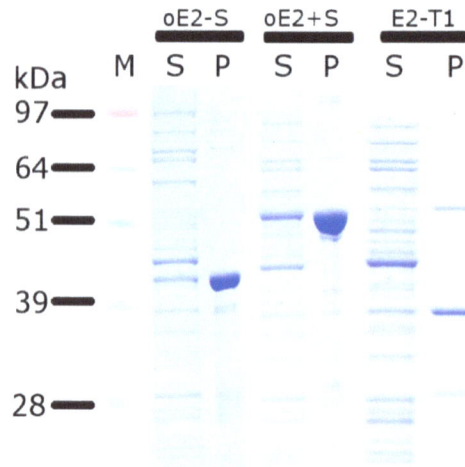

Figure 3: Pilot expression of E2 proteins at 4 hr; oE2-S, oE2+S and 2 hr; E2-T1. Crude extracts were sampled and separated into supernatant (S) and pellet (P).

3.2   Purification and Refolding

Optimisation of the purification and solubilisation system was initially performed with E2-T1 protein. Purification of E2-T1 from the soluble fraction was attempted using TALON resin. A step gradient of imidazole (50, 80, 100 and 150 mM) was used to determine the optimum elution profile. At 150 mM imidazole, E2-T1 was the major species eluted from the column. Although this protein was of high purity, the resultant yields were low (10 ng/L, data not shown).

The E2-T1 protein contained within the insoluble fraction was processed using BugBuster[TM] to produce highly pure E2-T1 protein. The E2-T1 protein was solubilised in a DTT-SDS buffer (50 mM Tris (pH6.8), 100 mM DTT, 1% SDS, 10% Glycerol). The volume of the re-solubilisation buffer was adjusted to ensure complete solubilisation, this volume ranged from 1-6 mL for E2-T1 and oE2-S/+S respectively. Refolding of E2-T1 protein was achieved by dialysis into 50 mM Tris (pH 7.0), 0.2% Igepal CA630 at room temperature. Refolded E2-T1 protein could be digested by SUMO protease resulting in removal of the SUMO tag (data not shown).

The codon optimised proteins (oE2-S & oE2+S), which were also expressed as predominantly insoluble proteins, were purified following the same procedure and also resulted in highly pure proteins. The expression yield of the oE2-S and oE2+S proteins was 100-150 mg/L of culture compared to 1-2 mg/L for E2-T1 (Figure 4). The relative purity of the predominant protein bands detected by Western blot hybridisation, were determined by densitometry to be 87, 93 and 82% for oE2-S, oE2+S and E2-T1 respectively.

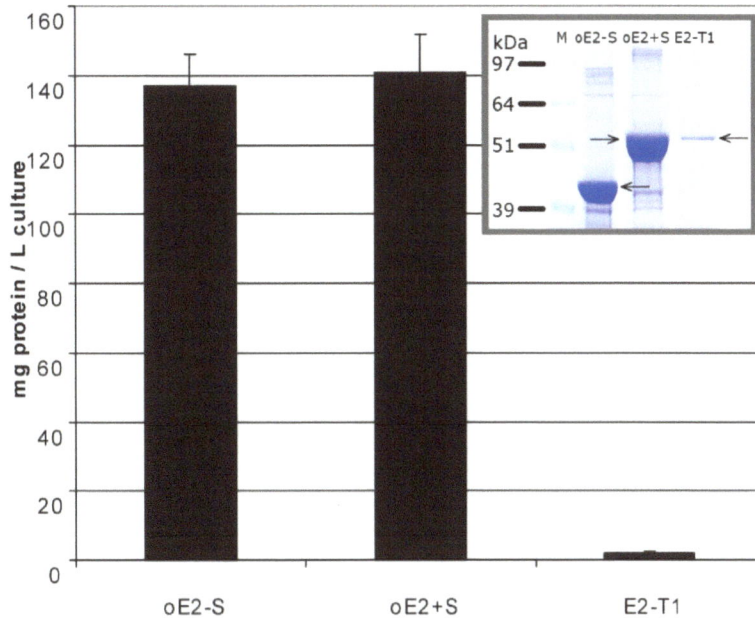

Figure 4: Expression levels of E2 proteins. Purified E2 proteins were analysed by protein assay and by PAGE (insert). Insert: M: SeeBlue® Plus2 MW standards, oE2-S, oE2+S, E2-T1.

3.3   Endotoxin Removal

Endotoxin assays measured by Limulus Amoebocyte Lysate (LAL) assay revealed levels ranging from 5.29 to 714.39 EU/mL (Table 4) for untreated batches of E2 proteins. Treatment by phase separation using Triton X-114 on the insoluble IB pellets resulted in 3 phases: an aqueous phase, a detergent phase and the IB pellet fraction. Analysis of all three phases by SDS-PAGE showed that the protein was retained in the IB pellet with no loss of protein in the aqueous or oil phases (Figure 5). The resulting Triton X-114 treated protein samples had greatly reduced endotoxin levels below 3 EU/mL (Table 4). Due to the validation methods used for the LAL test, an absolute reading below this minimal threshold value could not be determined. Proteins to be used in immunisation studies in mice should ideally have a level of < 3 EU/mL (Fifis *et al.*, 2004; Scheerlinck *et al.*, 2006) therefore this integrated method of endotoxin removal from the IB pellets was an efficient method of producing protein suitable for small animal studies.

3.4   Physical Properties

On purification and solubilisation, the resultant E2 proteins exhibit high stability, resisting both degradation and aggregation for up to 1 year at room temperature. The resistance to aggregation can be examined by zeta potential (ZP). ZP is indicative of the potential stability of a colloidal system; high absolute values indicate the capacity of the proteins to remain in solution. The ZP of the E2 proteins and the widely used ovalbumin (OVA; for comparison) are shown in Table 5.

Sample ID	Protein Concentration (ng/µL)	Endotoxin Level (EU/mL)
E2-T1 #1	200.80	110.32
E2-T1 #2	279.15	199.31
E2-T1 #3	265.32	29.91
E2-T1 #4	92.50	5.29
E2-T1 #6b *	113.34	< 3
E2-T1 #7b *	138.88	< 3
oE2-S #1	1496.00	714.39
oE2-S #2	1303.00	139.87
oE2-S #3 *	884.00	< 3
oE2-S #4 *	1018.00	< 3

Table 4: Purified protein concentrations and endotoxin levels. Triton X-114 treated samples are denoted with *.

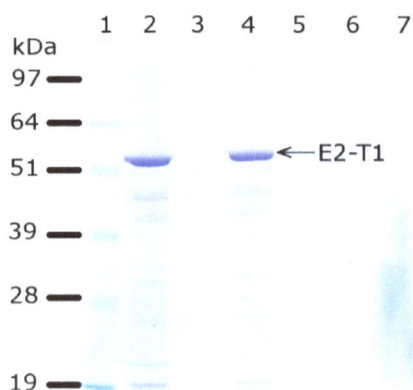

Figure 5: Protein fractions following endotoxin removal from E2-T1 IB by Triton X-114 extraction were separated by electrophoresis on 10% Bis-Tris gel and stained with Coomassie blue. Lane 1, SeeBlue® Plus2 MW standards; lane 2, IB pellets resuspended in PBS before Triton X-114 treatment; lane 3, aqueous layer post Triton X-114 treatment; lane 4, recovered IB pellet post Triton X-114 treatment; lane 5, Triton TX-114 layer.

Protein	Buffer	Zeta Potential (mV)
oE2-S	T-I	-25.7
oE2-S	PBS	-21.1
oE2+S	T-I	-16.45
E2-T1	T-I	-14.4
OVA	T-I	-4.5
OVA	PBS	-3.6

Table 5: Zeta potentials measurements of E2 proteins and OVA in 50 mM Tris (pH7.0), 0.2% Igepal CA630 (T-I) and PBS.

Although oE2+S and E2-T1 are identical polypeptides, they exhibit different zeta potentials. Further analysis of these proteins was performed by DLS to show size distribution. Size by intensity reflects relative intensity of each species, while size by mass (or volume) indicates actual percentages of each species. To determine the physical size of the proteins the data was analysed by the Zetasizer software. E2-T1 exhibits 3 distinct peaks; 10.7, 39.1 and 163.7 nm, the first peak of 10.72 nm accounts for 91.1% by mass, however oE2+S shows 2 major peaks; 15.5 and 62.0 nm accounting for 62.3% and 37.7% respectively (Figure 6A). oE2-S exhibits a peak at 7.1 nm, 100% by mass and a peak at 260.0 nm which does not account for a significant mass (Figure 6B).

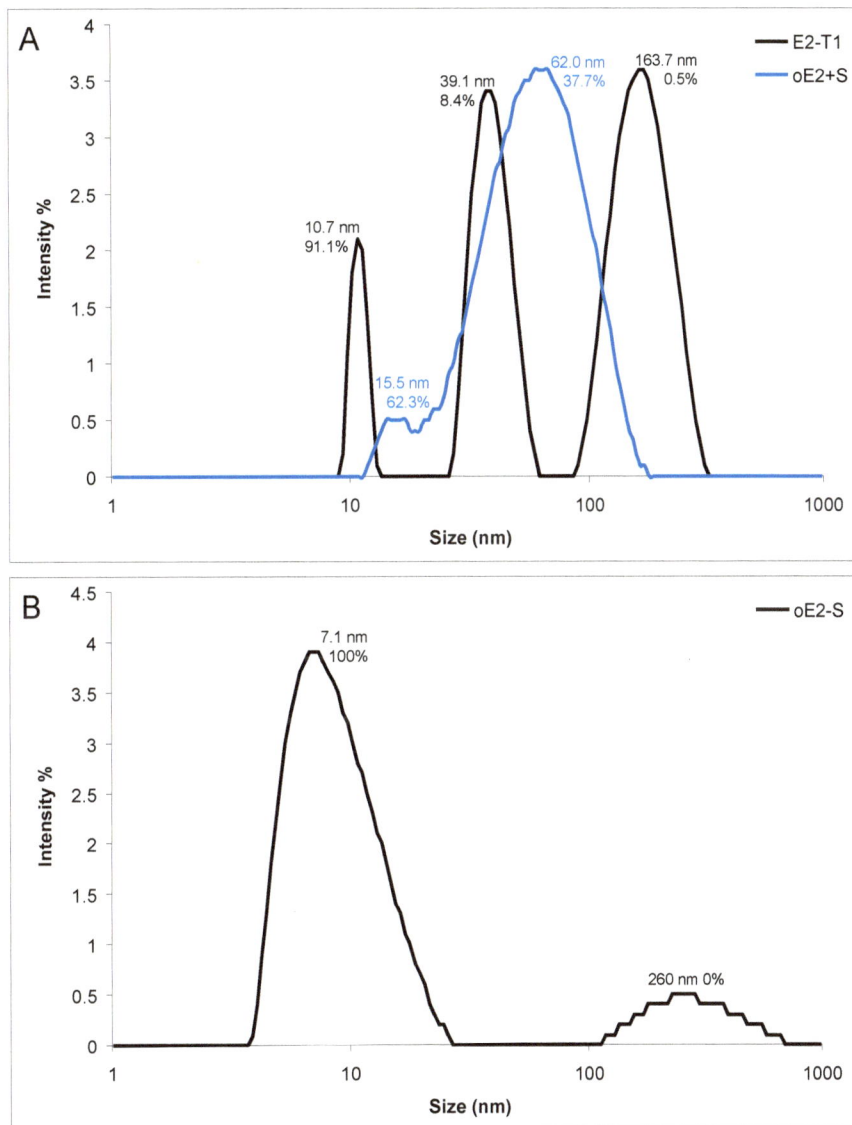

Figure 6: DLS analysis of E2 proteins. Data processing was performed for protein analysis. Diameter was determined by intensity as shown by the plots and by mass, as indicated by the percentages of the proteins at the indicated sizes. A: Comparison of the identical amino acid sequence proteins oE2+S and E2-T1. B: The optimised protein lacking the SUMO oE2-S.

DLS analyses of the proteins give the polydispersity index (PdI) of particles in solution which is an indication of the level of homogeneity of the particles. Higher values indicate a higher distribution of particle sizes and in the case of proteins the presence of aggregates. The PdI values of the E2 proteins are shown in Table 6, indicating oE2+S had the lowest amount of aggregation (PdI of 0.211), and E2-T1 the highest amount of aggregation (PdI of 0.501). From the graph it appeared that oE2-S exhibits the most consistent size.

Sample	Buffer	PdI
E2-T1	T-I	0.501
oE2-S	T-I	0.309
oE2-S	PBS	0.263
oE2+S	T-I	0.211

Table 6: DLS analysis of E2 proteins to determine Polydispersity index (PdI). Proteins solubilised in 50 mM Tris (pH7.0), 0.2% Igepal CA630 (T-I) or PBS.

3.5   Immune Responses

Western blot hybridisation analyses showed all three variants of solubilised E2 protein were recognised by both polyclonal and monoclonal E2-specific antisera. E2-T1, oE2-S and oE2+S proteins were recognised by antibodies raised against BVDV in sheep (804) as well as the BVDV-E2 monoclonal antibodies, mAb-157 and mAb-348 (Figure 7A). Sera raised in mice against E2-T1 (M1) detected both oE2-S and oE2+S. Sera raised against oE2-S in sheep, detected both oE2+S and E2-T1 (Figure 7B).

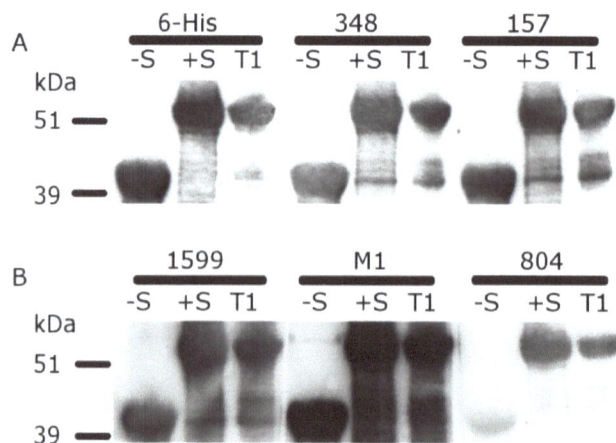

Figure 7: Western blot of E2 proteins. Equivalent amounts of protein (10 µg) were transferred to Hybond C membrane and visualised by ECL. Proteins: –S, oE2-S; +S, oE2+S, T1, E2-T1. Membrane probed with Anti 6-His, VMRD 348 mAb, VMRD 157 mAb, Sheep Sera 1599, Mouse Sera M1 & Sheep Sera 804.

Analysis of E2 as a potential subunit vaccine was conducted by comparison of the immune response to E2-T1 and oE2-S in mice. Mice were immunised with 50 µg of purified E2-T1 or oE2-S in combination with 10 μg of QuilA, subcutaneously in the tail base at 2 week intervals. The immune response was titrated to detect both humoral immunity by ELISA and cell-mediated immunity by ELISPOT.

ELISA assays conducted with mice sera from both oE2-S and E2-T1 immunised animals showed a good response after 2 injections with similar results seen in the response to both proteins with an antibody titre of greater than 10^4 observed. The response for E2-T1 is similar to the response seen in the preliminary trial (Cavallaro *et al.*, 2011). The final bleeds taken 2 weeks following the final vaccination also show no significant differences (Student's T-Test, $p < 0.1$) between oE2-S and E2-T1 (Figure 8).

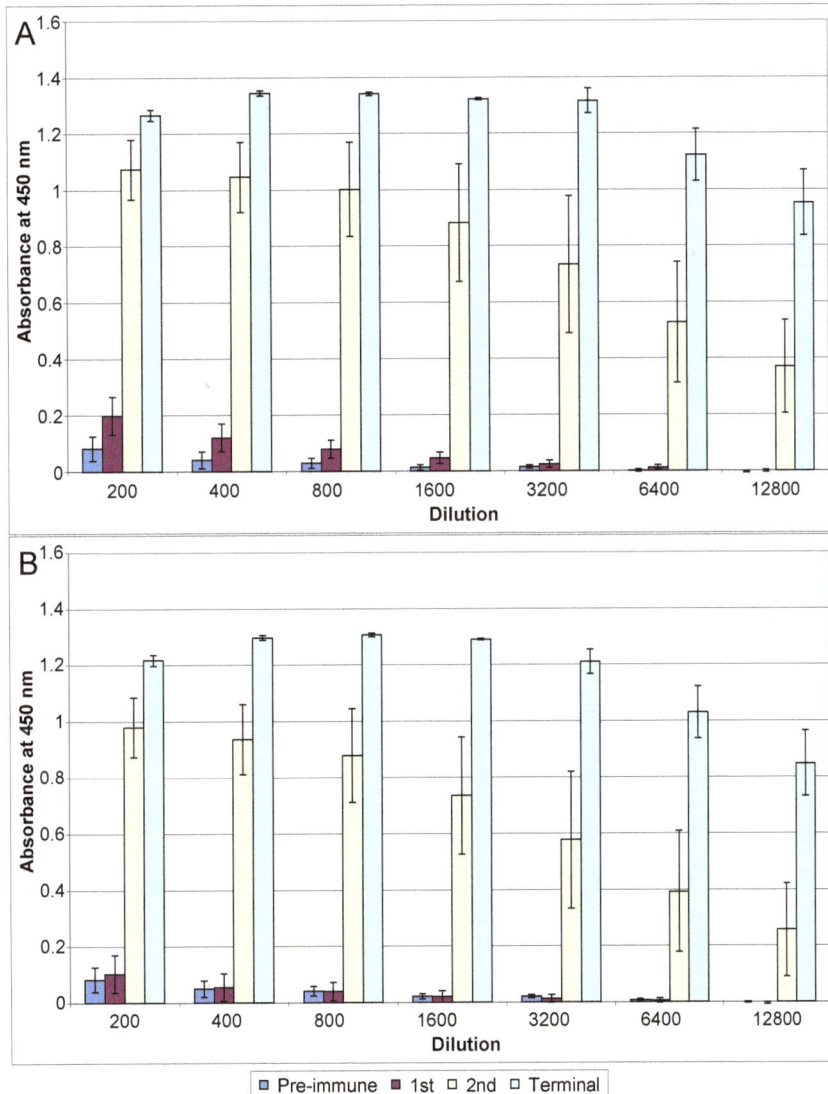

Figure 8: A. ELISA analysis of mice receiving three injections of oE2-S (A) or E2-T1 (B). Mice (n = 4) were injected with 50 μg oE2-S or E2-T1 with the addition of 10 μg QuilA at 2 week intervals. ELISA assays were performed using pre-immune sera and sera obtained two weeks following each injection, termed 1st, 2nd and terminal samples.

Splenocyte cell populations were used in CD8+ T cell interferon-γ ELISPOT assays to determine if there was a T-helper type 1 (Th1) cell-mediated immune response two weeks after the final immunisation. A very high cell-mediated response was seen for both oE2-S and E2-T1 compared to the unimmunised group (Figure 9). No reliable quantification was determined as the immune response exceeds the threshold for the detection software, as shown in Figure 9; the stimulated wells mainly show a continuous colour with few individual spots that can be detected. It is clear, however that a high response is present in the stimulated cells.

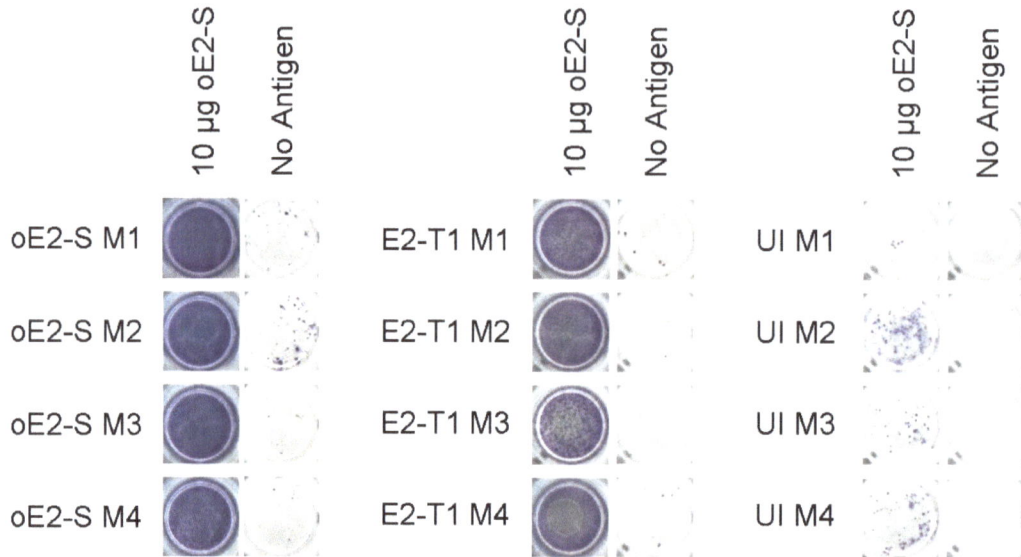

Figure 9: Response detected from antigen specific IFN-γ secretion by ELISPOT assay of murine splenocytes from oE2+QuilA and E2-T1+QuilA immunised mice and from unimmunised (UI) control mice. Splenocytes were stimulated *in vitro* with the oE2-S (10 μg) compared to unstimulated cells.

4   Discussion

We have previously shown the advantages of IB in facilitating efficient protein purification from *E. coli* (Cavallaro *et al.*, 2011). In the current study the yield of BVDV-E2 protein has been substantially increased by optimising the codon usage of the E2 open reading frame for *E. coli* expression to make the system more amenable for animal vaccine development. As cost is a major factor in the adoption of veterinary vaccines increasing the yield of the primary antigen yield is one way of making downstream processing such as endotoxin removal and protein refolding economically viable. By utilising codon optimisation we have increased the expression of E2 protein in *E. coli* 75-100 fold. The increase in yield reduces production cost, an important factor development of a subunit animal vaccine.

In vivo refolding studies of purified E2 have shown that intramolecular disulphide bonds form rapidly within 2.5 minutes and intermolecular disulfide bonds result in formation of E2 dimers (Branza-Nichita *et al.*, 2001). Since disulphide bonds are inefficiently formed in the reducing environment of the *E. coli* cytosol (Brondyk, 2009) and native E2 rapidly forms intramolecular disulphide bonds, misfolding of the nascent E2 polypeptides are likely to form an insoluble protein. Also, formation of intermolecular disulphide bonds within E2 proteins in the *E. coli* cytosol would lead to the formation of aggregates resulting in IB. In our study consistent and reproducible solubilisation of all E2 proteins was only achievable using a highly reducing buffer containing 100 mM DTT. The inclusion of DTT as a reducing agent in the re-suspension buffer would disrupt incorrectly formed disulphide bonds, and then during dialysis into DTT-free buffer, the disulphide bonds could reform in a confirmation that is more suitable for soluble protein.

Our analysis using the DiANNA disulphide prediction software indicates the formation of 8 disulphide bonds utilising 16 of the 17 cysteine amino acid residues present in E2 (Table 2). This hypothetical modelling, of course does not take into account any E2-E2 disulphide bonds that may form *in vitro* or E1-E2 and E2-E2 bonding *in vivo*. The presence of soluble aggregates in the final preparations of the E2 proteins also indicates that there may be disulphide bond formation between E2 molecules.

We had previously found refolding of E2-T1 to be successful in Tris based buffers, and the addition of the detergent Igepal CA630 (0.2%) was required to reduce aggregation. The PdI for E2-T1 which was refolded in Tris Buffer alone was 0.931 with of a lower value of PdI of 0.528 after the addition of the detergent (Cavallaro *et al.*, 2011). New analysis of the E2-T1 protein in 50 mM Tris, 0.2% Ipgepal CA630 shows the PdI to be 0.501. The optimised constructs were also dialysed with the addition of 0.2% Igepal CA630 to the Tris buffer and exhibited lower PdI values (0.263 and 0.211 for oE2-S and oE2+S respectively, Table 6) than that of E2-T1 (0.501, Table 6). Although the PdI values of oE2-S and oE2+S were lower than E2-T1, there was still some aggregation of the soluble proteins. The soluble aggregation could be due in part to the same intermolecular disulphide bond formation reported for native E2.

To utilise oE2-S as a stimulant in the ELISPOT assay, a solution of protein was required to be prepared in PBS. Previous attempts to dialyse soluble E2 proteins from 50 mM Tris, 0.2% Igepal CA630 to PBS were unsuccessful (data not shown), however dialysis of DTT solubilised protein was successful and the resultant protein displayed a comparative PdI value of 0.263 (Table 6) to oE2-S in Tris buffer (0.309). Interestingly, while E2 protein was soluble at room temperature and was successfully used as an antigen in the ELISPOT assay, it was found to form precipitates when stored at temperatures 4 °C and below. ZP measurements give an indication of the aggregation within a colloidal system. Absolute values above 30 are considered to be stable insofar that they will not form insoluble aggregates. The ZP of oE2-S in PBS is -21.1 mV as compared to -25.7 mV for oE2-S in 50 mM Tris, 0.2 Igepal CA630, which may account for why oE2-S in 50 mM Tris, 0.2 Igepal CA630 exhibits higher storage stability. We have found that oE2-S in PBS (directly after room temperature dialysis) remains soluble and stable at room temperature for periods > 1 year but not at lower temperatures of 4 and -20 °C. This indicates that E2 protein is sensitive to both buffer and temperature variations.

E2-T1 and oE2+S are identical polypeptides; however as proteins they exhibit different physical properties. Although the ZP values for both proteins were similar, E2-T1 (ZP of -14.4) and oE2+S (ZP of -16.45) (Table 5), the size distribution of E2-T1 and oE2+S were radically different. E2-T1 showed 3 distinct peaks, while oE2+S only exhibited 2 distinct peaks. By mass the majority of E2-T1 was 10.71 nm (91.1%), while oE2+S was found to be 15.5 nm (62.3%) and at 62 nm (37.7%). One explanation could be that the higher level of expression of oE2+S ultimately resulted in misfolded protein. It has been shown that rapid translation can affect protein folding and lead to proteins such as enzymes becoming inactive (Komar *et al.*, 1999). The difference in physical properties may also be related to the concentrations of the proteins obtained after purification and refolding, whereas oE2+S concentrations were usually 1.5 – 2 mg/mL, E2-T1 was much lower at 0.3 – 0.8 mg/mL.

Codon optimisation may result in high expression of proteins in *E. coli*, which can lead to a high stress situation where the proteins form insoluble IB (Cortazzo *et al.*, 2002; Sorensen and Mortensen, 2005). With the BVDV E2 proteins even relatively low level expression (1 mg/L culture) was found to lead to IB formation. By increasing the expression of E2 through utilising codon optimised constructs the protein yield increased and the protein remained insoluble. Both optimised constructs exhibit 60-75 fold increase in expressed protein yield. The absence of the 13 kDa SUMO tag did not affect the expression level. As E2-T1 and oE2+S have identical amino acid sequences, this indicates that the yield increase is due to the codon optimisation and no increase in expression can be attributed to the removal of the SU-MO tag.

Proteins expressed in *E. coli* systems are inherently contaminated with endotoxins. Endotoxin levels lower than 3 EU/mL of *E. coli* derived proteins have been reported to be safe, causing no adverse reactions in animal trials (Fifis *et al.*, 2004; Scheerlinck *et al.*, 2006). Six separate purified E2 samples from *E. coli* showed a range of endotoxin levels of 5.29, 29.91, 110.31, 139.87, 199.31 and 714.39 EU/mL (Table 4). These levels are considered unsuitable for testing E2 proteins in mice as a daily dose of 100 μL at 1.5 EU/mL has been determined to be safe (Malyala and Singh, 2008).

Commercially available techniques for endotoxin removal typically employ affinity columns and require buffer changes for washing and elution of the protein. Attempts to use ion exchange chromatography were discontinued due to consistently low recovery of E2-T1. We introduced a significantly innovative step for endotoxin removal from the *E. coli* IB by adding a Triton X-114 extraction step to the purification protocol prior to solubilisation and recovery of the target protein. Phase separation with Triton X-114 resulted in up to 600 fold reduction in the endotoxin levels of the E2-T1 preparations (Table 4). Likewise samples of oE2-S treated with Triton X-114 during the purification process, also resulted in reduction of endotoxin to <3 EU/ml. Importantly, using this method resulted in no detectable protein loss (Figure 5), as E2 proteins remained insoluble within the IB. This approach could be generally applicable for the efficient removal of endotoxins from other proteins expressed as predominantly IB preparations, by maintaining the IB in a buffer incompatible with the solubilisation of the target protein, while still facilitating endotoxin removal with Triton X-114.

We have shown that E2 proteins produced in *E. coli* were recognised by sheep sera (sample 804) and also by two BVDV-specific monoclonal antibodies 348 and 157 (Figure 7) indicating the usefulness of these E2 proteins for diagnostic applications such as monitoring the serological status of animals which are the natural host of BVDV. Sera raised against E2-T1 in mice detected the optimised proteins, oE2-S and oE2+S. Similarly sera from sheep immunised with oE2-S successfully detects E2-T1 and oE2+S. These results demonstrated that all three E2 protein variants are immunologically similar.

An important characteristic for a subunit vaccine is its ability to induce an immune response in animals. We have previously shown E2-T1 immunisation resulted in a significant humoral immune response in mice (Cavallaro *et al.*, 2011) . A comparable humoral immune response was seen when animals were immunised with oE2-S. A comparison between E2-T1 and oE2-S showed both proteins exhibit similar immune responses with titres exceeding 10^4. Statistical analysis of the responses using the Student's T-Test ($p < 0.1$) showed no significant differences in the immune responses. In addition to the humoral response, cell-mediated immunity was examined using a CD8+ T cell interferon-γ ELISPOT assays. As shown in Figure 9, a high response was observed in the stimulated cells for both E2-T1 and oE2-S, which exceeds 1600 SFU/million cells, a level which could not be accurately quantified as the spot density exceeds the threshold for the analysis software. By comparison the unstimulated cells exhibited levels of 4 – 200 SFU/million cells. Together these results demonstrated that the bacterially derived E2 proteins solubilised from IB can induce an excellent humoral and cell-mediated response in small animals, a highly advantageous attribute for a potential subunit vaccine.

5   Conclusion

The development of cost effective veterinary vaccines and diagnostics requires the use of efficient methods that enable the production of large quantities of immunogenic and non-toxic proteins. We have demonstrated that the level of protein production can be increased 60-75 fold through optimisation of the codon usage of the gene of interest to reflect that of *E. coli*. Utilising our previous expertise in exploiting the formation of IB for the purification and solubilisation of E2-T1, we have successfully expressed a higher yielding construct (oE2-S) utilising the elegant solution for endotoxin removal using Triton X-114 two-phase extraction. The optimised oE2-S, lacking the SUMO tag was shown to be highly immunogenic in mice giving both humoral and cell-mediated responses, comparable to the native codon usage E2-T1. The optimised oE2-S shows many advantages in yield and immunogenicity and is a giant step forward in the development of *E. coli* expressed E2 as a potential subunit vaccine candidate.

References

Adam, O., A. Vercellone, et al. (1995). *A Nondegradative Route for the Removal of Endotoxin from Exopolysaccharides. Analytical Biochemistry 225(2): 321-327.*

Aida, Y. and M. J. Pabst (1990). *Removal of endotoxin from protein solutions by phase separation using Triton X-114. Journal of Immunological Methods 132: 191-195.*

Alvarez, M., J. M. Bielsa, et al. (2007). *Compatibility of a live infectious bovine rhinotraheitis (IBR) marker vaccine and an inactivated bovine viral diarrhoea virus (BVDV) vaccine. Vaccine 25(36): 6613-6617.*

Bauermann, F. V., E. F. Flores, et al. (2012). *Antigenic relationships between Bovine viral diarrhea virus 1 and 2 and HoBi virus: possible impacts on diagnosis and control. Journal of Veterinary Diagnostic Investigation 24(2): 253-261.*

Bolin, S. R. and J. F. Ridpath (1996). *Glycoprotein E2 of bovine viral diarrhea virus expressed in insect cells provides calves limited protection from systemic infection and disease. Archives of Virology 141(8): 1463-1477.*

Branza-Nichita, N., D. Durantel, et al. (2001). *Antiviral effect of N-butyldeoxynojirimycin against bovine viral diarrhea virus correlates with misfolding of E2 envelope proteins and impairment of their association into E1-E2 heterodimers. Journal of Virology 75(8): 3527-3536.*

Brondyk, W. H. (2009). *Selecting an Appropriate Method for Expressing a Recombinant Protein. Methods in Enzymology 463: 131-147.*

Callan, R. J. (2002). *Bovine Viral Diarrhea Virus Control and Eradication [cited 10/06/12]. Colorado, Colorado State University*

Cavallaro, A. S., D. Mahony, et al. (2011). *Endotoxin-free purification for the isolation of Bovine Viral Diarrhoea Virus E2 protein from insoluble inclusion body aggregates. Microb Cell Fact 10: 57.*

Chen, D. Q. and D. E. Texada (2006). *Low-usage codons and rare codons of Escherichia coli. Gene Therapy and Molecular Biology 10A: 1-12.*

Chia, S. C., P. S. C. Leung, et al. (2001). *Fragment of Japanese encephalitis virus envelope protein produced in Escherichia coli protects mice from virus challenge. Microbial Pathogenesis 31(1): 9-19.*

Ciulli, S., E. Galletti, et al. (2009). Analysis of variability and antigenic peptide prediction of E2 BVDV glycoprotein in a mucosal-disease affected animal. Veterinary Research Communications 33 Suppl 1: 125-127.

Corbett, E. M., D. L. Grooms, et al. (2011). Use of sentinel serology in a Bovine viral diarrhea virus eradication program. Journal of Veterinary Diagnostic Investigation 23(3): 511-515.

Cortazzo, P., C. Cervenansky, et al. (2002). Silent mutations affect in vivo protein folding in Escherichia coli. Biochemical and Biophysical Research Communications 293(1): 537-541.

Craig, M. I., A. Venzano, et al. (2008). Detection of bovine viral diarrhoea virus (BVDV) nucleic acid and antigen in different organs of water buffaloes (Bubalus bubalis). Res Vet Sci 85(1): 194-196.

Das, D., F. Jacobs, et al. (2007). Differential expression of the Ebola virus GP(1,2) protein and its fragments in E-coli. Protein Expression and Purification 54(1): 117-125.

Demain, A. L. and P. Vaishnav (2009). Production of recombinant proteins by microbes and higher organisms. Biotechnology Advances 27(3): 297-306.

Deregt, D., P. A. van Rijn, et al. (1998). Monoclonal antibodies to the E2 protein of a new genotype (type 2) of bovine viral diarrhea virus define three antigenic domains involved in neutralization. Virus Research 57(2): 171-181.

Divers, T. J. and S. F. Peek (2008). Rebuhn's Diseases of Dairy Cattle. St Louis,USA, Saunders Elsevier.

Donofrio, G., E. Bottarelli, et al. (2006). Expression of bovine viral diarrhea virus glycoprotein E2 as a soluble secreted form in a mammalian cell line. Clinical and Vaccine Immunology 13(6): 698-701.

Duff, G. C. and M. L. Galyean (2007). Board-invited review: recent advances in management of highly stressed, newly received feedlot cattle. Journal of Animal Science 85(3): 823-840.

Ferre, F. and P. Clote (2005a). DiANNA: a web server for disulfide connectivity prediction. Nucleic Acids Research 33(Web Server issue): W230-232.

Ferre, F. and P. Clote (2005b). Disulfide connectivity prediction using secondary structure information and diresidue frequencies. Bioinformatics 21(10): 2336-2346.

Ferre, F. and P. Clote (2006). DiANNA 1.1: an extension of the DiANNA web server for ternary cysteine classification. Nucleic Acids Research 34(Web Server issue): W182-185.

Ferrer, F., S. C. Zoth, et al. (2007). Induction of virus-neutralizing antibodies by immunization with Rachiplusia nu per os infected with a recombinant baculovirus expressing the E2 glycoprotein of bovine viral diarrhea virus. Journal of Virological Methods 146(1-2): 424-427.

Fifis, T., P. Mottram, et al. (2004). Short peptide sequences containing MHC class I and/or class II epitopes linked to nano-beads induce strong immunity and inhibition of growth of antigen-specific tumour challenge in mice. Vaccine 23(2): 258-266.

Garcia-Fruitos, E. (2010). Inclusion bodies: a new concept. Microbial Cell Factories 9.

Gard, J. A., M. D. Givens, et al. (2007). Bovine viral diarrhea virus (BVDV): Epidemiologic concerns relative to semen and embryos. Theriogenology 68(3): 434-442.

Hessman, B. E., R. W. Fulton, et al. (2009). Evaluation of economic effects and the health and performance of the general cattle population after exposure to cattle persistently infected with bovine viral diarrhea virus in a starter feedlot. American Journal of Veterinary Research 70(1): 73-85.

Houe, H. (1999). Epidemiological features and economical importance of bovine virus diarrhoea virus (BVDV) infections. Veterinary Microbiology 64(2-3): 89-107.

Howard, C. J., M. C. Clarke, et al. (1989). Protection against respiratory infection with bovine virus diarrhoea virus by passively acquired antibody. Veterinary Microbiology 19(3): 195-203.

Howard, C. J., M. C. Clarke, et al. (1994). Systemic vaccination with inactivated bovine virus diarrhoea virus protects against respiratory challenge. Veterinary Microbiology 42(2): 171-179.

Hurley, J. C. (1995). Endotoxemia - Methods of Detection and Clinical Correlates. Clinical Microbiology Reviews 8(2): 268-292.

Kane, J. F. and D. L. Hartley (1988). Formation of recombinant protein inclusion bodies in Escherichia coli. Trends in Biotechnology 6: 95-101.

Komar, A. A., T. Lesnik, et al. (1999). Synonymous codon substitutions affect ribosome traffic and protein folding during in vitro translation. FEBS Letters 462(3): 387-391.

Liu, S. G., R. Tobias, et al. (1997). Removal of endotoxin from recombinant protein preparations. Clinical Biochemistry 30(6): 455-463.

Mahony, T. J., F. M. McCarthy, et al. (2005). Genetic analysis of bovine viral diarrhoea viruses from Australia. Veterinary Microbiology 106(1-2): 1-6.

Makrides, S. C. (1996). Strategies for achieving high-level expression of genes in Escherichia coli. Microbiological Reviews 60(3): 512-538.

Malyala, P. and M. Singh (2008). Endotoxin limits in formulations for preclinical research. Journal of Pharmaceutical Sciences 97(6): 2041-2044.

Marzocca, M. P., C. Seki, et al. (2007). Truncated E2 of bovine viral diarrhea virus (BVDV) expressed in Drosophila melanogaster cells: A candidate antigen for a BVDV ELISA. Journal of Virological Methods 144(1-2): 49-56.

McGowan, M., P. Kirkland, et al. (2008). Guidelines for the investigation and control of BVDV (bovine viral diarrhea virus of bovine pestivirus) in beef and dairy herds and feedlots.   Retrieved 3/1/09, from http://bvdvaustralia.com/documents/BVDV-Guidelines-Edition-2-May-2008.pdf.

Merck.   Bovilis   BVD.   [cited   16.04.12].   from   http://www.msd-animal-health.co.uk/Products_Public/Bovilis_BVD/020_Product_Datasheet.aspx.

Nelson, G., P. Marconi, et al. (2012). Immunocompetent truncated E2 glycoprotein of bovine viral diarrhea virus (BVDV) expressed in Nicotiana tabacum plants: A candidate antigen for new generation of veterinary vaccines. Vaccine 30(30): 4499-4504.

Niskanen, R. and A. Lindberg (2003). Transmission of Bovine Viral Diarrhoea Virus by Unhygienic Vaccination Procedures, Ambient Air, and from Contaminated Pens. The Veterinary Journal 165(2): 125-130.

Novartis.   (2006).   Fundamentals   of   BVD.   [cited   10/07/12].   from http://www.livestock.novartis.com/pdf/FinalBVDReport.pdf.

Pande, A., B. V. Carr, et al. (2005). The glycosylation pattern of baculovirus expressed envelope protein E2 affects its ability to prevent infection with bovine viral diarrhoea virus. Virus Research 114(1-2): 54-62.

Patterson, R., J. Nerren, et al. (2012). Yeast-surface expressed BVDV E2 protein induces a Th1/Th2 response in naive T cells. Developmental & Comparative Immunology 37(1): 107-114.

Pecora, A., M. S. Aguirreburualde, et al. (2012). Safety and efficacy of an E2 glycoprotein subunit vaccine produced in mammalian cells to prevent experimental infection with bovine viral diarrhoea virus in cattle. Veterinary Research Communications.

Petsch, D. and F. B. Anspach (2000). Endotoxin removal from protein solutions. Journal of Biotechnology 76(2-3): 97-119.

Ridpath, J. E., J. D. Neill, et al. (2003). Effect of passive immunity on the development of a protective immune response against bovine viral diarrhea virus in calves. American Journal of Veterinary Research 64(1): 65-69.

Sako, K., H. Aoyama, et al. (2008a). Carboline derivatives with anti-bovine viral diarrhea virus (BVDV) activity. Bioorganic and Medicinal Chemistry 16: 3780-3790.

Sako, K., H. Aoyama, et al. (2008b). Gamma-Carboline derivatives with anti-bovine viral diarrhea virus (BVDV) activity. Bioorganic & Medicinal Chemistry 16(7): 3780-3790.

Scheerlinck, J. P. Y., S. Gloster, et al. (2006). Systemic immune responses in sheep, induced by a novel nano-bead adjuvant. Vaccine 24(8): 1124-1131.

Schweizer, M. and E. Peterhans (2001). Noncytopathic bovine viral diarrhea virus inhibits double-stranded RNA-induced apoptosis and interferon synthesis. Journal of Virology 75(10): 4692-4698.

Sorensen, H. P. and K. K. Mortensen (2005). Advanced genetic strategies for recombinant protein expression in Escherichia coli. Journal of Biotechnology 115(2): 113-128.

Speed, M. A., D. I. C. Wang, et al. (1996). Specific aggregation of partially folded polypeptide chains: The molecular basis of inclusion body composition. Nature Biotechnology 14(10): 1283-1287.

Yilmaz, H., E. Altan, et al. (2012). Genetic diversity and frequency of bovine viral diarrhea virus (BVDV) detected in cattle in Turkey. Comparative Immunology Microbiology and Infectious Diseases 35(5): 411-416.

Zhou, Z., P. Schnake, et al. (2004). Enhanced expression of a recombinant malaria candidate vaccine in Escherichia coli by codon optimization. Protein Expression and Purification 34(1): 87-94.

Regulation of Adenovirus Alternative RNA Splicing by PKA, DNA-PK, PP2A and SR Proteins

Anne Katrine Kvissel
Department of Molecular Biology, Division for Diagnostics and Technology
Akershus University Hospital, Norway

Heidi Törmänen Persson
Department of Medical Biochemistry and Microbiology, Science for Life Laboratory
Uppsala University, Sweden

Anne Kristin Aksaas
Department of Nutrition
St. Olavs Hospital, Trondheim University Hospital, Norway

Göran Akusjärvi
Department of Medical Biochemistry and Microbiology, Science for Life Laboratory
Uppsala University, Sweden

Bjørn Steen Skålhegg
Department of Nutrition, Institute of Basic Medical Sciences
University of Oslo, Norway

1   General Introduction to RNA Splicing

The regulation of gene transcription, precursor-messenger RNA (pre-mRNA) splicing and mRNA export are highly complex processes in the eukaryotic cell and involve a tight regulation of protein-protein, protein-DNA and protein-RNA interactions in time and space. Human adenoviruses have been used extensively as a tool and a model system to study these processes. Adenovirus gene expression have been thoroughly mapped and shown to occur in a coordinated and sequential fashion. Directly following infection adenovirus produce a number of early regulatory proteins inducing the onset of genome replication and production of the late structural proteins by an intricate regulation of pre-mRNA splicing. The late phase proteins consist of at least 15 different gene products encoded from a single pre-mRNA originating from the major late transcription unit (MLTU). The MLTU produces five groups of mRNAs (L1–L5) that are combined into at least 20 alternatively spliced mRNAs whose expression is tightly regulated at the level of alternative splicing and 3'-end formation.

Over the last two decades it has become increasingly evident that reversible phosphorylation is crucial in regulating transcription, pre-mRNA splicing and RNA export during virus infections. Here we will present recent discoveries and discuss how signaling pathways involving cyclic 3', 5'-adenosine monophosphate (cAMP)-dependent protein kinase (PKA) and DNA-dependent protein kinase (DNA-PK) act to regulate pre-mRNA processing in adenovirus infected cells. We will also discuss how adenovirus, by recruiting protein phosphatase 2A (PP2A), controls the activity of the essential cellular serine/arginine-rich (SR) family of splicing factors in virus-infected cells. We will further review the known effects of PKA on SR protein activity and RNA splicing.

1.1   Spliceosome Assembly and Pre-mRNA Processing

In eukaryotes, the RNA transcribed from the DNA template is not a functional template for protein synthesis until it has undergone specific modifications of specific pre-mRNA. These processes are co-transcriptional events where regulatory factors assemble onto the DNA-dependent RNA polymerase (RNAP) II carboxyl-terminal domain (CTD) to assist in the conversion of the transcript into a mature mRNA (Hirose & Ohkuma, 2007). Pre-mRNA processing includes capping (the addition of a 7-methyl guanosine (m^7G) cap at the 5'-end), pre-mRNA splicing (removal of intervening non-coding sequences called introns), and 3'-end formation by cleavage and polyadenylation. The 5'- (m^7G) cap and the 3' poly(A) tail protect the mRNA from degradation by exonucleases, they facilitate transport from the nucleus to the cytoplasm and further promote recognition of the mRNA by the ribosome (Wakiyama *et al.*, 2000; Furuichi *et al.*, 1977; Sachs, 1993; Ford *et al.*, 1997; Coller *et al.*, 1998; Visa *et al.*, 1996).

1.2   Pre-mRNA Splicing

In 1977, Philip Sharp and Richard Roberts discovered the split gene concept of eukaryotic genes while working with adenovirus mRNA structures (Berget *et al.*, 1977; Chow *et al.*, 1977). During their attempts to map the position of individual mRNAs on the adenovirus chromosome, they discovered that the mRNAs expressed from the adenoviral MLTU lacked some internal sections present in the viral DNA genome. They concluded that the mRNAs contained discontinuous segments derived from multiple places in the viral genome. Soon after this discovery, scientists working in other systems were able to show that the split gene concept was not unique to adenovirus (Lewin, 1980).

A typical human gene consists of an average of 9 exons with a mean size of 145 nucleotides, separated by introns of at least ten times the exon size (Lander *et al*., 2001). In a constitutively spliced transcript, all exons are included and all introns are removed from the resulting mRNA (International Human Genome Sequencing Consortium, 2004). The process of alternative RNA splicing occurs in the same fashion. However, usage of strong and weak splice sites results in selective exclusion and/or inclusion of nucleotide sequences in the final mRNA. There are several known patterns of alternative RNA splicing (Matlin *et al*., 2005). They include exon skipping and cassette exon splicing, where an exon is independently included or excluded from the mRNA. This may result in the complete inclusion or loss of a functional protein domain. The use of alternative 5'- and 3'-splice sites, on the other hand, may result in shortened or extended exons, which typically lead to subtle changes in the protein activity and fine-tuning of the protein function. Finally, an intron can be retained in the mature mRNA and this may lead to an additional protein domain or an altered reading frame and a complete change in protein function. The complexity in mRNA outcome is further expanded by the usage of alternative promoters and/or poly(A) sites, which has an impact on the sequence composition of the start and/or end of an mRNA sequence. In a single pre-mRNA transcript several of these alternative splicing patterns may be used. Today it is known that alternative RNA splicing is not an unusual event but rather the ruling principle. In fact, in more than 90% of the nearly 25,000 human genes, at least one exon out of a multi-exon pre-mRNA is alternatively spliced (Wang *et al*., 2008).

1.3   Spliceosome Assembly

Pre-mRNA splicing is carried out by the multi megadalton ribonucleoprotein (RNP) complex called the spliceosome that is assembled *de novo* in a step-wise manner on each new intron to be removed (Wahl *et al*., 2009). The main components of the spliceosome are five small nuclear ribonucleoproteins (snRNPs) (U1, U2, U4, U5 and U6) where each of them consists of small nuclear RNA (snRNA) and at least seven common Sm-proteins and a variable number of particle-specific proteins (Will & Luhrmann, 2011). Splice site selection is dependent on interactions between *cis*-acting sequence elements in the RNA and several co-factors (*trans*-acting factors), which in turn recruit the spliceosome. The final splice site selection is thus dependent on multiple RNA-RNA interactions as well as interactions between RNA and protein (Collins & Guthrie, 2000) (Figure 1). The pre-mRNA sequence contains several conserved nucleotide sequences that are important for splice site recognition and spliceosome assembly. These include the 5'-splice site (at the exon-intron border), the branch point, the polypyrimidine tract and the 3'-splice site (at the intron-exon border).

Assembly of the spliceosome is initiated by recognition of the 5' splice sites by the U1 snRNP. The snRNA component in the U1 snRNP binds to the 5'-splice site sequence by base pairing. The polypyrimidine tract, which is a region of 10-50 nucleotides enriched in pyrimidines and positioned down stream of the branch point, interacts with the 65 kilodaltons (kDa) subunit (U2AF65) of the heterodimeric U2 snRNP auxiliary factor (U2AF), which also consists of a 35kDa subunit (U2AF35). U2AF binds preferentially to long pyrimidine tracts (strong splice sites) and U2AF35 stabilizes the interaction by binding to the AG dinucleotide (Wu *et al*., 1999; Zamore & Green, 1989; Kielkopf *et al*., 2001), however U2AF35 is reported not always to be present in the dimer (Ruskin *et al*., 1988; Guth *et al*., 1999). The binding of U2AF consequently recruits the U2snRNP to the branch point. The interaction of both U1 snRNP and U2AF with the 5' and 3' splice sites, respectively, is further stabilized by SR proteins, which are serine/arginine-rich proteins involved in the regulation of splice site selection in eukaryotic pre-

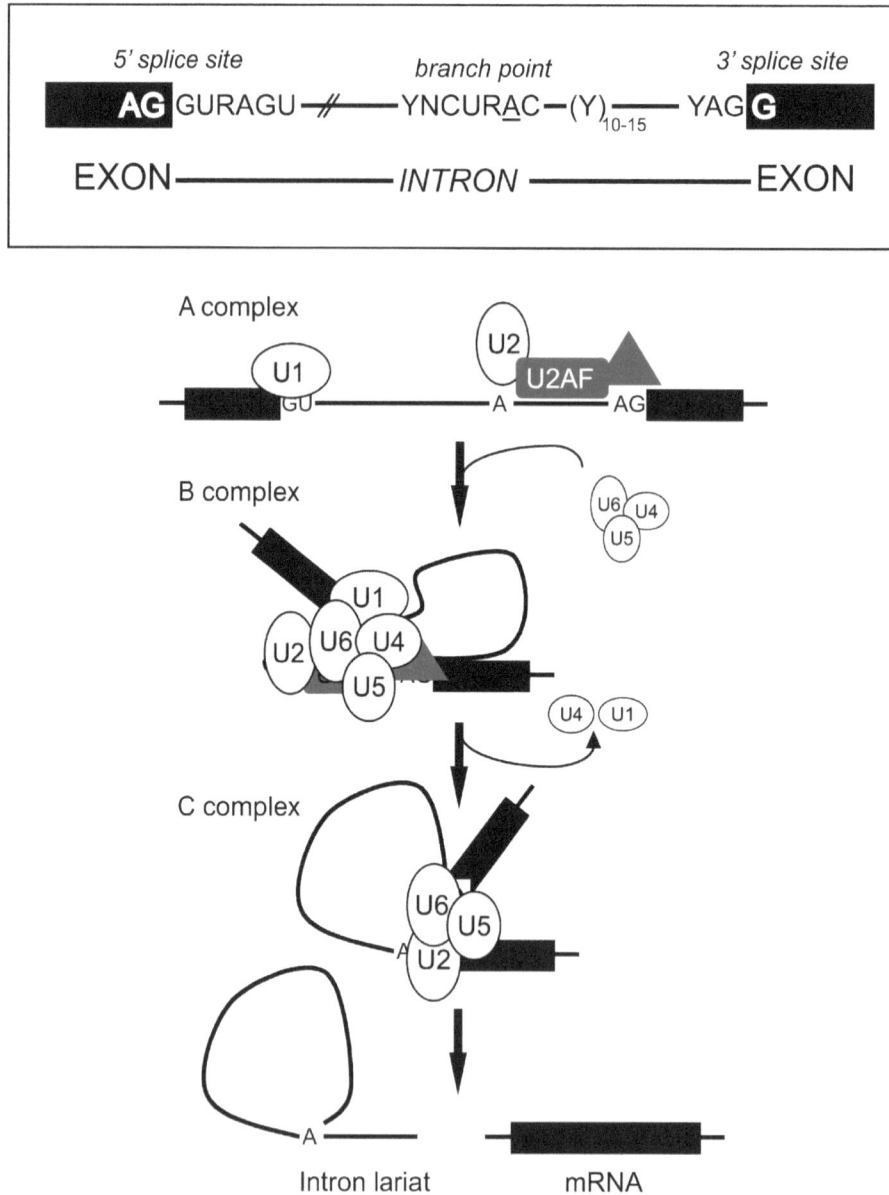

Figure 1: (Upper panel) Conserved sequences found at the exon-intron (5' splice site) and the intron-exon (3' splice site) borders and branch point of U2-type pre-mRNA introns. Exons are indicated by filled boxes and the intron by a thin line, unless specific nucleotide is specified. Y=pyrimidine (C or U), R=purine (G or A) and N=any nucleotide (A, U, G or C). The polypyrimidine tract is indicated by (Y)$_{10-15}$ and the branch point adenine is underlined (A). (Lower panel) Spliceosome assembly showing the U2AF heterodimer and the U snRNPs (U1, U2, U4, U5 and U6) assembling in a stepwise manner on the RNA. Formation of A, B and finally the catalytic C complex, where the transesterification reaction is completed, and the intron lariat and mRNA product are produced.

mRNA molecules (Tazi *et al.*, 2009). Next the U4/U6.U5 tri-snRNP is recruited, whereafter several steps of rearrangements form the catalytically active spliceosome, by which the intron is enzymatically released by a two-step process and the exons are joined together to form the mature intronless mRNA (Black, 2003; van der Feltz *et al.*, 2012).

1.4   Regulation of Constitutive and Alternative RNA Splicing

Alternative RNA splicing is regulated at many steps, from the level of the pre-mRNA sequence itself to the level of chromatin structure. Splicing factors binding to the pre-mRNA may recruit or hinder assembly of the splicing machinery by sterically promoting or blocking splice site usage. The degree to which splicing factors interact with the pre-mRNA is in some cases regulated through post-translational modifications. The next level of regulation occurs through coupling of RNA splicing to RNAP II transcription as well as the kinetics of transcription and RNA processing. This suggests that pre-mRNA splicing occurs co-transcriptionally. This is corroborated by the observation that the splicing machinery is physically linked to the transcriptional apparatus by interactions between splicing factors and the CTD in the largest protein subunit of RNAP II (Perales & Bentley, 2009). The CTD also has important roles for processes like 5´-end capping, splicing, and 3´-end cleavage and polyadenylation, which all are orchestrated by factors associating with the CTD (McCracken *et al.*, 1997b; McCracken *et al.*, 1997a). The importance of the transcription rate as a mean to regulate pre-mRNA splicing is demonstrated by the observation that if RNAP II is slowed down, exon inclusion is favored, whereas exon skipping is enhanced with a rapidly transcribing RNAP II (de la Mata *et al.*, 2003; Munoz *et al.*, 2009). Finally, the levels of spliceosomal components, intron size and competition between splices sites further determine the outcome of exon usage (Nilsen & Graveley, 2010).

The pre-mRNA sequence itself may conceal or expose splicing relevant sites depending on its secondary structure. *Cis*-acting elements are RNA sequences of about ten nucleotides that may promote or repress the usage of splice sites. Splicing enhancer sequences may reside in an exon or an intron and are named exonic splicing enhancer (ESE) or intronic splicing enhancer (ISE) sequences, respectively. Such sequences typically regulate the recognition and usage of weak splice sites. Their counterparts are exonic or intronic splicing silencer (ESS and ISS, respectively) which are sequences where complexes that repress the usage of a splice site may block the function of a competing ESE or looping out the alternative exon (Ghigna *et al.*, 2008). Recently, more than one hundred different ISEs were identified and clustered by sequence similarity (Wang *et al.*, 2012). It was shown that all ISEs functioned in multiple cell types and in heterologous introns. Interestingly, patterns of distribution and conservation across pre-mRNA regions were similar to those of ESSs. In addition, trans-factors of each ISE group were identified with six subgroups, whereas five of the groups are recognized by hnRNP H and hnRNP F, the sixth group is controlled by factors that either activate or supress splicing. This demonstrates how single elements, such as an ISE, function oppositely depending on location and binding factors.

Cis-regulatory elements are recognized by *trans*-acting co-factors. The concentration and activity of such *trans*-acting factors influence the splice pattern of a pre-mRNA and may be used to explain temporal and tissue specific splicing of a pre-mRNA (Chen & Manley, 2009). A well-studied group of *trans*-acting factors are the heterogenous nuclear ribonucleoproteins (hnRNPs) that may both facilitate and inhibit splice site usage by blocking U1 or U2 snRNP recruitment. They often recognize ISS or ESS sequences and hinder the recruitment of positive regulatory factors to a splice site (Black, 2003). Many of these factors are RNA-binding proteins (RBPs) which then are considered multifunctional regulators of

RNA splicing. RBPs contain one or several RNA recognition motifs (RRMs), which are common in nature and encoded by approximately 1% of all human genes (Cassola *et al.*, 2010). Since RNA-protein interactions are weak in general, stable binding requires several interaction points with one or several RRMs (Auweter *et al.*, 2006). RBPs bind to a selected set of target RNA sequences that are highly conserved through evolution (Cassola *et al.*, 2010; Voelker *et al.*, 2012).

Short non-coding RNAs are also involved in the regulation of pre-mRNA splicing. Their binding to the U1 and U2 snRNPs promotes exon inclusion, whereas blocking of the 3' and 5' splice sites, as well as targeting of ESS or ISS sequences, promotes exon skipping (Khanna & Stamm, 2010). Furthermore, about 50% of the pre-mRNA transcripts are alternatively polyadenylated. Hence, mRNA isoforms with different 3'- exonic sequences are generated that may have impact on the protein product, mRNA stability, localization as well as transport (Tian *et al.*, 2005). Recent studies have also revealed that regulation of alternative RNA splicing occurs via polymorphic chromatin structures and histone marks, where histone modifications, such as trimethylation of histone 3 at lysine 36 (H3K36me3) determines which exons to be used in splicing (Kolasinska-Zwierz *et al.*, 2009; Luco *et al.*, 2010). This is achieved by alterations in the positioning of the nucleosome and thereby the accessibility for RNAP II, transcription factors and other regulators (Luco *et al.*, 2011).

1.5   The SR Family of Splicing Factors

An important group of co-factors involved in RNA splicing is the SR family of splicing factors. SR proteins are essential splicing factors required at multiple steps in constitutive splicing and functioning as regulators of alternative RNA splicing (Bourgeois *et al.*, 2004). In 2010, based on the sequence properties of the known SR proteins, a novel SR-protein nomenclature was established. This concluded that there are 12 classical human SR proteins (Table 1) that contain one or two conserved RRMs and a C-terminal RS domain of at least 50 amino acids with an RS content above 40% (Manley & Krainer, 2010). They typically recognize and bind ESEs to recruit spliceosomal components such as U2AF, U1-70K or tri-snRNP to the splice sites (Ghosh & Adams, 2011). In addition, SR proteins can inhibit the binding of splicing repressor proteins to their silencer elements by binding to enhancer elements in close proximity (Solis *et al.*, 2008). SR proteins have together with the U1 snRNP also been shown to associate with RNAP II, suggesting an involvement in transcription-coupled regulation of splicing (Das *et al.*, 2007). Further, they can act as bridges bringing splice sites in close proximity. The RS domain is mainly believed to function as a protein-interaction surface for association with other proteins like other SR-or SR-related proteins in addition to spliceosomal components (Graveley, 2000; Kohtz *et al.*, 1994; Blencowe *et al.*, 1999; Teigelkamp *et al.*, 1997). Furthermore, the subcellular localization of SR proteins is controlled by the RS domain, which acts as a nuclear localization signal (Kataoka *et al.*, 1999; Lai *et al.*, 2000).

SR proteins also serve additional functions and participate in mRNA nuclear export, mRNA translation, micro RNA (miRNA) processing and nonsense-mediated mRNA decay (NMD) (Zhong *et al.*, 2009). The large average intron size in eukaryotic cells greatly increases the probability that aberrant splicing events take place. This may result in the integration of a nonsense (stop) codon (UAA, UAG, UGA) within the open reading frame. NMD is triggered by exon-junction complexes (EJCs; components of the assembled RNP) that are deposited during pre-mRNA processing and is the end point quality control that destroys mRNAs that are aberrantly spliced. If such RNAs contain a premature translational stop signal or lack a translation signal all together they are susceptible to NMD (Maquat, 2004). The overall importance of SR proteins for viability has been demonstrated in mice null-mutants for the SR-splicing

New protein/gene symbol	Synonyms
SRSF1	ASF, SF2, SRp30
SRSF2	SC35, PR264, SRp30b
SRSF3	SRp20
SRSF4	SRp75
SRSF5	SRp40, HRS
SRSF6	SRp55, B52
SRSF7	9G8
SRSF8	SRp46
SRSF9	SRp30c
SRSF10	TASR1, SRp38, SRrp40
SRSF11	p54, SRp54
SRSF12	SRrp35

Table 1: New and previous SR protein nomenclature (Manley & Krainer, 2010)

factors 1 through 3 (SRSF1, SRSF2 and SRSF3) where the mutations were shown to be embryonic lethal (Moroy & Heyd, 2007).

SR proteins are functionally regulated by post-translational modifications such as reversible phosphorylation (Kanopka *et al.*, 1998). The activity and the subcellular localization of SR proteins are coordinated by the SR-specific protein kinase (SRPK) and the cdc2-like kinase (CLK) families of kinases that phosphorylate multiple serines in the RS domain (Ghosh & Adams, 2011). Whereas phosphorylated SR proteins typically promote splicing, dephosphorylated SR proteins inhibit splice site recognition and spliceosome assembly. During the two-step splicing catalysis a sequential dephosphorylation of SR proteins occurs. Furthermore, it has been demonstrated that qualitative phosphorylation alone is not sufficient for full activity, as either hyper- or hypo-phosphorylation makes the SR proteins unable to support splicing (Graveley, 2000; Shepard & Hertel, 2009).

2 Extracellular-Dependent Regulation of RNA Processing

The impact of signal transduction in RNA processing has so far received little attention. However during recent years it has become increasingly evident that molecular changes mediated by signal transduction control splice site selection *in vivo*. Extracellular stimuli can affect alternative splicing through post-translational modifications of *trans*-acting regulatory factors. Known modifications of splicing factors are phosphorylation, acetylation, methylation and glycosylation (Edmond *et al.*, 2011; Rho *et al.*, 2007; Soulard *et al.*, 1993; Stamm, 2008).

The best characterized phosphorylation-events involved in RNA processing are those of the CTD in RNAP II and the SR family of splicing factors (Fluhr, 2008). SR proteins are phosphorylated through many signaling pathways, and whereas SRSF5 is phosphorylated in response to insulin stimulation (Patel *et al.*, 2005), SRSF1 and SRSF7 are phosphorylated upon stimulation by growth factors (Blaustein *et al.*, 2005). Some consequences of phosphorylation of SRSF1 through growth factor stimulation are increased affinity of SRSF1 for U1 70K snRNP, enhancement of pre-mRNA splicing and decreased nuclear export of SRSF1 (Cao *et al.*, 1997; Huang *et al.*, 2004). Phosphorylation is also believed to regulate SRSF1, 3,

4, 6, 7 and 10 shuttling between the nucleus and cytoplasm (Cazalla *et al.*, 2002; Sapra *et al.*, 2009). In fact, transport from the cytoplasm to the nucleus and nuclear localization of SR proteins requires cytoplasmic phosphorylation (Barbe *et al.*, 2008; Caceres *et al.*, 1997; Caceres *et al.*, 1998; Cowper *et al.*, 2001; Koizumi *et al.*, 1999; Lai *et al.*, 2000; Lai *et al.*, 2003; Ngo *et al.*, 2005; Sakashita & Endo, 2010). On the other side dephosphoryation mediates nuclear export of the SR proteins (Huang *et al.*, 2004; Lai & Tarn, 2004; Tenenbaum & Aguirre-Ghiso, 2005).

Despite the dependence of phosphorylation, it is also well established that nucleocytoplasmic shuttling of e.g. SRSF1 depends on its ability to bind RNA. Dysfunctional RNA binding causes SRSF1 to accumulate in the nucleus. In fact, for constitutive pre-mRNA splicing by SRSF1 both of its RRMs and the RS domain are involved. However, to induce alternative RNA splicing, especially 5'-splice site selection, the two RRMs alone are sufficient (Caceres & Krainer, 1993; Caceres *et al.*, 1997; Delestienne *et al.*, 2010; Tintaru *et al.*, 2007). To this end, it is interesting to note that Cho and colleagues (Cho *et al.*, 2011) demonstrate that hypo-phosphorylation of the RS domain in SRSF1 promotes self-association with its own RRM, preventing U1-70K binding. On the other hand, hyper-phosphorylation of the RS domain permits the formation of a ternary complex containing ESE, an SR protein and U1 snRNP. This report represents a clear example of how phosphorylation of the RS domain, e.g. in SRSF1, represents a key molecular switch from intra- to intermolecular interactions. This also demonstrates the requirement for a phosphorylation/dephosporylation cycle during pre-mRNA splicing.

Furthermore, RBPs, such as Signal transduction and activation of RNA (STAR) proteins, also contain proline-rich sequences that can bind to the Src homology (SH3) domains of signaling proteins. In addition, the RNA binding activity and oligomerization of the STAR protein Src-associated in mitosis 68 (SAM68) are inhibited by tyrosine phosphorylation, indicating that STAR proteins, and thus RBPs take part in linking signaling pathways to RNA metabolism (Chen *et al.*, 1997; Lasko, 2003; Wang *et al.*, 1995).

In addition to the well characterized kinases involved in splicing regulation, Clk/Sty and SRPK1, SR proteins are reversibly phosphorylated by other protein kinases such as mitogen-activated AKT kinase, DNA topoisomerase I and protein kinase A (PKA) and links pre-mRNA splicing to external regulation (Aksaas *et al.*, 2011a; Blaustein *et al.*, 2005; Kvissel *et al.*, 2007a; Patel *et al.*, 2005; Rossi *et al.*, 1996; Shi *et al.*, 2011; Gu *et al.*, 2011)

2.1 PKA and Its Multiple Functions in RNA Processing

Cyclic AMP is a key intracellular signaling molecule, which main function is to activate the cAMP-dependent protein kinases (PKA). PKA is a heterotetrameric holoenzyme, which contains a regulatory (R) subunit dimer and two catalytic (C) subunits. In human, two main forms of the R subunit are expressed, RI and RII, which make the basis for two major forms of PKA, PKAI and PKAII (Corbin *et al.*, 1975) . Four genes of the R subunit (RIα, RIβ, RIIα, RIIβ) and four different C subunits (Cα, Cβ, Cγ and PrKX) are expressed. The PKA holoenzyme is activated when four molecules of cAMP bind to the R subunit dimer, two to each R subunit, releasing two active C subunits (Skalhegg & Tasken, 2000).

PKA is a well-established regulator of gene expression, mainly through phosphorylation of transcription factors such as NF-κB, HSF1, CREB, CREM and AP-1 (Daniel *et al.*, 1998). Over the recent years it has become increasingly clear that PKA and related members of this signaling pathway are also involved in regulation of pre-mRNA splicing. This was initially demonstrated by the observation that the C subunit of PKA is located to splicing factor compartments (SFC) and promotes distal splicing of the adenoviral E1A minigene (Kvissel et al., 2007a). Moreover, it has been shown that PKA phosphorylation enhances binding of mRNA to the K homology (KH) domain of A-kinase anchoring protein (AKAP) 1 (Ginsberg et al., 2003; Ranganathan et al., 2002; Rogne et al., 2009). AKAPs are proteins which target PKA to distinct subcellular compartments and may also act as scaffolding proteins that coordinate multiple intracellular signals during physiological processes (Wong & Scott, 2004). Furthermore, recently it was demonstrated that the SR-related protein SFSR17A, is an AKAP that directly interacts with SRSF1 (Jarnaess et al., 2009; Mangs et al., 2006). SFSR17A1 and 2 are believed to dock the RIα subunit of PKA, and subsequently the C subunit, to SFCs.

The Polypyrimidine Tract Binding Protein (PTB), which is a splicing factor of the hnRNP protein family, is also phosphorylated by PKA. This phosphorylation event has not been shown to regulate pre-mRNA splicing directly, but leads to translocation of PTB from the cytoplasm into the nucleus (Xie et al., 2003). Furthermore, the cAMP/PKA pathway also regulates alternative splicing of the cyclin Ania-6a through dopamine stimulation. The Ania-6a promoter contains one cAMP-responsive element (CRE) and its gene expression is stimulated by forskolin and inhibited by the PKA specific inhibitor H89 (Berke et al., 2001). However, forskolin has an additional effect that may not be reflected by PKA activity on the alternative splicing pattern and inducement of the Ania-6a60 variant (Sgambato et al., 2003).

Furthermore, we recently demonstrated that the PKA C subunit phosphorylates several SR proteins, in particular SRSF1 (Kvissel et al., 2007a). PKA phosphorylation of SRSF1 in vitro has also been verified by others, and recently an interaction between the two proteins was reported by three independent reports including us (Aksaas et al., 2011a; Colwill et al., 1996; Gu et al., 2011; Shi et al., 2011). Whereas we also showed that PKA phosphorylation of SRSF1Ser[119] modulates its activity as a splicing enhancer protein, Gu and co-workers showed that PKA through interaction and phosphorylation of SRSF1 promotes exclusion of exons 14, 15 and 16 in Ca2+/calmodulin-dependent protein kinase IIδ (CaMKIIδ) (Gu et al., 2011).

The perhaps best studied example of PKA-regulated splicing is the alternative splicing of exon 10 in Tau. Tau is a neuronal protein associated with microtubules. Alternative splicing of exon 10 produces variants of Tau with three (3R) or four (4R) microtubule-binding repeats. Imbalance between these two Tau variants affects its functions in assembly and stabilization of microtubules and is associated with neurodegenerative diseases such as Alzheimer disease (Shi et al., 2008; Shi et al., 2011; Gu et al., 2012). PKA phosphorylation of SRSF1 enhances the inclusion of exon 10 in the Tau transcript. Furthermore, a recent paper has also identified SRSF7 as a new interaction partner and substrate for PKA C. SRSF7 do primarily suppress the inclusion of exon 10 in Tau. Up-regulation of PKA activity by forskolin prevents the exclusion of exon 10 by SRSF7 (Gu et al., 2012). Hence, PKA promotes exon 10 inclusion via two different splicing factors. Interestingly, phosphorylation of Ser[227], Ser[234] and Ser[238] in SRSF1 by dual specificity tyrosine-Y-phosphorylation regulated kinase 1A (Dyrk1A) suppresses the inclusion of the same exon.

Despite that PKA-dependent regulation of pre-mRNA splicing appears to be involved at several steps in splicing, it is not likely that PKA contributes to the pre-mRNA catalysis itself. This is supported by the fact that neither of the PKA R- or C subunits contains an RBD, nor are they known to bind RNA (Ranganathan et al., 2002). However, it is possible that PKA contributes to the regulation of spliceosome assembly directly or through interaction and phosphorylation of other proteins associated with the spliceosome. Recently it has been demonstrated that the PKA C subunit may be a scaffolding protein with multiple sites for protein interactions (Taylor et al., 2005). The role of PKA in regulating RBPs has been demonstrated in that it binds to and phosphorylates the G-patch and KOW motifs-containing protein (GPKOW). GPKOW, which is a nuclear protein, binds RNA and acts to coordinate dynamic protein-protein interactions of the human spliceosome during splicing (Hegele *et al.*, 2012). Using a yeast two-hybrid screen with the PKA C subunit Cβ2 as bait, we recently identified GPKOW as a PKA C subunit binding protein that can be phosphorylated by PKA at Ser[27] and Thr[316] *in vitro*. Moreover, site directed mutations of the PKA phosphorylation sites showed that the RNA-binding capacity of GPKOW was altered (Aksaas *et al.*, 2011b). This points to the fact that PKA-dependent regulation may involve alteration of effector proteins that interact with specific mRNA sequences. This is supported by other studies demonstrating the existence of a PKA/CaMKIV responsive element in exon 16 in the calcium/calmodulin-dependent protein kinase kinase 2 (CaMKK2) transcripts. This CAAAAAA sequence, which can be considered a parallel to the CRE element in DNA, also appears to be enriched in alternatively spliced exons (Li *et al.*, 2009).

Furthermore, it is well-established that PKA is able to regulate gene expression in general and it is now apparent that this may contribute to a change in the steady-state level of available regulatory factors for RNA processing. The mechanism by which PKA acts is however unknown, but the most likely possibility is that the C subunit phosphorylates *trans*-acting splicing regulators, such as SR proteins, hnRNP proteins and snRNP-associated factors. Such phosphorylation events may lead to alterations of subcellular localization, as well as the ability of various factors to interact with and to perform regulatory effects on RNA and protein functions. Furthermore, it is now clear that several kinases are involved in pre-mRNA splicing at different steps. For example, cGMP-dependent protein kinase (PKG) phosphorylates Ser[20] in Splicing factor 1 (SF1) and hence disrupts the interaction between SF1 and U2AF65, which results in inhibition of spliceosome assembly (Wang *et al.*, 1999).

2.2   DNA-PK and Its Functions in DNA Repair and Transcription

DNA-PK is a nuclear serine/threonine protein kinase that belongs to the super family of phosphatidylinositol 3-kinase-related kinases (PIKKs) (Lempiainen & Halazonetis, 2009). The PIKKs are conserved through evolution with homologues in many organisms from yeast to mammals. They are considered as atypical protein kinases due to the fact that their kinase domain has a low sequence similarity to other classical eukaryotic protein kinases and that they rather share common features with the lipid phosphatidyl inositol 3-kinase (PI3K) family of proteins (Manning *et al.*, 2002; Keith & Schreiber, 1995). Biochemical studies have shown that DNA-PK is a heterotrimeric enzyme composed of a catalytic subunit (DNA-PKcs) and two regulatory subunits Ku86 and Ku70 (Yaneva *et al.*, 1997; Gottlieb & Jackson, 1993). DNA-PK preferentially phosphorylates serine or threonine residues followed by a glutamine, (Ser/Thr-Gln-motif) (Collis *et al.*, 2005). The biological functions of PIKKs are diverse and involve responses to DNA damage, metabolism and cell growth control, regulation of NMD, transcriptional regulation and maintenance of telomere length (Lempiainen & Halazonetis, 2009; Woodard *et al.*, 1999; Neal & Meek, 2011).

The best characterized function of DNA-PK is its role in the double strand break repair (DSBR) system and non-homologous end-joining (NHEJ) pathway (Jackson & Jeggo, 1995). To repair double strand breaks (DSB) in the DNA, the Ku heterodimer recognizes the DSB and facilitates the recruitment of DNA-PKcs to the DNA. This DNA binding leads to activation of DNA-PK and further autophosphorylation of the catalytic subunit. Following this, DNA-PK dissociates and the DNA ends become accessible for the other components of the NHEJ, which in turn join and ligate the DNA ends (Neal & Meek, 2011; Lees-Miller *et al.*, 1990; Carter *et al.*, 1990).

DNA-PK has also been suggested to have a direct role in transcription. It phosphorylates transcription factors like Sp1, Oct-1, c-Myc, c-Jun and p53, thereby regulating their functions (Lees-Miller, 1996; Schild-Poulter *et al.*, 2007; Shieh *et al.*, 1997). Further, DNA-PK seems to be involved in regulation of the initiation step of transcription and has also been shown to interact with and phosphorylate the CTD of RNAP II. (Maldonado *et al.*, 1996; Peterson *et al.*, 1992; Woodard *et al.*, 1999). Interestingly, DNA-PK has been shown to induce phosphorylation of Ser^2 and Ser^7 in the heptapeptide repeat (Trigon *et al.*, 1998). The biological relevance of these phosphorylations is not understood, but it is known that Ser^2 phosphorylation is associated with RNAP II elongation and that Ser^7 phosphorylation stimulates cyclin-dependent kinase 9 (CDK9) phosphorylation of Ser^2 (Czudnochowski *et al.*, 2012). This is associated with enrichment of transcribed introns, which may suggest a link between pre-mRNA splicing and DNA-PK activity (Kim *et al.*, 2010).

3   The Adenovirus Model System

Virus-infected cells are widely used as model systems to study cell transformation, cell cycle control, gene regulation, pre-mRNA splicing and tumor formation. The viral genome is relatively small, can easily be modified and the gene products interfere with many of the biosynthetic machineries in the infected cell, including RNA processing. Adenoviruses are small non-enveloped linear double stranded DNA (dsDNA) viruses encoding for about 30 to 40 genes. The early viral genes are in general required to force the cell into S-phase, block apoptosis and initiate viral DNA replication and new virus progeny formation (Tauber & Dobner, 2001). To do this, the virus takes advantage of processes like alternative RNA splicing and polyadenylation to expand the coding capacity of the limited viral genome. Of specific interest for this review is the observation that the production and accumulation of the alternatively spliced and polyadenylated mRNAs are temporally regulated during the virus life cycle, producing distinct mRNA species at different time points during the infection (Akusjarvi, 2008).

3.1   The Major Late Transcription Unit (MLTU) and the L1 Model System

Activation of adenoviral gene expression is under a strict temporal control with an expression of early genes directly after infection, and late genes after the onset of viral genome replication. Studies of the MLTU have shown that the early-to-late switch in gene expression is controlled at the level of premature transcription termination, alternative splicing and choice of poly(A) site usage (Akusjarvi, 2008).

The MLTU produces a primary transcript of approximately 28,000 nucleotides. This transcript can be polyadenylated at five different positions, producing five families of mRNAs with co-terminal 3'-ends, termed L1 to L5 (Figure 2). Transcription of the MLTU is initiated at the major late promoter (MLP), which is activated within the first hours of infection and at this stage produces shortened transcripts that gradually pre-terminate between the L1- and the L3 poly(A) sites (Young, 2003; Shaw & Ziff, 1980). Even though a low percentage of transcription proceeds beyond the L3 poly(A) site, only the L1 poly(A) site is efficiently used at the early phase of infection. At this stage, only the L1 52,55K mRNA accumulates in the cytoplasm. After the onset of viral DNA replication transcription is extended and proceeds through to the L5 poly(A) site (Akusjarvi & Persson, 1981; Nevins & Wilson, 1981). The use of the L2-L5 poly(A) sites are temporally divided into two phases. At the intermediate phase, before the onset of late protein synthesis, a selective activation of the L4 poly(A) site is observable (Larsson *et al.*, 1992). When discovered, we attributed this finding to a selective control of poly(A) site usage. However, a recent study has suggested an interesting alternative mechanism, where the activation of L4 mRNA expression is controlled by a novel L4 specific promoter that becomes selectively activated at the intermediate time of virus infection (Morris & Leppard, 2009). During the late phase, when late protein synthesis has been initiated, mRNA expression from the L2, L3 and L5 poly(A) sites becomes activated (Larsson *et al.*, 1991; Larsson *et al.*, 1992).

The boost in mRNA accumulation seen late in infection is not only due to a shift in poly(A) site usage or an enhancement of the activity of the MLP, but is to a large extent caused by a temporal shift in alternative RNA splice site usage. For example, the MLTU transcripts use alternative splicing to produce approximately 20 different mRNAs. All spliced mRNAs contain a common 201 nucleotide long 5' noncoding sequence, called the tri-partite leader, which functions as translational enhancer in late virus infected cells (Dolph *et al.*, 1988). Splicing together the three first exons in the MLTU produces this leader sequence, which is further joined to the different coding exons down-stream in the MLTU. The mRNAs produced from the L1-L5 units are derived by alternative 3' splice site usage. A common 5' splice site at the third exon in the tripartite leader is spliced to multiple alternative 3' splice sites within each unit (Akusjarvi, 2008).

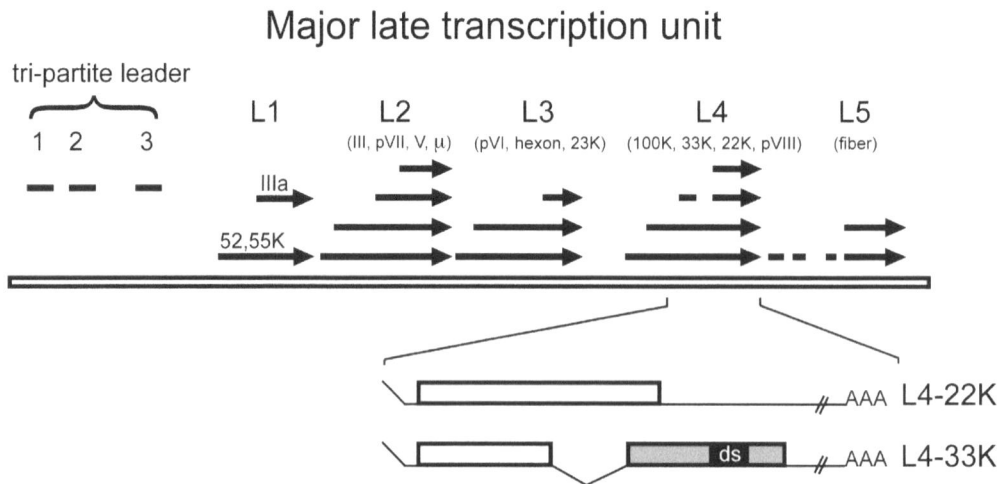

Figure 2: Schematic drawing showing the spliced structure of the mRNAs expressed from the MLTU. The common tri-partite leader is via RNA splicing connected to all of the variable last exons (symbolized as arrows). The five poly(A) sites, generating family units (L1-L5), are indicated by arrow heads. The 52,55K mRNA from the L1 unit is the only mRNA produced early during infection. Below, the blow up shows the organization of the L4-22K and L4-33K open reading frames, including the functional important ds region.

L1 is the only unit in the MLTU producing mRNAs both early and late during the virus life cycle. Thus, the 52,55K mRNA is produced both during the early and late phase, whereas the IIIa mRNA, which encodes for a structural protein that is interspersed between the hexons in the capsid (Akusjarvi &

Stevenin, 2003; Flint, 2004), is only produced at late times of infection. The 52,55K protein has a role in viral genome encapsidation by stabilizing the association of the viral genome with the preformed empty capsids. The functional reason for a temporal regulation of the expression of these proteins is unclear, but has been studied in tissue culture cell experiments. The results show that the loss of 52,55K protein or gain of IIIa protein early during infection does not have a detrimental effect on virus growth. However, the results suggested that the IIIa protein may have a regulatory role in L1 alternative splicing by suppressing 52,55K mRNA splicing in late infected cells (Molin *et al.*, 2002).

The L1 unit has been extensively used as a model transcript for studies of the temporal regulation of alternative RNA splicing. To date, it is known that it uses a common 5´ splice site and two competing 3´ splice sites to produce two mRNAs, the 52,55K mRNA (proximal 3' splice site), and the IIIa mRNA (distal 3' splice site) (Figure 3). Previous results have shown that the activation of the IIIa 3' splice site is not dependent on a *cis*-competition between the 52,55K and IIIa 3' splice sites *in vivo* (Gustin & Imperiale, 1998). Thus, inactivation of an ESE downstream of the 52,55K 3' splice site, did not affect the temporal activation of IIIa splice site usage at the late phase of infection.

Our mechanistic work has shown that IIIa splice site activation depends on two *cis*-acting elements in the transcript; the IIIa repressor element (3RE) and the IIIa virus infection-dependent splicing enhancer (3VDE) located in the intron just upstream of the IIIa 3' splice site (Figure 3).

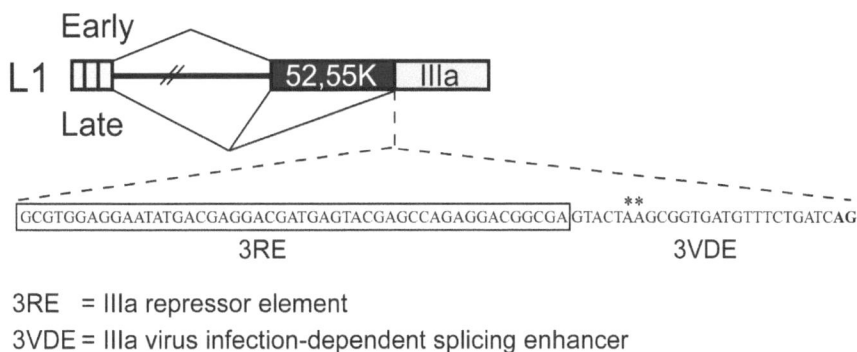

Figure 3: The temporal splicing pattern of the L1 unit with the regulatory *cis*-elements in the upstream IIIa intron. Boxes represent exons, the thick line an intron, and thin lines with hookes the region that is spliced out. The two adenosines at the branch point are indicated with asterisks (*) and the 3'splice site nucleotides are in bold.

3.1.1   Function of the 3RE and The Importance of SR Proteins in IIIa 3' Splice Site Activation

The 3RE is a 49 nucleotide long RNA segment located immediately upstream of the IIIa branch site that functions as a IIIa splicing repressor element. It binds classical SR protein splicing factors and this binding suppresses IIIa splice site usage by blocking U2 snRNP recruitment to the IIIa branch site (Kanopka *et al.*, 1996). The absence of IIIa splicing in early virus-infected cells can therefore, to a large extent, be explained by a direct inhibitory effect of the cellular SR proteins on IIIa 3' splice site usage. Interestingly, moving the 3RE from its natural intronic position to the IIIa second exon converts the 3RE from a splicing repressor element to a classical splicing enhancer element (Kanopka *et al.*, 1996). Collectively, these results suggest that the activity of SR proteins is sequence position-dependent. If they bind to an intron they may repress splicing whereas they may activate splicing from an exonic position.

Of the SR proteins, SRSF1, has been studied in more detail. The splicing enhancer and splicing repressor functions of SRSF1 has been separated and attributed to distinct domains in the protein in adenovirus splicing. The RS domain functions as the splicing enhancer domain (Graveley, 2000), whereas the second RRM (RRM2) is associated with a splicing repressor function (Dauksaite & Akusjarvi, 2002). The repressor activity of RRM2 appears to be a general effect since tethering of SRSF1-RRM2 at an intronic position in the rabbit β-globin pre-mRNA also resulted in splicing repression.

SR proteins binding to the 3RE do not block IIIa splicing by simply sterically hindering U2 snRNP recruitment to the IIIa branch site. Thus, tethering a bulky protein, markedly larger than SRSF1, at the position of the 3RE does not result in splicing repression, whereas tethering of a truncated SRSF1 protein encompassing only the SRSF1-RRM2 fragment was sufficient to reproduce the splicing repressor phenotype (Dauksaite & Akusjarvi, 2002). Further, the heptapeptide motif, SWQDLKD, which is completely conserved in SR proteins encompassing two RRMs, was shown to be essential for activity of the repressor domain (Dauksaite & Akusjarvi, 2002).

In the context of mini-gene constructs where the distance between the 52,55K and the IIIa 3' splice sites was shortened to 80 nucleotides, the 3RE functions simultaneously as a splicing repressor element for IIIa splicing and as a classical second exon splicing enhancer for 52,55K splicing (Kanopka et al., 1996). However, in the authentic L1 unit, the 3RE and the 52,55K 3' splice sites are separated by approximately 1200 nucleotides, and in this case the 3RE can not function as a 52,55K splicing enhancer element. Instead, it appears that the 52,55K 3'splice site has a separate ESE element located about 50-60 nucleotides downstream of the 52,55K 3' splice site that controls its activity (Gustin & Imperiale, 1998).

The adenovirus E4 open-reading-frame 4 (E4-ORF4) protein is a multifunctional viral regulator that has been shown to block E1A induced transcription activation (Muller et al., 1992; Kleinberger & Shenk, 1993; Bondesson et al., 1996), induce hypo-phosphorylation of various viral and cellular proteins (Kanopka et al., 1998; Muller et al., 1992) and regulate adenovirus alternative RNA splicing (Kanopka et al., 1998). In late-infected cells, the E4-ORF4 protein binds to the cellular protein phosphatase PP2A and thus induces SR protein dephosphorylation. This dephosphorylation reduces the binding of SR proteins to the 3RE, which relieves the repressive function on IIIa splicing and makes the branch point accessible for U2 snRNP recruitment (Kanopka et al., 1998). Interestingly, re-phosphorylation of SR proteins isolated from late adenovirus-infected cells restores their activity as splicing repressor proteins (Huang et al., 2002). Since SR proteins are essential for generic pre-mRNA splicing (Fu, 1995; Manley & Tacke, 1996), the virus-induced dephosphorylation results in an inhibition of splicing of pre-mRNAs with constitutive splicing signals (Kanopka et al., 1998). This mechanism may therefore contribute to the virus-induced inhibition of host cell gene expression seen late after infection.

It is also believed that the interaction between E4-ORF4 and PP2A is involved in selective p53-independent apoptosis in transformed cells (Marcellus et al., 1998; Shtrichman & Kleinberger, 1998), and G2/M arrest in yeast and mammalian cells (Kornitzer et al., 2001; Branton & Roopchand, 2001). Another consequence of SR protein dephosphorylation caused by the E4-ORF4 protein is activation of IIIa splicing, and the 3RE is required for this activation (Kanopka et al., 1998). Thus, deletion of the 3RE from the IIIa pre-mRNA increases basal IIIa splicing and eliminates the stimulatory effect of E4-ORF4 on splicing (Kanopka et al., 1998; Estmer et al., 2001). Conversely, transfer of the 3RE to the ß-globin pre-mRNA reduces basal ß-globin splicing but makes this transcript sensitive to E4-ORF4 activation of splicing (Estmer *et al.*, 2001).

E4-ORF4 has been shown to interact specifically with SRSF1 and SRSF9 (Estmer *et al.*, 2001). However, the interaction with SRSF9 does not correlate with E4-ORF4 induced activation of IIIa splicing, suggesting that SRSF1 is the primary target for E4-ORF4. Further, E4-ORF4 selectively interacts with the highly phosphorylated form of the SR protein, the form observed in uninfected and the early stage of virus infection. However, since all SR proteins, except SRSF3, appear to be hypo-phosphorylated in adenovirus infected HeLa nuclear extracts (Ad-NE) (Kanopka *et al.*, 1998), these results suggest that the E4-ORF4 induced SR protein dephosphorylation can not be the only mechanism controlling SR protein phosphorylation during infection. Interestingly, the *de novo* synthesis of the sphingolipid ceramide, at the late stage of an adenovirus infection, has been suggested to induce hypo-phosphorylation of SR proteins (Kanj *et al.*, 2006). In fact, previous work has shown that ceramide causes SR protein dephosphorylation through activation of the Protein phosphatase 1 (PP1) pathway (Chalfant *et al.*, 2001). Collectively, current results therefore may suggest that adenovirus uses both the E4-ORF4/PP2A and the ceramide/PP1 pathways to control SR protein function during a lytic infection.

During an adenovirus infection, the nucleus undergoes a dramatic restructuring resulting in the appearance of foci with zones of actively replicating genomes bordered by pools of viral ssDNA and nascent viral mRNA (Pombo *et al.*, 1994). During the late phase of infection, the splicing factor containing SFCs are rearranged from the speckled pattern seen in uninfected cells to ring-like structures that has been termed viral replication centers. These centers can be visualized as small spots increasing in amount over the course of the infection to finally spreading throughout the whole nucleus (Puvion-Dutilleul *et al.*, 1984; Pombo *et al.*, 1994). The area immediately surrounding the replication centers have been shown to be sites of viral transcription, and both snRNPs and SRSF1 (Aspegren *et al.*, 1998; Gama-Carvalho *et al.*, 2003; Pombo *et al.*, 1994) are recruited to these so-called peripheral replicative zones (Puvion-Dutilleul *et al.*, 1992; Bridge *et al.*, 1995). In the late phase of infection, when the viral mRNAs starts to accumulate in the cytoplasm, the snRNPs and splicing factors redistribute from the peripheral replicative zones to enlarged nuclear speckles that are distributed to the peripheral regions of the nucleus (Aspegren *et al.*, 1998; Gama-Carvalho *et al.*, 2003; Bridge *et al.*, 2003; James *et al.*, 2010). Although E4-ORF4 clearly has a regulatory function in RNA splicing, our results show that another viral factor, the L4-33K protein, which also is localized to viral replication centers during infection (Ostberg *et al.*, 2012) , is the key regulator of L1 alternative splicing (see below).

3.1.2   The 3VDE is the key element enhancing IIIa pre-mRNA splicing

Although the 3RE plays an important role in IIIa 3' splice site activation, collectively our data suggest that the 3VDE is the most critical element controlling IIIa pre-mRNA splicing. The 3VDE consists of the IIIa branch site, the weak pyrimidine tract and the 3' splice site AG (Figure 3). Mutations in the short IIIa pyrimidine tract effectively abolish IIIa splice site activation in Ad-NE (Muhlemann *et al.*, 2000; Muhlemann *et al.*, 1995). Further, the 3VDE is essential for regulated IIIa pre-mRNA splicing and sufficient to convert a heterologous transcript from a pre-mRNA that is repressed to a pre-mRNA that is activated in Ad-NE (Muhlemann *et al.*, 2000).

The IIIa 3' splice site does not efficiently bind the general splicing factor U2AF, and this recruitment is even further weakened in adenovirus–infected cells (Muhlemann *et al.*, 2000; Lutzelberger *et al.*, 2005; Muhlemann *et al.*, 1995). U2AF has a strong preference for binding to long pyrimidine rich sequences (Zamore *et al.*, 1992; Singh *et al.*, 1995). In general, splicing of pre-mRNAs that contain long prototypical polypyrimidine tracts are repressed in Ad-NE, while splicing of 3' splice sites, which have a weak sequence context, are enhanced. Weak 3' splice sites are typical for many of the late adenoviral introns (Tormanen *et al.*, 2006; Lutzelberger *et al.*, 2005; Muhlemann *et al.*, 1995) .

U2AF65 specifically binds to the pyrimidine tract whereas U2AF35 makes contact with the 3' splice site AG dinucleotide (Merendino *et al.*, 1999; Wu *et al.*, 1999). Introns with weak pyrimidine tracts that bind U2AF65 inefficiently require U2AF35 interaction with the 3' splice site AG to be functional, so-called AG-dependent introns. In contrast, 3' splice sites with strong pyrimidine tracts can splice without the contribution of U2AF35, so-called AG-independent introns. Interestingly, it appears that U2AF35 is not required for splicing in Ad-NE. Thus, the IIIa intron, which is an AG-dependent intron in uninfected cell extracts, becomes AG-independent in Ad-NE (Lutzelberger *et al.*, 2005). In fact, splicing of the IgM pre-mRNA, which have a 3' splice site that is characterized as weak with a short polypyrimidine tract, undergoes the first catalytic step of splicing in U2AF-depleted Ad-NE (Lutzelberger *et al.*, 2005). Taken together, it seems that spliceosome assembly might be U2AF-independent in late adenovirus-infected cells.

The mechanism by which the 3VDE activates IIIa splice site usage is not yet resolved. Available evidence is compatible with the model that splicing activation by the 3VDE operates through a novel U2AF-independent mechanism, or alternatively does not require stable binding of U2AF to the IIIa pyrimidine tract. However, U2 snRNP binding to the branch point is required for 3VDE function (Muhlemann *et al.*, 2000). In our working hypothesis we predict that a not yet identified component, the 3VDE interacting factor, 3VDF, replaces U2AF as the pyrimidine tract recognition factor, and participates in the recruitment of U2 snRNP to the IIIa branch site. As discussed below, the viral L4-33K protein appears to be the viral component of 3VDF.

3.2 L4-33K is a Virus-Encoded Alternative RNA Splicing Factor

As mentioned, the expression of the L4 unit of mRNAs precedes the activation of IIIa splicing and the accumulation of the full set of mRNAs from the MLTU. This burst in L4 mRNA accumulation results in the production of several proteins of which two are of special interest for this review: the L4-33K and L4-22K proteins. The L4-22K and L4-33K mRNAs differ in that the L4-33K mRNA has an additional intron removed (Figure 2). This splicing event causes a translational frame-shift resulting in the production of two related proteins that share the first 106 amino acids, but have unique C-terminal ends. The key observation that renewed the interest in L4-33K was the demonstration that this protein leads to cytoplasmic accumulation of late mRNAs, thus indicating that this protein is a key component for the early-to-late switch in adenovirus late gene expression (Farley *et al.*, 2004). Several previous reports have also indicated that L4-33K might be important and function as a virus assembly factor (Fessler & Young, 1999; Finnen *et al.*, 2001; Kulshreshtha *et al.*, 2004). Thus, by introducing stop codons in the unique C-terminal part of the protein, the production of infectious virus particles failed completely (Finnen *et al.*, 2001). In addition, L4-33K has been suggested to bind directly to the packaging domain of the viral genome and also to function as a transcription factor stimulating the MLP (Ali *et al.*, 2007).

It should also be mentioned that the L4-22K protein has similar functions, as it binds to the viral packaging sequence (Ostapchuk *et al.*, 2006) and appears to stimulate MLP transcription by binding to the enhancer element located approximately 100 nucleotides downstream of the MLP (Ostapchuk *et al.*, 2006; Morris & Leppard, 2009; Backstrom *et al.*, 2010). In addition, L4-22K stimulates accumulation of a selected set of late mRNAs (Morris & Leppard, 2009), suggesting a possible role for the protein in RNA processing. In conclusion, L4-22K and L4-33K seem to have redundant or complementary effects on late mRNA production, and both proteins appear to have important roles in the early-to-late switch in MLTU expression. However, the exact roles of the two proteins are still debated and will need further investigation. Despite this, it is well established that L4-33K has splicing enhancer activity and acts as a strong activator of L1 alternative splicing both *in vitro* and in transient transfection assays (Tormanen *et al.*, 2006; Backstrom *et al.*, 2010; Ostberg *et al.*, 2012). In fact L4-33K appears to be the key regulator of L1 alternative splicing since expression of this protein alone is sufficient to shift the L1 alternative splicing pattern to the same as observed in an adenovirus-infected cell (Tormanen *et al.*, 2006).

L4-33K activates L1-IIIa splicing primarily through the 3VDE making this protein the leading candidate of being the unknown 3VDF, or at least the viral component of the 3VDF. In agreement with this, L4-33K preferentially activates transcripts with weak 3' splice sites, the sequence context typical for many of the 3' splice sites in the MLTU that are activated at the late stage of infection (Tormanen *et al.*, 2006). The unique C-terminus of L4-33K is highly conserved between human and animal adenoviruses and has been shown to be the domain functioning as the L1-IIIa splicing enhancer domain *in vitro* (Tormanen *et al.*, 2006). Interestingly, this splicing domain contains a tiny RS repeat that is important for L4-33K function (Figure 4). Interestingly, this feature makes L4-33K slightly related to the SR family of splicing factors (Bourgeois *et al.*, 2004; Shepard & Hertel, 2009). However, it should be noted that L4-33K is not a classical SR protein, since the RS domain is much shorter than required (Manley & Krainer, 2010). A L4-33K deletion mutant lacking the tiny RS-repeat makes L4-33K unable to activate splicing (Tormanen *et al.*, 2006). Furthermore, substitution of the serines to glycines in the tiny RS-repeat suggested that the serines may serve redundant functions, and that Serine[192] is essential for the L4-33K splicing enhancer function (Tormanen *et al.*, 2006; Ostberg *et al.*, 2012). Interestingly, L4-33K localizes to the nuclear margin in uninfected cells. During infection the L4-33K protein relocalizes to the periphery of the viral replication centers. Further, deleting the tiny RS repeat or mutating Ser[192], results in a failure of the protein to redistribute to the viral replication centers (Ostberg *et al.*, 2012).

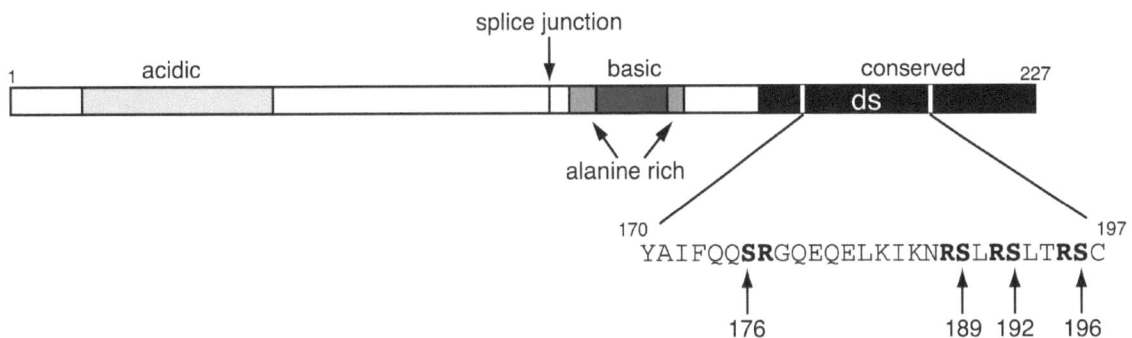

Figure 4: A schematic drawing of the L4-33K protein showing different motifs with an expansion of the 28 carboxyl-terminal amino acids corresponding to the so-called ds region. The tiny RS repeat is shown with bold amino acids in the sequence and the specific serines are indicated with their positional numbers.

To our knowledge there is only one report describing another protein with a functional tiny RS repeat. The human lamin B receptor protein has four small RS repeats that are phosphorylated by SRPK1, and this phosphorylation induces a conformational change in the protein that appears to be necessary for lamin B receptor interaction with histone H3 (Sellis *et al.*, 2012).

3.3   DNA-PK and PKA Phosphorylate L4-33K and Have Opposite Effects on L1 Alternative RNA Splicing

L4-33K is the major phosphoprotein expressed during an adenovirus infection (Axelrod, 1978). This has led to our search for protein kinases that phosphorylate L4-33K with the hope of establishing an experimental system where reversible phosphorylation controlling alternative RNA splicing could be studied. This has so far resulted in the identification of two cellular protein kinases, DNA-PK and PKA, that phosphorylates L4-33K and have opposite impact on L1 alternative splicing (Tormanen *et al.*, 2012).

The L4-33K protein specifically associates with DNA-PKcs in pull down assays, but more importantly also during a lytic adenovirus infection. This interaction did not involve the two Ku regulatory subunits. Also, the L4-33K protein is highly phosphorylated by DNA-PK *in vitro* in a double stranded DNA-independent manner. The Ku subunits are required for DNA-PKcs recruitment to DNA double strand breaks. The failure to find a binding between L4-33K and the Ku subunits is therefore in agreement with the observation that DNA-PK phosphorylation of L4-33K is double- tranded DNA-independent. This is an unusual but not unique property of DNA-PK (Zhang *et al.*, 2004; Yaneva *et al.*, 1997; Oyama *et al.*, 2009; Nock *et al.*, 2009). Although L4-33K is an excellent substrate for PKA phosphorylation *in vitro* a stable interaction between the two proteins could not be demonstrated (Tormanen *et al.*, 2012). The interaction may therefore be indirect or alternatively occur via a hit and run mechanism, which is not entirely unexpected, since a stable interaction between PKA and its substrate proteins has only been described for a handful of the more than hundred characterized PKA substrate proteins (Shabb, 2001). Interestingly, both protein kinases seem to phosphorylate L4-33K within the unique C-terminal splicing enhancer domain, suggesting that these phosphorylation events may have regulatory effects. In the case of DNA-PK the predominant phosphorylation was further shown to reside within a short peptide containing the tiny RS repeat, which is essential for function.

Perhaps the most interesting finding was that both kinases have a regulatory effect on the early to late shift in L1 alternative RNA splicing, with DNA-PK functioning as an inhibitor of the splicesite shift and PKA as an activator of L1-IIIa mRNA splicing. In these experiments, DNA-PKcs deficient cells showed a strong enhancement of L1-IIIa mRNA accumulation. These experiments were done using adenovirus infected cells. This adds another layer of complexity to the interpretation of the results since adenovirus encodes for additional proteins, like E4-ORF4 that may complicate the observed changes in the L1 splicing phenotype. Also, two other adenoviral proteins, E4-ORF3 and E4-ORF6, associate with DNA-PK. Thus, the linear adenovirus genome is recognized as a double stranded break by the Mre11-Rad50-Nbs1 (MRN) complex DNA repair system, leading to accumulation of concatemers of the viral genome (Weiden & Ginsberg, 1994; Weitzman & Ornelles, 2005). E4-ORF3 and E4-ORF6 by binding to DNA-PK block this genome concatenation (Weiden & Ginsberg, 1994; Boyer *et al.*, 1999). E4-ORF3 and E4-ORF6 also function as alternative RNA splicing factors *in vivo*. E4-ORF3 stimulates tripartite leader splicing by facilitating i-leader exon inclusion, whereas E4-ORF6 favors i-leader exon skipping (Nordqvist *et al.*, 1994). However, more recently we have reproduced the DNA-PKcs activation of L1-IIIa mRNA splicing in L4-33K transfection experiments (unpublished), making it more likely that the effect of DNA-PKcs on L4-33K activation of splicing is more direct. The effect of PKA on L4-33K activated L1-IIIa mRNA splicing is major. Although impressive, there are reasons to suspect that the PKA effect might be complex as a stable interaction could not be detected and that the multiple effects of PKA on RNA splicing in most cases seem to be mediated by intermediary factors. Therefore, PKA phosphorylation of L4-33K may, for example, change the subcellular localization of the protein or the ability of the protein to interact with other proteins or RNA, as is the case with GPKOW and SRSF1 rather than having a direct effect on L1 alternative splicing. These are examples of questions that need to be addressed experimentally to clarify the function of L4-33K in the control of alternative RNA splicing.

Surprisingly, PKA also had a marked effect on total L1 mRNA accumulation, suggesting a possible function of PKA as a MLP transcription factor. This effect on transcription was not expected since the MLP promoter does not contain an identifiable CRE binding site (Bosilevac *et al.*, 1998). However, it is known that the catalytic subunit of PKA activates other transcription factors, such as the p65 Rel component of the NFκB-complex (Zhong *et al.*, 1997) and Heat shock transcription factor 1 (HSF1) (Murshid *et al.*, 2010). Whether any of these factors, or other PKA regulated transcription factors, yet to be identified, regulate the MLP remains to be investigated.

The cAMP/PKA signaling pathway has previously been shown to play an important role at multiple stages of the adenovirus life cycle. For example, PKA has been shown to facilitate the microtubule-mediated nuclear targeting of the partially dismantled virus capsid (Suomalainen *et al.*, 2001). Further, the RIIα subunit of PKA interacts with the adenoviral EIA-12S protein, which appears to function as a viral AKAP. RIIα has been reported to be redistributed from the cytoplasm to the nucleus during infection and appears to be involved in EIA-12S-mediated activation of the adenoviral E2 promoter (Fax *et al.*, 2001). In addition, the adenoviral E1A, E2A, E3 and E4 promoters contain CRE elements and are PKA responsive (Gilchrist *et al.*, 1996). As discussed above, PKA, by phosphorylating L4-33K, probably contributes to the induction of the early to late shift in adenovirus gene expression. It is also noteworthy that that we have previously shown that the C- but not the R- subunit of PKA interacts with homologous to AKAP95 (HA95) (Han *et al.*, 2002). HA95 which is a nuclear protein, is involved in regulation of adenovirus E1A pre-mRNA splicing (Kvissel *et al.*, 2007b; Orstavik *et al.*, 2000).

Ad5 DNA replication has also been reported to be sensitive to PKA activity, as shown by the fact that the adenylyl cyclase activator forskolin enhances and the PKA inhibitor H-89 decreases viral DNA replication (Di & Chiorini, 2003). Interestingly, the Adeno-associated virus 2 (AAV2), which depend on a helper virus for a productive infection, inhibits adenovirus DNA replication by expressing two viral proteins Rep 78 and Rep 52. Rep78 and 52 both interact with the PKA C subunit via a domain similar to that of its endogenous nuclear inhibitor, PKI. This may suggest that they inhibit PKA enzyme activity and contribute to explain how AAV2 promotes its own replication (Di & Chiorini, 2003).

A possible link between DNA-PK and PKA has been reported for the Epstein Barr virus (EBV) protein EBNA-LP, which is a co-activator of EBNA-2-mediated transcription. EBNA-LP binds to several cellular proteins, including DNA-PKcs, HA95 and the PKA C subunit (Han *et al.*, 2002; Han *et al.*, 2001). It is therefore possible that HA95 in EBV infected cells may function as a scaffold for EBNA-LP, DNA-PKcs, PKA C and other proteins involved in virus-mediated transcriptional activation. Potentially a similar multiprotein complex orchestrated by L4-33K may exist in an adenovirus-infected cell. This is supported by the observation that over-expression of the PKA C subunit or HA95 down-regulates the expression of the EBV latent membrane protein 1 (LMP1) in EBV-infected cells. It has also been proposed that the PKA C subunit becomes localized to nuclear sites by HA95 and EBNA-LP where it can affect transcription from specific promoters (Han *et al.*, 2002). In addition, PKA appears to directly regulate DNA-PK localization by promoting the nuclear entry of DNA-PK, probably by phosphorylation of Ser[1790] (Huston *et al.*, 2008). In summary, it seems likely that large protein complexes exist, which are important in regulating the adenoviral life cycle, here illustrated by a potential PKA/DNA-PK/L4-33K regulatory loop.

3.4   A Model for the Regulation of IIIa 3' Splice Site Activation

Figure 5 shows a model integrating current knowledge of how IIIa 3' splice site activation might be controlled during an infection.

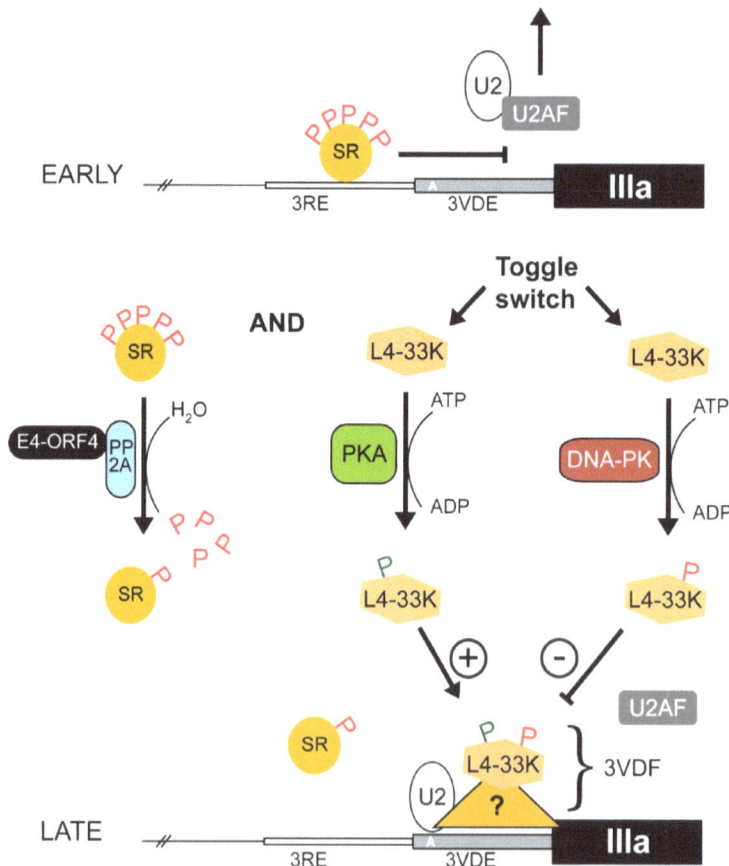

Figure 5: A hypothetical model for the temporal control of L1 alternative splicing. The black box represents the IIIa exon. Thin boxes, white and gray, indicate the position of the 3RE and 3VDE respectively, and the thin line the rest of the intron. Cellular factors are labelled accordingly SR proteins (SR), U2 snRNP (U2), U2 auxiliary factor (U2AF), Protein phosphatase 2A (PP2A), Protein kinase A (PKA), DNA-dependent protein kinase (DNA-PK), unknown protein of viral or host origin (?) and viral factors by their names. Phosphorylation is indicated by addition of phosphate group (P) to the substrate factor and dephosphorylation by loss of P.

At early times of infection highly phosphorylated SR proteins binds to the 3RE and block U2 snRNP recruitment to the IIIa branch site. Further, the IIIa pyrimidine tract is weak and does not efficiently bind U2AF. Late after infection, the E4-ORF4/PP2A protein complex induces a partial SR protein dephosphorylation, which relieves the inhibitory effect of SR proteins on IIIa splicing. Activation of IIIa splicing is further controlled by the key viral L4-33K protein, which form part of the 3VDF factor, which binds to the 3VDE and stimulates U2 snRNP recruitment to the IIIa 3' splice site. The composition of 3VDF is currently not known. Since we have not been able to demonstrate that L4-33K binds directly to the 3VDE we speculate that the 3VDF also contain an unknown cellular RNA binding factor that makes direct contact with the 3VDE. Considering the toggle switch-like mechanism described here for the PKA and DNA-PK regulated shifts in L1 alternative splicing, we appear to have a unique possibility to study the significance of reversible protein phosphorylation as a mechanism controlling alternative RNA splicing. For instance, we need to identify the critical amino acids phosphorylated by PKA and DNA-PK to be able to study the interplay between a positive and a negative phosphorylation event. How does this affect the structure of the protein? Are there additional protein kinases and protein phosphatases that have a regulatory role in L1 alternative splicing? The future presents us with several exiting possibilities that we are looking forward to explore.

Acknowledgements

The work done in our laboratories were made possible by generous grants from the Swedish Cancer Society, the Uppsala RNA Research Centre, EURASNET, The Norwegian Cancer Society, grants 419114 and 418817 and the Throne Holst Foundation, University of Oslo.

References

Aksaas, A. K., Eikvar, S., Akusjarvi, G., Skalhegg, B. S., & Kvissel, A. K. (2011a). Protein kinase a-dependent phosphorylation of serine 119 in the proto-oncogenic serine/arginine-rich splicing factor 1 modulates its activity as a splicing enhancer protein. Genes and Cancer, 2, 841-851.

Aksaas, A. K., Larsen, A. C., Rogne, M., Rosendal, K., Kvissel, A. K., & Skalhegg, B. S. (2011b). G-patch domain and KOW motifs-containing protein, GPKOW; a nuclear RNA-binding protein regulated by protein kinase A. J.Mol.Signal., 6, 10.

Akusjarvi, G. (2008). Temporal regulation of adenovirus major late alternative RNA splicing. Front Biosci., 13, 5006-5015.

Akusjarvi, G. & Persson, H. (1981). Controls of RNA splicing and termination in the major late adenovirus transcription unit. Nature, 292, 420-426.

Akusjarvi, G. & Stevenin, J. (2003). Remodelling of the host cell RNA splicing machinery during an adenovirus infection. Curr.Top.Microbiol.Immunol., 272, 253-286.

Ali, H., LeRoy, G., Bridge, G., & Flint, S. J. (2007). The adenovirus L4 33-kilodalton protein binds to intragenic sequences of the major late promoter required for late phase-specific stimulation of transcription. J.Virol., 81, 1327-1338.

Aspegren, A., Rabino, C., & Bridge, E. (1998). Organization of splicing factors in adenovirus-infected cells reflects changes in gene expression during the early to late phase transition. Exp.Cell Res., 245, 203-213.

Auweter, S. D., Oberstrass, F. C., & Allain, F. H. (2006). Sequence-specific binding of single-stranded RNA: is there a code for recognition? Nucleic Acids Res., 34, 4943-4959.

Axelrod, N. (1978). Phosphoproteins of adenovirus 2. Virology, 87, 366-383.

Backstrom, E., Kaufmann, K. B., Lan, X., & Akusjarvi, G. (2010). Adenovirus L4-22K stimulates major late transcription by a mechanism requiring the intragenic late-specific transcription factor-binding site. Virus Res., 151, 220-228.

Barbe, L., Lundberg, E., Oksvold, P., Stenius, A., Lewin, E., Bjorling, E. et al. (2008). Toward a confocal subcellular atlas of the human proteome. Mol.Cell Proteomics., 7, 499-508.

Berget, S. M., Moore, C., & Sharp, P. A. (1977). Spliced segments at the 5' terminus of adenovirus 2 late mRNA. Proc.Natl.Acad.Sci.U.S.A, 74, 3171-3175.

Berke, J. D., Sgambato, V., Zhu, P. P., Lavoie, B., Vincent, M., Krause, M. et al. (2001). Dopamine and glutamate induce distinct striatal splice forms of Ania-6, an RNA polymerase II-associated cyclin. Neuron, 32, 277-287.

Black, D. L. (2003). Mechanisms of alternative pre-messenger RNA splicing. Annu.Rev.Biochem., 72, 291-336.

Blaustein, M., Pelisch, F., Tanos, T., Munoz, M. J., Wengier, D., Quadrana, L. et al. (2005). Concerted regulation of nuclear and cytoplasmic activities of SR proteins by AKT. Nat.Struct.Mol.Biol., 12, 1037-1044.

Blencowe, B. J., Bowman, J. A., McCracken, S., & Rosonina, E. (1999). SR-related proteins and the processing of messenger RNA precursors. Biochem.Cell Biol., 77, 277-291.

Bondesson, M., Ohman, K., Manervik, M., Fan, S., & Akusjarvi, G. (1996). Adenovirus E4 open reading frame 4 protein autoregulates E4 transcription by inhibiting E1A transactivation of the E4 promoter. J.Virol., 70, 3844-3851.

Bosilevac, J. M., Gilchrist, C. A., Jankowski, P. E., Paul, S., Rees, A. R., & Hinrichs, S. H. (1998). Inhibition of activating transcription factor 1- and cAMP-responsive element-binding protein-activated transcription by an intracellular single chain Fv fragment. J.Biol.Chem., 273, 16874-16879.

Bourgeois, C. F., Lejeune, F., & Stevenin, J. (2004). Broad specificity of SR (serine/arginine) proteins in the regulation of alternative splicing of pre-messenger RNA. Prog.Nucleic Acid Res.Mol.Biol., 78, 37-88.

Boyer, J., Rohleder, K., & Ketner, G. (1999). Adenovirus E4 34k and E4 11k inhibit double strand break repair and are physically associated with the cellular DNA-dependent protein kinase. Virology, 263, 307-312.

Branton, P. E. & Roopchand, D. E. (2001). The role of adenovirus E4orf4 protein in viral replication and cell killing. Oncogene, 20, 7855-7865.

Bridge, E., Mattsson, K., Aspegren, A., & Sengupta, A. (2003). Adenovirus early region 4 promotes the localization of splicing factors and viral RNA in late-phase interchromatin granule clusters. Virology, 311, 40-50.

Bridge, E., Xia, D. X., Carmo-Fonseca, M., Cardinali, B., Lamond, A. I., & Pettersson, U. (1995). Dynamic organization of splicing factors in adenovirus-infected cells. J.Virol., 69, 281-290.

Caceres, J. F. & Krainer, A. R. (1993). Functional analysis of pre-mRNA splicing factor SF2/ASF structural domains. EMBO J., 12, 4715-4726.

Caceres, J. F., Misteli, T., Screaton, G. R., Spector, D. L., & Krainer, A. R. (1997). Role of the modular domains of SR proteins in subnuclear localization and alternative splicing specificity. J.Cell Biol., 138, 225-238.

Caceres, J. F., Screaton, G. R., & Krainer, A. R. (1998). A specific subset of SR proteins shuttles continuously between the nucleus and the cytoplasm. Genes Dev., 12, 55-66.

Cao, W., Jamison, S. F., & Garcia-Blanco, M. A. (1997). Both phosphorylation and dephosphorylation of ASF/SF2 are required for pre-mRNA splicing in vitro. RNA., 3, 1456-1467.

Carter, T., Vancurova, I., Sun, I., Lou, W., & DeLeon, S. (1990). A DNA-activated protein kinase from HeLa cell nuclei. Mol.Cell Biol., 10, 6460-6471.

Cassola, A., Noe, G., & Frasch, A. C. (2010). RNA recognition motifs involved in nuclear import of RNA-binding proteins. RNA.Biol., 7, 339-344.

Cazalla, D., Zhu, J., Manche, L., Huber, E., Krainer, A. R., & Caceres, J. F. (2002). Nuclear export and retention signals in the RS domain of SR proteins. Mol.Cell Biol., 22, 6871-6882.

Chalfant, C. E., Ogretmen, B., Galadari, S., Kroesen, B. J., Pettus, B. J., & Hannun, Y. A. (2001). FAS activation induces dephosphorylation of SR proteins; dependence on the de novo generation of ceramide and activation of protein phosphatase 1. J.Biol.Chem., 276, 44848-44855.

Chen, M. & Manley, J. L. (2009). Mechanisms of alternative splicing regulation: insights from molecular and genomics approaches. Nat.Rev.Mol.Cell Biol., 10, 741-754.

Chen, T., Damaj, B. B., Herrera, C., Lasko, P., & Richard, S. (1997). Self-association of the single-KH-domain family members Sam68, GRP33, GLD-1, and Qk1: role of the KH domain. Mol.Cell Biol., 17, 5707-5718.

Cho, S., Hoang, A., Sinha, R., Zhong, X. Y., Fu, X. D., Krainer, A. R. et al. (2011). Interaction between the RNA binding domains of Ser-Arg splicing factor 1 and U1-70K snRNP protein determines early spliceosome assembly. Proc.Natl.Acad.Sci.U.S.A, 108, 8233-8238.

Chow, L. T., Gelinas, R. E., Broker, T. R., & Roberts, R. J. (1977). An amazing sequence arrangement at the 5' ends of adenovirus 2 messenger RNA. Cell, 12, 1-8.

Coller, J. M., Gray, N. K., & Wickens, M. P. (1998). mRNA stabilization by poly(A) binding protein is independent of poly(A) and requires translation. Genes Dev., 12, 3226-3235.

Collins, C. A. & Guthrie, C. (2000). The question remains: is the spliceosome a ribozyme? Nat.Struct.Biol., 7, 850-854.

Collis, S. J., DeWeese, T. L., Jeggo, P. A., & Parker, A. R. (2005). The life and death of DNA-PK. Oncogene, 24, 949-961.

Colwill, K., Pawson, T., Andrews, B., Prasad, J., Manley, J. L., Bell, J. C. et al. (1996). The Clk/Sty protein kinase phosphorylates SR splicing factors and regulates their intranuclear distribution. EMBO J., 15, 265-275.

Corbin, J. D., Keely, S. L., & Park, C. R. (1975). The distribution and dissociation of cyclic adenosine 3':5'-monophosphate-dependent protein kinases in adipose, cardiac, and other tissues. J.Biol.Chem., 250, 218-225.

Cowper, A. E., Caceres, J. F., Mayeda, A., & Screaton, G. R. (2001). Serine-arginine (SR) protein-like factors that antagonize authentic SR proteins and regulate alternative splicing. J.Biol.Chem., 276, 48908-48914.

Czudnochowski, N., Bosken, C. A., & Geyer, M. (2012). Serine-7 but not serine-5 phosphorylation primes RNA polymerase II CTD for P-TEFb recognition. Nat.Commun., 3, 842.

Daniel, P. B., Walker, W. H., & Habener, J. F. (1998). Cyclic AMP signaling and gene regulation. Annu.Rev.Nutr., 18, 353-383.

Das, R., Yu, J., Zhang, Z., Gygi, M. P., Krainer, A. R., Gygi, S. P. et al. (2007). SR proteins function in coupling RNAP II transcription to pre-mRNA splicing. Mol.Cell, 26, 867-881.

Dauksaite, V. & Akusjarvi, G. (2002). Human splicing factor ASF/SF2 encodes for a repressor domain required for its inhibitory activity on pre-mRNA splicing. J.Biol.Chem., 277, 12579-12586.

de la Mata, M., Alonso, C. R., Kadener, S., Fededa, J. P., Blaustein, M., Pelisch, F. et al. (2003). A slow RNA polymerase II affects alternative splicing in vivo. Mol.Cell, 12, 525-532.

Delestienne, N., Wauquier, C., Soin, R., Dierick, J. F., Gueydan, C., & Kruys, V. (2010). The splicing factor ASF/SF2 is associated with TIA-1-related/TIA-1-containing ribonucleoproteic complexes and contributes to post-transcriptional repression of gene expression. FEBS J., 277, 2496-2514.

Di, P. G. & Chiorini, J. A. (2003). PKA/PrKX activity is a modulator of AAV/adenovirus interaction. EMBO J., 22, 1716-1724.

Dolph, P. J., Racaniello, V., Villamarin, A., Palladino, F., & Schneider, R. J. (1988). The adenovirus tripartite leader may eliminate the requirement for cap-binding protein complex during translation initiation. J.Virol., 62, 2059-2066.

Edmond, V., Moysan, E., Khochbin, S., Matthias, P., Brambilla, C., Brambilla, E. et al. (2011). Acetylation and phosphorylation of SRSF2 control cell fate decision in response to cisplatin. EMBO J., 30, 510-523.

Estmer, N. C., Petersen-Mahrt, S., Durot, C., Shtrichman, R., Krainer, A. R., Kleinberger, T. et al. (2001). The adenovirus E4-ORF4 splicing enhancer protein interacts with a subset of phosphorylated SR proteins. EMBO J., 20, 864-871.

Farley, D. C., Brown, J. L., & Leppard, K. N. (2004). Activation of the early-late switch in adenovirus type 5 major late transcription unit expression by L4 gene products. J.Virol., 78, 1782-1791.

Fax, P., Carlson, C. R., Collas, P., Tasken, K., Esche, H., & Brockmann, D. (2001). Binding of PKA-RIIalpha to the Adenovirus E1A12S oncoprotein correlates with its nuclear translocation and an increase in PKA-dependent promoter activity. Virology, 285, 30-41.

Fessler, S. P. & Young, C. S. (1999). The role of the L4 33K gene in adenovirus infection. Virology, 263, 507-516.

Finnen, R. L., Biddle, J. F., & Flint, J. (2001). Truncation of the human adenovirus type 5 L4 33-kDa protein: evidence for an essential role of the carboxy-terminus in the viral infectious cycle. Virology, 289, 388-399.

Flint, S. J. (2004). Principles of virology. (vols. 2nd ed.) Washington, D.C.: ASM Press.

Fluhr, R. (2008). Regulation of splicing by protein phosphorylation. Curr.Top.Microbiol.Immunol., 326, 119-138.

Ford, L. P., Bagga, P. S., & Wilusz, J. (1997). The poly(A) tail inhibits the assembly of a 3'-to-5' exonuclease in an in vitro RNA stability system. Mol.Cell Biol., 17, 398-406.

Fu, X. D. (1995). The superfamily of arginine/serine-rich splicing factors. RNA., 1, 663-680.

Furuichi, Y., LaFiandra, A., & Shatkin, A. J. (1977). 5'-Terminal structure and mRNA stability. Nature, 266, 235-239.

Gama-Carvalho, M., Condado, I., & Carmo-Fonseca, M. (2003). Regulation of adenovirus alternative RNA splicing correlates with a reorganization of splicing factors in the nucleus. Exp.Cell Res., 289, 77-85.

Ghigna, C., Valacca, C., & Biamonti, G. (2008). Alternative splicing and tumor progression. Curr.Genomics, 9, 556-570.

Ghosh, G. & Adams, J. A. (2011). Phosphorylation mechanism and structure of serine-arginine protein kinases. FEBS J., 278, 587-597.

Gilchrist, C. A., Orten, D. J., & Hinrichs, S. H. (1996). Evidence for the Role of Cyclic AMP-Responsive Elements in Human Virus Replication and Disease. J.Biomed.Sci., 3, 293-306.

Ginsberg, M. D., Feliciello, A., Jones, J. K., Avvedimento, E. V., & Gottesman, M. E. (2003). PKA-dependent binding of mRNA to the mitochondrial AKAP121 protein. J.Mol.Biol., 327, 885-897.

Gottlieb, T. M. & Jackson, S. P. (1993). The DNA-dependent protein kinase: requirement for DNA ends and association with Ku antigen. Cell, 72, 131-142.

Graveley, B. R. (2000). Sorting out the complexity of SR protein functions. RNA., 6, 1197-1211.

Gu, J., Shi, J., Wu, S., Jin, N., Qian, W., Zhou, J. et al. (2012). Cyclic AMP-dependent protein kinase regulates 9G8-mediated alternative splicing of tau exon 10. FEBS Lett., 586, 2239-2244.

Gu, Q., Jin, N., Sheng, H., Yin, X., & Zhu, J. (2011). Cyclic AMP-dependent protein kinase a regulates the alternative splicing of CaMKIIdelta. PLoS.One., 6, e25745.

Gustin, K. E. & Imperiale, M. J. (1998). Encapsidation of viral DNA requires the adenovirus L1 52/55-kilodalton protein. J.Virol., 72, 7860-7870.

Guth, S., Martinez, C., Gaur, R. K., & Valcarcel, J. (1999). Evidence for substrate-specific requirement of the splicing factor U2AF(35) and for its function after polypyrimidine tract recognition by U2AF(65). Mol.Cell Biol., 19, 8263-8271.

Han, I., Harada, S., Weaver, D., Xue, Y., Lane, W., Orstavik, S. et al. (2001). EBNA-LP associates with cellular proteins including DNA-PK and HA95. J.Virol., 75, 2475-2481.

Han, I., Xue, Y., Harada, S., Orstavik, S., Skalhegg, B., & Kieff, E. (2002). Protein kinase A associates with HA95 and affects transcriptional coactivation by Epstein-Barr virus nuclear proteins. Mol.Cell Biol., 22, 2136-2146.

Hegele, A., Kamburov, A., Grossmann, A., Sourlis, C., Wowro, S., Weimann, M. et al. (2012). Dynamic protein-protein interaction wiring of the human spliceosome. Mol.Cell, 45, 567-580.

Hirose, Y. & Ohkuma, Y. (2007). Phosphorylation of the C-terminal domain of RNA polymerase II plays central roles in the integrated events of eucaryotic gene expression. J.Biochem., 141, 601-608.

Huang, T. S., Nilsson, C. E., Punga, T., & Akusjarvi, G. (2002). Functional inactivation of the SR family of splicing factors during a vaccinia virus infection. EMBO Rep., 3, 1088-1093.

Huang, Y., Yario, T. A., & Steitz, J. A. (2004). A molecular link between SR protein dephosphorylation and mRNA export. Proc.Natl.Acad.Sci.U.S.A, 101, 9666-9670.

Huston, E., Lynch, M. J., Mohamed, A., Collins, D. M., Hill, E. V., MacLeod, R. et al. (2008). EPAC and PKA allow cAMP dual control over DNA-PK nuclear translocation. Proc.Natl.Acad.Sci.U.S.A, 105, 12791-12796.

International Human Genome Sequencing Consortium (2004). Finishing the euchromatic sequence of the human genome. Nature, 431, 931-945.

Jackson, S. P. & Jeggo, P. A. (1995). DNA double-strand break repair and V(D)J recombination: involvement of DNA-PK. Trends Biochem.Sci., 20, 412-415.

James, N. J., Howell, G. J., Walker, J. H., & Blair, G. E. (2010). The role of Cajal bodies in the expression of late phase adenovirus proteins. Virology, 399, 299-311.

Jarnaess, E., Stokka, A. J., Kvissel, A. K., Skalhegg, B. S., Torgersen, K. M., Scott, J. D. et al. (2009). Splicing factor arginine/serine-rich 17A (SFRS17A) is an A-kinase anchoring protein that targets protein kinase A to splicing factor compartments. J.Biol.Chem., 284, 35154-35164.

Kanj, S. S., Dandashi, N., El-Hed, A., Harik, H., Maalouf, M., Kozhaya, L. et al. (2006). Ceramide regulates SR protein phosphorylation during adenoviral infection. Virology, 345, 280-289.

Kanopka, A., Muhlemann, O., & Akusjarvi, G. (1996). Inhibition by SR proteins of splicing of a regulated adenovirus pre-mRNA. Nature, 381, 535-538.

Kanopka, A., Muhlemann, O., Petersen-Mahrt, S., Estmer, C., Ohrmalm, C., & Akusjarvi, G. (1998). Regulation of adenovirus alternative RNA splicing by dephosphorylation of SR proteins. Nature, 393, 185-187.

Kataoka, N., Bachorik, J. L., & Dreyfuss, G. (1999). Transportin-SR, a nuclear import receptor for SR proteins. J.Cell Biol., 145, 1145-1152.

Keith, C. T. & Schreiber, S. L. (1995). PIK-related kinases: DNA repair, recombination, and cell cycle checkpoints. Science, 270, 50-51.

Khanna, A. & Stamm, S. (2010). Regulation of alternative splicing by short non-coding nuclear RNAs. RNA.Biol., 7, 480-485.

Kielkopf, C. L., Rodionova, N. A., Green, M. R., & Burley, S. K. (2001). A novel peptide recognition mode revealed by the X-ray structure of a core U2AF35/U2AF65 heterodimer. Cell, 106, 595-605.

Kim, H., Erickson, B., Luo, W., Seward, D., Graber, J. H., Pollock, D. D. et al. (2010). Gene-specific RNA polymerase II phosphorylation and the CTD code. Nat.Struct.Mol.Biol., 17, 1279-1286.

Kleinberger, T. & Shenk, T. (1993). Adenovirus E4orf4 protein binds to protein phosphatase 2A, and the complex down regulates E1A-enhanced junB transcription. J.Virol., 67, 7556-7560.

Kohtz, J. D., Jamison, S. F., Will, C. L., Zuo, P., Luhrmann, R., Garcia-Blanco, M. A. et al. (1994). Protein-protein interactions and 5'-splice-site recognition in mammalian mRNA precursors. Nature, 368, 119-124.

Koizumi, J., Okamoto, Y., Onogi, H., Mayeda, A., Krainer, A. R., & Hagiwara, M. (1999). The subcellular localization of SF2/ASF is regulated by direct interaction with SR protein kinases (SRPKs). J.Biol.Chem., 274, 11125-11131.

Kolasinska-Zwierz, P., Down, T., Latorre, I., Liu, T., Liu, X. S., & Ahringer, J. (2009). Differential chromatin marking of introns and expressed exons by H3K36me3. Nat.Genet., 41, 376-381.

Kornitzer, D., Sharf, R., & Kleinberger, T. (2001). Adenovirus E4orf4 protein induces PP2A-dependent growth arrest in Saccharomyces cerevisiae and interacts with the anaphase-promoting complex/cyclosome. J.Cell Biol., 154, 331-344.

Kulshreshtha, V., Babiuk, L. A., & Tikoo, S. K. (2004). Role of bovine adenovirus-3 33K protein in viral replication. Virology, 323, 59-69.

Kvissel, A. K., Orstavik, S., Eikvar, S., Brede, G., Jahnsen, T., Collas, P. et al. (2007a). Involvement of the catalytic subunit of protein kinase A and of HA95 in pre-mRNA splicing. Exp.Cell Res., 313, 2795-2809.

Kvissel, A. K., Ramberg, H., Eide, T., Svindland, A., Skalhegg, B. S., & Tasken, K. A. (2007b). Androgen dependent regulation of protein kinase A subunits in prostate cancer cells. Cell Signal., 19, 401-409.

Lai, M. C., Lin, R. I., Huang, S. Y., Tsai, C. W., & Tarn, W. Y. (2000). A human importin-beta family protein, transportin-SR2, interacts with the phosphorylated RS domain of SR proteins. J.Biol.Chem., 275, 7950-7957.

Lai, M. C., Lin, R. I., & Tarn, W. Y. (2003). Differential effects of hyperphosphorylation on splicing factor SRp55. Biochem.J., 371, 937-945.

Lai, M. C. & Tarn, W. Y. (2004). Hypophosphorylated ASF/SF2 binds TAP and is present in messenger ribonucleoproteins. J.Biol.Chem., 279, 31745-31749.

Lander, E. S., Linton, L. M., Birren, B., Nusbaum, C., Zody, M. C., Baldwin, J. et al. (2001). Initial sequencing and analysis of the human genome. Nature, 409, 860-921.

Larsson, S., Kreivi, J. P., & Akusjarvi, G. (1991). Control of adenovirus alternative RNA splicing: effect of viral DNA replication on RNA splice site choice. Gene, 107, 219-227.

Larsson, S., Svensson, C., & Akusjarvi, G. (1992). Control of adenovirus major late gene expression at multiple levels. J.Mol.Biol., 225, 287-298.

Lasko, P. (2003). Gene regulation at the RNA layer: RNA binding proteins in intercellular signaling networks. Sci.STKE., 2003, RE6.

Lees-Miller, S. P. (1996). The DNA-dependent protein kinase, DNA-PK: 10 years and no ends in sight. Biochem.Cell Biol., 74, 503-512.

Lees-Miller, S. P., Chen, Y. R., & Anderson, C. W. (1990). Human cells contain a DNA-activated protein kinase that phosphorylates simian virus 40 T antigen, mouse p53, and the human Ku autoantigen. Mol.Cell Biol., 10, 6472-6481.

Lempiainen, H. & Halazonetis, T. D. (2009). Emerging common themes in regulation of PIKKs and PI3Ks. EMBO J., 28, 3067-3073.

Lewin, B. (1980). Structure and evolution of interrupted genes. Ann.N.Y.Acad.Sci., 354, 453-465.

Li, H., Liu, G., Yu, J., Cao, W., Lobo, V. G., & Xie, J. (2009). In vivo selection of kinase-responsive RNA elements controlling alternative splicing. J.Biol.Chem., 284, 16191-16201.

Luco, R. F., Allo, M., Schor, I. E., Kornblihtt, A. R., & Misteli, T. (2011). Epigenetics in alternative pre-mRNA splicing. Cell, 144, 16-26.

Luco, R. F., Pan, Q., Tominaga, K., Blencowe, B. J., Pereira-Smith, O. M., & Misteli, T. (2010). Regulation of alternative splicing by histone modifications. Science, 327, 996-1000.

Lutzelberger, M., Backstrom, E., & Akusjarvi, G. (2005). Substrate-dependent differences in U2AF requirement for splicing in adenovirus-infected cell extracts. J.Biol.Chem., 280, 25478-25484.

Maldonado, E., Shiekhattar, R., Sheldon, M., Cho, H., Drapkin, R., Rickert, P. et al. (1996). A human RNA polymerase II complex associated with SRB and DNA-repair proteins. Nature, 381, 86-89.

Mangs, A. H., Speirs, H. J., Goy, C., Adams, D. J., Markus, M. A., & Morris, B. J. (2006). XE7: a novel splicing factor that interacts with ASF/SF2 and ZNF265. Nucleic Acids Res., 34, 4976-4986.

Manley, J. L. & Krainer, A. R. (2010). A rational nomenclature for serine/arginine-rich protein splicing factors (SR proteins). Genes Dev., 24, 1073-1074.

Manley, J. L. & Tacke, R. (1996). SR proteins and splicing control. Genes Dev., 10, 1569-1579.

Manning, G., Whyte, D. B., Martinez, R., Hunter, T., & Sudarsanam, S. (2002). The protein kinase complement of the human genome. Science, 298, 1912-1934.

Maquat, L. E. (2004). Nonsense-mediated mRNA decay: splicing, translation and mRNP dynamics. Nat.Rev.Mol.Cell Biol., 5, 89-99.

Marcellus, R. C., Lavoie, J. N., Boivin, D., Shore, G. C., Ketner, G., & Branton, P. E. (1998). The early region 4 orf4 protein of human adenovirus type 5 induces p53-independent cell death by apoptosis. J.Virol., 72, 7144-7153.

Matlin, A. J., Clark, F., & Smith, C. W. (2005). Understanding alternative splicing: towards a cellular code. Nat.Rev.Mol.Cell Biol., 6, 386-398.

McCracken, S., Fong, N., Rosonina, E., Yankulov, K., Brothers, G., Siderovski, D. et al. (1997a). 5'-Capping enzymes are targeted to pre-mRNA by binding to the phosphorylated carboxy-terminal domain of RNA polymerase II. Genes Dev., 11, 3306-3318.

McCracken, S., Fong, N., Yankulov, K., Ballantyne, S., Pan, G., Greenblatt, J. et al. (1997b). The C-terminal domain of RNA polymerase II couples mRNA processing to transcription. Nature, 385, 357-361.

Merendino, L., Guth, S., Bilbao, D., Martinez, C., & Valcarcel, J. (1999). Inhibition of msl-2 splicing by Sex-lethal reveals interaction between U2AF35 and the 3' splice site AG. Nature, 402, 838-841.

Molin, M., Bouakaz, L., Berenjian, S., & Akusjarvi, G. (2002). Unscheduled expression of capsid protein IIIa results in defects in adenovirus major late mRNA and protein expression. Virus Res., 83, 197-206.

Moroy, T. & Heyd, F. (2007). The impact of alternative splicing in vivo: mouse models show the way. RNA., 13, 1155-1171.

Morris, S. J. & Leppard, K. N. (2009). Adenovirus serotype 5 L4-22K and L4-33K proteins have distinct functions in regulating late gene expression. J.Virol., 83, 3049-3058.

Muhlemann, O., Kreivi, J. P., & Akusjarvi, G. (1995). Enhanced splicing of nonconsensus 3' splice sites late during adenovirus infection. J.Virol., 69, 7324-7327.

Muhlemann, O., Yue, B. G., Petersen-Mahrt, S., & Akusjarvi, G. (2000). A novel type of splicing enhancer regulating adenovirus pre-mRNA splicing. Mol.Cell Biol., 20, 2317-2325.

Muller, U., Kleinberger, T., & Shenk, T. (1992). Adenovirus E4orf4 protein reduces phosphorylation of c-Fos and E1A proteins while simultaneously reducing the level of AP-1. J.Virol., 66, 5867-5878.

Munoz, M. J., Perez Santangelo, M. S., Paronetto, M. P., de la Mata, M., Pelisch, F., Boireau, S. et al. (2009). DNA damage regulates alternative splicing through inhibition of RNA polymerase II elongation. Cell, 137, 708-720.

Murshid, A., Chou, S. D., Prince, T., Zhang, Y., Bharti, A., & Calderwood, S. K. (2010). Protein kinase A binds and activates heat shock factor 1. PLoS.One., 5, e13830.

Neal, J. A. & Meek, K. (2011). Choosing the right path: does DNA-PK help make the decision? Mutat.Res., 711, 73-86.

Nevins, J. R. & Wilson, M. C. (1981). Regulation of adenovirus-2 gene expression at the level of transcriptional termination and RNA processing. Nature, 290, 113-118.

Ngo, J. C., Chakrabarti, S., Ding, J. H., Velazquez-Dones, A., Nolen, B., Aubol, B. E. et al. (2005). Interplay between SRPK and Clk/Sty kinases in phosphorylation of the splicing factor ASF/SF2 is regulated by a docking motif in ASF/SF2. Mol.Cell, 20, 77-89.

Nilsen, T. W. & Graveley, B. R. (2010). Expansion of the eukaryotic proteome by alternative splicing. Nature, 463, 457-463.

Nock, A., Ascano, J. M., Jones, T., Barrero, M. J., Sugiyama, N., Tomita, M. et al. (2009). Identification of DNA-dependent protein kinase as a cofactor for the forkhead transcription factor FoxA2. J.Biol.Chem., 284, 19915-19926.

Nordqvist, K., Ohman, K., & Akusjarvi, G. (1994). Human adenovirus encodes two proteins which have opposite effects on accumulation of alternatively spliced mRNAs. Mol.Cell Biol., 14, 437-445.

Orstavik, S., Eide, T., Collas, P., Han, I. O., Tasken, K., Kieff, E. et al. (2000). Identification, cloning and characterization of a novel nuclear protein, HA95, homologous to A-kinase anchoring protein 95. Biol.Cell, 92, 27-37.

Ostapchuk, P., Anderson, M. E., Chandrasekhar, S., & Hearing, P. (2006). The L4 22-kilodalton protein plays a role in packaging of the adenovirus genome. J.Virol., 80, 6973-6981.

Ostberg, S., Tormanen, P. H., & Akusjarvi, G. (2012). Serine 192 in the tiny RS repeat of the adenoviral L4-33K splicing enhancer protein is essential for function and reorganization of the protein to the periphery of viral replication centers. Virology, In press.

Oyama, S., Yamakawa, H., Sasagawa, N., Hosoi, Y., Futai, E., & Ishiura, S. (2009). Dysbindin-1, a schizophrenia-related protein, functionally interacts with the DNA- dependent protein kinase complex in an isoform-dependent manner. PLoS.One., 4, e4199.

Patel, N. A., Kaneko, S., Apostolatos, H. S., Bae, S. S., Watson, J. E., Davidowitz, K. et al. (2005). Molecular and genetic studies imply Akt-mediated signaling promotes protein kinase CbetaII alternative splicing via phosphorylation of serine/arginine-rich splicing factor SRp40. J.Biol.Chem., 280, 14302-14309.

Perales, R. & Bentley, D. (2009). "Cotranscriptionality": the transcription elongation complex as a nexus for nuclear transactions. Mol.Cell, 36, 178-191.

Peterson, S. R., Dvir, A., Anderson, C. W., & Dynan, W. S. (1992). DNA binding provides a signal for phosphorylation of the RNA polymerase II heptapeptide repeats. Genes Dev., 6, 426-438.

Pombo, A., Ferreira, J., Bridge, E., & Carmo-Fonseca, M. (1994). Adenovirus replication and transcription sites are spatially separated in the nucleus of infected cells. EMBO J., 13, 5075-5085.

Puvion-Dutilleul, F., Pedron, J., & Cajean-Feroldi, C. (1984). Identification of intranuclear structures containing the 72K DNA-binding protein of human adenovirus type 5. Eur.J.Cell Biol., 34, 313-322.

Puvion-Dutilleul, F., Roussev, R., & Puvion, E. (1992). Distribution of viral RNA molecules during the adenovirus type 5 infectious cycle in HeLa cells. J.Struct.Biol., 108, 209-220.

Ranganathan, G., Phan, D., Pokrovskaya, I. D., McEwen, J. E., Li, C., & Kern, P. A. (2002). The translational regulation of lipoprotein lipase by epinephrine involves an RNA binding complex including the catalytic subunit of protein kinase A. J.Biol.Chem., 277, 43281-43287.

Rho, J., Choi, S., Jung, C. R., & Im, D. S. (2007). Arginine methylation of Sam68 and SLM proteins negatively regulates their poly(U) RNA binding activity. Arch.Biochem.Biophys., 466, 49-57.

Rogne, M., Stokka, A. J., Tasken, K., Collas, P., & Kuntziger, T. (2009). Mutually exclusive binding of PP1 and RNA to AKAP149 affects the mitochondrial network. Hum.Mol.Genet., 18, 978-987.

Rossi, F., Labourier, E., Forne, T., Divita, G., Derancourt, J., Riou, J. F. et al. (1996). Specific phosphorylation of SR proteins by mammalian DNA topoisomerase I. Nature, 381, 80-82.

Ruskin, B., Zamore, P. D., & Green, M. R. (1988). A factor, U2AF, is required for U2 snRNP binding and splicing complex assembly. Cell, 52, 207-219.

Sachs, A. B. (1993). Messenger RNA degradation in eukaryotes. Cell, 74, 413-421.

Sakashita, E. & Endo, H. (2010). SR and SR-related proteins redistribute to segregated fibrillar components of nucleoli in a response to DNA damage. Nucleus., 1, 367-380.

Sapra, A. K., Anko, M. L., Grishina, I., Lorenz, M., Pabis, M., Poser, I. et al. (2009). SR protein family members display diverse activities in the formation of nascent and mature mRNPs in vivo. Mol.Cell, 34, 179-190.

Schild-Poulter, C., Shih, A., Tantin, D., Yarymowich, N. C., Soubeyrand, S., Sharp, P. A. et al. (2007). DNA-PK phosphorylation sites on Oct-1 promote cell survival following DNA damage. Oncogene, 26, 3980-3988.

Sellis, D., Drosou, V., Vlachakis, D., Voukkalis, N., Giannakouros, T., & Vlassi, M. (2012). Phosphorylation of the arginine/serine repeats of lamin B receptor by SRPK1-insights from molecular dynamics simulations. Biochim.Biophys.Acta, 1820, 44-55.

Sgambato, V., Minassian, R., Nairn, A. C., & Hyman, S. E. (2003). Regulation of ania-6 splice variants by distinct signaling pathways in striatal neurons. J.Neurochem., 86, 153-164.

Shabb, J. B. (2001). Physiological substrates of cAMP-dependent protein kinase. Chem.Rev., 101, 2381-2411.

Shaw, A. R. & Ziff, E. B. (1980). Transcripts from the adenovirus-2 major late promoter yield a single early family of 3' coterminal mRNAs and five late families. Cell, 22, 905-916.

Shepard, P. J. & Hertel, K. J. (2009). The SR protein family. Genome Biol., 10, 242.

Shi, J., Qian, W., Yin, X., Iqbal, K., Grundke-Iqbal, I., Gu, X. et al. (2011). Cyclic AMP-dependent Protein Kinase Regulates the Alternative Splicing of Tau Exon 10: A MECHANISM INVOLVED IN TAU PATHOLOGY OF ALZHEIMER DISEASE. J.Biol.Chem., 286, 14639-14648.

Shi, J., Zhang, T., Zhou, C., Chohan, M. O., Gu, X., Wegiel, J. et al. (2008). Increased dosage of Dyrk1A alters alternative splicing factor (ASF)-regulated alternative splicing of tau in Down syndrome. J.Biol.Chem., 283, 28660-28669.

Shieh, S. Y., Ikeda, M., Taya, Y., & Prives, C. (1997). DNA damage-induced phosphorylation of p53 alleviates inhibition by MDM2. Cell, 91, 325-334.

Shtrichman, R. & Kleinberger, T. (1998). Adenovirus type 5 E4 open reading frame 4 protein induces apoptosis in transformed cells. J.Virol., 72, 2975-2982.

Singh, R., Valcarcel, J., & Green, M. R. (1995). Distinct binding specificities and functions of higher eukaryotic polypyrimidine tract-binding proteins. Science, 268, 1173-1176.

Skalhegg, B. S. & Tasken, K. (2000). Specificity in the cAMP/PKA signaling pathway. Differential expression,regulation, and subcellular localization of subunits of PKA. Front Biosci., 5, D678-D693.

Solis, A. S., Shariat, N., & Patton, J. G. (2008). Splicing fidelity, enhancers, and disease. Front Biosci., 13, 1926-1942.

Soulard, M., Della, V., V, Siomi, M. C., Pinol-Roma, S., Codogno, P., Bauvy, C. et al. (1993). hnRNP G: sequence and characterization of a glycosylated RNA-binding protein. Nucleic Acids Res., 21, 4210-4217.

Stamm, S. (2008). Regulation of alternative splicing by reversible protein phosphorylation. J.Biol.Chem., 283, 1223-1227.

Suomalainen, M., Nakano, M. Y., Boucke, K., Keller, S., & Greber, U. F. (2001). Adenovirus-activated PKA and p38/MAPK pathways boost microtubule-mediated nuclear targeting of virus. EMBO J., 20, 1310-1319.

Tauber, B. & Dobner, T. (2001). Adenovirus early E4 genes in viral oncogenesis. Oncogene, 20, 7847-7854.

Taylor, S. S., Kim, C., Vigil, D., Haste, N. M., Yang, J., Wu, J. et al. (2005). Dynamics of signaling by PKA. Biochim.Biophys.Acta, 1754, 25-37.

Tazi, J., Bakkour, N., & Stamm, S. (2009). Alternative splicing and disease. Biochim.Biophys.Acta, 1792, 14-26.

Teigelkamp, S., Mundt, C., Achsel, T., Will, C. L., & Luhrmann, R. (1997). The human U5 snRNP-specific 100-kD protein is an RS domain-containing, putative RNA helicase with significant homology to the yeast splicing factor Prp28p. RNA., 3, 1313-1326.

Tenenbaum, S. A. & Aguirre-Ghiso, J. (2005). Dephosphorylation shows SR proteins the way out. Mol.Cell, 20, 499-501.

Tian, B., Hu, J., Zhang, H., & Lutz, C. S. (2005). A large-scale analysis of mRNA polyadenylation of human and mouse genes. Nucleic Acids Res., 33, 201-212.

Tintaru, A. M., Hautbergue, G. M., Hounslow, A. M., Hung, M. L., Lian, L. Y., Craven, C. J. et al. (2007). Structural and functional analysis of RNA and TAP binding to SF2/ASF. EMBO Rep., 8, 756-762.

Tormanen, H., Backstrom, E., Carlsson, A., & Akusjarvi, G. (2006). L4-33K, an adenovirus-encoded alternative RNA splicing factor. J.Biol.Chem., 281, 36510-36517.

Tormanen, P. H., Aksaas, A. K., Kvissel, A. K., Punga, T., Engstrom, A., Skalhegg, B. S. et al. (2012). Two Cellular Protein Kinases, DNA-PK and PKA, Phosphorylate the Adenoviral L4-33K Protein and Have Opposite Effects on L1 Alternative RNA Splicing. PLoS.One., 7, e31871.

Trigon, S., Serizawa, H., Conaway, J. W., Conaway, R. C., Jackson, S. P., & Morange, M. (1998). Characterization of the residues phosphorylated in vitro by different C-terminal domain kinases. J.Biol.Chem., 273, 6769-6775.

van der Feltz, C., Anthony, K., Brilot, A., & Pomeranz Krummel, D. A. (2012). Architecture of the Spliceosome. Biochemistry (Mosc)., 10, In press.

Visa, N., Izaurralde, E., Ferreira, J., Daneholt, B., & Mattaj, I. W. (1996). A nuclear cap-binding complex binds Balbiani ring pre-mRNA cotranscriptionally and accompanies the ribonucleoprotein particle during nuclear export. J.Cell Biol., 133, 5-14.

Voelker, R. B., Erkelenz, S., Reynoso, V., Schaal, H., & Berglund, J. A. (2012). Frequent gain and loss of intronic splicing regulatory elements during the evolution of vertebrates. Genome Biol.Evol., 4, 659-674.

Wahl, M. C., Will, C. L., & Luhrmann, R. (2009). The spliceosome: design principles of a dynamic RNP machine. Cell, 136, 701-718.

Wakiyama, M., Imataka, H., & Sonenberg, N. (2000). Interaction of eIF4G with poly(A)-binding protein stimulates translation and is critical for Xenopus oocyte maturation. Curr.Biol., 10, 1147-1150.

Wang, E. T., Sandberg, R., Luo, S., Khrebtukova, I., Zhang, L., Mayr, C. et al. (2008). Alternative isoform regulation in human tissue transcriptomes. Nature, 456, 470-476.

Wang, L. L., Richard, S., & Shaw, A. S. (1995). P62 association with RNA is regulated by tyrosine phosphorylation. J.Biol.Chem., 270, 2010-2013.

Wang, X., Bruderer, S., Rafi, Z., Xue, J., Milburn, P. J., Kramer, A. et al. (1999). Phosphorylation of splicing factor SF1 on Ser20 by cGMP-dependent protein kinase regulates spliceosome assembly. EMBO J., 18, 4549-4559.

Wang, Y., Ma, M., Xiao, X., & Wang, Z. (2012). Intronic splicing enhancers, cognate splicing factors and context-dependent regulation rules. Nat.Struct.Mol.Biol., 19, 1044-1052.

Weiden, M. D. & Ginsberg, H. S. (1994). Deletion of the E4 region of the genome produces adenovirus DNA concatemers. Proc.Natl.Acad.Sci.U.S.A, 91, 153-157.

Weitzman, M. D. & Ornelles, D. A. (2005). Inactivating intracellular antiviral responses during adenovirus infection. Oncogene, 24, 7686-7696.

Will, C. L. & Luhrmann, R. (2011). Spliceosome structure and function. Cold Spring Harb.Perspect.Biol., 3, a003707.

Wong, W. & Scott, J. D. (2004). AKAP signalling complexes: focal points in space and time. Nat.Rev.Mol.Cell Biol., 5, 959-970.

Woodard, R. L., Anderson, M. G., & Dynan, W. S. (1999). Nuclear extracts lacking DNA-dependent protein kinase are deficient in multiple round transcription. J.Biol.Chem., 274, 478-485.

Wu, S., Romfo, C. M., Nilsen, T. W., & Green, M. R. (1999). Functional recognition of the 3' splice site AG by the splicing factor U2AF35. Nature, 402, 832-835.

Xie, J., Lee, J. A., Kress, T. L., Mowry, K. L., & Black, D. L. (2003). Protein kinase A phosphorylation modulates transport of the polypyrimidine tract-binding protein. Proc.Natl.Acad.Sci.U.S.A, 100, 8776-8781.

Yaneva, M., Kowalewski, T., & Lieber, M. R. (1997). Interaction of DNA-dependent protein kinase with DNA and with Ku: biochemical and atomic-force microscopy studies. EMBO J., 16, 5098-5112.

Young, C. S. (2003). The structure and function of the adenovirus major late promoter. Curr.Top.Microbiol.Immunol., 272, 213-249.

Zamore, P. D. & Green, M. R. (1989). Identification, purification, and biochemical characterization of U2 small nuclear ribonucleoprotein auxiliary factor. Proc.Natl.Acad.Sci.U.S.A, 86, 9243-9247.

Zamore, P. D., Patton, J. G., & Green, M. R. (1992). Cloning and domain structure of the mammalian splicing factor U2AF. Nature, 355, 609-614.

Zhang, S., Schlott, B., Gorlach, M., & Grosse, F. (2004). DNA-dependent protein kinase (DNA-PK) phosphorylates nuclear DNA helicase II/RNA helicase A and hnRNP proteins in an RNA-dependent manner. Nucleic Acids Res., 32, 1-10.

Zhong, H., SuYang, H., Erdjument-Bromage, H., Tempst, P., & Ghosh, S. (1997). The transcriptional activity of NF-kappaB is regulated by the IkappaB-associated PKAc subunit through a cyclic AMP-independent mechanism. Cell, 89, 413-424.

Zhong, X. Y., Wang, P., Han, J., Rosenfeld, M. G., & Fu, X. D. (2009). SR proteins in vertical integration of gene expression from transcription to RNA processing to translation. Mol.Cell, 35, 1-10.

Environmental Resistance Development to Influenza Antivirals – and the Return to Humans

Josef D. Järhult

Department of Medical Sciences
Uppsala University, Sweden

1   Introduction

Influenza A is a major health concern in both human and veterinary medicine. Viruses of human and avian origin are linked through the exchange of genetic material, e.g. the reassortment process that can form pandemic viruses in humans. There is growing evidence that the active substance of the neuraminidase inhibitor (NAI) oseltamivir (Tamiflu®) is stable and it can be detected in aquatic environments when oseltamivir is widely used. Low levels of the active substance induce resistance in influenza A virus in mallards, the natural influenza reservoir. If resistance is established in viruses circulating among wild birds, there is a risk of an oseltamivir-resistant pandemic or highly-pathogenic avian influenza (HPAI) virus through reassortment or direct transmission. The connection is displayed in Figure 1 and has previously been described (Jarhult, 2012). This chapter aims to review the current knowledge in this field, to identify gaps in the knowledge and to point out important future research areas.

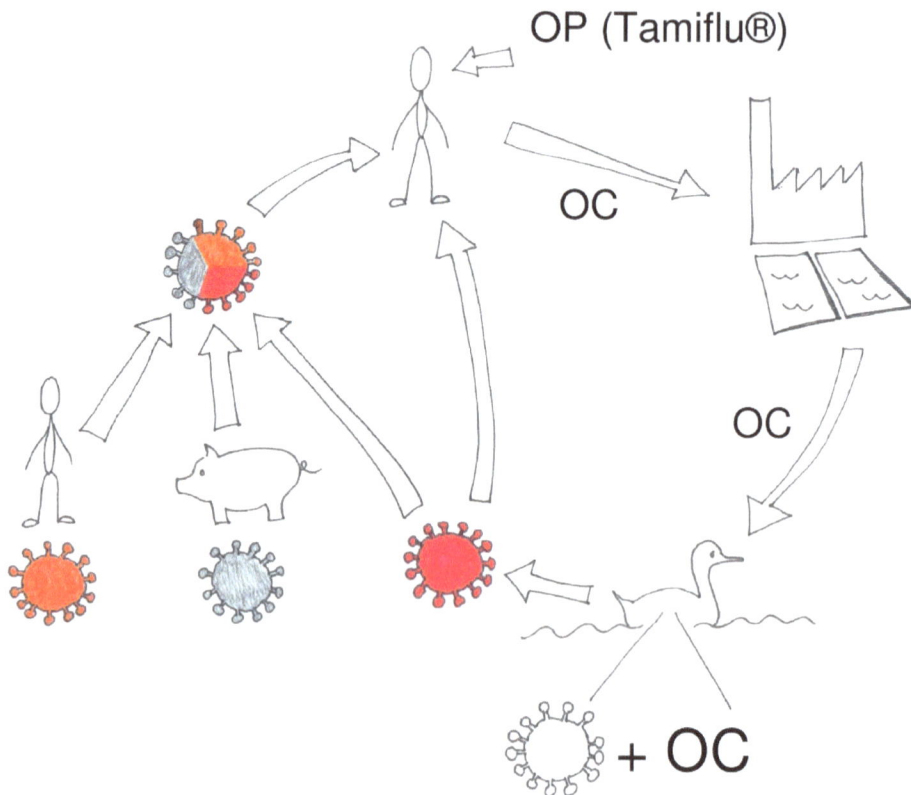

Figure 1: The possible connection of environmental levels of oseltamivir, resistance development and influenza A viruses of avian and human origin. OC=oseltamivir carboxylate, OP=oseltamivir phosphate. Illustration kindly provided by S.J. Järhult.

2   Influenza Pandemics

During the last century, influenza A viruses have caused four pandemic outbreaks. In 1918-1920, the "Spanish Flu" H1N1 pandemic killed at least 50 million, perhaps up to 100 million people (Johnson &

Mueller, 2002). There has been a controversy regarding the genetic origin of the Spanish Flu, with some authors claiming a direct transmission of an avian virus (Taubenberger & Morens, 2006; Taubenberger *et al.*, 2005). However, phylogenetic evidence strongly suggests that the 1918 pandemic strain was the result of a reassortment of human, avian and possibly swine viruses (Smith *et al.*, 2009). The 1957 H2N2 "Asian Flu" and the 1968 H3N2 "Hong Kong Flu" pandemics were both milder than the 1918 pandemic and caused much less mortality. They were the results of reassortments of human and avian viruses. Little is known about the sequences of swine viruses at that time and thus the involvement of swine viruses in the reassortant cannot be precluded (Guan *et al.*, 2010). The recent A/H1N1 "Swine Flu" pandemic was a result of reassortment events in swine. The neuraminidase (NA) and the matrix genes were derived from the Eurasian avian-like swine H1N1 lineage while the remaining six gene segments had their origin in North American triple reassortant lineages. Human, avian and classical swine viruses contributed the genes that were derived from the North America triple reassortants (Smith *et al.*, 2009b).

3   Influenza in Birds

Influenza A virus is a zoonosis, the natural hosts are wetland birds, mostly Anseriformes (ducks, geese, swans) and Charadriiformes (gulls, terns, waders) (Olsen *et al.*, 2006; Webster *et al.*, 1992). Dabbling ducks such as the mallard (*Anas platyrhyncos*), are particularly well suited for the perpetuation of influenza viruses in several aspects. They feed in shallow water which facilitates spread via the fecal – oral route (Webster *et al.*, 1992). Furthermore, they congregate in flocks, have a large population size, migrate to interact with new individuals and every year new, immunologically naïve juveniles are added to the population. Influenza A viruses are well adapted to aquatic environments; some viral strains can remain infective for well over a year at 4°C but only for days at 37°C (Brown *et al.*, 2009). Dabbling ducks are considered the major natural reservoir of influenza A viruses (Olsen *et al.*, 2006).

Most viruses circulating among wild birds are low-pathogenic (low-pathogenic avian influenza, LPAI) viruses. The prevalence of LPAI viruses among dabbling ducks vary with season with a higher percentage of birds infected during fall migration. One contributing factor to this variation is the high proportion of non-immune juveniles in the fall. There are also geographic differences; a study from Sweden found 15% infected mallards during fall and 4 % in the springtime (Wallensten *et al.*, 2007), whereas data from North America show a higher fall prevalence but a lower spring prevalence (Webster *et al.*, 1992). 16 of 17 HA and all 9 NA variants of influenza A viruses discovered so far have been found in birds and most of them in dabbling ducks. Exceptions are H13 and H16 that are predominantly isolated from gulls and terns (Fouchier *et al.*, 2005) and H17 that has been found in bats (Tong *et al.*, 2012). Most subtypes of LPAI viruses have a large geographical spread, possibly through migration. H14 and H15 are exceptions, being mostly isolated in Russia and Australia (Kawaoka *et al.*, 1990; Rohm *et al.*, 1996). Phylogenetically, LPAI viruses studied so far belong to either the Eurasian or the North American lineage (Schafer *et al.*, 1993). However, several findings of viruses with a lineage-mixed genome have been reported (Makarova *et al.*, 1999; Wahlgren *et al.*, 2008; Wallensten *et al.*, 2005) indicating that the separation is not complete. Hence, the naturally circulating gene pool of LPAI viruses in wild birds can be considered large and variable in several aspects.

LPAI in dabbling ducks has a mild clinical course but has some effects on the host. For example, in an infection experiment a slight, short-lasting increase in body temperature was observed (Jourdain *et al.*, 2010), the migration of LPAI-infected swans was delayed (van Gils *et al.*, 2007) and mallard hens had a transient decrease in egg production (Laudert *et al.*, 1993). Interestingly, a recent study found mallards in normal body condition more sensitive to LPAI infection when compared to mallards -10% and -20% in body weight (Arsnoe *et al.*, 2011). This is contradictory to the hypothesis that birds in worse body condition would be more sensitive to infection. LPAI infection in ducks is located mainly in the gastrointestinal tract (Brojer *et al.*, in press; Webster *et al.*, 1978).

4   Treatment and Prophylaxis of Influenza

There are two different strategies regularly used in the treatment and prophylaxis of influenza A: antiviral drugs and vaccines.

Vaccines are an effective way to prevent influenza. A trivalent vaccine containing antigens from H1N1, H3N2 and B strains is the standard preventive measure for seasonal influenza (Centers For Disease Control (CDC), 2011). In a pandemic scenario, the rapid mass-production of vaccines is problematic as most production techniques still depend on embryonated hen eggs. According to the Global Action Plan developed by WHO, the goal in a pandemic situation is to have produced 2 billion doses 6 months after a vaccine candidate is available. However, in a WHO study evaluating the 2009 pandemic it was demonstrated that in 6 months, only 534 million doses had been produced and that it took 5 months from the identification of the pandemic A/H1N1 virus strain until the first vaccines were available. Furthermore, the supply of vaccines to developing countries is especially hard to accomplish; this is problematic as a severe pandemic is expected to hit particularly hard in those countries (Partridge & Kieny, 2010).

The antiviral drugs mostly used for influenza are admantanes and neuraminidase inhibitors (NAIs). The admantanes, amantadine and rimantadine, block the M2 protein and thus inhibit viral replication at an early stage (Wang *et al.*, 1993). However, due to a massive development of resistance both in human and avian strains (Ilyushina *et al.*, 2005; Nelson *et al.*, 2009) the clinical use of admantanes has virtually stopped. Another disadvantage of admantanes is their high rate of adverse events such as nausea, insomnia and hallucinations (Jefferson *et al.*, 2006).

4.1   Neuraminidase Inhibitors (NAIs)

The NAIs inhibit the viral enzyme NA that is needed for the release of newly formed virions from the infected host cell (Nayak *et al.*, 2004) but also for the process of viral entry through the airways of the host by cutting mucoproteins (Matrosovich *et al.*, 2004). The possibility to decrease viral entry in the airway epithelium through hindering of NA binding may contribute to the successfulness of NAI prophylaxis (Hayden *et al.*, 1996). There are two commercially available NAIs worldwide: oseltamivir (Tamiflu®) and zanamivir (Relenza®). Two more substances, perimivir and lanamivir, are available in some regions and more substances of the class are in the pipeline of drug production.

4.1.1   Oseltamivir

Oseltamivir is administered orally as a prodrug, oseltamivir phosphate (OP) due to the poor bioavailability of the active substance oseltamivir carboxylate (OC). OP is readily absorbed and rapidly converted to OC by esterases, mainly in the liver. More than 75% of an oral dose reaches the circulation as OC. The active metabolite is then excreted from the body in unchanged form predominantly via the urine (Sweetman). OC is likely as poorly absorbed in the intestine of ducks as in the intestine of humans. However, as the LPAI infection in ducks takes place in the intestine, replicating virus and OC co-exist, potentially enabling resistance to develop. Oseltamivir has been extensively stockpiled; e.g. the US had 40 million treatment regimens in stock as of April 2009 (Patel & Gorman, 2009). Worldwide, more than 220 million treatment courses have been stockpiled, and the shelf life has been extended to 7 years (Wan Po *et al.*, 2009). As the mass-production of vaccines is a process of several months, antiviral drugs are the only option in the early phase of a pandemic. Thus, oseltamivir is a cornerstone of pandemic preparedness plans all over the world.

OC is stable in the aqueous phase and is not removed or degraded in normal sewage treatment plants (STPs) (Fick *et al.*, 2007). Persistence of oseltamivir in surface water ranged from non-detectable degradation to a half-life of 53 days in another study (Accinelli *et al.*, 2010). Thus, there is reason to believe that OC is present in the aquatic environment near STPs when oseltamivir is used extensively. Japan has had the highest per-capita consumption of oseltamivir during several seasonal influenza outbreaks. In one study, it was estimated that more than 10 million treatment courses – corresponding to almost 10% of the population – were used during the 2004-2005 season (Tashiro *et al.*, 2009). The manufacturer Roche estimated that 6 million people out of 16 million infected with influenza used the drug during the same season (F. Hoffman - La Roche Ltd, 2005).

A study on water from the Yodo River system in Japan during the influenza season 2007-2008 demonstrated OC levels of up to 58 ng/L (Söderstrom *et al.*, 2009). This correlated well with levels estimated from data on oseltamivir consumption. During the influenza season 2008-2009, another study in the same area measured levels of OC in river water up to 190 ng/L and in outlets from STPs up to 293 ng/L (Ghosh *et al.*, 2010). Very limited sampling for OC has been performed in aquatic environments, thus higher levels can exist under circumstances yet to be examined. Furthermore, both studies were performed during seasonal influenza outbreaks; during a pandemic, usage and thus environmental levels of OC are expected to be considerably higher, reaching µg/L-levels. This is exemplified by a Norwegian study in which OC levels in the outlet of a STP during the 2009 pandemic were measured to more than 1.4 µg/L (Leknes *et al.*, 2012). A study from Germany also suggests discharge from pharmaceutical industries as a potential source of OC (Prasse *et al.*, 2010).

4.1.2 Zanamivir

Zanamivir cannot be administered orally but is inhaled or more rarely used in an intravenous formulation. Little is known about the degradation of zanamivir in aquatic environments and in STP processes. However, the chemical similarity to OC makes it probable that also zanamivir is stable under those conditions. Studies from the manufacturer show that the substance is stable in water (half-life >1 year) and not biodegradable (<1% degradation in active sludge for 28 days) (Glaxo Smith Kline, 2004). After inhalation of zanamivir, 4-20% of the dose (the normal daily dose for inhalation is 20 mg) reaches the circulation and is excreted unchanged via the urine (Sweetman). About 80% of the dose is deposited in the oropharynx (Cass *et al.*, 1999); most of which is probably swallowed and excreted in unchanged form in feces (zanamivir has a low bioavailability of about 2%) (Sweetman). The most frequently used dose of intravenous zanamivir is 1200 mg daily. However, this formulation is not yet commercially available, but a phase III trial comparing 600 mg or 1200 mg of intravenous zanamivir daily to oseltamivir is under way.

5   Resistance to Neuraminidase Inhibitors

When the NAIs were introduced, resistance development was not considered a practical problem. Resistant viruses were observed after drug pressure assays e.g. in cell lines and in 4% of volunteers in an early study of oseltamivir (Gubareva *et al.*, 2001), but the mutants had severely reduced viral fitness. Therefore, it was deduced that resistance development to NAIs interfered too much with the key function of NA to be a problem *in vivo*. However, resistance was observed also in clinical isolates and in some settings it reached considerable levels as in the study by Kiso *et al* where 14% of Japanese children carried resistant viruses after oseltamivir treatment (Kiso *et al.*, 2004).

There are 19 amino-acid residues that are well conserved among NAs of all subtypes. They are divided into *catalytic* residues involved in the interaction of the substrate and the active site of NA (R118, D151, R152, R224, E276, R292, R371 and Y406) and *framework* residues important for the structure and stabilization of the active site (E119, R156, W178, S179, D198, I222, E227, H274, E277, N294 and E425) (Colman *et al.*, 1983). Resistance could potentially arise from a mutation at or near any of those residues and many are previously described (Ferraris & Lina, 2008).

The mutation H274Y, conferring resistance to oseltamivir, was rarely seen in clinical practice until the influenza season 2007-2008. That season, H274Y was observed in seasonal H1N1 viruses, first in Norway and then in the rest of Europe (Meijer *et al.*, 2009). Low percentages of H274Y was reported from the rest of the world 2007-2008, but in the next season 2008-2009, resistant viruses constituted the absolute majority worldwide (Moscona, 2009). There was no correlation to the use of oseltamivir (Kramarz *et al.*, 2009; Moscona, 2009).

It has been demonstrated that an influenza A/H1N1 virus in mallards exposed to low levels of OC in their sole water source develops resistance through acquisition of the mutation H274Y (Jarhult *et al.*, 2011). H274Y was detected when the ducks were subjected to 1µg/L of OC and mutants quickly outnumbered the wild-type virus at 80 µg/L. The IC_{50} difference between wild-type isolates (2-4 nM) and H274Y isolates (400-700 nM) is consistent with findings in human clinical isolates (Rameix-Welti *et al.*, 2008). As µg/L-levels of OC are expected in the environment, the experimental conditions correspond to a realistic scenario. This means that oseltamivir resistance could be induced in influenza A viruses of wild ducks when the drug is widely used, but this is only true for limited periods of time during pandemic or seasonal influenza outbreaks. As earlier *in vitro* studies have indicated a decreased viral fitness in strains with NAI resistance mutations the question arises: Will the resistance prevail when OC disappears from the environment?

In this sense, it is interesting to study the results from isolations in embryonated hen eggs of a sample with mixed genotype (i.e. a virus population consisting of both wild-type and H274Y) from the mallard study (Jarhult *et al.*, 2011). During the replication process in the eggs, no OC is present and hence there is no drug pressure. Two different isolations gave rise to one wild-type and one H274Y-positive isolate which demonstrates that either genotype can dominate the replication and outcompete the other. This is not a true fitness test but still a good indication that the fitness of the wild-type and the mutant are not dramatically different when H274Y is induced in a randomly chosen virus from a wild mallard in Sweden. Sweden uses oseltamivir conservatively and the sampling was performed in a rural area on an island by the seaside. Therefore, this strain cannot possibly have been exposed to any drug pressure around the time of sampling. Another interesting fact is the accumulation of H274Y in seasonal influenza A/H1N1 in the seasons 2007-2008 and 2008-2009. As there was no correlation between the spread of resistance and the use of oseltamivir (Kramarz *et al.*, 2009; Moscona, 2009), i.e. the drug pressure, the

H274Y mutant must have been fit enough to outcompete the wild-type strain(s). It has been demonstrated that this is probably due to compensatory, "permissive" mutations (V234M and R222Q) which restore the decreased surface expression of NA caused by H274Y (Bloom *et al.*, 2010). Another study has also demonstrated a compensatory effect on NA activity in H274Y mutants by D344N (Collins *et al.*, 2009). Thus, it seems that the genetic makeup of the virus strain where resistance mutations such as H274Y develop will determine whether the mutation results in a decreased viral fitness or not.

5.1   Resistance in Wild Birds

The probability of a virus strain carrying a permissive genetic makeup appears to be higher in LPAI viruses of dabbling ducks than in human influenza viruses. This is because dabbling ducks are the natural reservoir of influenza A viruses [10] meaning that many more strains co-circulate at a given time and that there is a larger genetic variation. For example, the sensitivity to oseltamivir in avian A/H1N1 viruses showed a much larger variation when compared to mammalian viruses (Stoner *et al.*). The analysis of sequences from the NCBI database in the mallard study (Jarhult *et al.*, 2011) revealed that H274Y has been reported in wild birds, though rarely. H274Y has been found both in H5N1 and H1N1 viruses - interestingly, the H1N1 isolate originated from a duck in Minto Flats in Interior Alaska, a habitat with high densities of nesting ducks. The interior of Alaska is scarcely populated and oseltamivir use is negligible, thus there is no drug pressure. The occurrence of H274Y under these circumstances further supports the idea that H274Y does not require drug pressure to prevail when present in a virus with a suitable genetic makeup.

6   Spread of Influenza from Birds to Humans

Influenza A viruses can spread from birds to humans in two distinctly different ways. Two or more strains from birds, humans and/or other mammals like swine can form a human-adapted virus with pandemic potential through reassortment. Another way of transfer is through a direct transmission of an avian virus to humans – also termed *de novo* introduction. HPAI can be transmitted directly from birds to humans but so far a very high infectious dose has been required and transmission has mostly been observed in people in close contact with infected birds. The mortality in human HPAI H5N1 infection is 59% according to the cumulative number of cases and deaths reported to WHO since 2003 (WHO, 2012). There have been few reports of human-to-human transmission of HPAI and none of sustained transmission.

An oseltamivir-resistant pandemic where an NA gene containing resistance mutation(s) has been recruited from an avian virus is an alarming example of the reassortment route. It would render stockpiles of oseltamivir useless and make the treatment and prophylaxis parts of pandemic preparedness plans very difficult to accomplish.

Another possibility is that oseltamivir resistance is established in the pool of circulating HPAI viruses with the risk that such a virus acquires human-to-human transmissibility. This possibility is highlighted by the recent demonstration from two independent research groups that a modified HPAI H5N1 virus can be transmissible between ferrets. A group led by Kawaoka combined the HA gene from a HPAI H5N1 virus with the remaining genome from a human pandemic A/H1N1 virus. This resulted in a ferret-transmissible virus, although it caused a less severe disease in the animals compared to the wild-type virus. In total, four mutations in combination with reassortment were needed to allow transmission between mammals (Imai *et al.*, 2012). Fouchier's research group introduced three mutations in a HPAI H5N1 virus and serially passaged this virus in ferrets. After ten passages, viruses evolved with the capability to spread between ferrets without direct contact. Only two more mutations were consistently found in those viruses, indicating that five mutations altogether may be enough to confer airborne transmission of a HPAI H5N1 in mammals. The ferret-transmissible virus was lethal after intratracheal inoculation but less pathogenic than the wild-type H5N1 virus, suggesting that some of the pathogenicity may be lost in the process of adaptation to mammals (Herfst *et al.*, 2012). Surveillance data reveal that numerous viruses have been isolated from birds that lack three mutations of the Imai *et al*-virus and four mutations of the Herfst *et al*-virus. A mathematical model indicates that the remaining mutations could evolve in a single mammalian host (Russell *et al.*, 2012). The dual-use principle has sparked an intense debate on the biosecurity aspects of these experiments demonstrating the impact of the issue (Fauci & Collins, 2012; Frankel, 2012; Lipsitch *et al.*, 2012; Wolinetz, 2012). In conclusion, the genetic barrier for direct transmission appears to be lower than previously thought, stressing the risk associated to resistance development in HPAI viruses circulating among wild birds.

To study resistance development in influenza viruses of treated patients is important. However, there are good reasons to complement these studies by investigating the role of antivirals in the environment and resistance development in wild birds because:

1. The size and diversity of the influenza gene pool among wild birds is overwhelming compared to the pool of circulating human influenza viruses. At any given time, more or less only three different strains circulate among humans. In wild birds, almost all subtypes described to date have been found. Furthermore, there are two distinct genetic lineages and there is a constant circulation of virus year-round and a large proportion of the population is exchanged each year, adding non-immune juveniles. Thus, it is perhaps more common that resistance develops in treated humans, but it is more probable in the bird population that a resistance mutation occurs in a virus with a suitable genetic makeup.

2. If resistance spreads to humans via a reassortment event causing a pandemic or a human-adapted HPAI virus, the consequences are far worse than if it arises in a strain already circulating in the human population. In the latter case there is already some immunity in the population and the resistant virus is likely a more harmless circulating seasonal strains (like the development of H274Y in the former seasonal A/H1N1 virus). In the former case, preparedness plans rely on oseltamivir both as an attempt to blanket the outbreak and as treatment and prophylaxis especially during the first wave.

7   Clinical Consequences of Resistance

Generally, resistance in influenza is a problem to physicians especially when treating immunosuppressed patients. Numerous reports exist on resistant viruses recovered from such individuals. An interesting example is the finding of I222R in a pandemic A/H1N1 virus isolated from an immunocompromised Dutch patient (van der Vries *et al.*, 2011). This mutation caused resistance to all available NAIs and as the circulating pandemic A/H1N1 virus is already resistant to admantanes, there are no treatment options left in this case.

In the event of an oseltamivir-resistant pandemic with morbidity in the same magnitude as the Spanish Flu, the consequences are almost unimaginable – e.g. ventilator capacity in intensive care units would quickly be outnumbered. The same goes for the scenario of a HPAI virus capable of human-to-human spread and retaining pathogenicity.

8   Strategies to Lower Environmental Levels of OC

A promising means to reduce OC levels in the environment is to increase the degradation through ozonization. A study from Japan demonstrated that the addition of ozonization as a tertiary treatment in a STP increased the removal of OC to >90% (Ghosh *et al.*, 2010). Apart from increasing the degradation of OC, the ozonization process has the potential to reduce the outlet of antibiotics and other pharmaceuticals.

However, the most important measure remains a prudent use of antiviral drugs. The effect of NAIs in healthy people suffering a seasonal influenza infection is limited; oseltamivir 75 mg twice daily or a corresponding dose in children shortens duration of symptoms with approximately one day (Jefferson *et al.*, 2012). On the contrary, in immunosuppressed patients there is growing evidence that a combination therapy is favorable. *In vitro* and *in vivo* experimental data suggest an additive or synergistic effect and a decrease in resistance development and therefore the use of combination therapy is increasingly advocated (Govorkova & Webster, 2010; Hoopes *et al.*, 2011; Nguyen *et al.*, 2010; Nguyen *et al.*, 2012). To strictly limit the use in the young and healthy in non-pandemic periods and to consider combination therapy for those with a suppressed immune defense appears to be a reasonable strategy.

Apart from limiting the use of NAIs, the development of new anti-influenza drugs is essential. However, it is crucial to consider the risk of resistance development – including what happens in the environment – and to limit the use of new drugs from the beginning. Each new antiviral, or antibiotic, has a limited life span which is heavily dependent on its use.

9   Future Research

There are several aspects discussed in this chapter that deserve further attention including the following:

1. To learn more about OC in the environment. Studies performed so far are few and small. A global approach including pandemic periods is desirable. The environmental perspective discussed here needs to be applied on zanamivir and other NAIs and antivirals including those in the pipeline of drug development.

2. To extend the knowledge of the influenza situation among wild birds. This concerns influenza ecology in general and the resistance situation in particular. An extensive screening for influenza viruses and resistance mutations among wild birds in different parts of the world is important, also to follow the development over time. Genotypic analysis might not always be sufficient; to some extent the screening should be complemented with phenotypic methods to detect decreased sensitivity to NAIs that does not correlate with previously described resistance mutations.

3. To broaden the understanding of influenza resistance development in dabbling ducks exposed to NAIs. It is crucial to study if, and how, resistance mutations are affected by decreasing levels of OC and thus how resistance prevails in between influenza outbreaks. To date, only one subtype

of influenza A virus is examined in the sense of resistance development under low drug pressure of OC. It is still unknown how environmental levels of OC affect the large and important phylogenetic N2-group of NAs that have distinct resistance mutations. Low level exposure studies in dabbling ducks should be performed also with other NAIs, particularly zanamivir, to look for potential environmental resistance development.

4. To further assess the genetic barrier to human-to-human transmission of HPAI viruses. Special surveillance focus should be put on regions with circulating viruses genetically close to achieving mammalian transmission and intermediate mammalian hosts. Deep sequencing should be employed to better understand resistance development at the quasispecies level. To estimate the risk of human adaptation of HPAI viruses is important in the sense of pandemic preparedness in general, but it also has implications for the potential spread of a resistant HPAI virus.

10   Summary

OC is present in the aquatic environment during seasonal influenza outbreaks. Thus, the natural influenza reservoir, dabbling ducks, can be exposed to the substance. Furthermore, an influenza A/H1N1 virus in mallards subjected to low, environmental-like, concentrations of OC develops oseltamivir resistance through acquisition of the resistance mutation H274Y. Therefore, there is reason to believe that resistance development occurs in influenza A viruses of wild ducks when oseltamivir is used widely. The occurrence of H274Y in influenza viruses isolated from wild birds and the fact that H274Y became established in the pre-pandemic seasonal human H1N1 virus support the thought that once induced, oseltamivir resistance can prevail if present in a virus with a suitable, permissive genetic makeup. Through reassortment or direct transmission, oseltamivir resistance can spread to a human-adapted influenza virus with pandemic potential, threatening to disable oseltamivir, a cornerstone in pandemic preparedness planning (Figure 2). In a bigger perspective, this chapter exemplifies that antiviral drugs, like antibiotics, have a limited life span due to resistance development. The substances can have complex environmental effects that include humans, necessitating a broad, multi-disciplinary research approach.

References

Accinelli, C., Sacca, M. L., Fick, J., Mencarelli, M., Lindberg, R. & Olsen, B. (2010). Dissipation and Removal of Oseltamivir (Tamiflu) in Different Aquatic Environments. Chemosphere, 79(8), 891-897.

Arsnoe, D. M., Ip, H. S. & Owen, J. C. (2011). Influence of Body Condition on Influenza A Virus Infection in Mallard Ducks: Experimental Infection Data. PLoS One, 6(8), e22633.

Bloom, J. D., Gong, L. I. & Baltimore, D. (2010). Permissive Secondary Mutations Enable the Evolution of Influenza Oseltamivir Resistance. Science, 328(5983), 1272-1275.

Brojer, C., Jarhult, J. D., Muradrasoli, S., Soderstrom, H., Olsen, B. & Gavier-Widén, D. (in press). Pathobiology and Virus Shedding of Low-Pathogenic Avian Influenza Virus (A/H1N1) Infection in Mallards Exposed to Oseltamivir. Journal of Wildlife Diseases.

Brown, J. D., Goekjian, G., Poulson, R., Valeika, S. & Stallknecht, D. E. (2009). Avian Influenza Virus in Water: Infectivity Is Dependent on pH, Salinity and Temperature. Veterinary Microbiology, 136(1-2), 20-26.

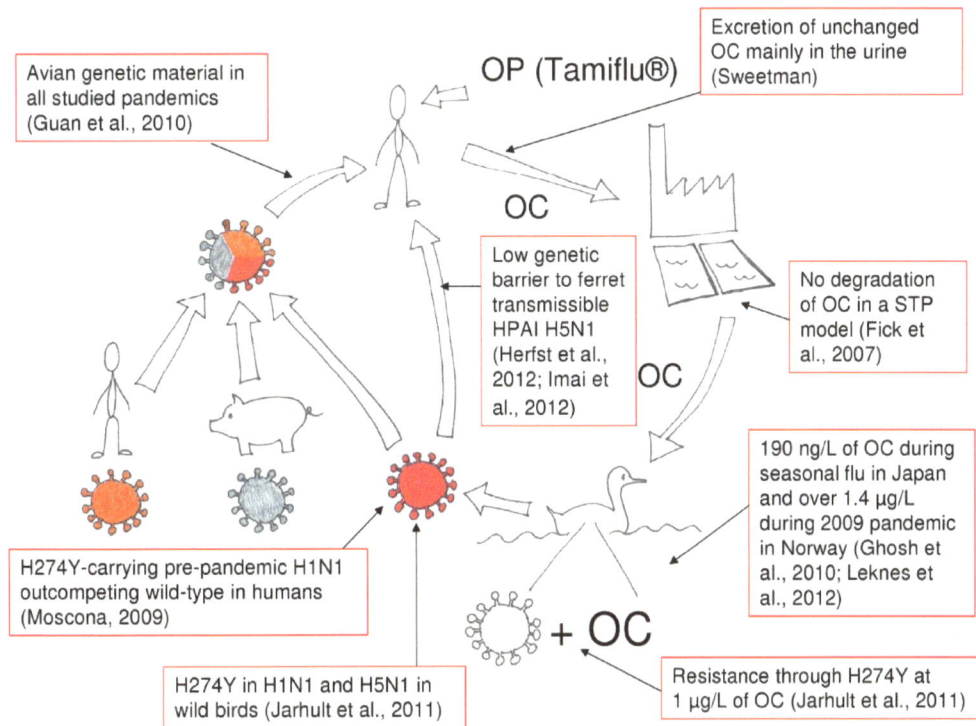

Figure 2: Graphic summary of studies regarding the connection of environmental levels of oseltamivir, resistance development and influenza A viruses of avian and human origin. OC=oseltamivir carboxylate, OP=oseltamivir phosphate. Illustration by S.J. Järhult.

Cass, L. M., Brown, J., Pickford, M., Fayinka, S., Newman, S. P., Johansson, C. J. & Bye, A. (1999). Pharmacoscinti-graphic Evaluation of Lung Deposition of Inhaled Zanamivir in Healthy Volunteers. Clinical Pharmacokinetics, 36 Suppl 1, 21-31.

Centers For Disease Control (CDC). (2011). Prevention and Control of Influenza with Vaccines: Recommendations of the Advisory Committee on Immunization Practices (ACIP), 2011. Morbidity and Mortality Weekly Report, 60(33), 1128-1132.

Collins, P. J., Haire, L. F., Lin, Y. P., Liu, J., Russell, R. J., Walker, P. A., Martin, S. R., Daniels, R. S., Gregory, V., Skehel, J. J., Gamblin, S. J. & Hay, A. J. (2009). Structural Basis for Oseltamivir Resistance of Influenza Viruses. Vaccine, 27(45), 6317-6323.

Colman, P. M., Varghese, J. N. & Laver, W. G. (1983). Structure of the Catalytic and Antigenic Sites in Influenza Virus Neuraminidase. Nature, 303(5912), 41-44.

F. Hoffman - La Roche Ltd. (2005). Further Expansion of Tamiflu Manufacturing Capacity. http://www.roche.com/med-cor-2005-10-18.

Fauci, A. S. & Collins, F. S. (2012). Benefits and Risks of Influenza Research: Lessons Learned. Science, 336(6088), 1522-1523.

Ferraris, O. & Lina, B. (2008). Mutations of Neuraminidase Implicated in Neuraminidase Inhibitors Resistance. Journal of Clinical Virology, 41(1), 13-19.

Fick, J., Lindberg, R. H., Tysklind, M., Haemig, P. D., Waldenstrom, J., Wallensten, A. & Olsen, B. (2007). Antiviral Oseltamivir Is Not Removed or Degraded in Normal Sewage Water Treatment: Implications for Development of Resistance by Influenza A Virus. PLoS One, 2(10), e986.

Fouchier, R. A., Munster, V., Wallensten, A., Bestebroer, T. M., Herfst, S., Smith, D., Rimmelzwaan, G. F., Olsen, B. & Osterhaus, A. D. (2005). Characterization of a Novel Influenza A Virus Hemagglutinin Subtype (H16) Obtained from Black-Headed Gulls. Journal of Virology, 79(5), 2814-2822.

Frankel, M. S. (2012). Regulating the Boundaries of Dual-Use Research. Science, 336(6088), 1523-1525.

Ghosh, G. C., Nakada, N., Yamashita, N. & Tanaka, H. (2010). Occurrence and Fate of Oseltamivir Carboxylate (Tamiflu) and Amantadine in Sewage Treatment Plants. Chemosphere, 81(1), 13-17.

Ghosh, G. C., Nakada, N., Yamashita, N. & Tanaka, H. (2010). Oseltamivir Carboxylate, the Active Metabolite of Oseltamivir Phosphate (Tamiflu), Detected in Sewage Discharge and River Water in Japan. Environmental Health Perspective, 118(1), 103-107.

Glaxo Smith Kline. (2004). Relenza Diskhaler - Safety Data Sheet. http://www.msds-gsk.com/11057406.pdf.

Govorkova, E. A. & Webster, R. G. (2010). Combination Chemotherapy for Influenza. Viruses, 2, 1510-1529.

Guan, Y., Vijaykrishna, D., Bahl, J., Zhu, H., Wang, J. & Smith, G. J. (2010). The Emergence of Pandemic Influenza Viruses. Protein & Cell, 1(1), 9-13.

Gubareva, L. V., Kaiser, L., Matrosovich, M. N., Soo-Hoo, Y. & Hayden, F. G. (2001). Selection of Influenza Virus Mutants in Experimentally Infected Volunteers Treated with Oseltamivir. Journal of Infectious Diseases, 183(4), 523-531.

Hayden, F. G., Treanor, J. J., Betts, R. F., Lobo, M., Esinhart, J. D. & Hussey, E. K. (1996). Safety and Efficacy of the Neuraminidase Inhibitor GG167 in Experimental Human Influenza. Journal of the American Medical Association, 275(4), 295-299.

Herfst, S., Schrauwen, E. J., Linster, M., Chutinimitkul, S., de Wit, E., Munster, V. J., Sorrell, E. M., Bestebroer, T. M., Burke, D. F., Smith, D. J., Rimmelzwaan, G. F., Osterhaus, A. D. & Fouchier, R. A. (2012). Airborne Transmission of Influenza A/H5N1 Virus between Ferrets. Science, 336(6088), 1534-1541.

Hoopes, J. D., Driebe, E. M., Kelley, E., Engelthaler, D. M., Keim, P. S., Perelson, A. S., Rong, L., Went, G. T. & Nguyen, J. T. (2011). Triple Combination Antiviral Drug (TCAD) Composed of Amantadine, Oseltamivir, and Ribavirin Impedes the Selection of Drug-Resistant Influenza a Virus. PLoS One, 6(12), e29778.

Ilyushina, N. A., Govorkova, E. A. & Webster, R. G. (2005). Detection of Amantadine-Resistant Variants among Avian Influenza Viruses Isolated in North America and Asia. Virology, 341(1), 102-106.

Imai, M., Watanabe, T., Hatta, M., Das, S. C., Ozawa, M., Shinya, K., Zhong, G., Hanson, A., Katsura, H., Watanabe, S., Li, C., Kawakami, E., Yamada, S., Kiso, M., Suzuki, Y., Maher, E. A., Neumann, G. & Kawaoka, Y. (2012). Experimental Adaptation of an Influenza H5 HA Confers Respiratory Droplet Transmission to a Reassortant H5 HA/H1N1 Virus in Ferrets. Nature, 486(7403), 420-428.

Jarhult, J. D., Muradrasoli, S., Wahlgren, J., Soderstrom, H., Orozovic, G., Gunnarsson, G., Brojer, C., Latorre-Margalef, N., Fick, J., Grabic, R., Lennerstrand, J., Waldenstrom, J., Lundkvist, A. & Olsen, B. (2011). Environmental Levels of the Antiviral Oseltamivir Induce Development of Resistance Mutation H274Y in Influenza A/H1N1 Virus in Mallards. PLoS One, 6(9), e24742.

Jarhult, J. D. (2012). Oseltamivir (Tamiflu((R))) in the Environment, Resistance Development in Influenza A Viruses of Dabbling Ducks and the Risk of Transmission of an Oseltamivir-Resistant Virus to Humans - a Review. Infection Ecology and Epidemiology, 2, 18385.

Jefferson, T., Demicheli, V., Rivetti, D., Jones, M., Di Pietrantonj, C. & Rivetti, A. (2006). Antivirals for Influenza in Healthy Adults: Systematic Review. Lancet, 367(9507), 303-313.

Jefferson, T., Jones, M. A., Doshi, P., Del Mar, C. B., Heneghan, C. J., Hama, R. & Thompson, M. J. (2012). Neuraminidase Inhibitors for Preventing and Treating Influenza in Healthy Adults and Children. Cochrane Database of Systematic Reviews, 1, CD008965.

Johnson, N. P. & Mueller, J. (2002). Updating the Accounts: Global Mortality of the 1918-1920 "Spanish" Influenza Pandemic. Bulletin of the History of Medicine, 76(1), 105-115.

Jourdain, E., Gunnarsson, G., Wahlgren, J., Latorre-Margalef, N., Brojer, C., Sahlin, S., Svensson, L., Waldenstrom, J., Lundkvist, A. & Olsen, B. (2010). Influenza Virus in a Natural Host, the Mallard: Experimental Infection Data. PLoS One, 5(1), e8935.

Kawaoka, Y., Yamnikova, S., Chambers, T. M., Lvov, D. K. & Webster, R. G. (1990). Molecular Characterization of a New Hemagglutinin, Subtype H14, of Influenza A Virus. Virology, 179(2), 759-767.

Kiso, M., Mitamura, K., Sakai-Tagawa, Y., Shiraishi, K., Kawakami, C., Kimura, K., Hayden, F. G., Sugaya, N. & Kawaoka, Y. (2004). Resistant Influenza A Viruses in Children Treated with Oseltamivir: Descriptive Study. Lancet, 364(9436), 759-765.

Kramarz, P., Monnet, D., Nicoll, A., Yilmaz, C. & Ciancio, B. (2009). Use of Oseltamivir in 12 European Countries between 2002 and 2007-Lack of Association with the Appearance of Oseltamivir-Resistant Influenza A(H1N1) Viruses. Eurosurveillance, 14(5), 19112.

Laudert, E. A., Sivanandan, V. & Halvorson, D. A. (1993). Effect of Intravenous Inoculation of Avian Influenza Virus on Reproduction and Growth in Mallard Ducks. Journal of Wildlife Diseases, 29(4), 523-526.

Leknes, H., Sturtzel, I. E. & Dye, C. (2012). Environmental Release of Oseltamivir from a Norwegian Sewage Treatment Plant During the 2009 Influenza A (H1N1) Pandemic. Science of the Total Environment, 414, 632-638.

Lipsitch, M., Plotkin, J. B., Simonsen, L. & Bloom, B. (2012). Evolution, Safety, and Highly Pathogenic Influenza Viruses. Science, 336(6088), 1529-1531.

Makarova, N. V., Kaverin, N. V., Krauss, S., Senne, D. & Webster, R. G. (1999). Transmission of Eurasian Avian H2 Influenza Virus to Shorebirds in North America. Journal of General Virology, 80, 3167-3171.

Matrosovich, M. N., Matrosovich, T. Y., Gray, T., Roberts, N. A. & Klenk, H. D. (2004). Neuraminidase Is Important for the Initiation of Influenza Virus Infection in Human Airway Epithelium. Journal of Virology, 78(22), 12665-12667.

Meijer, A., Lackenby, A., Hungnes, O., Lina, B., van-der-Werf, S., Schweiger, B., Opp, M., Paget, J., van-de-Kassteele, J., Hay, A. & Zambon, M. (2009). Oseltamivir-Resistant Influenza Virus A (H1N1), Europe, 2007-08 Season. Emerging Infectious Diseases, 15(4), 552-560.

Moscona, A. (2009). Global Transmission of Oseltamivir-Resistant Influenza. New England Journal of Medicine, 360(10), 953-956.

Nayak, D. P., Hui, E. K. & Barman, S. (2004). Assembly and Budding of Influenza Virus. Virus Research, 106(2), 147-165.

Nelson, M. I., Simonsen, L., Viboud, C., Miller, M. A. & Holmes, E. C. (2009). The Origin and Global Emergence of Adamantane Resistant A/H3N2 Influenza Viruses. Virology, 388(2), 270-278.

Nguyen, J. T., Hoopes, J. D., Le, M. H., Smee, D. F., Patick, A. K., Faix, D. J., Blair, P. J., de Jong, M. D., Prichard, M. N. & Went, G. T. (2010). Triple Combination of Amantadine, Ribavirin, and Oseltamivir Is Highly Active and Synergistic against Drug Resistant Influenza Virus Strains in Vitro. PLoS One, 5(2), e9332.

Nguyen, J. T., Smee, D. F., Barnard, D. L., Julander, J. G., Gross, M., de Jong, M. D. & Went, G. T. (2012). Efficacy of Combined Therapy with Amantadine, Oseltamivir, and Ribavirin in Vivo against Susceptible and Amantadine-Resistant Influenza A Viruses. PLoS One, 7(1), e31006.

Olsen, B., Munster, V. J., Wallensten, A., Waldenstrom, J., Osterhaus, A. D. & Fouchier, R. A. (2006). Global Patterns of Influenza A Virus in Wild Birds. Science, 312(5772), 384-388.

Partridge, J. & Kieny, M. P. (2010). Global Production of Seasonal and Pandemic (H1N1) Influenza Vaccines in 2009-2010 and Comparison with Previous Estimates and Global Action Plan Targets. Vaccine, 28(30), 4709-4712.

Patel, A. & Gorman, S. E. (2009). Stockpiling Antiviral Drugs for the Next Influenza Pandemic. Clinical Pharmacology & Therapeutics, 86(3), 241-243.

Prasse, C., Schlusener, M. P., Schulz, R. & Ternes, T. A. (2010). Antiviral Drugs in Wastewater and Surface Waters: A New Pharmaceutical Class of Environmental Relevance? Environmental Science & Technology, 44(5), 1728-1735.

Rameix-Welti, M. A., Enouf, V., Cuvelier, F., Jeannin, P. & van der Werf, S. (2008). Enzymatic Properties of the Neuraminidase of Seasonal H1N1 Influenza Viruses Provide Insights for the Emergence of Natural Resistance to Oseltamivir. PLoS Pathogens, 4(7), e1000103.

Rohm, C., Zhou, N., Suss, J., Mackenzie, J. & Webster, R. G. (1996). Characterization of a Novel Influenza Hemagglutinin, H15: Criteria for Determination of Influenza A Subtypes. Virology, 217(2), 508-516.

Russell, C. A., Fonville, J. M., Brown, A. E., Burke, D. F., Smith, D. L., James, S. L., Herfst, S., van Boheemen, S., Linster, M., Schrauwen, E. J., Katzelnick, L., Mosterin, A., Kuiken, T., Maher, E., Neumann, G., Osterhaus, A. D., Kawaoka, Y., Fouchier, R. A. & Smith, D. J. (2012). The Potential for Respiratory Droplet-Transmissible A/H5N1 Influenza Virus to Evolve in a Mammalian Host. Science, 336(6088), 1541-1547.

Schafer, J. R., Kawaoka, Y., Bean, W. J., Suss, J., Senne, D. & Webster, R. G. (1993). Origin of the Pandemic 1957 H2 Influenza A Virus and the Persistence of Its Possible Progenitors in the Avian Reservoir. Virology, 194(2), 781-788.

Smith, G. J., Bahl, J., Vijaykrishna, D., Zhang, J., Poon, L. L., Chen, H., Webster, R. G., Peiris, J. S. & Guan, Y. (2009). Dating the Emergence of Pandemic Influenza Viruses. Proceedings of the National Academy of Sciences USA, 106(28), 11709-11712.

Smith, G. J., Vijaykrishna, D., Bahl, J., Lycett, S. J., Worobey, M., Pybus, O. G., Ma, S. K., Cheung, C. L., Raghwani, J., Bhatt, S., Peiris, J. S., Guan, Y. & Rambaut, A. (2009). Origins and Evolutionary Genomics of the 2009 Swine-Origin H1N1 Influenza A Epidemic. Nature, 459(7250), 1122-1125.

Stoner, T. D., Krauss, S., DuBois, R. M., Negovetich, N. J., Stallknecht, D. E., Senne, D. A., Gramer, M. R., Swafford, S., DeLiberto, T., Govorkova, E. A. & Webster, R. G. (2010). Antiviral Susceptibility of Avian and Swine Influenza Virus of the N1 Neuraminidase Subtype. Journal of Virology, 84(19), 9800-9809.

Sweetman, S. Martindale: The Complete Drug Reference [Online]. http://www.medicinescomplete.com.

Soderstrom, H., Jarhult, J. D., Olsen, B., Lindberg, R. H., Tanaka, H. & Fick, J. (2009). Detection of the Antiviral Drug Oseltamivir in Aquatic Environments. PLoS One, 4(6), e6064.

Tashiro, M., McKimm-Breschkin, J. L., Saito, T., Klimov, A., Macken, C., Zambon, M. & Hayden, F. G. (2009). Surveillance for Neuraminidase-Inhibitor-Resistant Influenza Viruses in Japan, 1996-2007. Antiviral Therapy, 14(6), 751-761.

Taubenberger, J. K. & Morens, D. M. (2006). 1918 Influenza: The Mother of All Pandemics. Emerging Infectious Diseases, 12(1), 15-22.

Taubenberger, J. K., Reid, A. H., Lourens, R. M., Wang, R., Jin, G. & Fanning, T. G. (2005). Characterization of the 1918 Influenza Virus Polymerase Genes. Nature, 437(7060), 889-893.

Tong, S., Li, Y., Rivailler, P., Conrardy, C., Castillo, D. A., Chen, L. M., Recuenco, S., Ellison, J. A., Davis, C. T., York, I. A., Turmelle, A. S., Moran, D., Rogers, S., Shi, M., Tao, Y., Weil, M. R., Tang, K., Rowe, L. A., Sammons, S., Xu, X., Frace, M., Lindblade, K. A., Cox, N. J., Anderson, L. J., Rupprecht, C. E. & Donis, R. O. (2012). A Distinct Lineage of Influenza A Virus from Bats. Proceedings of the National Academy of Sciences USA, 109(11), 4269-4274.

Wahlgren, J., Waldenstrom, J., Sahlin, S., Haemig, P. D., Fouchier, R. A., Osterhaus, A. D., Pinhassi, J., Bonnedahl, J., Pisareva, M., Grudinin, M., Kiselev, O., Hernandez, J., Falk, K. I., Lundkvist, A. & Olsen, B. (2008). Gene Segment Reassortment between American and Asian Lineages of Avian Influenza Virus from Waterfowl in the Beringia Area. Vector Borne Zoonotic Diseases, 8(6), 783-790.

Wallensten, A., Munster, V. J., Elmberg, J., Osterhaus, A. D., Fouchier, R. A. & Olsen, B. (2005). Multiple Gene Segment Reassortment between Eurasian and American Lineages of Influenza A Virus (H6N2) in Guillemot (Uria Aalge). Archives of Virology, 150(8), 1685-1692.

Wallensten, A., Munster, V. J., Latorre-Margalef, N., Brytting, M., Elmberg, J., Fouchier, R. A., Fransson, T., Haemig, P. D., Karlsson, M., Lundkvist, A., Osterhaus, A. D., Stervander, M., Waldenstrom, J. & Olsen, B. (2007). *Surveillance of Influenza A Virus in Migratory Waterfowl in Northern Europe.* Emerging Infectious Diseases, 13(3), 404-411.

van der Vries, E., Veldhuis Kroeze, E. J., Stittelaar, K. J., Linster, M., Van der Linden, A., Schrauwen, E. J., Leijten, L. M., van Amerongen, G., Schutten, M., Kuiken, T., Osterhaus, A. D., Fouchier, R. A., Boucher, C. A. & Herfst, S. (2011). *Multidrug Resistant 2009 A/H1N1 Influenza Clinical Isolate with a Neuraminidase I223R Mutation Retains Its Virulence and Transmissibility in Ferrets.* PLoS Pathogens, 7(9), e1002276.

van Gils, J. A., Munster, V. J., Radersma, R., Liefhebber, D., Fouchier, R. A. & Klaassen, M. (2007). *Hampered Foraging and Migratory Performance in Swans Infected with Low-Pathogenic Avian Influenza A Virus.* PLoS One, 2(1), e184.

Wan Po, A. L., Farndon, P. & Palmer, N. (2009). *Maximizing the Value of Drug Stockpiles for Pandemic Influenza.* Emerging Infectious Diseases, 15(10), 1686-1687.

Wang, C., Takeuchi, K., Pinto, L. H. & Lamb, R. A. (1993). *Ion Channel Activity of Influenza A Virus M2 Protein: Characterization of the Amantadine Block.* Journal of Virology, 67(9), 5585-5594.

Webster, R. G., Bean, W. J., Gorman, O. T., Chambers, T. M. & Kawaoka, Y. (1992). *Evolution and Ecology of Influenza A Viruses.* Microbiological Reviews, 56(1), 152-179.

Webster, R. G., Yakhno, M., Hinshaw, V. S., Bean, W. J. & Murti, K. G. (1978). *Intestinal Influenza: Replication and Characterization of Influenza Viruses in Ducks.* Virology, 84(2), 268-278.

WHO. (2012). *Cumulative Number of Confirmed Human Cases for Avian Influenza A(H5N1) Reported to WHO, 2003-2012.* http://www.who.int/influenza/human_animal_interface/EN_GIP_20120810CumulativeNumberH5N1cases.pdf.

Wolinetz, C. D. (2012). *Implementing the New U.S. Dual-Use Policy.* Science, 336(6088), 1525-1527.

Epidemiology, Clinical Manifestations and Long Term Outcomes of a Major Outbreak of Chikungunya: A South Asian Experience

Sajitha C. Weerasinghe
The National Hospital of Sri Lanka, Colombo, Sri Lanka

Senanayake A.M. Kularatne
Department of Medicine, Faculty of Medicine
University of Peradeniya, Peradeniya, Sri Lanka

Champika M. Gihan
Department of Obstetrics and Gynaecology
University of Peradeniya, Peradeniya, Sri Lanka

1   Introduction

Chikungunya, a crippling mosquito-borne disease caused by the Chikungunya virus that recently emerged as a significant public health problem in Sri Lanka (Ministry of Healthcare and Nutrition, Sri Lanka, 2007). In February 2005, Chikungunya infection hit islands of the southern Indian Ocean affecting up to 200 000 inhabitants. Affected islands were Comoro, Mauritius, Seychelles and Reunion islands. Then it has spread to India in 2006 resulting in 1.38 million symptomatic illnesses in Central and southern India (Chastel, 2005; Parola *et al*., 2006; Kalantri *et al*., 2006; Ligon, 2006; Taubitz & Cramer, 2007; Hapuarachchi *et al*., 2010). The worst affected was Reunion Island where 35% of its inhabitants were affected by the epidemic (Simon *et al*., 2007).

First isolated in Tanzania in 1953, Chikungunya virus belongs to the family Togaviridae, genus Alphavirus with three genotypes: East African, West African and Asian (Kalantri *et al*., 2006; Pialoux *et al*., 2007). A study showed that the recent epidemic in South-East Asia was due to five genetically distinct subpopulations of chikungunya virus strains belonging to East, Central and South African (ECSA) lineage and were evolutionarily more related to Indian strain (Hapuarachchi *et al*., 2010).

Chikungunya is a zoonotic disease and the life cycle involves primates and *Aedes* mosquitoes (Higgs, 2006). Chikungunya virus has been associated with the urban *Aedes* mosquito in Asian countries in an epidemiologic cycle resembling that of dengue, no animal reservoir, direct human-to-human transmission by urban mosquitoes, and the potential risk of major epidemics (Parola *et al*., 2006). The mosquito was originally indigenous to Southeast Asia, the Western Pacific, and the Indian Ocean. Mainly because of transportation of dormant eggs in tires, it has spread to Africa, the Middle East, Europe and the Americas (Gratz, 2004).

The acute disease is self- limiting and only symptomatic treatment is necessary. However, the chronic phase is crippling for varying time periods. There is no effective vaccine to prevent the disease, so that mosquito control is the appropriate strategy to control and to contain the infection (Charrel *et al*., 2007). A few studies have examined the chronic phase of the illness but the overall picture and natural history were not well documented (Simon *et al*., 2007; Pialoux *et al*., 2007; Kennedy *et al*., 1980; Brighton *et al*., 1983). Thus, studying a cohort of patients from an affected community with close follow up for a long period would certainly elucidate more information about the infection.

The disease struck Sri Lanka in mid October 2006 affecting many parts of the Island and there were isolated pockets of high incidence of infection (Ministry of Healthcare and Nutrition, Sri Lanka, 2007; Ministry of Healthcare and Nutrition, Sri Lanka, 2006). One such area was Galagedara-Madige, a village in Kandy District, Sri Lanka, which was the focus of our study (Kularatne 2012). In this village a substantial number of inhabitants were affected by the epidemic and large numbers have been suffering from its chronic complications even six months after the infection. The objectives of the study were to describe the epidemiology, clinical picture, complications, outcome and natural history of the chikungunya infection among all households of the village.

2   Methods

2.1   Subject Enrolment

We carried out a household survey in Galagedara – Madige, the index village of the study situated in Kandy District, Sri Lanka, during a period of three weeks from May to June 2007. At that time seven months had elapsed from the onset of the epidemic in the village. The village has been exclusively inhabited by Sri Lankan Muslims with high population density. The households of surrounding villages of Galagedara – Madige were also interviewed for comparison of results.

Ethical clearance was obtained from the Ethical Committee, Faculty of Medicine, University of Peradeniya, Sri Lanka. Permission to interview people in the village was sought from the local health authorities, Deputy Director of Health Services and Medical Officer of Health – Galagedara.

2.2 Data Collection

Interviewers were three qualified medical graduates (including the authors) who first underwent familiarization with the data collection sheet and the format of interview. A structured, interviewer-completed questionnaire was used for the data collection. In order to avoid inter-observer variation, a common format was agreed upon after deliberations amongst the team members.

The questionnaire consisted of two parts viz. 'Family Data Sheet' and 'Individual Data Sheet'. Part one, 'Family Data Sheet' was used to collect the demographic data (name, age, gender, contact details, number of family members) of the family and part two, 'Individual Data Sheet' was used to compile data with respect to each patient who presently suffers from chikungunya or had a previous attack. Part two of the questionnaire contained details such as onset of the disease, clinical features, disability state, non-arthritic complications and past medical history. Where available, the patient's clinical notes were inspected to gather more details. Individuals with Chronic Arthritic Disability were followed up periodically in the field at 6, 12, 24 and 36 months till June 2010. All the family members and the patients were interviewed individually by the interviewers.

2.3 Diagnosis of Cases and Disability

Though, viral diagnostic tests are used for the confirmation of the infection, its availability in an outbreak is limited [5]. Hence, reliance on clinical data and circumstantial evidence was stressed. While interviewing the individuals, diagnosis of cases was made clinically, considering the epidemiological and circumstantial evidence. Clinical, laboratory and serology records were also examined for confirmation of the diagnosis, since local doctors had documented the diagnosis during the epidemic. Validation of clinical diagnosis was made based on published data from Kandy district, Sri Lanka during the same periods [16]. Diagnosis of chronic arthritic disability was made on clinical grounds, if the patient was having or had arthritic disability for more than 14 days after the defervescence of the acute illness. Also the other chronic complications such as carpal tunnel syndrome and post-viral fatigue syndrome were recorded during the interview.

2.4 Statistical Analysis

All the data collected were coded and computerized using Microsoft Excel Software (Microsoft Office 2007 Package). Analysis of the data was done using the statistical package, SPSS version 17.0 for Windows.

Calculation of frequencies and percentages was the first step in the analysis of the demographic data. The associations between rates of chikungunya infection and the demographic data were then analyzed using the Chi – square test and 'Student's" t-test. The correlation coefficients between the number of patients per family and the number of individuals in the family were also calculated. The Chi – square test was used to analyze the association between demographic data and acute illness, disability, carpal tunnel syndrome and relapses.

3   Results

3.1   Basic Epidemiological Analysis

Of the 1832 individuals interviewed in the study, 1001 (55%) were from Galagedara – Madige (Study village) and the rest 831 (45%) were from the neighboring village of Galagedara – Madige(Control group). Of the 1001 individuals of Madige, 513 (51%) were infected with chikungunya compared to 47 (6%) cases in the control group (p=0.000) during the outbreak of chikungunya in the region from October 2006 to May 2007. The incidence of cases had peaked during December 2006 to January 2007 in the study village-Madige (see Figure 1).

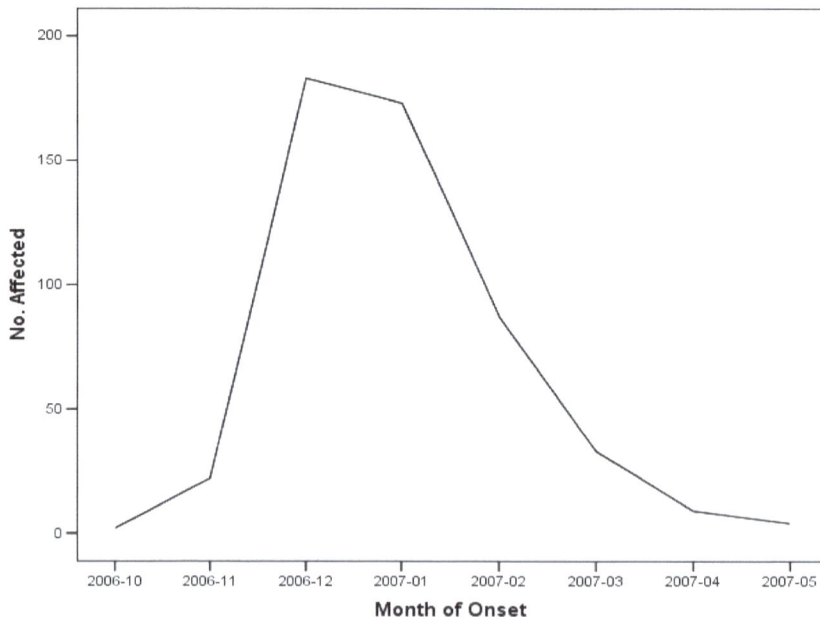

Figure 1: Temporal Relationship of Chikungunya Incidence in Madige

There were 199 families living in Madige and of them 159 (80%) families were affected during the epidemic. There was a positive correlation between the numbers of individuals affected per family with the total number of family members (Pearson's correlation coefficient = 0.497, p=0.01) (see Figure 2). The study sample of Madige (1001) comprised 485 (49%) males and 516 (52%) females (see Table 1).

Of the affected 513(51%) people, 237 (46%) were males and 276 (54%) were females (p=0.144) whilst   160 (31%) were house wives, 120 (23%) were school students and 100 (20%) were businessmen. The incidence of the disease had increased with increasing age, and peaked at 40- 50 years with the lowest incidence in children as shown in Table 2. The mean age of the affected group and the non-affected group was 35 years (range 1 – 90) and 26 years (range 1 – 98) years (p=0.000) respectively.

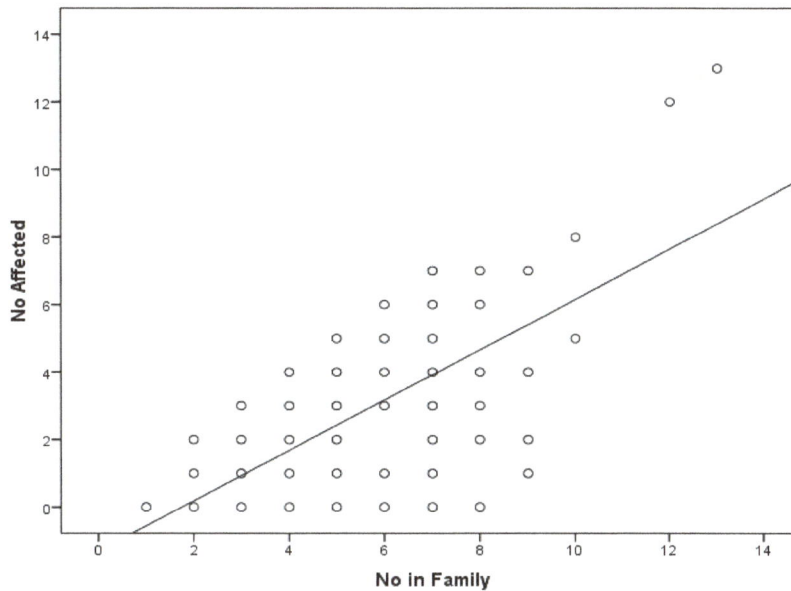

Figure 2: Relationship between numbers of affected per family and number of individuals per family.

Variable [N]		Male %	Female %	p Value [a]
Population of Madige (1001)		485(48)	516(52)	
Affected people in Madige (513)		237(46)	276(54)	0.144
Triad of symptoms (61)		17(28)	44(72)	0.002
Arthralgia (430)		191(44)	239(56)	0.560
Arthritis (233)		86(37)	147(63)	0.000
Chronic Arthritic Disability (230)		94(41)	136(59)	0.029
Carpal Tunnel Syndrome				
	Present	22	88	0.000
	Absent	214	184	
Relapses				
	Present	68	105	0.000
	Absent	166	167	

a - χ^2 statistics

Table 1: Gender based analysis of features.

Categorized Age	Chikungunya Fever [N, %] *				Total
	Infected		Non Infected		
0 - 12	93	38%	152	62%	245
13 – 22	74	45%	91	55%	165
23 – 32	81	51%	78	49%	159
33 – 42	80	58%	57	42%	137
43 – 52	76	62%	47	38%	123
53 – 62	54	59%	38	41%	92
63 – 72	41	71%	17	29%	58
73 – 82	12	67%	6	33%	18
83 – 92	2	67%	1	33%	3
93 – 102	0	0%	1	100%	1
Total	513	51%	488	49%	1001

Count, % within categorized Age

Table 2: Incidence of Chikungunya infection by age group.

3.2   Analysis of Acute Illness

Of the triad of clinical features (fever, rash and joint disease) used for the diagnosis of Chikungunya infection, 100 (20%) had the rash, 233 (46%) had polyarthritis and 430 (85%) had arthralgia. Of the patients with the entire triad (61), the majority were females (p=0.002), but the incidence of arthralgia did not show a significant gender based difference (p=0.56) (see Table 1).

Among the Chikungunya affected 513, there was a single death and details of the postmortem could not be traced. Of the remaining 512, 233(46%) had polyarthritis comprising 86 (37%) males and 147 (54%) females (p=0.000). Of them, 107(46%) had arthritis along with fever while 114 (49%) had arthritis at the deferversence and 12 (5%) had arthritis before the onset of fever. Involvement of joints during the acute phase showed more involvement of weight- bearing joints; ankle 173(74%), knee joint 96(41%) and feet 75(32%) than other joints; wrist 34(14%) and back 7(3%).

3.3   Analysis of Chronic Arthritic Disability

Of the 512 Chikungunya affected group, 230 (45%) had chronic arthritic disability (CAD) that comprised 99% of patients who had initial acute polyarthritis with female preponderance (p=0.029) (see Table1). Distribution of the joint involvement was the same as in acute arthritis with persistent disability in the weight-bearing joints. The proportion with CAD had increased with advancing age as shown in Table 3.

Considering the first two age categories, the proportion who had CAD was 10 % and 27 % respectively and this difference was significant (p=0.005).The mean ages for the CAD group and the non-disability group were 44years (range 2 – 90) and 27 years (range 1- 90) (p=0.000) respectively. Waxing and waning of chronic arthritis was reported by 204(89%) patients and the commonest cause of relapses was work-related activity.

Age Category	With Disability [N,%]		Without Disability [N,%]		Total
0 - 12	9	9.9	82	90.1	91
13 - 22	20	27.0	54	73.0	74
23 - 32	35	43.2	46	56.8	81
33 - 42	44	55.7	35	44.3	79
43 - 52	46	60.5	30	39.5	76
53 - 62	36	67.9	17	32.1	53
63 - 72	31	75.6	10	24.4	41
73 - 82	8	66.7	4	33.3	12
83 - 92	1	50.0	1	50.0	2

Table 3: Distribution of chronic arthritic disability in age groups.

Of the 230 who complained of CAD 102 (44%) had recovered from the disability state (Recovered group- 20% of 512 patients with chikungunya) whilst 128 (56%) had persisting disability (persistent group) at the time of the interview. The mean duration of the disability in the recovered group was 141 days (range 30 – 210 days). The severity of arthritic disability was graded as pain, pain with swelling, limitation of movements, limitation of function and bed ridden.. Out these five categories pain in the joints was the commonest CAD and it was found in 59 % followed by limitation of function (31%) of the patients. The outcome of the persistent group will be assessed periodically over next three years.

Of the 512 with chikungunya, 34(7%) patients gave a past-history of arthritic condition. Out of them 21 (64%) had an exacerbation of arthritis with Chikungunya infection and 12 (36%) patients remained quiescent (p=0.037). Also 18 (53%) of them had disability and 16 (47%) did not have disability (p=0.454).

The Carpal Tunnel Syndrome (CTS) was the commonest non-arthritic complication following the Chikungunya infection (see Table 4).

Complication	Number Affecte [N,%]	
Carpal Tunnel Syndrome	110	21.5
Post Viral Fatigue Syndrome	8	1.6
Thrombophlebitis	2	0.4
Respiratory Tract Infections	4	0.8
Calf Swelling	1	0.2
Facial Swelling	3	0.6

Table 4: Non – arthritic complications among Chikungunya affected patients.

The proportion with CTS had increased with the age. In the age group of 0 – 12 years there were no reported cases of CTS whilst the incidence increased with age: in 13 – 22 y group 5%, 33 – 42y group 31%, 43 – 52y group 37%, and 53 – 62 y group 36%. Furthermore, the incidence of CTS had significantly increased in females, in patients with past-history of arthritis and in the chronic arthritic disability group (sees Tables 5 and 6).

	With Relapses		Without Relapses		p Value
Mean Age	44.1		29.9		0.000[b]
Cause of Relapse (N,%)					
Work related	122	73	46	27	
Off NSAIDs[c]	44	26	124	74	
Cold environment	38	23	130	77	

a - χ^2 statistics

b - "Student's" t-test

c - Non-Steroidal Anti-inflammatory Drugs

Table 5: Analysis of the Relapses of Chronic Disabling Arthritis (N =173) (75% out of CDA 230 Patients).

		Carpal Tunnel Syndrome		χ^2 Value	p Value
		Present	Absent		
Past - Arthritis	Present	16	18	14.121	0.000
	Absent	94	384		
Chronic Arthritic Disability	Present	84	146	56.069	0.000
	Absent	26	253		

Table 6: Analysis of Carpal Tunnel Syndrome

Subjects with CAD were followed up at 6 12, 24 and 36 months following the acute clinical illness. The numbers with the CAD are as follows – 230(100%), 41(17.8%), 22(9.5%) and 14(6.1%) respectively (see Figure 3). For the recovered group, CAD category and the prevalence are given in Table 7.

4   Discussion

This survey describes the pattern of spread, prevalence of long term sequels and the natural history of chikungunya infection which swept across a hamlet in central Sri Lanka during the recent outbreak of the disease. This village is a compact mass of houses which is inhabited only by the Sri Lankan Muslim community who prefers to live as close extended family and this fact would have contributed to the higher incidence of the disease compared to the neighboring villages. The peak of the infection lasted two months bringing the life in the whole village to a standstill with economic difficulties. The infection was peaked during the December 2006 and January 2007 period. The reason may be rainfall pattern in Sri Lanka. December to February is the Northeast -monsoon season, which is one of the major rainfall seasons in for the country. (Department of Meteorology Sri Lanka, 2012)

We found that the infection had affected more adults than children and a concurrent sharp rise of the incidence within households of big families. Figure 2, shows the relationship between the number of inhabitants in the family (household index) and the number affected. Hence, the alarming rapidity of spread of the infection is an epidemiological feature to be investigated. This could be due to the easy spread of this mosquito borne disease with the higher population density.

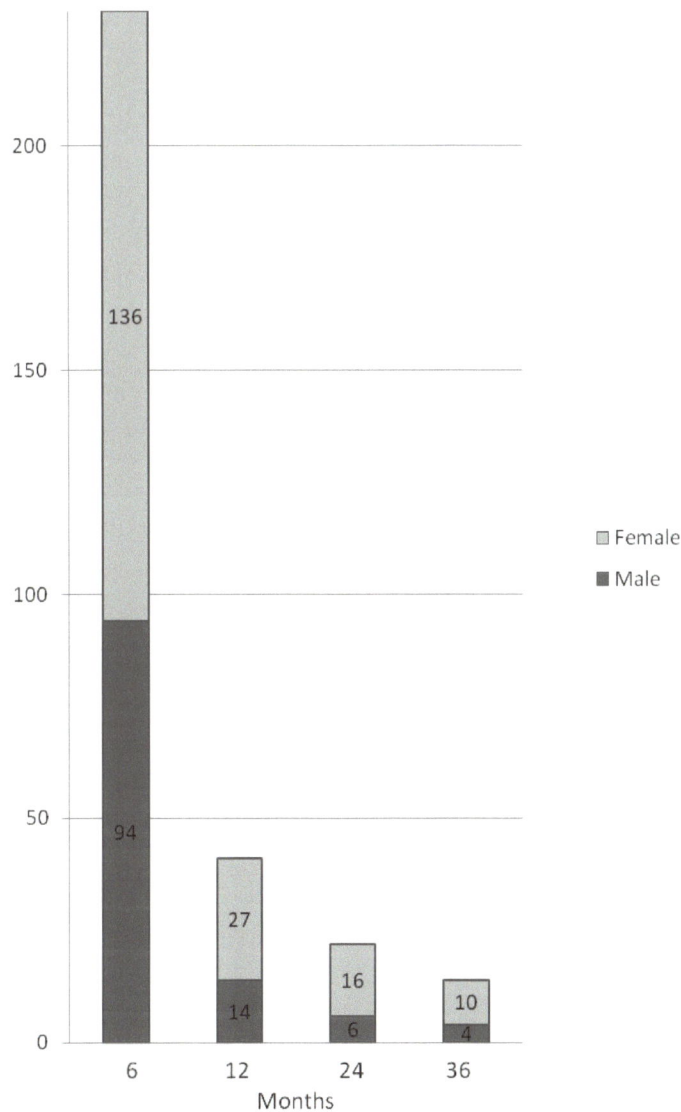

Figure 3: Number of individuals with chronic arthritic disability (CAD) at follow up

Disability	Number affected [N,%]	
Pain	60	59
Pain and Swelling	8	8
Limitation of Movement	2	2
Limitation of Function	32	31
Bed Ridden	0	0

Table 7: Chronic arthritic disability (CAD) scores analysis of the recovered group. (N = 102, 44.3% of total CAD)

Morbidity was more among females as they outnumbered the males in acute polyarthritis, chronic arthritic disability (CAD), Carpal Tunnel Syndrome (CTS) and relapses of arthritis (Table 1). The exact reason for the higher prevalence of disease morbidity is not known and it should be investigated in the future.

Polyarthralgia was the dominant symptom in the acute stage of the illness and only about 20% gave a history of a skin rash. Acute polyarthritis affected 45% of the cohort and of them 50% of patients had developed arthritis with the defervescence. Furthermore, weight-bearing joints were more affected. Interestingly, 99% of patients with acute polyarthritis had progressed to CAD which was characterized by waxing and waning in severity and very often exacerbated by physical activities (Table 4). The acute arthritis and CAD were much less in the paediatric age group (p=0.001) and what made them less susceptible to these complications is an open-ended question. The duration of the CAD varied from 30 – 210 days in the recovered group accounting for 44% of CAD, but the balance 56%, classified as persistent group would probably continue with symptoms for hitherto unknown period. At the end of three years of follow up of CAD, we found 6.1% were still suffering with with debilities.

The reason why the study population had significant arthritic complications is an unanswered question and it needs further research, focusing on genetic studies or HLA studies to identify any predisposition. The CTS was the commonest non – arthritic complication (22%) in our study and this was commoner in females (p=0.001) and a smaller proportion of patients had symptoms suggestive of a post-viral fatigue syndrome.

Chikungunya virus is not a stranger to Sri Lanka as the first epidemic was reported in the early 1960s, followed by quiescence until the current epidemic which started in mid October 2006 (Ministry of Healthcare and Nutrition, Sri Lanka, 2007; Munasinghe et al., 1966). There were more than 37, 000 cases were reported in first few months from different parts of the island but this was a tip of the iceberg due to underreporting (Ministry of Healthcare and Nutrition, Sri Lanka, 2007). Devastating outbreaks occurred in pockets of close communities and one such a hotspot was the index village of our study. Viral transmission from human to human through direct contact with highly viremic blood was postulated in France (Parola, 2006).

The disese is transmitted by Aedes mosquito, which is the vector of Dengue fever and Chikungunya, found in Sri Lanka.(Kularatne et al., 2009). It is an urban mosquito and breeds in clear water. However, overcrowding of houses would have led to poor hygiene and prevalence of mosquito breeding sites. A study done in India showed that high population density, lack of adequate vector control and poor hygiene was important risk factors in the population (Saxena, 2006).

In the acute illness, we recorded skin manifestation in 20% of cases, but other studies had observed 40-50% involvement of skin (Ligon, 2006; Brighton, 1983). More data are available on arthritis that had affected 73-80% patients in some published series and had chronically persisted 4 months and 3 years in 33% and 10% of patients respectively (Ligon, 2006 ; Pialoux et al., 2007 ; Brighton, 1983). Furthermore, in a series of 47 travelers returning to France 38(81%) had chronic peripheral rheumatism affecting mainly ankle, wrist, fingers and toes after the 10th day of illness contrary to the findings of our series where 44% of patients had chronic arthritic debility mainly affecting weight bearing joints (Simon et al., 2007). Further, the same study showed a preponderance of arthritis to previously injured joints, similar to our observation where there was a significant association between past - arthritis and the CAD. Among the non – arthritic complications, CTS was the commonest complication (n=110, 22%). A previous study showed that 10 out of 47 patients had CTS (Simon et al., 2007), but further analysis of the CTS has not been done. We found the incidence of CTS was more associated with females, chikungunya arthritis, past medical history of arthritic conditions (Table 6) and age.

Interestingly the outbreak of chikungunya in1965 had reported less joint disease and non arthritic complications than the current series (Munasinghe *et al.*, 1966). Furthermore, re-emerged infection appeared to be more severe than the past disease (Pialoux *et al.*, 2007). Plausible explanations for the increased morbidity of the current infection include mutations of the virus, absence of herd immunity, lack of vector control and globalization of travel and trade (Ligon, 2006 ; Pialoux *et al.*, 2007). Sri Lanka records high incidence of chikungunya among the regions during the ongoing epidemic in the Indian Ocean. A large number was affected during the epidemic and they are still suffering from its chronic complications. This has affected the activities of daily living and the well being of the substantial number of people in the community. Unfortunately, there is no evidence based-treatment policy for the management of CAD except for its natural healing and alleviation of symptoms. Hence, proper understanding of the pathophysiology of chronic disability and development of an effective treatment regimen would be an urgent task.

Acknowledgements

The authors would like to acknowledge Prof. S.N.Arseculeratne for the valuable comments.

References

Brighton, S. W., Prozesky, O. W., de la Harpe, A. L. (1983). Chikungunya virus infection. A retrospective study of 107 cases. South African Medical Journal, 63 (9), 313-315.

Charrel, R. N., Lamballerie, X., Raoult, D. (2007). Chikungunya Outbreaks — The Globalization of Vector borne Diseases," The New England Journal of Medicine, 356, 769-771.

Chastel, C. (2005). Chikungunya virus: its recent spread to the southern Indian Ocean and Reunion Island. Bulletin de l'Académie nationale de médecine, 189 (8), 1827-1835.

Department of Meteorology Sri Lanka. (2012). Climate in Sri Lanka.

Gratz, N.G. (2004). Critical review of the vector status of Aedes albopictus. Med Vet Entomol, 18 (3), 215-27.

Hapuarachchi, H.C., Lee-Ching Ng, Bandara, K.B.A.T., et al. (2010). Re-emergence of Chikungunya virus in South-east Asia: virological evidence from Sri Lanka and Singapore. Journal of General Virology 91 (4), 1067–1076.

Higgs, S. (2006). The 2005-2006 Chikungunya epidemic in the Indian Ocean. Vector borne and zoonotic diseases, 6 (2), 115-116.

Kalantri, S.P., Joshi, R., Riley, L.W. (2006). Chikungunya epidemic: an Indian Perspective. The National medical journal of India, 19 (6), 315-322.

Kennedy, A. C., Fleming, J., Solomon, L. (1980). Chikungunya viral arthropathy: a clinical description. The Journal of Rheumatology, 7 (2), 231-236.

Kularatne, S. A., Gihan, M.C., Weerasinghe, S. C., Gunasena, S. (2009). Concurrent outbreaks of Chikungunya and Dengue fever in Kandy, Sri Lanka, 2006-07: a comparative analysis of clinical and laboratory features. Postgraduate medical journal, 85 (1005), 342-346.

Kularatne, Senanayake A. M., Weerasinghe, Sajitha C., Gihan, Champika et al. (2012). Epidemiology, Clinical Manifestations, and Long-Term Outcomes of a Major Outbreak of Chikungunya in a Hamlet in Sri Lanka, in 2007: A Longitudinal Cohort Study. J Trop Med, 2012: 639178. doi: 10.1155/2012/639178.

Ligon, B. L. (2006). Reemergence of an unusual disease: the chikungunya epidemic. Seminars in pediatric infectious diseases, 17 (2), 99-104.

Ministry of Healthcare and Nutrition, Sri Lanka (2007). Investigation of the outbreak of Chikungunya fever – 2006/7 Sri Lanka. Retrieved from http://www.epid.gov.lk/pdf/chikungunya/OBOFCHIGYA.pdf.

Ministry of Healthcare and Nutrition, Sri Lanka. (2006). Ministry News Latter 2006. Retrieved from http://www.epid.gov.lk.

Ministry of Healthcare and Nutrition, Sri Lanka. (2007). Brief account of the situation regarding the suspected outbreak of Chikungunya in Sri Lanka. Retrieved from http://www.epid.gov.lk/pdf/chikungunya/Message_in_chikungunya_24_11_06.pdf

Munasinghe, D. R., Amarasekera, P. J., Fernando, F. O. C. (1966). An Epidemic of Dengue- like fever in Ceylon (Chikungunya) – A clinical and Haematological Study. The Ceylon Medical Journal, 11 (4) 129-142.

Parola, P., de Lamballerie, X., Jourdan J., et al. (2006). Novel chikungunya virus variant in travellers returning from Indian Ocean islands. Emerging Infectious Diseases, 12 (10), 1493- 1499.

Pialoux, G., Gaüzère, B. A., Jauréguiberry, S., Strobel, M. (2007). Chikungunya, an epidemic arbovirosis. The Lancet Infectious Diseases, 7 (5), 319-327.

Retrieve from http://www.meteo.gov.lk/index.php?option=com_content&view=article&id=106&Itemid=81&lang=en.

Saxena, S. K., Singh, M., Mishra, N., Lakshmi, V. (2006). Resurgence of chikungunya virus in India: an emerging threat. Euro Surveillance- European communicable disease bulletin, 11 (8), E060810.2.

Simon, F., Parola, P., Grandadam M., et al. (2007). Chikungunya infection: an emerging rheumatism among travelers returned from Indian Ocean islands. Report of 47 cases. Medicine (Baltimore), 86 (3), 123-137.

Taubitz, W., Cramer, J. P. (2007). Chikungunya fever in travelers: clinical presentation and course. Clinical Infectious Diseases, 45 (1), e1-4.

Mokola Virus (MOKV) in Southern Africa: A Review of Genetic, Epidemiologic and Surveillance Studies

Claude Sabeta

OIE Rabies Reference Laboratory

Agricultural Research Council – Onderstepoort Veterinary Institute, Pretoria, South Africa

Baby Phahladira

OIE Rabies Reference Laboratory

Agricultural Research Council – Onderstepoort Veterinary Institute, Pretoria, South Africa

1   Introduction

Isolations of MOKV are rare but in southern Africa (specifically South Africa and Zimbabwe), this unusual *Lyssavirus* variant has been recovered in cats and a dog. The initial isolation of this *Lyssavirus* variant was in a domestic cat near Durban (South Africa) in 1970 and subsequent isolations occurred thereafter in the 1980s in Zimbabwe and many years later in the 1990s and 2000s in South Africa. To date, a total of 26 viruses from the African continent (South Africa n=9 & Zimbabwe n=8) have been confirmed as MOKV either during lyssavirus surveillance or routine rabies diagnostics. Here, we review the genetic and antigenic data of selected MOKVs recovered from the southern African countries of Zimbabwe and South Africa. Interestingly, the majority of MOKVs were isolated from hosts that had previously been immunized against rabies, underlining the limited spectrum of protection provided by inactivated rabies virus (RABV) vaccines against some African lyssaviruses. Although appropriate diagnostic tools and targeted surveillance coupled with accurate reporting systems for MOKV are key for its control, there may be a need to increase the spectrum of protection of current vaccines and biologicals to include the unusual lyssaviruses encountered in Africa and other potentially emerging lyssavirus variants. However, the continual isolation of MOKVs in domestic cats is speculative of the existence of a reservoir host species amongst bats or rodents.

For thousands of years, rabies was considered as a single entity transmitted via the bite of a rabid animal, but it was only at the turn of the 20th century that the causative agent of this fatal zoonotic disease was actually shown to be a virus (Steele, 1975). Rabies is probably one of the oldest but certainly the most feared disease known in medical history (Charlton, 1988; Wiktor, 1985; Brown, 2011). Once the virus has successfully established infection in a host, the disease is inevitably fatal in all warm-blooded vertebrates including humans (King & Turner, 1993), making it a disease of great public health significance (Smith & Seidel, 1993). Despite the availability of biologicals for rabies control, human deaths still occur globally but mainly in the developing nations of Africa (24 000 human deaths annually) and Asia (31 000 human deaths annually) (Knobel *et al.*, 2005), although the number could be as high as 75 000 human fatalities. At least 95% of these human deaths are dog-mediated with most being recorded in children under the age of 15 years.

Rabies is caused by members of the *Lyssavirus* genus in the *Rhabdoviridae* family, order *Mononegavirales*. These viruses are highly neurotropic and are characterized by negative-sense and RNA stranded genomes that contain five genes encoding for the nucleocapsid protein (N), phosphoprotein (P), the polymerase (L), the envelope matrix protein (M) and the glycoprotein (G) (Tordo & Kouknetzoff, 1993; Tordo *et al.*, 1997). The N, P and L proteins assemble to form a ribonucleoprotein aggregate (RNP). The L protein functions as an RNA-dependent RNA polymerase together with the P protein (a cofactor) for polymerase activity. On the other hand, the genomic RNA is encapsidated by the N protein, together with P and L, and this acts as a functional template for both transcription and replication processes.

2   Lyssavirus Taxonomy

Currently, the *Lyssavirus* genus is composed of 12 species (ICTV Official Taxonomy: Updates since the 8th Report, 2009) (Fauquet *et al.*, 2004), and all with the exception of MOKV, are associated with infection in a variety of chiropteran species. Spillover of a bat lyssavirus to terrestrial mammals is believed to have occurred at least 500 years ago highlighting an important host-switch event in *Lyssavirus* evolution (Badrane & Tordo, 2001). *Lyssavirus* species that include Lagos bat virus (LBV), Mokola virus (MOKV) and Duvenhage virus (DUVV) are exclusive to the African continent and were initially discovered in West Africa lending support to the belief that West Africa is probably the birthplace of lyssaviruses. Within the African continent, and similar to many other parts of the globe (Europe, North and South America), Classical rabies virus type species (RABV) is the most prevalent lyssavirus strain maintained in terrestrial wildlife. In southern Africa, RABV is maintained in (black-backed & side-striped jackal spp. *Canis adustus* and *Canis mesomelas sp.*, bat-eared fox *Otocyon megalotis*) and domestic dog populations (Nel & Markotter, 2007; Swanepoel *et al.*, 1993; Bingham *et al.*, 1999a, b).

Rabies-related viruses consisting of *Lagos bat virus*, *Mokola virus*, *Duvenhage virus*, the *Shimoni Bat Virus* (SHIBV) (Kuzmin *et al.*, 2010) and *Ikoma virus* (IKOV) (Marston *et al.*, 2012a, 2012b), have all been recovered from a variety of host species in Africa. In Europe, the *European Bat Lyssavirus* type-1 (EBLV-1) and type-2 (EBLV-2) as well as *Bokeloh Bat Lyssavirus* (BBLV) were identified from specific regions of the continent (Davis *et al.*, 2005). The *Australian bat Lyssavirus* (ABLV) was initially confirmed in 1996 (Gould *et al.*, 1998) and since then, there have been several isolations including two fatal human cases (Allworth *et al.*, 1996; Hanna *et al.*, 2000). Several bat-associated lyssaviruses have been reported from Eurasia. These are *Aravan virus* (ARAV) in Kyrgystan (Botvinkin *et al.*, 2003), *Khujand virus* (KHUV) in Tajikistan (Kuzmin *et al.*, 2003; 2005), *Irkut virus* (IRKV) in Eastern Siberia (Botvinkin *et al.*, 2003). The most recent lyssavirus isolated from this region is the *West Caucasian Bat virus* (WCBV) from a bat in Russia (Kuzmin *et al.*, 2005; 2008).

More recently, an assessment of pathogenic, phylogenetic and immunogenic properties of lyssaviruses in a mouse model of rabies segregated members of the *Lyssavirus* genus into 2 phylogroups, namely phylogroups I and II. Phylogroup I is composed of members that are highly pathogenic to mice when inoculated via both the intracerebral (i.c.) and intramuscular (i.m) routes, whereas phylogroup II (composed of MOKV, LBV and IKOV) is pathogenic via the i.c. route (Badrane *et al.*, 2001). These observations seem to suggest that phylogroup II members may be less of a public health threat in comparison to those in phylogroup I. From previous studies undertaken using a mouse model, both MOKV and LBV appeared less pathogenic when inoculated i.m. unlike when introduced through the i.c. route. These results (obtained by Badrane *et al.*, 2001) have since been refuted by Markotter (2007). In the latter studies (Markotter, 2007; Markotter *et al.*, 2008) it was demonstrated that certain viruses in phylogroup II (LBV and MOKV) possess the same pathogenicity effect as those from phylogroup I particularly for classical RABVs in both mice and in shrews (Kemp *et al.*, 1973). Based on the general criterion for phylogroup I and II (Badrane *et al.*, 2001), it appears WCBV does not belong to either group and is clearly the most phylogenetically divergent *Lyssavirus* compared to RABV and exhibits limited relatedness to LBVs and MOKVs (Weyer *et al.*, 2008). As WCBV could not be included into either of these phylogroups, it was suggested to be an independent phylogroup III (Hanlon *et al.*, 2005; Kuzmin *et al.*, 2005).

In the early 1970s, it became apparent that rabies-related viruses were indeed capable of causing encephalitis in man as well as other mammalian species (Meredith, 1971; Bourhy *et al.*, 1990). Firstly, LBV was recovered from mature megachiropteran frugivorous bat species (*Eidolon helvum*) during a survey for rabies in this bat species on Lagos Island in Nigeria (Boulger & Porterfield, 1958). This *Lyssavirus* species was subsequently isolated in laboratory mice from a pool of brains and salivary glands of male fruit bats that had been collected from a tree roost. The (LBV) isolate in question was only confirmed many years later, following the isolation of another distant *Lyssavirus* species, MOKV. The two

(LBV and MOKV) had similar serological properties to classical RABV and only then was the LBV isolate shown to be indeed a Rhabdovirus (Shope *et al.*, 1970). Subsequent isolations of LBV were made in a common frugivorous *Micropterus pusillus* bat near Bangui in the Central African Republic (Sureau *et al.*, 1977; 1980).

During a dog rabies outbreak in rabies-endemic KwaZulu/Natal Province of South Africa (see map of South Africa, Figure 1) in June 1980, two accidental virus isolations from unidentified bats (designated SA2 and SA3) were made, followed by a further 7 isolations, primarily from large fruit-eating bats *Epomophorus wahlbergi*. Another virus isolate was recovered from a domestic cat (designated SA30) from the same geographical region, that had contracted rabies despite previous vaccinations (described in Schneider, 1982; Schneider *et al.*, 1985). The fact that the cat (SA30) contracted rabies despite having received anti-rabies vaccines bears testimony to the inability of current rabies vaccines to fully protect against this group of lyssaviruses. The LBV epizootic in and around Durban was probably caused by the common epauletted fruit bat, although only one bat was conclusively identified as such (Crick *et al.*, 1982; Schneider *et al.*, 1985). Animal experiments with one of the LBV isolates on laboratory rodents and vervet monkeys produced fatal rabies-like encephalitis (Meredith, unpublished). A description of LBV epidemiology involving recent LBV isolates in South Africa is described elsewhere (Markotter *et al.*, 2006a; 2006b; Markotter, 2007).

MOKV was initially isolated from shrews (*Crocidura* sp.) in Mokola district near Ibadan, in Nigeria in 1968 (Boulger & Porterfield, 1958). Subsequently, MOKV was recovered from two human patients in the same country, one of which was fatal (Familusi & Moore, 1972; Familusi *et al.*, 1972; Kemp *et al.*, 1972). Two arthropod-borne rhabdoviruses, Obhodhiang and Kotonkan, were initially placed in the same serogroup as classical RABV based on limited antigenic cross-reactivity with MOKV. This led to a proposal that the evolutionary pathway for the rabies-related viruses could in actual fact include arthropod-borne Obhodhiang and Kotonkan viruses as progenitors through MOKV (Harrison *et al.*, 1970). Therefore the origin of lyssaviruses has been centred on the "insect origin" hypothesis where it was suggested that insect rhabdoviruses gave rise to lyssaviruses after transmission to insectivorous bats (Shope, 1982; Badrane & Tordo, 2001). Incidentally, MOKV is the only lyssavirus capable of replicating in insect cells (Buckley, 1975; Aitken, 1984). There are however no MOKV insect-derived isolates that have been obtained in nature. Rigorous serological and gene sequencing studies (Kuzmin *et al.*, 2005) demonstrated that Obhodhiang and Kotonkan viruses actually belong to Ephemeroviruses.

In 1970, a domestic cat from the beach resort of Umhlanga rocks near Durban South Africa was diagnosed with rabies (later confirmed to be MOKV in 1981) (Foggin, 1988), and subsequently MOKV was confirmed in shrews in Cameroon in 1974 (Le Gonidec *et al.*, 1978), in a rodent in the Central African Republic in 1983 (Saluzzo *et al.*, 1984), and during the unique outbreak in domestic cats in Zimbabwe (Foggin, 1988). In 1989, MOKV was isolated from a cat in Ethiopia (Mebatsion *et al.*, 1992). From April 1981 to May 1982 and during a unique epizootic in the Bulawayo region in southern Zimbabwe (Figure 1), the brains of 6 domestic cats, one of which had previously been vaccinated with a rabies vaccine (Foggin, 1988), were found to be infected with atypical rabies viruses. The isolation of MOKVs in Bulawayo appears to be the first report of this *Lyssavirus* species from central or southern Africa and the first from domestic animals (Foggin, 1982; 1983). The nervous symptoms displayed by these cats were not of the furious rabies type although aggression was at times evident. Further to the MOKVs isolations in the early 1980s in Zimbabwe, it was only in 2001 that another MOKV was confirmed retrospectively from a cat from this country (Bingham *et al.*, 2001).

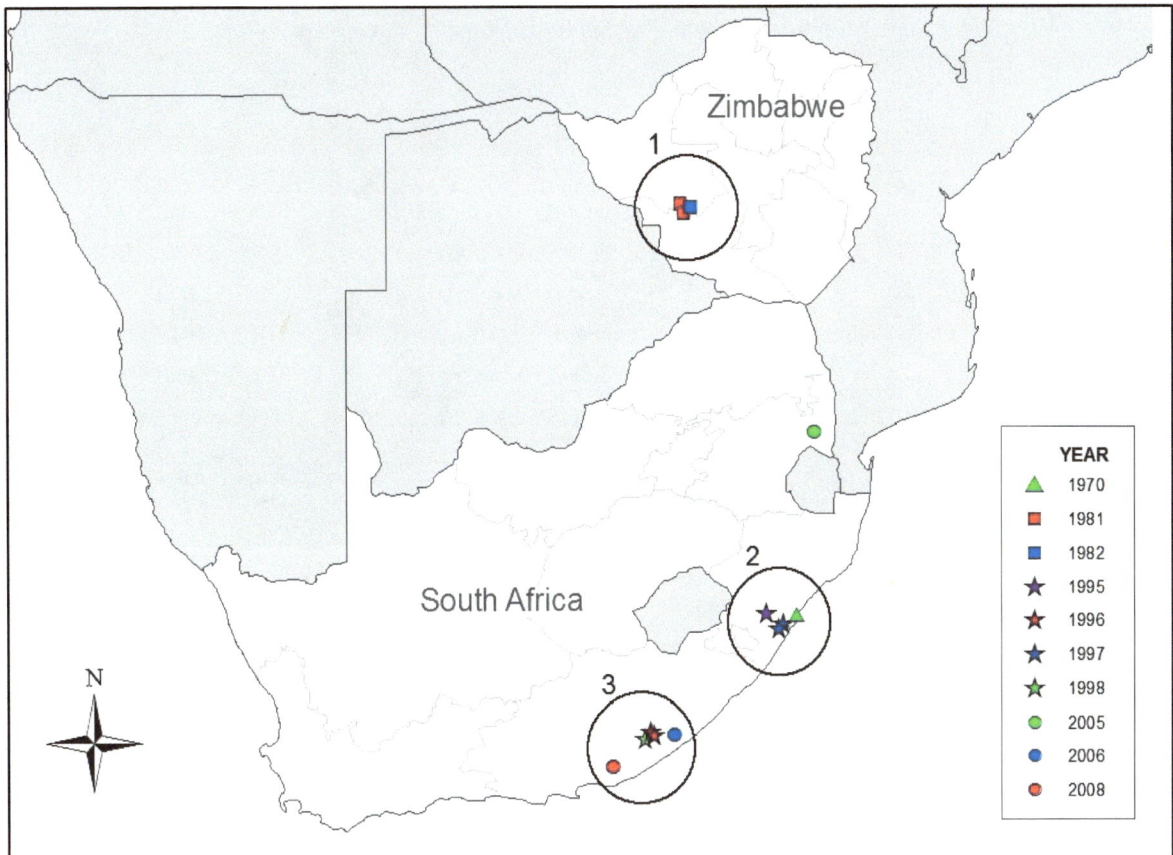

Figure 1: Map of Zimbabwe and South Africa showing the geographical locations where MOKV isolates have been recovered. The numbers correlate with the clades shown in Figure 2: 1 = ZIM 1, 2 = RSA1 and 3 = RSA2.

After the Umhlanga isolate of 1970, no further isolations of MOKV were made in South Africa until 1995 (Meredith *et al.*, 1996). In the MOKV isolations of the 1990s, 5 cases and all from domestic cats were made from different localities in two adjacent provinces of South Africa, namely the KwaZulu/Natal and Eastern Cape provinces respectively. The first isolation was in Mdantsane (East London), the second one was 15 km to the north east from where the first cat was found, the third 5 km north of East London, the fourth from Pinetown (near Durban) in 1997, and lastly the fifth from Pietermaritzburg (near Durban) in 1998 (Von Teichman *et al.*, 1998). Three of these cats had previously been vaccinated against rabies as per the South African government regulations that require pets to be vaccinated at three months of age and thereafter one more time during the next 9 months. Unlike symptoms due to classical RABV infection, cats that succumbed to MOKV infection from Zimbabwe in the 1980 outbreak were not aggressive (Von Teichman *et al.*, 1998). The three most recent MOKV cases in South Africa (in the 2000s) involved one case of MOKV infection in a domestic dog from Mpumalanga, the first such reported case in a dog for South Africa and the African continent (Sabeta *et al.*, 2007). The second was made in a domestic cat in East London, the host species from which all of the previous isolates from South Africa were recovered. The third and most recent case of MOKV (in 2008) was associated with a human contact in Grahamstown (Sabeta *et al.*, 2010). At least 25 isolations of this lyssavirus have since been recovered throughout Africa (in Cameroon, the Central African Republic, Ethiopia, South Africa and Zimbabwe) (see Table 1).

Locality & country of isolation	Year of isolation	Host source of isolate	Reference
Ibadan, Nigeria	1968	Shrew (*Crocidura* sp.)	Shope *et al.*, 1970
Ibadan, Nigeria	1968	Shrew (*Crocidura* sp.)	Shope *et al.*, 1970
Ibadan, Nigeria	1968	Shrew (*Crocidura* sp.)	Shope *et al.*, 1970
Ibadan, Nigeria	1968	Human (*Homo sapiens*)	Kemp *et al.*, 1972
Ibadan, Nigeria	1968	Shrew (*Crocidura* sp.)	Kemp *et al.*, 1972
Umhlanga, South Africa	1970	Cat (*Felis domesticus*)	Nel *et al.*, 2000
Ibadan, Nigeria	1971	Human (*Homo sapiens*)	Kemp *et al.*, 1972
Yaounde, Cameroon	1974	Shrew (*Crocidura* sp.)	Le Gonidec *et al.* 1978
Bangui, Central African Republic	1981	Rodent (*Lophuromys sikapusi*)	Salluzo *et al.*, 1984
Bulawayo, Zimbabwe	1981	Cat (*Felis domesticus*)	Foggin, 1988
Bulawayo, Zimbabwe	1981	Cat (*Felis domesticus*)	Foggin, 1988
Bulawayo, Zimbabwe	1981	Cat (*Felis domesticus*)	Foggin, 1988
Bulawayo, Zimbabwe	1981	Cat (*Felis domesticus*)	Foggin, 1988
Bulawayo, Zimbabwe	1981	Cat (*Felis domesticus*)	Foggin, 1988
Bulawayo, Zimbabwe	1982	Cat (*Felis domesticus*)	Foggin, 1988
Bulawayo, Zimbabwe	1982	Cat (*Felis domesticus*)	Foggin, 1988
Addis Ababa, Ethiopia	1989-1990	Cat (*Felis domesticus*)	Mebatsion *et al.*, 1992
Selous, Zimbabwe	1982	Cat (*Felis domesticus*)	Bingham *et al.*, 2001
Mdantsane, South Africa	1995	Cat (*Felis domesticus*)	Meredith *et al.*, 1996
East London, South Africa	1996	Cat (*Felis domesticus*)	von Teichman *et al.*, 1998
Yellow Sands, South Africa	1996	Cat (*Felis domesticus*)	von Teichman *et al.*, 1998
Pinetown, South Africa	1997	Cat (*Felis domesticus*)	von Teichman *et al.*, 1998
Pietermaritzburg, South Africa	1998	Cat (*Felis domesticus*)	von Teichman *et al.*, 1998
Nkomazi, South Africa	2005	Dog (*Canis lupus familiaris*)	Sabeta *et al.*, 2007
East London, South Africa	2006	Cat (*Felis domesticus*)	Sabeta *et al.*, 2007
Grahamstown, South Africa	2008	Cat (*Felis domesticus*)	Sabeta *et al.*,2010

Table 1: Table illustrates the epidemiological information of all MOKVs isolated to date on the African continent

There were problems associated with the diagnosis of the early MOKV cases. For instance an acetone–fixed brain smear of the 1970 MOKV displayed atypical staining on the fluorescent antibody test (FAT) (Dean *et al.*, 1996). For this reason it was stored and only confirmed to be MOKV in the mid-1980s using antigenic typing. During that time, initial diagnosis of MOKVs using the FAT with the standard rabies conjugate produced dull fluorescence due to the poor fluorescence obtained with the FAT and misdiagnosis of other MOKVs or rabies-related viruses was highly likely. Today, the initial diagnosis is now carried out using high quality polyclonal conjugate generated against both rabies (Street *ala-bama Duferrin*, SAD: phylogroup I) and MOKVs (phylogroup II) purified nucleocapsid proteins (fluorescein isothiocyanate (FITC)-labelled polyclonal conjugate). After conjugation of FITC to the hyperimmuneserum against members of both phylogroups, the anti-lyssavirus conjugate is then capable of detecting all four African lyssaviruses (rabies, LBV, MOKV, IKOV and DUVV), thus covering the whole spectrum of lyssaviruses commonly found globally (Badrane *et al.*, 2001). Molecular methods capable of differentiating lyssaviruses have been developed and are now available (Foord *et al.*, 2006; Hayman *et al.*, 2011; Wakeley *et al.*, 2005) and these ideally should complement targeted surveillance, particularly in those countries with a large biological diversity as in sub-Saharan Africa (Coertse *et al.*, 2010).

Four isolations of another rabies-related virus, DUVV, have so far been made in South Africa (n=3) and Zimbabwe (n=1), and all with the exception of the Zimbabwean isolate, were associated with human deaths (Meredith *et al.*, 1971; Paweska *et al.*, 2006; Van Eeden *et al.*, 2011). The DUVV isolates have been recovered from an insectivorous bat probably *Nycteris* sp.

3   Antigenic and Genetic Characterization of MOKV Isolates

Over the last 40 years, antigenic and genetic techniques for characterizing pathogens have been developed and are now employed in many laboratories globally. Indeed, genetic characterization of *Lyssavirus* species has facilitated and improved the understanding of rabies epidemiology, prevention, treatment and prompted the development of new and novel laboratory techniques for rabies diagnosis. Before the advent of nucleotide sequencing, broad coverage of lyssavirus typing was achieved by antigenic typing.

Monoclonal antibodies (Mabs) produced by hybridisation of mouse myeloma cells with splenocytes of rabies-immunised BALB/C mice and directed against the envelope G, N and P of the virus demonstrated antigenic differences (Wiktor & Koprowski, 1980; Nadin-Davis *et al.*, 2011). Mabs have therefore been successfully used in the diagnosis of lyssaviruses, particularly in strain differentiation and selection of antigenic variants. In the case of Zimbabwean and South African lyssaviruses, Mabs were used for characterization of some isolates in cell culture and with an indirect immunofluorescent test (Wiktor & Koprowski, 1980, Schneider 1982; Schneider *et al.*, 1985; Vincent *et al.*, 1988; Bussereau *et al.*, 1988). Using this tool, lyssaviruses were differentiated and the degree of antigenic variation established among vaccine strains and field isolates of the RABV. At the Wistar Institute (in the USA), results of monoclonal antibody typing confirmed that the Bulawayo (Zimbabwean) isolates which gave atypical fluorescence on the initial FAT were in actual fact MOKVs. Some five years later, researchers at the Federal Research Institute for Animal Diseases (Germany) demonstrated the parallel existence of MOKV and DUVV among lyssaviruses of bat and terrestrial animals from the same region (Schneider *et al.*, 1985).

At the OIE Rabies Reference Laboratory (ARC-OVI, South Africa) and using panels of Mabs provided by the Canadian Food Inspection Agency (CFIA, Canada), several studies have been undertaken using both the anti-N (see Table 2) and anti-P Mabs (Nadin-Davis *et al.*, 2000; 2011). For instance, in a retrospective study on lyssaviruses collected between 1983 and 1997 from various areas of Zimbabwe and diagnosed as rabies by the FAT, one isolate gave a reaction pattern characteristic of MOKV (21846) (Bingham *et al.*, 2001). The most recent study (Nadin Davis *et al.*, 2011) utilized a new panel of 21 Mabs reactive with the P protein of MOKV. Reactivity of the anti-P Mabs identified Mabs that were cross-reactive to all members of the *Lyssavirus* genus. Within this panel of Mabs, discrimination between RABV, DUVV and phylogroup II viruses (LBV and MOKV) were clearly distinguishable and most importantly a single Mab was found to discriminate between LBV and MOKV. Some of the Mabs described herein together with other anti-P Mabs could therefore be useful for discriminating and diagnosing rabies and rabies-related viruses in Africa.

	Canid rabies	Mongoose rabies	LBV	MOKV	DUVV
*1C5	-	-	-	-	-
B7	+++	var	-	-	-
26BE2	+++	var	-	-	-
32GD12	var	var	-	-	-
**38HF2	+++	+++	+++	+++	+++
M612	-	-	+++	-	-
M837	-	-	-	-	+++
M850	-	var	-	-	+++
M853	+++	-	-	-	+++
M1001	-	-	-	+++	-
M1335	-	var	-	var	-
M1386	-	+++	-	-	-
M1400	-	var	-	-	-
M1407	++	var	-	-	-
M1412	++	var	-	-	-
M1494	-	var	-	-	+++

*1C5 is the negative control and **38HF2 the positive control and reacts with all lyssaviruses
Key: - no reactivity, +++ - reactivity with the Mab, var – Mab may react with some lyssaviruses

Table 2: Reactivity patterns of southern African rabies lyssaviruses against a panel of 16 N-Mabs.

A partial region of the highly conserved N gene has been used for genotyping, and in the case of MOKV isolates from Zimbabwe and South Africa, three genetic lineages (branch supporting the isolates with a 99% bootstrap value) (Figure 2), with an average 6% nucleotide sequence divergence (Nel et al., 2000) were delineated. Similar phylogenies were obtained via comparisons of partial or complete N gene sequences (Bourhy et al., 1993; Kuzmin et al., 2005), G gene (Badrane & Tordo, 2001), P gene (Nadin-Davis & Real, 2011) and L gene (Bourhy et al., 2005; Van Zyl et al., 2010). For instance, Van Zyl (2008), when analyzing full length gene sequence dataset of MOKVs, found that this group of viruses displayed up to 11.9% nucleotide difference. In these analyses, reconstructed trees with the NJ method utilizing a partial (405nt) and a complete gene sequence (1353nt) both displayed similar topologies. The tree generated from the full length set though provided better resolution, with bootstrap support of ≥70% for the majority of clades, compared to partial N sequence data.

Phylogenetically, the divergence of the viruses into three different lineages (Figure 2) indicates active cycles and significant evolutionary changes which probably occurred independently, albeit in close geographical proximity – a few hundred kilometers apart. This observation further highlights the general lack of our understanding of the epidemiology of MOKV facing rabies researchers. Indeed, the genetic studies on MOKVs from both southern African countries demonstrated that viruses from Zimbabwe are indeed different from those from the southern African neighbour. The large genetic diversity amongst such a very small group of viruses is intriguing and may indicate the long periods that this *Lyssavirus* variant has taken to evolve. Such a phenomenon is typical of RNA viruses as they adapt to changing host environments (Morimoto *et al.*, 1998) that may promote the emergence of new pathogens.

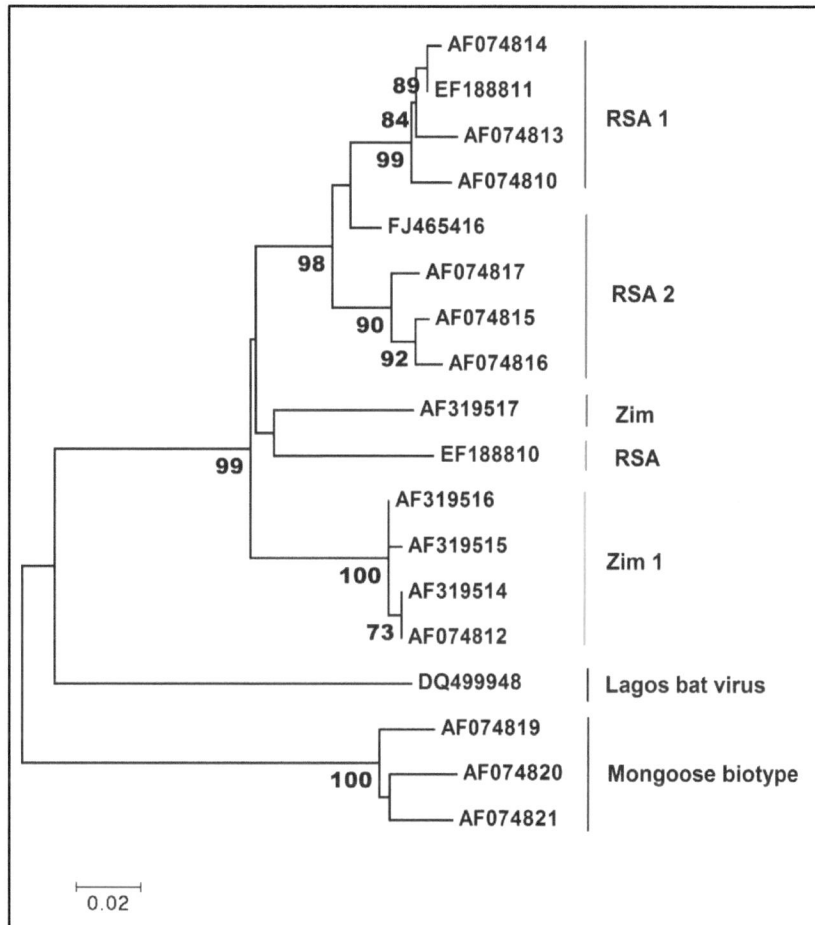

Figure 2: A neighbor-joining tree showing genetic relationships of Mokola viruses from Zimbabwe and South Africa derived from nucleotide sequences of a partial region of the nucleoprotein (N) gene generated using algorithms in MEGA version 4.0 (Kumar *et al.*, 2004). The Genbank accession numbers are shown on the tree branches as well as in Table 3. Bootstrap values determined with 1000 replicates are shown on the nodes. The scale shows nucleotide substitutions per site.

Country	Isolate number	Accession number	Reference
South Africa	112/96	AF074810	Nel *et al.*, 2000
South Africa	322/96	AF074813	Nel *et al.*, 2000
South Africa	543/95	AF074814	Nel *et al.*, 2000
South Africa	229/97	AF074815	Nel *et al.*, 2000
South Africa	252/97	AF074816	Nel *et al.*, 2000
South Africa	M420/90	AF074819	Nel *et al.*, 2000
South Africa	256/90	AF074820	Nel *et al.*, 2000
South Africa	m710/90	AF074821	Nel *et al.*, 2000
South Africa	071/98	AF074817	Nel *et al.*, 2000
South Africa	700/70	FJ465416	Van Zyl, 2008
South Africa	404/05	EF188810	Sabeta *et al.*, 2007
South Africa	173/06	EF188811	Sabeta *et al.*, 2007
Zimbabwe	13270/82	AF319514	Nel *et al.*, 2000
Zimbabwe	12341/81	AF319515	Nel *et al.*, 2000
Zimbabwe	12574/81	AF319516	Nel *et al.*, 2000
Zimbabwe	21846/93	AF319517	Nel *et al.*, 2000
Zimbabwe	Zim/82	AF074812	Nel *et al.*, 2000
South Africa	Mongoose2004	DQ499948	Markotter, 2007

Table 3: Genbank accession numbers of viruses used in the reconstruction of the phylogenetic tree.

4   Surveillance Studies: Cross-Reactivity and Cross-Protection

The epidemiology of rabies-related viruses demonstrates the limited number of isolations of both MOKV and LBV across Africa. This is most likely attributed to the specific responses to isolations of these viruses rather than their prevalence or distribution. For instance, a survey was undertaken to identify the host reservoir of MOKV shortly after the identification of MOKVs in South Africa in 1996. In this survey, 75 rodents were captured in the coastal areas and these comprised shrews (of the *Crocidura* and *Sunchus* sp., n = 10) and the rest were found in varying numbers of the species: *Otomys* sp., *Rhabdomys pumilio*, *Dasymus incomtus*, *Mus musculus*, *Mus minutoides*, *Praomys natalensis*, *Rattus rattus* and unidentified gerbils, possibly brantsii (Von Teichman *et al.*, unpublished). The collected viscera and brain material from every specimen was tested using the mouse inoculation test (MIT) and serum samples drawn from each rodent analysed using the fluorescent inhibitory microtest as described by Zalan *et al* (1979). The overall result of the survey was rather disappointing as there was no indication of the origin of the MOKV from this coastal part of South Africa. From the early identifications in the late 1960s, it appears that MOKV appears to be widely spread amongst shrews and possibly other rodents, which in West and Central Africa are common domestic commensals and that these animals would seem to be the most likely source of infection for humans.

Previous *in vitro* studies used a field isolate (MOKV173/06), that was later adapted and grown on neuroblastoma cells via three passages, to assess virus neutralizing antibody (VNAs) levels to MOKV in a fluorescent antibody virus neutralization test (FAVNT) as described by Cliquet *et al.*, (1998). The panel of test sera (n = 40; cats = 13 and dogs = 27), had previously been shown to neutralize CVS (Challenge Virus Standard, ATCC VR959) (at $100TCID_{50}$/ml, laboratory rabies strain) demonstrating adequate responses to rabies vaccination. The studies demonstrated that all with the exception of a single dog serum 1:81 dilution to MOKV and 1:729 to CVS, had neutralising activities of 1:3 dilution, similar to the negative reference serum (Anses, France). These results together with other experimental evidence to date lend support to the fact that the currently used inactivated rabies vaccines do not cross-protect against both MOKV and LBV (Foggin, 1988; Badrane *et al.*, 2001; Brookes *et al.*, 2005; Nel 2005). The first MOKV vaccine, a recombinant baculovirus expressing the MOKV glycoprotein (Tordo *et al.*, 1993) showed promise and elicited a protective immunological response in mice. Since then DNA vaccines and recombinants were also shown to protect against MOKV, but could not fully protect using a single immunisation (Nel *et al.*, 2003).

In a lentiviral pseudotype (pt) neutralisation assay, surrogate viruses were used and anti-rabies VNA responses in vaccine recipients determined (Wright *et al.*, 2009). Unfortunately, VNAs to MOKV were not established due to the unavailability of anti-sera to MOKV. However, in subsequent investigations (Wright *et al.*, 2010) demonstrated a similar seroprevalence of LBV and MOKV antibodies in Ghanaian *E. helvum*, similar to those found by Hayman *et al.*, (2008a) and Kuzmin *et al.*, (2008). Naturally, some of the ptMOKV neutralisation observed in these studies could be due cross-reaction with LBV VNAs as confirmed in some reports in Kenya and Nigeria (Dzikwi *et al.*, 2010, Aghomo *et al.*, 1990; Kuzmin *et al.*, 2008; Nel and Rupprecht, 2007). Bats appear to harbour antibodies to many viral pathogens including Lyssaviruses and Henipaviruses (Hayman *et al.*, 2008b). Interestingly, MOKV infections have never been reported in bats, however this should not be ruled out. There is thus a need for further surveillance and seroprevalence studies to elucidate the true distribution and host reservoirs of LBV, MOKV and other African lyssaviruses.

Rabies vaccines are not fully protective against MOKV. This has been demonstrated experimentally and in circumstantial situations. Challenge protection tests in mice (Foggin, 1988) showed little protection to a Zimbabwean MOKV in comparison to protection against CVS, but the human infection/protection scenario remains unknown. The fact that there is no vaccine protective against MOKV has generated substantial interest. These observations further confirm the lack of cross-protection of currently used vaccines against MOKV and LBV *Lyssavirus* species, is consistent with those from previous studies (Foggin, 1982; 1983; Badrane *et al.*, 2001; Wright *et al.*, 2008; Nel *et al.*, 2003; Koprowski *et al.*, 1985). For instance, Fekadu and co-workers at the Centers for Disease Control (CDC, USA) concluded that rabies vaccines protect against DUVV (Fekadu *et al.*, 1988).

Cross-protection between lyssavirus species within either phylogroup is possible given the shared antigenic sites in the G protein gene. Weyer and co-workers (2008) using recombinant vaccinia viruses that expressed single and dual copies of the G protein genes of RABV, MOKV and WCBV demonstrated that single antigen expressing the G gene of each of the lyssaviruses introduced via the i.m. route, that is, RABV, MOKV and WCBV protected mice against lethal challenge. In the process, the animals mounted measurable VNAs by day 7 post-vaccination.

DNA-mediated immunisation with G segments from various *Lyssavirus* species have demonstrated the potential for such vaccines to protect against all the members within the *Lyssavirus* genus (Bahloul *et al.*, 1998; Jallet *et al.*, 1999). Clearly, the approach may increase the spectrum of efficacy of conventional rabies vaccines, but the market for these vaccines is limited and the costs could be prohibitive. In studies undertaken by Koprowski and co-workers (1985), seven lyssaviruses isolated from human victims and grown on BHK cells via 3 passages demonstrated distinct differences in reactivity patterns with a limited panel of Mabs. In this case, 36 Mabs specific for the N and 44 for the G antigen of the virus were used. The differences were observed on both the N and the G antigens of the virus. Through the use of the 36-Mab panel, it was shown that antigenic similarities existed between all MOKVs isolated with that isolated in Nigeria. Secondly, it was observed that mice immunised by rabies vaccines prepared from CVS or PV-II strains of the rabies virus were fully protected against challenge with viruses isolated from persons initially infected by dogs and cats.

5   Conclusions

The foregoing discussion and the isolation of MOKV from a wide range of host species including shrews, a dog, domestic cats and a rodent demonstrate the ability of this and other lyssaviruses to cross species barriers and the potential for MOKV to establish itself in a new host range. One of the most important and unanswered questions in *Lyssavirus* epidemiology though is what the reservoir host for MOKV is. All we know is that the majority of the MOKV isolations from southern Africa were made from domestic mammals (Von Teichman *et al.*, 1998), although those from elsewhere in Africa were from shrews, a rodent and humans (Familusi & Moore, 1972). Foggin (1988) suggested that MOKV could be naturally confined to wildlife reservoir hosts and its presence is only recognized during surveys as in the case of the Bulawayo outbreak (Zimbabwe), when they are transmitted to domestic animals and humans. It is therefore possible that the reservoir host species will likely be found among the shrews, rodents and even bats, these being mammalian species that cats interact with. The presence of VNA to MOKV in sera of animals tested during surveys for rabies-related viruses could support the existence of a population of such a reservoir host amongst rodents. Results of these surveys showed that sera from some of these animals, mainly rodents and a side-striped jackal, had neutralizing activity against MOKV but not classical rabies.

Screening of dog sera at random in Nigeria demonstrated a low incidence of serum antibodies to MOKV (Aghomo *et al.*, 1990). Other species namely cattle, goats, pigs, birds as well as frugivorous bats have demonstrated positive serological results. Encounters with MOKV are indeed rare events and prior to this review only 26 isolates are known to have existed at one time or another. It is noteworthy that over the last 2 decades, all the MOKV isolates have been described from South Africa. The lack of rabies surveillance in many African countries in comparison to South Africa which boasts an active surveillance is therefore evident. There are likely many other MOKV cases that have not been recognized given the limited surveillance.

Phylogenetically, the divergence of the MOKVs into different lineages indicates active cycles underpinning evolutionary changes which appear to have occurred independently, albeit in close geographical proximity. Our lack of understanding of the epidemiology of MOKV is again highlighted, but the argument for a reservoir host(s) amongst small terrestrial animals of limited range seems to be supported by a body of evidence generated over the past 40 years. The public health implications of rabies-related African lyssaviruses especially MOKV has been documented by various scientists. Human infections with this *Lyssavirus* species are extremely rare leading some to argue that indeed lyssaviruses (from phylogroup II) are not a major public health threat. This fact should however not be ignored – but in the absence of a vaccine against MOKV, one should emphasise that the potential threat be recognised by all laboratory workers including researchers, veterinarians, wildlife personnel, gamekeepers and pet owners.

A better understanding of the epidemiology of these viruses is vital and can only be brought about by improved and integrated surveillance and awareness strategies.

References

Aghomo, H.O., Tomori, O., Oduye, O.O. and Rupprecht, C.E. (1990). Detection of Mokola virus antibodies in fruit bats (Eidolon helvum) from Nigeria. J Wildl Dis., 48 (2), 264.

Aitken, T.H.G., Kowalski, R.W., Beaty, B.J., Buckley, S.M., Wright, J.D., Shope, R.E. and Miller, B.R. (1984). Arthropod studies with rabies-related Mokola virus. Am J Trop Med Hyg., 33(5), 945-952.

Allworth, A., Murray, K., and Morgan, J. (1996). A human case of encephalitis due to a lyssavirus recently identified in fruit bats. Com Dis Intell., 20, 504.

Amengual, B., Whitby, J.E., King, A., Serra Cobo, J., and Bourhy, H. (1997). Evolution of European bat lyssaviruses. J Gen Virol., 78, 2319-2328.

Badrane, H. and Tordo, N. (2001). Host switching in the Lyssavirus history from the Chiroptera to Carnivora orders. J Virol., 17, 8096–8114.

Badrane, H., Bahloul, C., Perrin, P., and Tordo N. (2001). Evidence of two lyssavirus phylogroups with distinct pathogenicity and immunogenicity. J Virol., 75 (7), 3268-3276.

Bahloul, C., Jacob, Y., Tordo, N. and Perrin, P. (1998). DNA-based immunisation for exploring the enlargement of immunological cross-reactivity against the Lyssaviruses. Vaccine., 16(4):417-425.

Bingham, J., Foggin, C.M., Wandeler, A.I., and Hill, F.W. (1999a). The epidemiology of rabies in Zimbabwe. 1. Rabies in dogs (Canis familiaris). Onderstepoort J Vet Res., 66(1), 1-10.

Bingham, J., Foggin, C.M., Wandeler, A.I., and Hill, F.W. (1999b). The epidemiology of rabies in Zimbabwe. 2. Rabies in jackals (Canis adustus and Canis mesomelas). Onderstepoort J Vet Res., 66(1):11-23.

Bingham, J., Javangwe, S., Sabeta, C.T., Wandeler, A.I., and Nel, L.H. (2001). Report of isolations of unusual lyssaviruses (rabies and Mokola virus) identified retrospectively from Zimbabwe. J S Afr Vet Assoc., 72(2), 92-94.

Botvinkin, A.D., Poleschuk, E.M., Kuzmin, I.V., Borisova, T.I., Gazaryan, S.V., Yager, P., and Rupprecht, C.E. (2003). Novel lyssaviruses isolated from bats in Russia. Emerg Infect Dis., 9(12), 1623-5.

Boulger, L.R., and Porterfield, J.S. (1958). Isolation of a virus from Nigerian fruit bats. Trans. R. Soc. Trop. Med. Hyg., 52, 421-424.

Bourhy, H., Kissi, B., and Tordo, N. (1990). From rabies to rabies-related viruses. Vet. Micro., 23(1-4), 115-128.

Bourhy, H., Kissi, B., and Tordo, N. (1993). Molecular diversity of the Lyssavirus genus. Virology., 194(1), 70-81.

Bourhy, H., Cowley, J.A., Larrous, F., Holmes, E.C., and Walker, P.J. (2005). Phylogenetic relationships among rhabdoviruses inferred using the L polymerase gene. J Gen Virol., 86, 2849-58

Brookes, S.M., Parsons, G., Johnson, N., McElhinney, L.M., and Fooks, A.R. (2005). Rabies human diploid cell vaccine elicits cross-neutralising and cross-protecting immune responses against European and Australian bat lyssaviruses. Vaccine., 23, 4101-4109.

Brown, K. (2011). In: Mad dogs and Meerkats – A history of resurgent rabies in Southern Africa. Ohio University Press Series in Ecology and History. (Ed. Webb, J.L.A.).

Buckley, S.M. (1975). Arbovirus infection of vertebrate and insect cell cultures, with special emphasis on Mokola, Obodhiang and Kotonkan viruses of the rabies serogroup. An NY Acad Sci., 266, 241-250.

Bussereau, F., Vincent, J., Coudrier, D., and Sureau, P. (1988). Monoclonal antibodies to Mokola virus for Identification of Rabies and Rabies-Related Viruses. J Clin Microbiol., 26(12), 2489-2494.

Charlton, K.M. (1988). The pathogenesis of rabies. In: Rabies. (Eds. Campbell, J.M. and Charlton, K.M.). Kluwer Academic Publishers, Boston.

Cliquet, F., Aubert, M., and Sagne, L. (1998). Development of a fluorescent antibody virus neutralisation test (FAVN test) for the quantitation of rabies-neutralising antibody. J Immunol Methods., 212, 79-87.

Coertse, J., Weyer, J., Nel, L.H., and Markotter, W., (2010). Improved PCR methods for the detection of African rabies and rabies-related lyssaviruses. J Clin Microbiol., 48, 3949-3955.

Crick, J., Tignor, G.H., and Moreno, K. (1982). A new isolate of Lagos bat virus from the Republic of South Africa. Trans. Roy. Soc. Trop. Med and Hyg., 76, 211-213.

Davis, P.L., Holmes, E.C., Larrous, F., Van der Poel,W.H.M., Thornehoj, K., Alonso, W.J., and Bourhy, H. (2005). Phylogeography, Population Dynamics and Molecular evolution of European bat lyssaviruses. J Virol., 79, 10487-10497.

Dean, D.J., Abelseth, M.K., and Atanasiu, P., (1996). 'The fluorescent antibody test'. In: Laboratory techniques in rabies. (Eds. F.X. Meslin, M.M. Kaplan, & H. Koprowski). World Health Organization, Geneva (pp. 88-95).

Dzikwi, A.A., Kuzmin, I.I., Umoh, J.U., Kwaga, J.K.P., Ahmad, A.A., and Rupprecht, C.E. (2010). Evidence of Lagos Bat Virus circulation among Nigerian Fruit Bats. J Wildl Dis., 46(1), 267-271.

Familusi, J.B., and Moore, D.L. (1972). Isolation of a rabies-related virus from the cerebrospinal fluid. Afr J Med Sci., 3, 93-96.

Familusi, J.B., Osunkoya, B.O., Moore, D.L., Kemp, G.E., Fabiyi, A., and Moore, D.L. (1972). A fatal human infection with Mokola virus. Am J Trop Med Hyg., 21, 959-963.

Fauquet, C.M., Mayo, M.A., Maniloff, J., Desselberger, U., and Ball, L.A. (2004). Virus Taxonomy: the classification and nomenclature of viruses. The eight report of the International Committee on Taxonomy of Viruses. San Diego: Academic Press (pp. 623-631).

Fekadu, M., Shaddock, J.H., Sandelin, D.W., and Smith, J.S. (1988). Efficacy of rabies vaccines against Duvenhage virus isolated from European house bats (Eptesicus serotinus), classic rabies and rabies-related viruses. Vaccine. 6(6), 533-9.

Foggin, C.M. (1988). Rabies and rabies-related viruses in Zimbabwe: historical, virological and ecological aspects. [Doctoral dissertation]. Harare (Zimbabwe): University of Zimbabwe.

Foggin, C.M. (1982). Atypical rabies virus in cats and a dog in Zimbabwe. Vet. Rec., 110, 338.

Foggin, C.M. (1983). Mokola virus infections in cats and a dog in Zimbabwe. Vet. Rec., 113, 115.

Foord, A.J., Heine, H.G., Pritchard, L.I., Lunt, R.A., Newberry, K.M., Rootes, C.L., and Boyle, D.B. (2006). Molecular diagnosis of Lyssaviruses and sequence comparison of Australian bat Lyssavirus samples. Aust. Vet. J., 84(7), 225-230.

Gould, A.R., Hyatt, A.D., Lunt, R., Kattenbelt, J.A., Hengsberger, S., and Blacksell, S.D. (1998). Characterisation of a novel lyssavirus isolated from Pteropid bats in Australia. Virus Res., 54, 164-187.

Hanna, J.N., Cerney, J.K., Smith, G.A., Tannenberg, E.G., Deverill, J.E., Botha, J.A., Serafin, I.L., Harrower, B.J., Fitzpatrick, P.F., and Searle, J.W. (2000). Australian bat lyssavirus infection: a second human case, with a long incubation period. Med J Aust., 172(12), 597-599.

Hanlon, C.A., Kuzmin, I.V., Blanton, J.D., Weldon, W.C., Manangan, J.S. and Rupprecht CE. (2005). Efficacy of rabies biologics against new lyssaviruses from Eurasia. Virus Res., 111(1), 44–54

Harrison AK, Causey OR, Kemp G.E., Simpson, D.I.H. and Moore, D.L. (1970). Two African viruses serologically and morphologically related to rabies virus. J of Virol., 6, 690-692.

Hayman, D.T., Fooks, A.R., Horton, D., Suu-Ire, R., Breed, A.C., Cunningham, A.A., and Wood, J.L. (2008a). Antibodies against Lagos bat virus in megachiroptera from West Africa. Emerg Infect Dis., 14(6), 926-8.

Hayman, D.T.S., Suu-Ire, R., Breed, A.C., McEachern, J.A., Wang, L., Wood, J., and Cunningham, A.A. (2008b). Evidence of Henipavirus Infection in West African fruit bats. Plos One., 3(7), 1-7.

Hayman, D.T.S., Banyard, A.C., Wakeley, P.R., Harkess, G. et al., Marston, D., Wood, J.L.N., Cunningham, A.A. and Fooks, A.R. (2011). A universal real-time assay for the detection of Lyssaviruses. J. Virol., Meth. 177, 87-93.

Jallet, C., Jacob, Y., Bahloul, C., Drings, A., Desmezieres, E., Tordo, N., and Perrin, P. (1999). Chimeric lyssavirus glyco-proteins with increased immunological potential. J of Virol., 73(1), 225-33.

Kemp, G.E., Causey, O.R., Moore, D.L., Odelola, A., and Fabiyi, A. (1972). Mokola virus. Further studies on IbAn 27377, a new rabies-related etiologic agent of zoonosis in Nigeria. Am J Trop Med Hyg., 21, 356-359.

Kemp, G.E., Moore, D.L., Isoun, T.T., and Fabiyi, A. (1973). Mokola virus: experimental infection and transmission studies with the shrew, a natural host. Arch Gesamte Virusforrsch., 43(3), 242-250.

King, A.A., and Turner, G.S. (1993). Rabies – a review. J Comp Pathol., 108, 1-39.

Knobel, D. L., Cleveland, S., Coleman, P. G., Fèvre, E. M., Meltzer, M. I., Miranda, M.E.G., Shaw, A., Zinsstag, J., and Meslin, F. X. (2005). Re-evaluating the burden of rabies in Africa and Asia. Bull World Health Organ., 83, 360-368.

Koprowski, H., Wiktor, T.J., and Abelseth, M.K. (1985). Cross-reactivity and cross-protection: Rabies Variants and Rabies-Related Viruses. In: "Rabies in the Tropics". (Eds. E. Kuwert et al.,). (pp. 30-39).

Kumar, S., Tamura, K., and Nei, M. (2004). MEGA3: Integrated software for Molecular Evolutionary Genetics Analysis and sequence alignment. Brief Bioinform., 5, 150-163.

Kuzmin, I.V., Orciari, L.A., Arai, Y.T., Smith, J.S., Hanlon, C.A., Kameoka, Y., and Rupprecht, C.E. (2003). Bat lyssaviruses (Aravan and Khujand) from Central Asia: phylogenetic relationships according to N, P and G gene sequence. Virus Res., 97, 65-79.

Kuzmin, I.V., Hughes, G.J., Botvinkin, A.D., Orciari, L.A., and Rupprecht, C.E. (2005). Phylogenetic relationships of Irkut and West Caucasian bat viruses within the lyssavirus genus and suggested quantitative criteria based on the N gene sequence for lyssaviruses genotype definition. Virus Res., 111, 28-43.

Kuzmin, I.V., Wu, X., Tordo, N. and Rupprecht, C.E. (2008). Complete genomes of Aravan, Khujand, Irkut and West Caucasian bat viruses, with special attention to the polymerase gene and non473 coding regions. Virus Res., 136(1-2), 81-90.

Kuzmin, I.V., Mayer, A.E., Niezgoda, M., Markotter, W., Agwanda, B., Breiman, R.F., and Rupprecht, C.E. (2010). Shimoni bat virus, a new representative of the Lyssavirus genus. Virus Res., 149(2), 197-210.

Le Gonidec, G., Rickenbach, A., Robin, Y., and Heme, G. (1978). Isolation of a strain of Mokola virus in Cameroon. Annu Microbiol.. 129(2), 245-9.

Markotter, W., Kuzmin, I., Rupprecht, C.E., Randles, J., Sabeta, C.T., Wandeler, A.I., and Nel, L.H. (2006a). Isolation of Lagos bat Virus from water mongoose. Emerg Infect Dis., 12(12), 5-14.

Markotter, W., Randles, J., Sabeta, C.T., Wandeler, A.I., Taylor, P.J., and Nel, L.H. (2006b). Recent Lagos bat virus isolations from bats (suborder Megachiroptera) in South Africa. Emerg Infect Dis., 12, 504-506.

Markotter, W. (2007). Molecular Epidemiology and pathogenesis of Lagos bat virus, a rabies-related virus specific to Africa. PhD thesis, University of Pretoria, South Africa.

Markotter, W., Van Eeden, C., Kuzmin, I.V., Rupprecht, C.E., Paweska, J.T., Swanepoel, R., Fooks, A.R., Sabeta, C.T., Cliquet, F., and L.H. Nel. (2008). Epidemiology and pathogenicity of African lyssaviruses. Dev. Biol., 131, 317-325.

Marston, D.A., Horton, D.L., Ngeleja, C., Hampson, K., McElhinney, L.M., Banyard, A.C. Haydon, D., Cleaveland, S., Ruppreht, C.E., Bigambo, M., Fooks A.R., and Lembo, T. (2012a). Ikoma lyssavirus, highly divergent novel lyssavirus in an African civet. Emerg. Infect. Dis., 18(4), 664-7.

Marston, D.A., Ellis, R.J., Horton, D.L., Kuzmin, I.V., Wise, E.L., McElhinney, L.M., Banyard, A.C., Ngeleja, C., Keyyu, J., Cleaveland, S., Lembo, T., Rupprecht, C.E., and Fooks, A.R. (2012b). Complete genomic sequence of Ikoma Lyssavirus. J Virol., 86(18), 10242-3.

Mebatsion, T., Cox, J.H., and Frost, J.W. (1992). Isolation and characterisation of 115 street rabies virus isolates from Ethiopia by using monoclonal antibodies: identification of 2 isolates of Mokola and Lagos Bat viruses. J Infect Dis., 166, 972-977.

Meredith, C.D., Rossouw, A.P., and Van Praag Koch, H. (1971). An unusual case of human rabies thought to be of Chiropteran origin. S Afr Med J., 45, 767-769.

Meredith, C.D., Nel, L.H., and Von Teichman, B.F. (1996). A further isolation of Mokola virus in South Africa. Vet Rec. 138, 119-120.

Morimoto, K., Hooper, D.C., Carbough, H., Fu, Z.F., Koprowski, H., and Dietzchold, B. 1998. Rabies virus quasi-species : implications for pathogenesis. Proc. Natl. Acad. Sc., 9, 3152-3156.

Nadin-Davis, S.A., Sheen, M., Abdel-Malik, M., Elmgren, L., Armstrong, J., and Wandeler, A.I. (2000). A panel of monoclonal antibodies targeting the rabies virus phosphoprotein identifies a highly variable epitope of value for sensitive strain discrimination. J Clin Microbiol., 38(4), 1397-403.

Nadin-Davis, S.A., Elmgren, L., Sheen, M., Sabeta, C., and Wandeler, A.I. (2011). Generation and characterisation of a panel of anti-phosphoprotein monoclonal antibodies directed against Mokola virus. Virus Res., 160, 238-245.

Nadin-Davis, S.A., and Real, L.A. (2011). Molecular phylogenetics of the lyssaviruses--insights from a coalescent approach. Adv Virus Res., 79, 203-38.

Nel, L., Jacobs, J., Jaftha, J., von Teichman, B., and Bingham, J. (2000). New cases of Mokola virus infection in South Africa: a genotypic comparison of Southern African virus isolates. Virus Genes., 20(2), 103-106.

Nel, L.H., Niezgoda, M., Hanlon, C.A., Morril, P.A., Yager, P.A., and Rupprecht, C.E. (2003). A comparison of DNA vaccines for the rabies-related virus, Mokola. Vaccine., 21(19-20), 2598-606.

Nel, L.H., (2005). Vaccines for lyssaviruses other than rabies. Expert Rev Vaccines., 4(4), 533-540.

Nel, L. H., and Rupprecht, C. E. (2007). Emergence of Lyssaviruses in the Old World: the case of Africa. In : Wildlife and emerging zoonotic diseases: the biology, circumstances and consequences of cross-species transmission. (Eds. Childs J E, Mackenzie J S, Richt J A). Springer-Verlag, Berlin, Germany (pp. 161-193).

Nel, L. H., and Markotter, W. (2007) Lyssaviruses. Critical Rev. in Microbiology., 33, 301–324.

Paweska, J.T., Blumberg, L., Liebenberg, C., Hewlett, R.H., Grobbelaar, A.A., Leman, P.A., Croft, J.E., Nel, L.H., Nutt, L., and Swanepoel, R. (2006). Fatal human infection with rabies-related Duvenhage virus, South Africa. Emerg Infect Dis., 12, 1965-1967.

Sabeta, C.T., Markotter, W., Mohale, D.K., Shumba, W., Wandeler, A.I. and Nel, L.H. (2007). Mokola virus in domestic mammals, South Africa. Emerg Infect Dis., 13(9), 1371-1373.

Sabeta, C., Blumberg, L., Miyen, J., Mohale, D., Shumba, W., and Wandeler, A.I. (2010). Mokola virus involved in a human contact (South Africa). FEMS Immunol. Med. Microbiol., 58, 85-90.

Saluzzo JF, Rollin PE, Daugard C, Digoutte JP, Georges AJ. Sureau P. (1984). Premier isolement du virus Mokola a partir d'une rongeur (Lophuromys sikapusi). Annales de Institut Pasteur Vir., 135E, 57-66.

Schneider, L.G. (1982). Antigenic Variants of Rabies Virus. Comp. Immun. Microbiol. Infect., 5(1-3), 101-107.

Schneider, L.G., Barnard, B.J.H., and Schneider, H.P. (1985). Application of monoclonal antibodies for epidemiological investigations and oral vaccination studies. I-African viruses. In: "Rabies in the Tropics". (Eds. E. Kuwert et al.,). (pp. 47-53).

Shope, R.E., Murphy, F.A., Harrison, A.K., Causey, O.R., Kemp, G.E., Simpson, D.I.H., and Moore, D.L. (1970). Two African viruses serologically and morphologically related to rabies virus. J Virol., 6, 690-692.

Shope, R.E. (1982). Rabies-related viruses. The Yale J of Biol. And Med., 55, 271-275.

Smith, J.S. and Seidel, H.D. (1993). Rabies – a new look at an old disease. Pro. Med Virol. Barsel Karger., 40, 82-106.

Steele, J.H. (1975). History of rabies. In ed. G.M. Baer. The Natural History of Rabies Vol 1. New York Academic Press (pp.1-29).

Sureau, P., Germain, M., Herve, J.P., Geoffroy, B., Cornet, J.P., Heme, G., and Robin, Y. (1977). Isolent du virus Lagos bat en empire Centrafricain. Bulletin de la Societe de Pathologie Exotique., 70, 467-470.

Sureau, P., Tignor, G.H., and Smith, A.L. (1980). Antigenic characterisation of the Bangui strain (ANCB-672d) of Lagos bat virus. Ann. Virol. (Inst. Pasteur)., 131E, 25-32.

Swanepoel, R., Barnard, B.J., Meredith, C.D., Bishop, G.C., Brückner, G.K., Foggin, C.M., and Hübschle, O.J. (1993). Rabies in southern Africa. Onderstepoort J Vet Res., 60(4), 325-46.

Tordo, N. and Kouknetzorff, A. (1993). The rabies virus genome: An overview. Onderstepoort J Vet Res., 60, 263-269.

Tordo, N., Bourhy, H., Sather, S., and Ollo, R. (1993). Structure and expression in baculovirus of the Mokola virus glycoprotein: an efficient recombinant vaccine. Virology., 194, 59-69.

Tordo, N., Charlton, K. and Wandeler, A. (1997). Rhabdoviruses: rabies. In: Topley and Wilson's Principles of bacteriology, virology and immunity. 9th edition. (Eds. W.W.C. Topley, Wilson, G.S., and Collies, L). London (pp. 665-692).

Van Zyl, N. (2008). Molecular Epidemiology of African mongoose rabies and Mokola virus. MSc thesis submitted the University of Pretoria, South Africa.

Van Zyl, N., Markotter, W., and Nel, L.H. (2010). Evolutionary history of African mongoose rabies. Virus Res., 150(1-2), 93-102.

Van Eeden, C., Markotter, W., and Nel, L.H., (2011). Molecular phylogeny of Duvenhage virus. S Afr J Sci., 107, 1-5.

Vincent, J., Bussereau, F., and Sureau, P. (1988). Immunological relationships betweeen rabies virus and rabies-related viruses studied with monoclonal antibodies to Mokola virus. Ann. Ins. Pasteur., 157-173.

Von Teichman, B.F., de Koker, W.C., Bosch, S.J.E., Bishop, G.C., Meredith, C.D., and Bingham, J. (1998). Mokola virus infection: description of recent South African cases and a review of the virus epidemiology. J S Afr Vet Assoc., 69(4), 169-171.

Wakeley, P.R., Johnson, N., McElhinney, L.M., Marston, D., Sawyer, J., and Fooks, A.R. (2005). Development of a real-time, TaqMan reverse transcription-PCR assay for detection and differentiation of lyssavirus genotypes 1, 5, and 6. J Clin Microbiol., ;43(6):2786-92.

Weyer, J., Kuzmin, I., V., Rupprecht, C.E., and Nel, L.H. (2008). Cross-protective and cross-reactive immune responses to recombinant vaccinia viruses expressing full-length lyssavirus glycoprotein genes. Epidemiol Infect., 136(5), 670-8.

Wiktor, T.J., and Koprowski, H. (1980). Antigenic Variants of Rabies virus. J. Exp Med., 152, 99-112.

Wiktor, T.J. (1985). Historical aspects of rabies. In: World's debt to Pasteur. Allan R Liss. Inc (pp. 141-151).

Wright, E., McNabb, S., Goddard, T., Horton, D., Lembo, T., Nel, L.H., Weiss, R., Cleaveland, S., and Fooks, A.R. (2009). A robust lentiviral pseudotype neutralisation assay for in-field serosurveillance of rabies and lyssaviruses in Africa. Vaccine., 27, 7178-7186.

Wright, E., Hayman, D.T.S., Vaughan, A., Temperton, N.J., Wood, J., Cunningham, A.A., Suu-Ire, R., Weiss, R., and Fooks, A.R. (2010). Virus neutralising activity of African fruit bat (Eidolon helvum) sera against emerging lyssaviruses. Virology., 408, 183-189.

Zalan, E., Wilson, C., and Pukitis, D. (1979). A microtest for quantification of rabies virus neutralising antibodies. J. Biol. Stand., 7, 213-220.

HCV Helicase as a Therapeutic Target

Adil A. Shah
Department of Biological and Biomedical Sciences
Aga Khan University, Karachi, Pakistan

Sammer Siddiqui
Department of Biological and Biomedical Sciences
Aga Khan University, Karachi, Pakistan

Syed H. Ali
Department of Biological and Biomedical Sciences
Aga Khan University, Karachi, Pakistan

1   Introduction

In the past few decades, hepatitis C virus (HCV) has emerged as an infection with serious ramifications, leading to major paradigm shifts in global healthcare. It is estimated that 170 million individuals worldwide are infected with HCV, with the highest rate of infection in Asia, where 83 million people are reported be infected with this virus (Martinson *et al.*, 1996, 2000). Areas where the HCV endemic threatens to spill out into the general population include West Africa, Indian Subcontinent, West Central Africa, Central Africa and Southeast Asia (Simmonds *et al.*, 1994; Stuyver *et al.*, 1994; Tokita *et al.*, 1994a, 1994b, 1995; Mellor *et al.*, 1996; Ruggieri *et al.*, 1996). Of the individuals who develop chronic hepatitis C infection, 10-20% eventually develop chronic liver disease and other associated complications (World Health Report 1996 (World Health Organisation 1996). An estimated 22% of the cases of hepatocellular cancer around the world can be attributed to HCV infection. The effect of HCV infection on health systems and the resulting socio-economic burden has been especially aggravating in high risk regions of the world. To date, no vaccine is available for HCV. Development of a vaccine against this virus remains a challenge because of the rapid rate of HCV evolution. The current recommended treatment for HCV combines pegylated interferon-α (IFN-α) and a broad spectrum antiviral drug, Ribavirin. While involving considerable side effects, such a regimen has been shown to be only moderately effective in combating HCV infection, with considerable variation across the HCV genotypes (Fried *et al.*, 2002; Hadziyannis *et al.*, 2004). Hence, more effective therapeutic options need to be identified which should preferably incorporate a short treatment duration and low toxicity profile. Additionally, in developing countries high cost of combination therapy and its limited availability restrict the access of this treatment for the HCV infected individuals. Therefore, developing new treatment that is less costly and more readily available is the need of the hour.

In recent years, HCV-encoded non-structural-3 (NS3) protein has emerged as a promising target for novel drugs. In this chapter, we will discuss the advances that have been made toward developing new drugs that inhibit the HCV NS3 activity. We will give a brief overview of the HCV-mediated disease, the viral life cycle and the involvement of various viral proteins in it. We will then review the various approaches and analyses carried out so far in exploring the potential of HCV NS3 as an anti-viral drug target.

2   HCV Genome

The hepatitis C virus (HCV) is a single-stranded, positive-sense RNA virus belonging to the Flaviviridae family. HCV genome consists of an open reading frame (ORF) flanked on either side by non-translated regions (NTR) that serve to initiate translation of the ORF. The ORF encodes a single poly-protein that is then further cleaved. The ~3000 amino acid long poly-protein is cleaved into three structural (C, E1 and E2) and seven non-structural (p7, NS2, NS3, NS4A, NS4B, NS5A and NS5B) proteins (Brass *et al.*, 2006) (Fig.1). Each of these proteins have been assigned roles in the HCV life cycle (Table 1), and most of them have been implicated in contributing to the pathogenesis of HCV infection. These aspects are discussed below in detail.

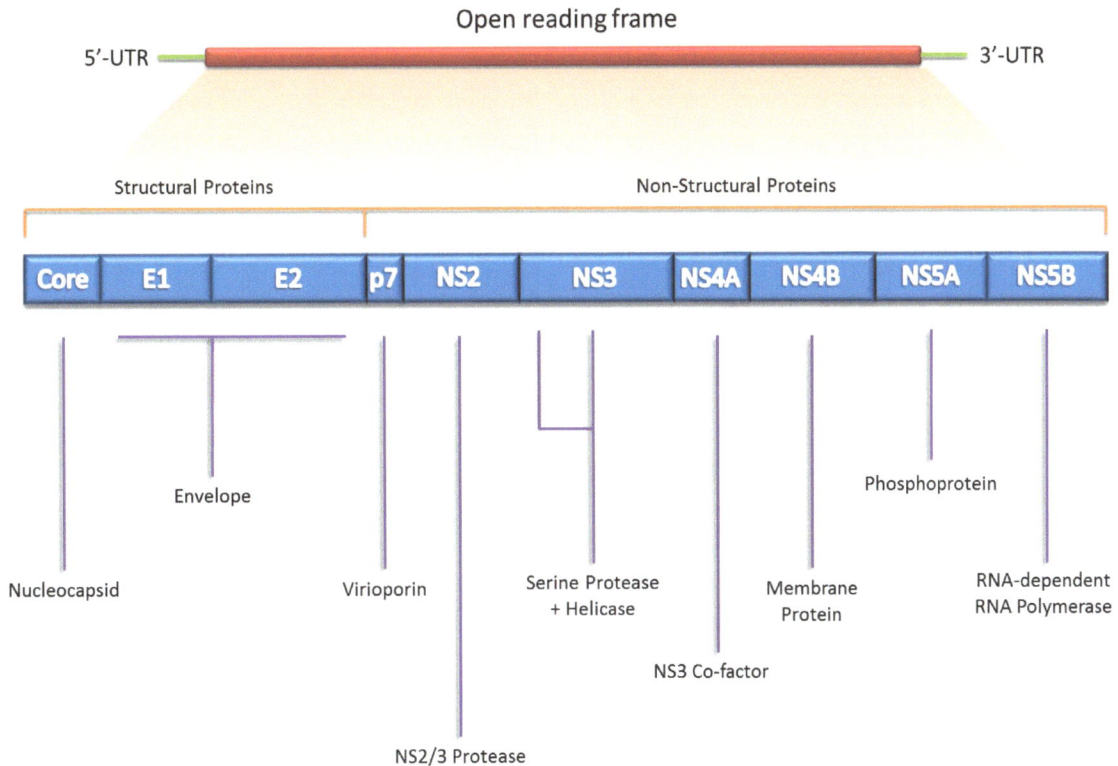

Figure 1: Structure of the HCV-genome. This viral genome contains a single open reading frame (ORF) encoding a polyprotein, which is processed into at least 10 proteins; three structural proteins and seven non-structural.

Structural Proteins	Function
Core Protein Nucleocapsid	Carcinogenesis and suppression of host immune response
E1/E2	Envelope Glycoproteins
Non-structural Proteins	**Function**
p7	Poly-protein processing and viral assembly
NS2/ NS3	NS2/NS3 Protease
NS3	Helicase
NS3/NS4A	Serine Protease
NS4B	Formation of Replication Complex
NS5B	RNA dependent RNA polymerase

Table 1: HCV-encoded proteins and their roles in the virus' life cycle.

3   HCV Pathogenesis

HCV mainly infects the hepatocytes, B-lymphocytes and dendritic cells. The human immune system plays an important role in the immuno-pathogenesis and progression of HCV infection. The T-cell-released inflammatory cytokines are the main stimuli in the development of host antiviral immune response (Boyer and Marcellin 2000). However, these cytokines also have an inhibitory effect on the immune system and favor the persistence of HCV infection (Coope *et al.*, 1999). The activated cytotoxic T cell response may eventually cause inflammation, which may ultimately lead to destruction and fibrosis of hepatocytes and liver parenchyma, contributing to progressive live damage (Shimotohno 2000).

Viral proteins play a role in the progression of HCV infection. The HCV Core protein is an RNA binding protein that condenses to form the viral capsid. Once in the cell it is aggressively involved in the activation of the Ras/Raf kinase pathway and of transcription factor NFκB. The Core also plays a role in inducing apoptosis by modulating the caspase 8 activity (Van Antwerp *et al.*, 1996; Aoki *et al.*, 2000; Lai & Ware 2000). Domain 1 of the Core protein carries a nuclear localization signal (NLS) and binds RNA while Domain 2 is responsible for its interaction with the endoplasmic reticulum, mitochondrial membranes and liposomes (Chang *et al.*, 1994; Suzuki *et al.*, 2005). Through modulation of *c-myc* and *c-fos* genes, the HCV Core is capable of affecting viral promoter transcription (Ray *et al.*, 1995). HCV core also contributes to liver steatosis by affecting lipid metabolism (Barba *et al.*, 1997; Moriya *et al.*, 1997; Moriya *et al.*, 1998; Asselah *et al.*, 2006). The HCV proteins E1 and E2 are part of the viral envelope. Besides facilitating viral entry into the cell cytoplasm, glycoprotein E2 inhibits protein kinase R (Taylor *et al.*, 1999; Bartosch *et al.*, 2003; Nielsen *et al.*, 2004). These glycoproteins harbor hyper-variable regions which serve as mutational hotspots and allow the virus to escape an immune response. The HCV NS4A protein contributes to HCV-mediated pathogenesis by inhibiting the host cell protein translation and by altering the production of interferon type-1 (Foy *et al.*, 2003; Nomura-Takigawa *et al.*, 2006). The NS4B has a myriad of functions, including NF-κB signaling activation (Kato *et al.*, 2000), reduction in host protein synthesis, and augmentation of IL-8 production (Florese *et al.*, 2002), that contribute to viral pathogenesis. The nonstructural protein, NS3, is also thought to contribute to hepato-carcinogenesis. The NS3 forms a complex with p53 (Ishido & Hotta 1998; Deng *et al.*, 2006), which significantly suppresses the p53-mediated transcriptional activation. This also lead to the repression of p53-mediated transcription of p21 which suppresses the apoptotic pathways in the cell (Kwun *et al.*, 2001). The NS3 is also known to play a role in the advancement of hepatocellular carcinoma (HCC) by enhancing the HCV replication through the activation of the Ras/Raf/MAPK/c-Myc signaling pathway. In fact, 30% cancers are reported to occur through the activation of this pathway (Zhang *et al.*, 2012).

4   HCV Life Cycle

The LDL receptor (LDL-R), tetraspanin protein CD81 (found on the surface of hepatocytes and numerous other cell types), scavenger receptor class B type I (SR-BI), and claudin-1 are the known host cell receptors for HCV (Pileri *et al.*, 1998; Agnello *et al.*, 1999; Scarsell *et al.*, 2002; Evans *et al.*, 2007). The first step of viral replication is the attachment of infectious particle to the host cell. Following that, HCV enters the cell through specific interactions between viral attachment proteins and host cell surface receptors. The host CD81 has been identified as a HCV receptor on the basis of its strong interaction with viral E2 protein (Pileri *et al.*, 1998). The HCV E2 is the major envelope glycoprotein thought to be responsible for initiating viral attachment to the host cell. The other route of entry for HCV, as well as for other members of Flaviviridae family, into host cell is through binding to low-density lipoprotein (LDL) receptors (Thomssen *et al.*, 1992). Based on experimental data, it has been proposed that HCV particles associate with LDL-Rs in order to gain entry into the host cell (Agnello *et al.*, 1999; Monazahian *et al.*, 1999).

Following receptor-mediated endocytosis, the positive-strand of HCV is released into the host cell cytoplasm (Fig.2). The translation of HCV RNA is initiated at its 5' end, using an RNA element known as internal ribosome entry site (Shimoik *et al.*, 2009).The resulting polyprotein travels through the rough endoplasmic reticulum (rER) where it undergoes co- and post-translational processing by host cell signalases and two viral proteinases (Lin *et al.*, 1994). The host signal peptidases process the core-NS2 region which is cleaved at the C-E1, E1-E2, E2-p7 and p7-NS2 junctions (Fig.1). At the carboxy terminus of the core protein, a second post- translational cleavage takes place, removing the E1 signal sequence by an as yet unidentified cellular enzyme (Hussy *et al.*, 1996). Post-translational processing of NS2 and NS3 is a rapid reaction, accomplished by the NS2-3 proteinase (Santolini *et al.*, 1995). Processing of the NS3-5B region is mediated by the NS3 proteinase with the protein junctions cleaved in the following order: NS3-4A, NS5A-B, NS4A-B, and NS4B-5A. The HCV NS5B is the key enzyme responsible for catalyzing the synthesis of minus- and plus-stranded RNA (Bartenschlager and Lohmann 2000).

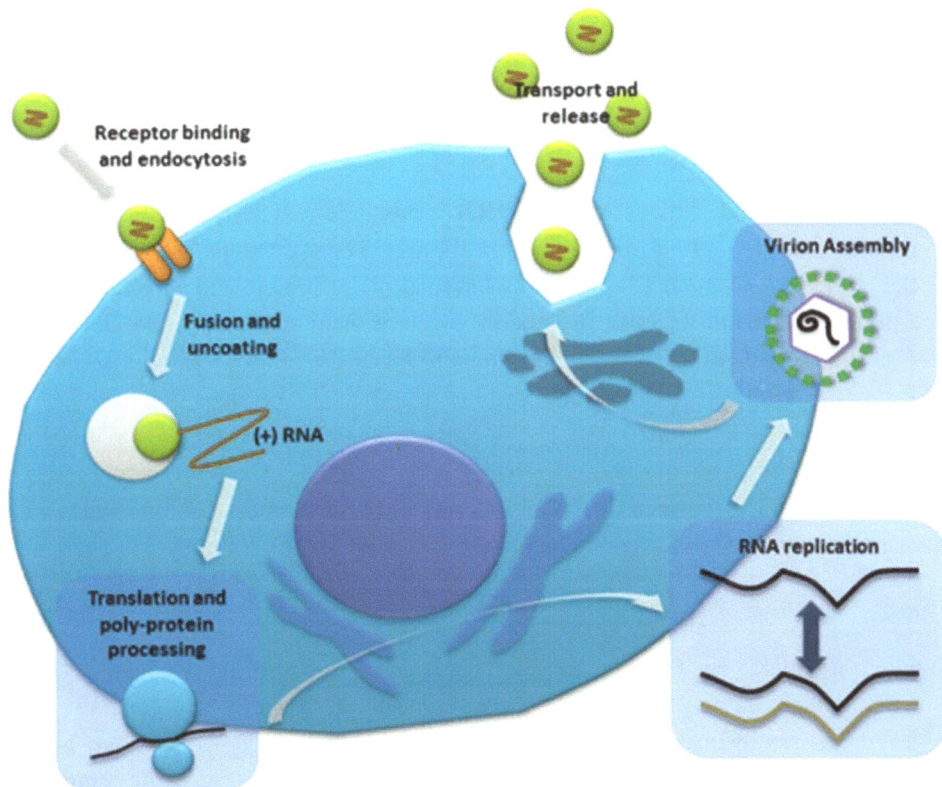

Figure 2: The HCV life cycle. After the virus enters the host cell through receptor-mediated endocytosis, the viral RNA is translated into a polyprotein. Functional and structural viral proteins are generated after post-translational processing of the polyprotein. These proteins then help in the replication of viral genome as well as in the further synthesis of viral proteins. The replicated genome is finally packed into the complete virion particle which is released from the host cell.

Following its synthesis, the positive-strand RNA is encapsulated with the newly synthesized structural proteins and is most likely enveloped while budding out of the lumen of the rER. The packaging of the HCV RNA genome into newly synthesized virions is probably mediated by specific interactions between sequences within the 5'-UTR of the HCV genome and the core protein. Such binding not only allows selective packaging of the plus-stranded genome but also appears to repress translation, suggesting a potential mechanism to switch from translation-replication to assembly. Finally, infectious virions are thought to be released by transport through the Golgi compartment and are exported via the constitutive secretory pathway (Shimoike *et al.*, 1999) (Fig.2).

5   NS3 Helicase

All helicases fall into two basic categories: those that encircle and form rings around DNA and/or RNA and those that do not. However, both ring and non-ring helicases interact with a single strand of the double-helical structure of DNA. The helicase either shifts from the 3'-end to 5'-end or from the 5'-end to the 3'-end on the DNA or RNA strand it binds. As a consequence, a 5'-3' helicase would bind the 5'-end of the single-stranded DNA tail while a 3'-5' helicase will attach itself to the 3'-end of a single-stranded DNA tail. HCV helicase is a non-ring helicase (Tai *et al.*, 1996; Morris *et al.*, 2002); a member of the superfamily-II (SF2) DExH helicase (Kim *et al.*, 1998).

5.1   NS3 Structure

The NS3 helicase must exist as a dimer to unwind RNA; monomeric NS3 has little or no activity (Wong and Lohman 1992, Cho *et al.*, 1998; Locatelli *et al.*, 2002). Three domains are revealed in the crystal structure of the HCV NS3. Domain 1 lies at the N-terminal of the protein and encompasses 181 residues of the serine protease. Domain 2 lies in the middle of the protein structure while Domain 3 at the C-terminal is 456 amino acid residues in length. Domain 3 has the helicase activity (Kim *et al.*, 1998) whereas ATP binds to a site that lies between domains 1 and 2. The residues implicated in binding and subsequent hydrolysis of ATP include K210, D290, E291, and H293 from domain 1, and Q460 and R467 from domain 2. The poly(dU) oligonucleotide (visualized in yellow; Fig.3) representing the helicase substrate threads through NS3 in between domain 3 and the other two domains. The residues that have significant interaction with this oligonucleotide include W510, T269, E493, R393, T411, T450, and H369.

5.2   ATP-Binding Site

The ATP binding site in NS3 is situated at the interface between domain 1 and domain 2 (Fig.3). Domain 1 consists of a phosphate binding loop (P-loop), conserved in all helicases and generally known as the 'Walker A box' (super family2 helicase motif I) (Walker *et al.*, 1982). Proteins that have the Walker type, NTP binding sites interact with ATP using a phosphate binding loop (P-loop) with a conserved Lysine (K210 in NS3) residue. The 'Walker B motif' (super family2 helicase motif II) in helicases, harbors an acidic residue, Aspartate (D290 in NS3), which interacts with positively charged divalent metal cations and the phosphates of ATP (Frick *et al.*, 2007). In helicases, another conserved basic residue near the P-loop is glutamate (E291 in NS3) required to activate the water molecule needed for ATP hydrolysis (Fric *et al.*, 2007).

Several Arginine residues, acting as arginine fingers, are present in domain 2 and also line the ATP binding cleft. These are part of a conserved region and include Arginines R467, R462 and R464 in NS3. Residue R467 regulates the host arginine methyltransferase (Duong *et al.*, 2005). Site-directed mutagenesis of this R467 with Lysine or Alanine leads to a significant impairment of the protein's ability to unwind DNA, with a concurrent 10-fold decrease in ATPase activity (Kim *et al.*, 1997; Kwong *et al.*, 2000).

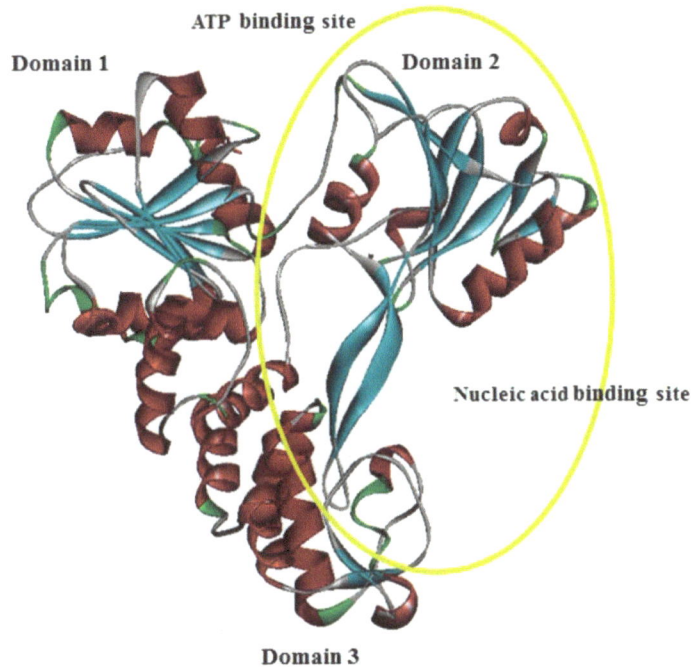

Figure 3: Structure of NS3. The three domains of NS3 marked in the crystal structure of the protein. In the crystal structure, the ATP binding site is located in domain1 whereas the nucleic acid binding site is in between domain 2 and 3 (marked by the yellow circle). Adapted and modified from (123) (PDB ID:1A1V).

5.3   Nucleic Acid Binding Site

In the NS3 structure, the cleft separating the subdomains 1 and 2 is known to bind DNA oligonucleotides, and is also responsible for accommodating one strand of RNA (Kim *et al.*, 1998; Mackintosh *et al.*, 2006) (Fig.3). The key residues involved in RNA binding are Trp (W501), Glu (E493) and Arg (R393). The most significant residue in this cleft is W501, which stacks like a bookend between the nucleic acid bases and locks the protein in position. The residue is critical for both RNA unwinding and HCV RNA replication (Lam and Frick 2006). Another key residue is E493, which must be protonated for the helicase to be optimally active. The residue R393 is essential for holding the DNA in the cleft by an arginine clamp which is centered on W393. This clamp rotates upon ATP binding, releasing the nucleic acid and allowing the protein to translocate (Lam *et al.* 2003). Site-directed mutagenesis studies have also revealed the significance of residues Thr-269 and Thr-411 in NS3 function, demonstrating that mutation of the two residues leads to the elimination of ATPase activity and a complete loss of helicase activity (Lin and Kim 1999).

5.4   NS3 Function

There exists much debate regarding the true nature of HCV helicase's role in RNA unwinding. The failure to elucidate the nature of the helicase structure while it interacts with RNA seems to fuel this debate. Two models have been proposed for the mechanism of RNA unwinding by the NS3 helicase. The helicase either functions a) as a monomer like an inchworm (Kim *et al.*, 1998) or, b) as a dimer which rolls down the nucleic acid (Cho *et al.*, 1998). The crystal structure of HCV NS3 was solved after the protein was first purified (Kim *et al.*, 1998). It is a 67 kDa tri-functional protein (Love *et al.*, 1996), with a helicase domain on the C-terminal and a protease domain at the N-terminal, NS3 has the unique capability to not only cleave viral self-proteins but to unwind DNA and/or RNA during viral replication. The enzyme has (d)NTPase and RNA/DNA helicase activities that allow it to translocate along the nucleic acid substrate (Kim *et al.*, 1998; Levin *et al.*, 2005; Frick, 2007). The full length NS3 is more proficient at unwinding DNA when compared to a truncated NS3 with an intact helicase domain. The non-covalent pairing of NS3 with NS4A allows NS3 helicase to function as a serine protease with the NS4A co-factor providing the activation subunit for the NS3 catalytic subunit (Zhang *et al.*, 2005). The principal role of HCV NS3 is to initiate RNA replication and to unwind stable stem loop structures as well as positive and negative strand termini of HCV RNA (Banerjee and Dasgupta 2001). It is postulated that it may also have a role in removing stable RNA secondary structures and may also be involved in the displacement of bound proteins that might interfere with RNA synthesis throughout the process of virion replication (Kolykhalov *et al.*, 2000). Finally, NS3 may also be required for the dissociation of the replicative form into negative and positive strands of HCV RNA.

As an enzyme with a significant role to play in the viral life cycle, the NS3 helicase is considered a potential and attractive target for the anti-HCV drugs. For the past 15 years, NS3 has been studied as a possible drug target against HCV (Frick 2007). Drugs that target unwinding activity of a helicase might act in a variety of ways which include prevention of ATP binding or hydrolysis by inhibiting ATPase activity, or blocking nucleic acid binding and thus inhibiting the unwinding process, etc. (Borowski *et al.* 2003; Gordon & Keller 2005; Krawczyk *et al.*, 2009). A few nucleic acid competitive inhibitors have been reported in the literature; however, most of these inhibitors have disappointingly low potency, undesirable pharmacokinetic properties and/or toxicity (Phoon *et al.*, 2001; Chen *et al*, 2009). The ATP and RNA-binding sites of NS3 helicase have been the focus of many studies investigating potential drug targets against HCV.

6   NS3 Inhibitors

The NS3 helicase of HCV is an obvious choice for a drug target, owing to its pivotal role in the virus' life cycle. The inhibitors tried against NS3, so far, are nucleic acid analogs and antibodies.

6.1   Nucleoside Analogs

It is postulated that the nucleoside analogs interact with the conserved Walker sequences on the helicase protein. There is also the possibility of the existence of a second site, as reported by Porter *et al.* (1998), that these analogs can bind to, in addition to the Walker sequence. Locatelli *et al.* (2002) have been able to demonstrate cooperative binding of nucleotides to HCV helicase, thereby further supporting the notion that there exists a second binding site for nucleotides. It appears that the said second binding site may be highly specific than the binding site between domain 1 and domain 2. Locatelli *et al.* (2002) were also able to demonstrate the certain NTPs facilitated unwinding more efficiently than others. Some (d)NTPs such as dATP, were found to be potent inhibitors of unwinding and poor substrates for the enzyme. Once again, this phenomenon can be explained by the presence of a binding site more specific to NTP binding compared to the catalytic site.

Some examples of the nucleoside analogs include ring expanded nucleosides and nucleotides, ribavirin triphosphate and 5'-O-(4-fluorosulphonylbenzoy)-esters of ribavirin, adenosine, guanosine and inosine. Other compounds that resemble nucleoside bases and have been found to inhibit helicases in related viruses include tetrachlorobenzotriazole (TCBT) and tetrabromobenzotriazole (TBBT) (Borowski *et al.*, 2003).

6.2 ATP Binding Inhibitors

Hu and coworkers (Chen *et al.*, 2009) have reported a number of compounds that could bind to NS3 at the Walker A site. In these studies, molecular modeling was employed to identify the compound, Soluble Blue Ht (Protein Database ID:2ZJO) (Fig.4a), that exhibited the maximum binding affinity for NS3 helicase. The binding of Blue Ht prevents the NS3 helicase from binding to and hydrolyzing ATP. This compound directly interacts with the lysine K210 (which is required for ATP hydrolysis) and aspartate D290 (Fig.5). Another study has reported that ATP mimetics, such as ADP.BeF3 (Fig.4b), also make similar interactions with the same residues present in the ATP binding domain of NS3 (Fig.5) (Gu and Rice 2010).

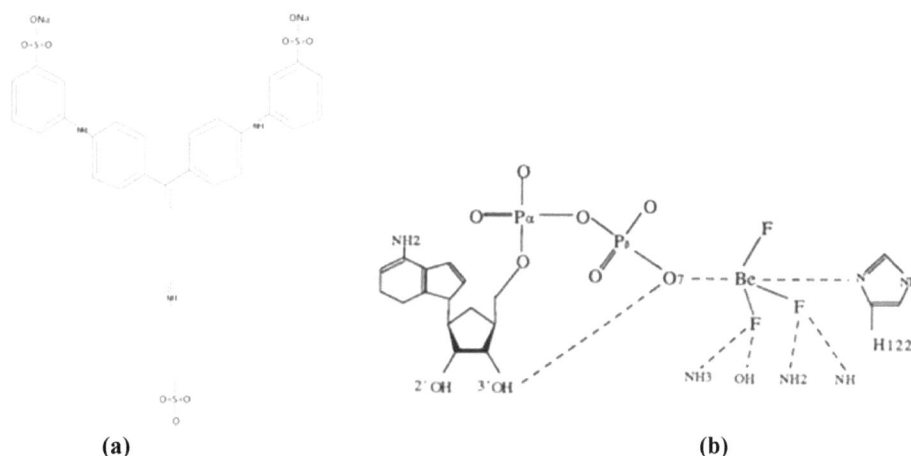

(a)   (b)

Figure 4: ATP binding inhibitors. Structures of a) Soluble Blue Ht and b) ADP.BeF3

6.3 Nucleic Acid-based Inhibitors

The SELEX (systemic evolution of ligands by exponential amplification) procedure has been employed to develop RNA-based inhibitors for HCV helicase. With this technique, RNA libraries were screened and RNA molecules were selected that showed tight binding with and inhibition of helicase activity (Fukuda *et al.*, 2004). In another approach, new RNA aptamer were reported which showed high affinity for, and inhibition of, the NS3 helicase portion (Banerjee and Dasgupta 2001, Hwang *et al.*, 2004).

To date, only a few compounds have been shown to sufficiently inhibit NS3 helicase by targeting the nucleic acid binding cleft. Few NS3 inhibitors have been reported to compete for the nucleic acid binding site but have been found to be of meek potency with a less than optimal pharmacokinetic profile, while exhibiting toxicity to the cells. Maga and co-workers (Maga *et al.*, 2005) described a series of quinoline and quinoxaline derivatives that inhibited HCV helicase activity by competing with the nucleic

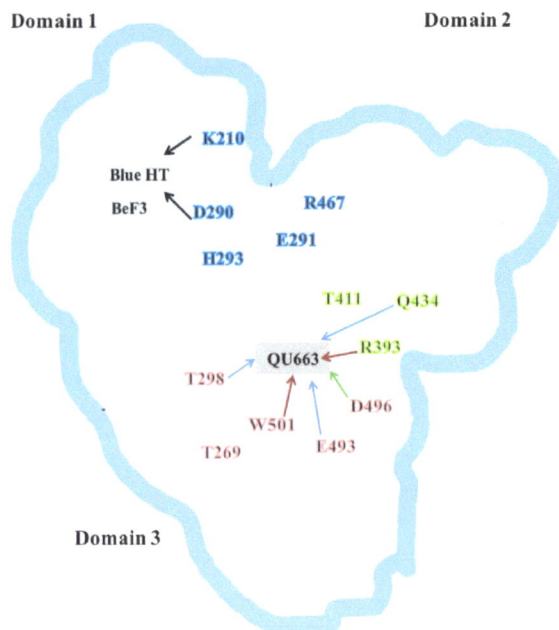

Figure 5: Amino acid residues in the three domains of NS3 which interact with the inhibitors of ATP (Blue Ht and BeF3) and nucleic acid (QU663) binding. The amino acids in blue are implicated in the interaction with ATP binding inhibitors; K210 and D290 being directly involved in the interaction. The amino acids in red and green are involved in the interaction with QU663; with W501 and R393 making direct interactions with the inhibitor (red arrows). The residues T298, E493 and Q434 interact with the inhibitor through H-bonding, whereas D496 makes ionic interactions (blue arrows). Residues T269 and 411 are located in conserved region of nucleic acid binding site and have a role to play in the unwinding activity.

acid without affecting the ATPase activity. Through the use of inhibition assays and docking and molecular modeling, Maga *et al.* (2005) were able to identify QU663 as an important inhibitor of nucleic acid binding (Fig.6). Docking studies have shown that QU663 binds NS3 helicase in place of the RNA substrate, interacting with residues W501 and R393, important for, respectively, nucleic acid binding and helicase activity.

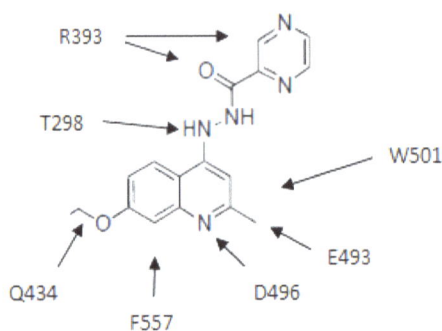

Figure 6: Structure of QU663. A quinoline derivative inhibitor of HCV Helicase (80). Amino acid residues of the helicase and their respective interactions with various portions of QU663 are indicated with arrows.

The new inhibitor QU663 showed remarkable interactions with the helicase enzyme region, with the salient features observed as follows: (i) polarized ð-ð interactions with W501 and F557 through the substituted quinoline ring, (ii) the negatively polarized oxygen of the hydrazide moiety and a cation-ð interaction involving the pyrazine ring with the R393 (iii) an ionic interaction with D496 through the protonated quinoline nitrogen, and (iv) H-bonding with T298, Q434, and E493 (Fig.5 and 6). QU663 binding to NS3 successfully blocks helicase function in a competitive manner, without affecting the ATPase activity.

A small peptide inhibitor has also been reported that can possibly interact with the known RNA-binding cleft of HCV helicase. This is a 14 amino acid-long peptide (p14) and has a sequence similar to HCV helicase arginine finger (SF2 helicase motif IV). The peptide p14 has the ability to inhibit HCV helicase-catalyzed DNA unwinding with an IC50 of 200 μM. It has also been shown to inhibit the replication of HCV replicons in culture cells with an IC50 of 83 μM (Borowski *et al.*, 2008).

6.4   Antibodies

Antibody mediated inhibition of HCV helicase is possibly the most promising new approach in developing anti-HCV therapy. Most, if not all, HCV patients mount a humoral response against HCV and are able to produce antibodies against HCV proteins, including the antibodies against NS3 protein, some of which are capable of binding to the helicase domain of NS3 (Chen *et al.*, 1998).

In order to successfully introduce anti-NS3 antibodies in infected cells they are transfected with the gene expressing a portion of an antibody reactive against NS3. There are two methods to achieve this: One way to introduce a functional anti-NS3 antibody into infected cells is to use single chain fragment (ScFv) antibodies. A linker protein connects the heavy chain to the light chain, both of which have interacting variable domains. A collection of human antibody expressing gene fragments is first created using polymerase chain reaction (PCR). Plasma cells extracted from infected patients are used to achieve this goal. Using various methods, from this amplified pool the antibodies are expressed and those reacting with NS3 helicase are purified (Tessmann *et al.*, 2002). ScFv's that bind HCV helicase have also been constructed by splicing together the variable domains of anti-HCV monoclonal antibodies (Zhang *et al.*, 2000; Sullivan *et al.*, 2002). After expression and purification, several of these recombinant proteins have been shown to inhibit HCV helicase-catalyzed DNA unwinding (Sullivan *et al.*, 2002; Artsaenko *et al.*, 2003).

6.5   Inhibitors targeting unknown sites

Here we discuss compounds found to be effective HCV helicase inhibitors based on in vitro assays. The binding sites for these compounds on the helicase have, however, not been elucidated so far. Among these, Tropolone derivatives are known to have antimicrobial, antifungal, antiviral and insecticidal properties. Reportedly, Tropolones also function as selective inhibitors of ribonuclease activity of the HIV reverse transcriptase (Budihas *et al.*, 2005) and have been shown to inhibit HCV helicase-catalyzed DNA unwinding. These compounds consist of a seven-member tropolone ring system, 3,7-dibromo-5-morpholinomethyltropolone (DBMTr), which is a potent inhibitor of HCV helicase. DBMTr has an IC50 of 17.6 μM and shows no effect on the ATPase activity of NS3. The low toxicity profile of DBMtr on yeast cells may permit its use on other eukaryotic tissues as well (Boguszewska-Chachulska *et al.*, 2006).

Stankiewicz-Drogon *et al.* (2008) have screened several acridone derivatives which had potent anticancer and antiviral activities. These compounds were also found to be inhibitors of HCV helicase DNA unwinding activity and HCV replication. Among these, compounds 20 (9-oxo-9,10-dihydro-acridine-4-

carboxylic acid pyridin-4-ylamide) and 27 (9-oxo-9,10-dihydro-acridine-4-carboxylic acid pyridin-2-ylamide) acted as the most potent inhibitors of HCV helicase-catalyzed DNA unwinding, with IC50s of 9 and 4 µM, respectively. Another derivative, acridone-carboxylates, is postulated to interact with the DNA substrate, showing inhibition of T7 RNA polymerase-catalyzed RNA synthesis as well the HCV replicon synthesis.

Structure-activity relationship analyses have led to the design and synthesis of Ceestatin, a member of epoxides, which happens to be a strong helicase inhibitor. Ceestatin has been found to exert its antiviral effects against HCV through inhibition of the host cofactor HMG-CoA synthase (Peng et al., 2007). Li et al. recently reported a series of potent HCV helicase inhibitors, synthesized from the main part of the yellow dye primuline. The dye has the ability to inhibit HCV helicase's ability to unwind DNA but does not exert its actions by binding to the helicase DNA substrate. These compounds exhibit a remarkable ability to inhibit viral helicase in a variety of ways; (i) by inhibiting NS3 helicase activity, (ii) by inhibiting RNA unwinding catalyzed by NS3, and (iii) by inhibiting the NS3 protease function (Ndjomou et al., 2012). Several groups have also reported non-nucleoside-based inhibitors for HCV helicase. These include piperidine derivative, heterocyclic carboxamide, anthracyclin antibiotics (Borowski et al., 2002), trifluoperazine (Borowski et al., 2002) and aminophenylbenzimidazole derivatives (Phoon et al., 2001). Many of these compounds can intercalate with nucleic acid and act by mechanisms yet to be deciphered.

6.6   Fluoroquinolones

The fluoroquinolones are a synthetic class of antimicrobial drugs derived from antimalarial drugs mepacrine and chloroquine (Wise and Phillips 2000). Nalidixic acid, the first quinolone, was synthesized in 1962 from the antimalarial drug chloroquine (Table 2) (Andriole 2005). Nalidixic acid is a naphthyridine derivative used against urinary tract infection and due to its narrow spectrum and poor serum concentration, limited to Enterobacteriacae (Tillotson 1996). The advancement in quinolones drug research was initially reported in 1980 by Koga et al. (1980). They introduced newer drugs with improved absorption and activity and structural modification at position 6 (addition of Fluorine). This new class of drugs, carryinh a Fluorine at position 6, were generally termed as the Fluoroquinolones.

Fluoroquinolones developed later, such as Pipemidic acid, Oxolinic acid and Cinoxacin, were reported to have greater potency and valuable advantages as compared to their precursor Nalidixic acid (Ringel et al., 1967; Holmes et al., 1974; Peters et al., 1979). Since then, more than 10,000 new quinolone-based derivatives have been patented. The generational terms have been used to classify the fluoroquinolones on the basis of their broad antimicrobial spectrum and toxicity profile. According to this system, flouoroquinolones have been classified into four generations (Ball 2003, Andriole 2005). First generation compounds have activity against aerobic gram-negative bacteria. Second generation quinolones are the true fluoroquinolone and possess improved activity against gram-negative and moderate against gram-positive. Third generation agents have prolonged potency against gram-positive and anaerobes. Fourth-generation drugs provide significant coverage against anaerobes (Bolon 2009) (Table 2).

Fluoroquinolone group are the most dynamic, broad-spectrum antibiotics. The new members of this group have wide-range bactericidal activity (Jones and Pfaller 2000), outstanding oral bioavailability (Robson 1992), excellent tissue accessibility (Gerding and Hitt 1989), and acceptable safety profiles. Figure 7 shows the pharmacophore of fluoroquinolone. The functional groups on this pharmacophore have been assigned various features:

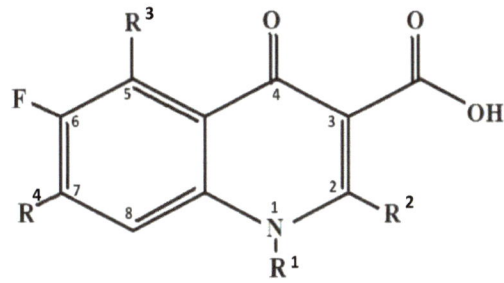

Figure 7: Fluoroquinolone pharmacophore.

No.	Name	Structure	Grouping
1	Nalidixic Acid		First Generation
2	Cinoxacin		
3	Flumequine		
4	Ciprofloxacin		Second Generation
5	Enoxacin		
6	Fleroxacin		

7	Lomefloxacin		
8	Norfloxacin		
9	Ofloxacin		
10	Balofloxacin		
11	Pefloxacin		
12	Levofloxacin		Third Generation
13	Sparfloxacin		
14	Moxifloxacin		Fourth Generation

Table 2: Classification and structures of Fluoroquinolones

6.6.1   Position 1

This position is important for binding of drug with the enzyme-DNA complex and making hydrophobic interactions with the major groove of DNA (Domagala 1994).

6.6.2   Position 2

This site is very near to the site where the gyrase or topoisomerase can bind. The addition of any bulky group at this site will inhibit the transport and result in low microbiological activity (Llorente *et al.*, 1996).

6.6.3   Position 3 and 4

These are linked with each other by carboxylic acid group and the keto group. These positions are crucial for gyrase binding to fluoroquinolones (Tillotson, 1996).

6.6.4   Position 5

This site has the ability to control potency. At this position, the small groups which are electron-donating in nature (such as amino, hydroxyl or methyl) are found to confer increased in vitro antibacterial activity against gram-positive pathogens (Yoshida *et al.*, 1996).

6.6.5   Position 6

The presence of fluorine group at this position surprisingly improves antimicrobial activity (Koga *et al.*, 1980).

6.6.6   Position 7

This position has 5 or 6 membered nitrogen heterocycles. This is considered as the site where DNA gyrase directly interacts with the drug (Ma *et al.*, 1999).

6.6.7   Position 8

The nitrogen or halogen atom at this position might produce clinically valuable drugs. The precise modifications at this site may alter the original target of fluoroquinolone. For example, substitution of hydrogen (as in ciprofloxacin), or fused ring (benzoxazine bridge between C-8 and N-1; as in Ofloxacin and Levofloxacin), can confer high activity against topoisomerase but little against DNA gyrase (Ahmed and Daneshtalab).

7   Mechanism of Action of Fluoroquinolones

Fluoroquinolones interfere with bacterial cell replication, transcription, and DNA repair by disabling two bacterial enzymes crucial to these processes, namely DNA gyrase (formerly topoisomerase II) and topoisomerase IV. Both of these enzymes help in the unwinding of bacterial DNA, thus playing a crucial role in DNA replication, transcription, etc. Fluoroquinolones bind to the enzyme–DNA complex, causing a conformational change in the enzyme. The fluoroquinolone traps the enzyme on the DNA as a fluoroquinolone–enzyme–DNA complex, inhibiting further DNA replication. The process of complex formation inhibits bacterial DNA replication, preventing cell growth and eventually leading to a bacteriostatic effect.

7.1   Antimicrobial Activity of Fluoroquinolones

Anaerobes are generally resistant to fluoroquinolones. Ofloxacin and Ciprofloxacin inhibit gram negative cocci and bacilli at low concentrations, however, little activity has been noticed against streptococci (Pneumococcus and Enterococci), and therefore these drugs may not be effective against respiratory tract infections. Levofloxacin (the L-isomer of Ofloxacin) and Sparfloxacin are more active against staphylo-coccus and streptococcus than Ciprofloxacin and Ofloxacin. Fluoroquinolones are active against intracel-lular pathogens such as Legionella, and Chlamydia. Fluoroquinolones activity extends against some My-cobacteria, including Mycobacterium tuberculosis (MTB) and Mycobacterium intermedium (MI)/Mycobacterium avian (MA) complex (Blondeau *et al.*, 2000).

7.2   Antiviral Activity of Fluoroquinolones

Fluoroquinolones inhibit the topoisomerase catalytic sequence by covalently coupling with the cleaved DNA. The fundamental composition of the quinolone-gyrase-DNA complex has been elucidated to some extent. Many viruses encode a helicase enzyme which plays an essential role in their genome replication. Functionally, viral helicase is homologous to bacterial gyrase, both enzymes catalyzing the unwinding of nucleic acid substrates. Based on this functional homology, it was hypothesized that inhibitors of bacteri-al gyrase, fluoroquinolones, can also inhibit viral helicase by a similar mechanism. Initial experiments that tested this hypothesis showed that Ofloxacin had inhibitory activity against vaccinia virus, but not against herpes simplex and influenza viruses (Ikeda *et al.*, 1987). The L-isomer of Ofloxacin (DR-3355) was later reported to shield cells form HIV-1 mediated cytolysis; the surviving cells showed lost expres-sion of the CD4 antigen, and were found incapable of producing infectious virion particles (Nozaki-Renard *et al.*, 1990).

   In clinical trials, fluoroquinolones have been found effective against DNA (Josephson *et al.* 2006) as well as RNA (Negro *et al.*, 1998; Kojima *et al.*, 2002) viruses. Replication as well as cytopathic effect of BK virus was shown to be inhibited by fluoroquinolones nalidixic acid and oxolinic acid (Portolani *et al.*, 1988). Similar studies in simian virus 40 (SV40) have shown inhibitory effect of several fluoroquin-olones on viral replication in cell culture. Using an in vitro assay, the same study also showed that the ability of SV40 T antigen helicase to dissociate a double-stranded DNA substrate was inhibited by all the fluoroquinolones tested in this analysis (Ali *et al.*, 2007). Recently, Khan *et al.* (2012) were able to show that in a panel of 12 fluoroquinolones, all the tested drugs inhibited the replication of hepatitis C replicon as well as the virion production in cell culture. Using the molecular beacon helicase assay, the same study also showed that the HCV NS3 helicase was inhibited by all the fluoroquinolones tested. Several new derivatives containing the basic quinolone carboxylic acid template and diverse lipophilic substituents have been patented as antiviral agents. Most of these compounds have proven activities against Human Immunodeficiency Virus-1 (HIV-1) and appear to be effective in the therapy and prophylaxis of Acquired Immune Deficiency Syndrome (AIDS) (Cecchetti *et al.*, 2000).

   Fluoroquinolones bearing piperazinyl and oxo substitutions at positions 7 and 8 have proven to be promising anti-viral complexes. Compound K-12 represses HIV-1 and HIV-2 transcription in persistently infected cells at levels that do not impede the propagation and viability of host cells. Moreover, in diseas-es caused by retroviruses, such as HIV-1, HIV-2 and Moloney murine sarcoma virus, K-12 has a role in preventing viral infections caused by Herpes virus saimiri, Cytomegalovirus, Varicella zoster virus and Herpes simplex virus types 1 and 2 (Witvrouw *et al.*, 1998). Another, fluoroquinolone derivative, K-37, has been found to deter HIV-1 replication. It demonstrated improved activity against persistently infected cells than the parental compound, K-12. K-37 represses RNA-dependent trans-initiation, involving HIV Tat protein (Okamoto *et al.*, 2000). Structure/activity relationship-based experiments have led to the discovery of a number of fascinating complexes with striking anti-viral selectivity indexes. While the antiviral efficacy of these compounds has been demonstrated against a broad range of viruses, their potential against HCV remains to be explored.

8   Concluding Remarks

Considering that over 200 million people are infected with HCV around the world, it is imperative to continue investigations for anti-HCV therapy options that are affordable, accessible, and have fewer side effects. For many years, unavaialability of a cell culture system and of animal models that could sustain HCV replication impeded research toward the discovery of anti-HCV drugs. With the new developments in those directions, we now have the *in vitro* cell culture as well as mouse models that may be exploited in anti-HCV discovery. The HCV NS3 helicase represents a relatively unexplored viral protein that may prove to be a potent drug target. A combinatorial approach involving crystallography, molecular dynamics, and *in vitro* enzyme assays should be employed to discover new chemical derivatives targeting NS3. The inhibitors found promising in this phase of the experiments should be tested on the available animal models. Similarly, a more multi-disciplinary approach needs to be developed for designing clinical trials. It is important to design the trials in a rigorous, open-minded approach that is closely inspired by the *in vitro* studies.

References

Hepatitis C--global prevalence (update). (2000). Wkly Epidemiol Rec 75(3): 18-19.

Agnello, V., G. Abel, M. Elfahal, G. B. Knight and Q. X. Zhang (1999). "Hepatitis C virus and other flaviviridae viruses enter cells via low density lipoprotein receptor." Proc Natl Acad Sci U S A 96(22): 12766-12771.

Ahmed, A. and M. Daneshtalab "Nonclassical biological activities of quinolone derivatives." J Pharm Pharm Sci 15(1): 52-72.

Ali, S. H., A. Chandraker and J. A. DeCaprio (2007). "Inhibition of Simian virus 40 large T antigen helicase activity by fluoroquinolones." Antivir Ther 12(1): 1-6.

Andriole, V. T. (2005). "The quinolones: past, present, and future." Clin Infect Dis 41 Suppl 2: S113-119.

Aoki, H., J. Hayashi, M. Moriyama, Y. Arakawa and O. Hino (2000). "Hepatitis C virus core protein interacts with 14-3-3 protein and activates the kinase Raf-1." J Virol 74(4): 1736-1741.

Artsaenko, O., K. Tessmann, M. Sack, D. Haussinger and T. Heintges (2003). "Abrogation of hepatitis C virus NS3 helicase enzymatic activity by recombinant human antibodies." J Gen Virol 84(Pt 9): 2323-2332.

Asselah, T., L. Rubbia-Brandt, P. Marcellin and F. Negro (2006). "Steatosis in chronic hepatitis C: why does it really matter?" Gut 55(1): 123-130.

Ball, P. (2003). "Adverse drug reactions: implications for the development of fluoroquinolones." J Antimicrob Chemother 51 Suppl 1: 21-27.

Banerjee, R. and A. Dasgupta (2001). "Specific interaction of hepatitis C virus protease/helicase NS3 with the 3'-terminal sequences of viral positive- and negative-strand RNA." J Virol 75(4): 1708-1721.

Barba, G., F. Harper, T. Harada, M. Kohara, S. Goulinet, Y. Matsuura, G. Eder, Z. Schaff, M. J. Chapman, T. Miyamura and C. Brechot (1997). "Hepatitis C virus core protein shows a cytoplasmic localization and associates to cellular lipid storage droplets." Proc Natl Acad Sci U S A 94(4): 1200-1205.

Bartenschlager, R. and V. Lohmann (2000). "Replication of hepatitis C virus." J Gen Virol 81(Pt 7): 1631-1648.

Bartosch, B., J. Dubuisson and F. L. Cosset (2003). "Infectious hepatitis C virus pseudo-particles containing functional E1-E2 envelope protein complexes." J Exp Med 197(5): 633-642.

Blondeau, J. M., R. Laskowski, J. Bjarnason and C. Stewart (2000). "Comparative in vitro activity of gatifloxacin, grepafloxacin, levofloxacin, moxifloxacin and trovafloxacin against 4151 Gram-negative and Gram-positive organisms." Int J Antimicrob Agents 14(1): 45-50.

Boguszewska-Chachulska, A. M., M. Krawczyk, A. Najda, K. Kopanska, A. Stankiewicz-Drogon, W. Zagorski-Ostoja and M. Bretner (2006). "Searching for a new anti-HCV therapy: synthesis and properties of tropolone derivatives." Biochem Biophys Res Commun 341(2): 641-647.

Bolon, M. K. (2009). "The newer fluoroquinolones." Infect Dis Clin North Am 23(4): 1027-1051, x.

Borowski, P., J. Deinert, S. Schalinski, M. Bretner, K. Ginalski, T. Kulikowski and D. Shugar (2003). "Halogenated benzimidazoles and benzotriazoles as inhibitors of the NTPase/helicase activities of hepatitis C and related viruses." Eur J Biochem 270(8): 1645-1653.

Borowski, P., M. V. Heising, I. B. Miranda, C. L. Liao, J. Choe and A. Baier (2008). "Viral NS3 helicase activity is inhibited by peptides reproducing the Arg-rich conserved motif of the enzyme (motif VI)." Biochem Pharmacol 76(1): 28-38.

Borowski, P., A. Niebuhr, H. Schmitz, R. S. Hosmane, M. Bretner, M. A. Siwecka and T. Kulikowski (2002). "NTPase/helicase of Flaviviridae: inhibitors and inhibition of the enzyme." Acta Biochim Pol 49(3): 597-614.

Borowski, P., S. Schalinski and H. Schmitz (2002). "Nucleotide triphosphatase/helicase of hepatitis C virus as a target for antiviral therapy." Antiviral Res 55(3): 397-412.

Boyer, N. and P. Marcellin (2000). "Pathogenesis, diagnosis and management of hepatitis C." J Hepatol 32(1 Suppl): 98-112.

Brass, V., D. Moradpour and H. E. Blum (2006). "Molecular virology of hepatitis C virus (HCV): 2006 update." Int J Med Sci 3(2): 29-34.

Budihas, S. R., I. Gorshkova, S. Gaidamakov, A. Wamiru, M. K. Bona, M. A. Parniak, R. J. Crouch, J. B. McMahon, J. A. Beutler and S. F. Le Grice (2005). "Selective inhibition of HIV-1 reverse transcriptase-associated ribonuclease H activity by hydroxylated tropolones." Nucleic Acids Res 33(4): 1249-1256.

Cecchetti, V., C. Parolin, S. Moro, T. Pecere, E. Filipponi, A. Calistri, O. Tabarrini, B. Gatto, M. Palumbo, A. Fravolini and G. Palu (2000). "6-Aminoquinolones as new potential anti-HIV agents." J Med Chem 43(20): 3799-3802.

Chang, S. C., J. H. Yen, H. Y. Kang, M. H. Jang and M. F. Chang (1994). "Nuclear localization signals in the core protein of hepatitis C virus." Biochem Biophys Res Commun 205(2): 1284-1290.

Chen, C. S., C. T. Chiou, G. S. Chen, S. C. Chen, C. Y. Hu, W. K. Chi, Y. D. Chu, L. H. Hwang, P. J. Chen, D. S. Chen, S. H. Liaw and J. W. Chern (2009). "Structure-based discovery of triphenylmethane derivatives as inhibitors of hepatitis C virus helicase." J Med Chem 52(9): 2716-2723.

Chen, M., M. Sallberg, A. Sonnerborg, L. Jin, A. Birkett, D. Peterson, O. Weiland and D. R. Milich (1998). "Human and murine antibody recognition is focused on the ATPase/helicase, but not the protease domain of the hepatitis C virus nonstructural 3 protein." Hepatology 28(1): 219-224.

Cho, H. S., N. C. Ha, L. W. Kang, K. M. Chung, S. H. Back, S. K. Jang and B. H. Oh (1998). "Crystal structure of RNA helicase from genotype 1b hepatitis C virus. A feasible mechanism of unwinding duplex RNA." J Biol Chem 273(24): 15045-15052.

Cooper, S., A. L. Erickson, E. J. Adams, J. Kansopon, A. J. Weiner, D. Y. Chien, M. Houghton, P. Parham and C. M. Walker (1999). "Analysis of a successful immune response against hepatitis C virus." Immunity 10(4): 439-449.

Deng, L., M. Nagano-Fujii, M. Tanaka, Y. Nomura-Takigawa, M. Ikeda, N. Kato, K. Sada and H. Hotta (2006). "NS3 protein of Hepatitis C virus associates with the tumour suppressor p53 and inhibits its function in an NS3 sequence-dependent manner." J Gen Virol 87(Pt 6): 1703-1713.

Domagala, J. M. (1994). "Structure-activity and structure-side-effect relationships for the quinolone antibacterials." J Antimicrob Chemother 33(4): 685-706.

Duong, F. H., V. Christen, J. M. Berke, S. H. Penna, D. Moradpour and M. H. Heim (2005). "Upregulation of protein phosphatase 2Ac by hepatitis C virus modulates NS3 helicase activity through inhibition of protein arginine methyltransferase 1." J Virol 79(24): 15342-15350.

Evans, M. J., T. von Hahn, D. M. Tscherne, A. J. Syder, M. Panis, B. Wolk, T. Hatziioannou, J. A. McKeating, P. D. Bieniasz and C. M. Rice (2007). "Claudin-1 is a hepatitis C virus co-receptor required for a late step in entry." Nature 446(7137): 801-805.

Florese, R. H., M. Nagano-Fujii, Y. Iwanaga, R. Hidajat and H. Hotta (2002). "Inhibition of protein synthesis by the non-structural proteins NS4A and NS4B of hepatitis C virus." Virus Res 90(1-2): 119-131.

Foy, E., K. Li, C. Wang, R. Sumpter, Jr., M. Ikeda, S. M. Lemon and M. Gale, Jr. (2003). "Regulation of interferon regulatory factor-3 by the hepatitis C virus serine protease." Science 300(5622): 1145-1148.

Frick, D. N. (2007). "The hepatitis C virus NS3 protein: a model RNA helicase and potential drug target." Curr Issues Mol Biol 9(1): 1-20.

Frick, D. N., S. Banik and R. S. Rypma (2007). "Role of divalent metal cations in ATP hydrolysis catalyzed by the hepatitis C virus NS3 helicase: magnesium provides a bridge for ATP to fuel unwinding." J Mol Biol 365(4): 1017-1032.

Fried, M. W., M. L. Shiffman, K. R. Reddy, C. Smith, G. Marinos, F. L. Goncales, Jr., D. Haussinger, M. Diago, G. Carosi, D. Dhumeaux, A. Craxi, A. Lin, J. Hoffman and J. Yu (2002). "Peginterferon alfa-2a plus ribavirin for chronic hepatitis C virus infection." N Engl J Med 347(13): 975-982.

Fukuda, K., T. Umehara, S. Sekiya, K. Kunio, T. Hasegawa and S. Nishikawa (2004). "An RNA ligand inhibits hepatitis C virus NS3 protease and helicase activities." Biochem Biophys Res Commun 325(3): 670-675.

Gerding, D. N. and J. A. Hitt (1989). "Tissue penetration of the new quinolones in humans." Rev Infect Dis 11 Suppl 5: S1046-1057.

Gordon, C. P. and P. A. Keller (2005). "Control of hepatitis C: a medicinal chemistry perspective." J Med Chem 48(1): 1-20.

Gu, M. and C. M. Rice (2010). "Three conformational snapshots of the hepatitis C virus NS3 helicase reveal a ratchet translocation mechanism." Proc Natl Acad Sci U S A 107(2): 521-528.

Hadziyannis, S. J., H. Sette, Jr., T. R. Morgan, V. Balan, M. Diago, P. Marcellin, G. Ramadori, H. Bodenheimer, Jr., D. Bernstein, M. Rizzetto, S. Zeuzem, P. J. Pockros, A. Lin and A. M. Ackrill (2004). "Peginterferon-alpha2a and ribavirin combination therapy in chronic hepatitis C: a randomized study of treatment duration and ribavirin dose." Ann Intern Med 140(5): 346-355.

Holmes, D. H., P. W. Ensminger and R. S. Gordee (1974). "Cinoxacin: effectiveness against experimental pyelonephritis in rats." Antimicrob Agents Chemother 6(4): 432-436.

Hussy, P., H. Langen, J. Mous and H. Jacobsen (1996). "Hepatitis C virus core protein: carboxy-terminal boundaries of two processed species suggest cleavage by a signal peptide peptidase." Virology 224(1): 93-104.

Hwang, B., J. S. Cho, H. J. Yeo, J. H. Kim, K. M. Chung, K. Han, S. K. Jang and S. W. Lee (2004). "Isolation of specific and high-affinity RNA aptamers against NS3 helicase domain of hepatitis C virus." RNA 10(8): 1277-1290.

Ikeda, S., M. Yazawa and C. Nishimura (1987). "Antiviral activity and inhibition of topoisomerase by ofloxacin, a new quinolone derivative." Antiviral Res 8(3): 103-113.

Ishido, S. and H. Hotta (1998). "Complex formation of the nonstructural protein 3 of hepatitis C virus with the p53 tumor suppressor." FEBS Lett 438(3): 258-262.

Jones, R. N. and M. A. Pfaller (2000). "In vitro activity of newer fluoroquinolones for respiratory tract infections and emerging patterns of antimicrobial resistance: data from the SENTRY antimicrobial surveillance program." Clin Infect Dis 31 Suppl 2: S16-23.

Josephson, M. A., J. W. Williams, A. Chandraker and P. S. Randhawa (2006). "Polyomavirus-associated nephropathy: update on antiviral strategies." Transpl Infect Dis 8(2): 95-101.

Kato, N., H. Yoshida, S. K. Ono-Nita, J. Kato, T. Goto, M. Otsuka, K. Lan, K. Matsushima, Y. Shiratori and M. Omata (2000). "Activation of intracellular signaling by hepatitis B and C viruses: C-viral core is the most potent signal inducer." Hepatology 32(2): 405-412.

Khan, I. A., S. Siddiqui, S. Rehmani, S. U. Kazmi and S. H. Ali (2012). "Fluoroquinolones inhibit HCV by targeting its helicase." Antivir Ther 17(3): 467-476.

Kim, D. W., J. Kim, Y. Gwack, J. H. Han and J. Choe (1997). "Mutational analysis of the hepatitis C virus RNA helicase." J Virol 71(12): 9400-9409.

Kim, J. L., K. A. Morgenstern, J. P. Griffith, M. D. Dwyer, J. A. Thomson, M. A. Murcko, C. Lin and P. R. Caron (1998). "Hepatitis C virus NS3 RNA helicase domain with a bound oligonucleotide: the crystal structure provides insights into the mode of unwinding." Structure 6(1): 89-100.

Koga, H., A. Itoh, S. Murayama, S. Suzue and T. Irikura (1980). "Structure-activity relationships of antibacterial 6,7- and 7,8-disubstituted 1-alkyl-1,4-dihydro-4-oxoquinoline-3-carboxylic acids." J Med Chem 23(12): 1358-1363.

Kojima, H., K. D. Kaita, K. Hawkins, J. Uhanova and G. Y. Minuk (2002). "Use of fluoroquinolones in patients with chronic hepatitis C virus-induced liver failure." Antimicrob Agents Chemother 46(10): 3280-3282.

Kolykhalov, A. A., K. Mihalik, S. M. Feinstone and C. M. Rice (2000). "Hepatitis C virus-encoded enzymatic activities and conserved RNA elements in the 3' nontranslated region are essential for virus replication in vivo." J Virol 74(4): 2046-2051.

Krawczyk, M., M. Wasowska-Lukawska, I. Oszczapowicz and A. M. Boguszewska-Chachulska (2009). "Amidinoanthracyclines - a new group of potential anti-hepatitis C virus compounds." Biol Chem 390(4): 351-360.

Kwong, A. D., J. L. Kim and C. Lin (2000). "Structure and function of hepatitis C virus NS3 helicase." Curr Top Microbiol Immunol 242: 171-196.

Kwun, H. J., E. Y. Jung, J. Y. Ahn, M. N. Lee and K. L. Jang (2001). "p53-dependent transcriptional repression of p21(waf1) by hepatitis C virus NS3." J Gen Virol 82(Pt 9): 2235-2241.

Lai, M. M. and C. F. Ware (2000). "Hepatitis C virus core protein: possible roles in viral pathogenesis." Curr Top Microbiol Immunol 242: 117-134.

Lam, A. M. and D. N. Frick (2006). "Hepatitis C virus subgenomic replicon requires an active NS3 RNA helicase." J Virol 80(1): 404-411.

Lam, A. M., D. Keeney and D. N. Frick (2003). "Two novel conserved motifs in the hepatitis C virus NS3 protein critical for helicase action." J Biol Chem 278(45): 44514-44524.

Levin, M. K., M. Gurjar and S. S. Patel (2005). "A Brownian motor mechanism of translocation and strand separation by hepatitis C virus helicase." Nat Struct Mol Biol 12(5): 429-435.

Lin, C. and J. L. Kim (1999). "Structure-based mutagenesis study of hepatitis C virus NS3 helicase." J Virol 73(10): 8798-8807.

Lin, C., B. D. Lindenbach, B. M. Pragai, D. W. McCourt and C. M. Rice (1994). "Processing in the hepatitis C virus E2-NS2 region: identification of p7 and two distinct E2-specific products with different C termini." J Virol 68(8): 5063-5073.

Llorente, B., F. Leclerc and R. Cedergren (1996). "Using SAR and QSAR analysis to model the activity and structure of the quinolone-DNA complex." Bioorg Med Chem 4(1): 61-71.

Locatelli, G. A., S. Spadari and G. Maga (2002). "Hepatitis C virus NS3 ATPase/helicase: an ATP switch regulates the cooperativity among the different substrate binding sites." Biochemistry 41(32): 10332-10342.

Love, R. A., H. E. Parge, J. A. Wickersham, Z. Hostomsky, N. Habuka, E. W. Moomaw, T. Adachi and Z. Hostomska (1996). "The crystal structure of hepatitis C virus NS3 proteinase reveals a trypsin-like fold and a structural zinc binding site." Cell 87(2): 331-342.

Ma, Z., D. T. Chu, C. S. Cooper, Q. Li, A. K. Fung, S. Wang, L. L. Shen, R. K. Flamm, A. M. Nilius, J. D. Alder, J. A. Meulbroek and Y. S. Or (1999). "Synthesis and antimicrobial activity of 4H-4-oxoquinolizine derivatives: consequences of structural modification at the C-8 position." J Med Chem 42(20): 4202-4213.

Mackintosh, S. G., J. Z. Lu, J. B. Jordan, M. K. Harrison, B. Sikora, S. D. Sharma, C. E. Cameron, K. D. Raney and J. Sakon (2006). "Structural and biological identification of residues on the surface of NS3 helicase required for optimal replication of the hepatitis C virus." J Biol Chem 281(6): 3528-3535.

Maga, G., S. Gemma, C. Fattorusso, G. A. Locatelli, S. Butini, M. Persico, G. Kukreja, M. P. Romano, L. Chiasserini, L. Savini, E. Novellino, V. Nacci, S. Spadari and G. Campiani (2005). "Specific targeting of hepatitis C virus NS3 RNA helicase. Discovery of the potent and selective competitive nucleotide-mimicking inhibitor QU663." Biochemistry 44(28): 9637-9644.

Martinson, F. E., K. A. Weigle, I. K. Mushahwar, D. J. Weber, R. Royce and S. M. Lemon (1996). "Seroepidemiological survey of hepatitis B and C virus infections in Ghanaian children." J Med Virol 48(3): 278-283.

Mellor, J., E. A. Walsh, L. E. Prescott, L. M. Jarvis, F. Davidson, P. L. Yap and P. Simmonds (1996). "Survey of type 6 group variants of hepatitis C virus in Southeast Asia by using a core-based genotyping assay." J Clin Microbiol 34(2): 417-423.

Monazahian, M., I. Bohme, S. Bonk, A. Koch, C. Scholz, S. Grethe and R. Thomssen (1999). "Low density lipoprotein receptor as a candidate receptor for hepatitis C virus." J Med Virol 57(3): 223-229.

Moriya, K., H. Fujie, Y. Shintani, H. Yotsuyanagi, T. Tsutsumi, K. Ishibashi, Y. Matsuura, S. Kimura, T. Miyamura and K. Koike (1998). "The core protein of hepatitis C virus induces hepatocellular carcinoma in transgenic mice." Nat Med 4(9): 1065-1067.

Moriya, K., H. Yotsuyanagi, Y. Shintani, H. Fujie, K. Ishibashi, Y. Matsuura, T. Miyamura and K. Koike (1997). "Hepatitis C virus core protein induces hepatic steatosis in transgenic mice." J Gen Virol 78 (Pt 7): 1527-1531.

Morris, P. D., A. K. Byrd, A. J. Tackett, C. E. Cameron, P. Tanega, R. Ott, E. Fanning and K. D. Raney (2002). "Hepatitis C virus NS3 and simian virus 40 T antigen helicases displace streptavidin from 5'-biotinylated oligonucleotides but not from 3'-biotinylated oligonucleotides: evidence for directional bias in translocation on single-stranded DNA." Biochemistry 41(7): 2372-2378.

Ndjomou, J., R. Kolli, S. Mukherjee, W. R. Shadrick, A. M. Hanson, N. L. Sweeney, D. Bartczak, K. Li, K. J. Frankowski, F. J. Schoenen and D. N. Frick (2012). "Fluorescent primuline derivatives inhibit hepatitis C virus NS3-catalyzed RNA unwinding, peptide hydrolysis and viral replicase formation." Antiviral Res 96(2): 245-255.

Negro, F., P. J. Male, L. Perrin, E. Giostra and A. Hadengue (1998). "Treatment of chronic hepatitis C with alpha-interferon plus ofloxacin in patients not responding to alpha-interferon alone." J Hepatol 29(3): 369-374.

Nielsen, S. U., M. F. Bassendine, A. D. Burt, D. J. Bevitt and G. L. Toms (2004). "Characterization of the genome and structural proteins of hepatitis C virus resolved from infected human liver." J Gen Virol 85(Pt 6): 1497-1507.

Nomura-Takigawa, Y., M. Nagano-Fujii, L. Deng, S. Kitazawa, S. Ishido, K. Sada and H. Hotta (2006). "Non-structural protein 4A of Hepatitis C virus accumulates on mitochondria and renders the cells prone to undergoing mitochondria-mediated apoptosis." J Gen Virol 87(Pt 7): 1935-1945.

Nozaki-Renard, J., T. Iino, Y. Sato, Y. Marumoto, G. Ohta and M. Furusawa (1990). "A fluoroquinolone (DR-3355) protects human lymphocyte cell lines from HIV-1-induced cytotoxicity." AIDS 4(12): 1283-1286.

Okamoto, H., T. P. Cujec, M. Okamoto, B. M. Peterlin, M. Baba and T. Okamoto (2000). "Inhibition of the RNA-dependent transactivation and replication of human immunodeficiency virus type 1 by a fluoroquinoline derivative K-37." Virology 272(2): 402-408.

Peng, L. F., S. S. Kim, S. Matchacheep, X. Lei, S. Su, W. Lin, W. Runguphan, W. H. Choe, N. Sakamoto, M. Ikeda, N. Kato, A. B. Beeler, J. A. Porco, Jr., S. L. Schreiber and R. T. Chung (2007). "Identification of novel epoxide inhibitors of hepatitis C virus replication using a high-throughput screen." Antimicrob Agents Chemother 51(10): 3756-3759.

Peters, G., H. Freiesleben, R. Marre, H. Metz, H. Tannenberg and G. Pulverer (1979). "[Antibacterial in-vitro activity of pipemidic acid and nalidixic acid (author's transl)]." Dtsch Med Wochenschr 104(26): 946-948.

Phoon, C. W., P. Y. Ng, A. E. Ting, S. L. Yeo and M. M. Sim (2001). "Biological evaluation of hepatitis C virus helicase inhibitors." Bioorg Med Chem Lett 11(13): 1647-1650.

Pileri, P., Y. Uematsu, S. Campagnoli, G. Galli, F. Falugi, R. Petracca, A. J. Weiner, M. Houghton, D. Rosa, G. Grandi and S. Abrignani (1998). "Binding of hepatitis C virus to CD81." Science 282(5390): 938-941.

Porter, D. J. (1998). "Inhibition of the hepatitis C virus helicase-associated ATPase activity by the combination of ADP, NaF, MgCl2, and poly(rU). Two ADP binding sites on the enzyme-nucleic acid complex." J Biol Chem 273(13): 7390-7396.

Portolani, M., P. Pietrosemoli, C. Cermelli, A. Mannini-Palenzona, M. P. Grossi, L. Paolini and G. Barbanti-Brodano (1988). "Suppression of BK virus replication and cytopathic effect by inhibitors of prokaryotic DNA gyrase." Antiviral Res 9(3): 205-218.

Ray, R. B., L. M. Lagging, K. Meyer, R. Steele and R. Ray (1995). "Transcriptional regulation of cellular and viral promoters by the hepatitis C virus core protein." Virus Res 37(3): 209-220.

Ringel, S. M., F. J. Turner, F. L. Lindo, S. Roemer, B. A. Direnga and B. S. Schwartz (1967). "Oxolinic acid, a new synthetic antimicrobial agent. II. Bactericidal rate and resistance development." Antimicrob Agents Chemother (Bethesda) 7: 480-485.

Robson, R. A. (1992). "Quinolone pharmacokinetics." Int J Antimicrob Agents 2(1): 3-10.

Ruggieri, A., C. Argentini, F. Kouruma, P. Chionne, E. D'Ugo, E. Spada, S. Dettori, S. Sabbatani and M. Rapicetta (1996). "Heterogeneity of hepatitis C virus genotype 2 variants in West Central Africa (Guinea Conakry)." J Gen Virol 77 (Pt 9): 2073-2076.

Santolini, E., L. Pacini, C. Fipaldini, G. Migliaccio and N. Monica (1995). "The NS2 protein of hepatitis C virus is a transmembrane polypeptide." J Virol 69(12): 7461-7471.

Scarselli, E., H. Ansuini, R. Cerino, R. M. Roccasecca, S. Acali, G. Filocamo, C. Traboni, A. Nicosia, R. Cortese and A. Vitelli (2002). "The human scavenger receptor class B type I is a novel candidate receptor for the hepatitis C virus." EMBO J 21(19): 5017-5025.

Shimoike, T., S. A. McKenna, D. A. Lindhout and J. D. Puglisi (2009). "Translational insensitivity to potent activation of PKR by HCV IRES RNA." Antiviral Res 83(3): 228-237.

Shimoike, T., S. Mimori, H. Tani, Y. Matsuura and T. Miyamura (1999). "Interaction of hepatitis C virus core protein with viral sense RNA and suppression of its translation." J Virol 73(12): 9718-9725.

Shimotohno, K. (2000). "Hepatitis C virus and its pathogenesis." Semin Cancer Biol 10(3): 233-240.

Simmonds, P., A. Alberti, H. J. Alter, F. Bonino, D. W. Bradley, C. Brechot, J. T. Brouwer, S. W. Chan, K. Chayama, D. S. Chen and et al. (1994). "A proposed system for the nomenclature of hepatitis C viral genotypes." Hepatology 19(5): 1321-1324.

Stankiewicz-Drogon, A., L. G. Palchykovska, V. G. Kostina, I. V. Alexeeva, A. D. Shved and A. M. Boguszewska-Chachulska (2008). "New acridone-4-carboxylic acid derivatives as potential inhibitors of hepatitis C virus infection." Bioorg Med Chem 16(19): 8846-8852.

Stuyver, L., W. van Arnhem, A. Wyseur, F. Hernandez, E. Delaporte and G. Maertens (1994). "Classification of hepatitis C viruses based on phylogenetic analysis of the envelope 1 and nonstructural 5B regions and identification of five additional subtypes." Proc Natl Acad Sci U S A 91(21): 10134-10138.

Sullivan, D. E., M. U. Mondelli, D. T. Curiel, V. Krasnykh, G. Mikheeva, P. Gaglio, C. B. Morris, S. Dash and M. A. Gerber (2002). "Construction and characterization of an intracellular single-chain human antibody to hepatitis C virus non-structural 3 protein." J Hepatol 37(5): 660-668.

Suzuki, R., S. Sakamoto, T. Tsutsumi, A. Rikimaru, K. Tanaka, T. Shimoike, K. Moriishi, T. Iwasaki, K. Mizumoto, Y. Matsuura, T. Miyamura and T. Suzuki (2005). "Molecular determinants for subcellular localization of hepatitis C virus core protein." J Virol 79(2): 1271-1281.

Tai, C. L., W. K. Chi, D. S. Chen and L. H. Hwang (1996). "The helicase activity associated with hepatitis C virus non-structural protein 3 (NS3)." J Virol 70(12): 8477-8484.

Taylor, D. R., S. T. Shi, P. R. Romano, G. N. Barber and M. M. Lai (1999). "Inhibition of the interferon-inducible protein kinase PKR by HCV E2 protein." Science 285(5424): 107-110.

Tessmann, K., A. Erhardt, D. Haussinger and T. Heintges (2002). "Cloning and molecular characterization of human high affinity antibody fragments against Hepatitis C virus NS3 helicase." J Virol Methods 103(1): 75-88.

Thomssen, R., S. Bonk, C. Propfe, K. H. Heermann, H. G. Kochel and A. Uy (1992). "Association of hepatitis C virus in human sera with beta-lipoprotein." Med Microbiol Immunol 181(5): 293-300.

Tillotson, G. S. (1996). "Quinolones: structure-activity relationships and future predictions." J Med Microbiol 44(5): 320-324.

Tokita, H., H. Okamoto, P. Luengrojanakul, K. Vareesangthip, T. Chainuvati, H. Iizuka, F. Tsuda, Y. Miyakawa and M. Mayumi (1995). "Hepatitis C virus variants from Thailand classifiable into five novel genotypes in the sixth (6b), seventh (7c, 7d) and ninth (9b, 9c) major genetic groups." J Gen Virol 76 (Pt 9): 2329-2335.

Tokita, H., H. Okamoto, F. Tsuda, P. Song, S. Nakata, T. Chosa, H. Iizuka, S. Mishiro, Y. Miyakawa and M. Mayumi (1994a). "Hepatitis C virus variants from Vietnam are classifiable into the seventh, eighth, and ninth major genetic groups." Proc Natl Acad Sci U S A 91(23): 11022-11026.

Tokita, H., S. M. Shrestha, H. Okamoto, M. Sakamoto, M. Horikita, H. Iizuka, S. Shrestha, Y. Miyakawa and M. Mayumi (1994b). "Hepatitis C virus variants from Nepal with novel genotypes and their classification into the third major group." J Gen Virol 75 (Pt 4): 931-936.

Van Antwerp, D. J., S. J. Martin, T. Kafri, D. R. Green and I. M. Verma (1996). "Suppression of TNF-alpha-induced apoptosis by NF-kappaB." Science 274(5288): 787-789.

Walker, J. E., M. Saraste, M. J. Runswick and N. J. Gay (1982). "Distantly related sequences in the alpha- and beta-subunits of ATP synthase, myosin, kinases and other ATP-requiring enzymes and a common nucleotide binding fold." EMBO J 1(8): 945-951.

Wise, R. and I. Phillips (2000). "Towards a common susceptibility testing method?" J Antimicrob Chemother 45(6): 919-920.

Witvrouw, M., D. Daelemans, C. Pannecouque, J. Neyts, G. Andrei, R. Snoeck, A. M. Vandamme, J. Balzarini, J. Desmyter, M. Baba and E. De Clercq (1998). "Broad-spectrum antiviral activity and mechanism of antiviral action of the fluoroquinolone derivative K-12." Antivir Chem Chemother 9(5): 403-411.

Wong, I. and T. M. Lohman (1992). "Allosteric effects of nucleotide cofactors on Escherichia coli Rep helicase-DNA binding." Science 256(5055): 350-355.

World Health Report 1996 (World Health Organisation, G. (1996). J Commun Dis 28(3): 215-219.

Yoshida, T., Y. Yamamoto, H. Orita, M. Kakiuchi, Y. Takahashi, M. Itakura, N. Kado, S. Yasuda, H. Kato and Y. Itoh (1996). "Studies on quinolone antibacterials. V. Synthesis and antibacterial activity of chiral 5-amino-7-(4-substituted-3-amino-1-pyrrolidinyl)-6- fluoro-1,4-dihydro-8-methyl-4-oxoquinoline-3-carboxylic acids and derivatives." Chem Pharm Bull (Tokyo) 44(7): 1376-1386.

Yu, J., W. Cheng, C. Bustamante and G. Oster (2010). "Coupling translocation with nucleic acid unwinding by NS3 helicase." J Mol Biol 404(3): 439-455.

Zhang, C., Z. Cai, Y. C. Kim, R. Kumar, F. Yuan, P. Y. Shi, C. Kao and G. Luo (2005). "Stimulation of hepatitis C virus (HCV) nonstructural protein 3 (NS3) helicase activity by the NS3 protease domain and by HCV RNA-dependent RNA polymerase." J Virol 79(14): 8687-8697.

Zhang, Q., R. Gong, J. Qu, Y. Zhou, W. Liu, M. Chen, Y. Liu, Y. Zhu and J. Wu (2012). "Activation of the Ras/Raf/MEK pathway facilitates hepatitis C virus replication via attenuation of the interferon-JAK-STAT pathway." J Virol 86(3): 1544-1554.

Zhang, Z. X., U. Lazdina, M. Chen, D. L. Peterson and M. Sallberg (2000). "Characterization of a monoclonal antibody and its single-chain antibody fragment recognizing the nucleoside Triphosphatase/Helicase domain of the hepatitis C virus nonstructural 3 protein." Clin Diagn Lab Immunol 7(1): 58-63.

Considerations in the Management of HCV-related Thrombocytopenia with Eltrombopag

Fazal-i-Akbar Danish
Quaid-e-Azam University, Islamabad, Pakistan

Saeeda Yasmin
Department of General Surgery
Shifa International Hospital, Islamabad, Pakistan

1   Introduction

Hepatitis C virus (HCV) infection is estimated to have chronically infected 160 million individuals worldwide (Lavanchy, 2011). HCV is known to cause thrombocytopenia even in the absence of overt hepatic disease (Pyrsopoulos & Reddy, 2001; Cacoub *et al.*, 2000) and is considered a surrogate marker for the severity of liver disease (Afdhal *et al.*, 2008). It is sometimes the *only* manifestation of viral hepatitis. Chiao *et al.* (2009) suggested that HCV infection is associated with an increased risk of developing chronic immune thrombocytopenic purpura (CITP) (HR, 1.8; 95% CI, 1.4 – 2.3). Similarly, Pockros *et al.* (2002) retrospectively estimated that the prevalence of CITP among their HCV patients was much greater than would be expected by chance ($P < .00001$). Conversely, many cross-sectional studies have reported positive HCV serology (up to 20%) in patients with a clinical diagnosis of CITP (Garcia-Suarez *et al.*, 2000; Sakuraya *et al.*, 2002). The documented severity of thrombocytopenia in different studies has been highly variable; may range from mild to severe. Thrombocytopenia is a well known *relative* contraindication for the initiation of antiviral therapy in HCV-infected patients. Thrombocytopenia may also result in the postponement of many invasive procedures that CLD patients may need to undergo like percutaneous, transjugular or laparoscopic liver biopsy, paracentesis, thoracentesis, radiofrequency ablation (RFA) or partial hepatectomy for hepatocellular carcinoma (HCC). Latter group of patients may also need to undergo splenectomy especially if the platelet counts are < 50,000/μL. Mild (> 75,000/μL – < 150,000/μL) to moderate (50,000/μL – 75,000/μL) thrombocytopenia is only rarely associated with any bleeding complications (Afdhal *et al.*, 2008). Doing invasive procedures in the background of severe thrombocytopenia (< 50,000/μL) however may be associated with significant morbidity necessitating repeated platelet transfusions in the peri-operative period (Giannini *et al.*, 2006; McCullough, 2000; Tripodi & Mannucci, 2007). Platelet transfusions are generally effective for only a few hours; moreover, these may be associated with multiple potential complications like febrile non-hemolytic & allergic reactions, platelet refractoriness (due to HLA alloimmunization), iron overload (with chronic repeated transfusions), need for hospitalization, risk of infection and cost (McCullough, 2000; Perrotta & Snyder, 2001). This explains the need & rationality to have an alternative therapeutic option to help raise the platelet counts when needed. Different therapeutic strategies have been suggested & tried to treat HCV-related thrombocytopenia in different studies with variable success rates (generally disappointing) (Nurden *et al.*, 2009). Recent introduction of 2nd generation thrombopoietin-receptor (TPO-R) agonists has opened up a novel way to treat thrombocytopenia. FDA approved Eltrombopag and Romiplostim in CITP patients' refractory to at least one standard treatment in 2008.

2   Cause-effect Relationship between HCV Infection & Thrombocytopenia

In areas of high HCV seroprevalence, it is generally recommended that if a patient presents with thrombocytopenia & has one or more risk factors for HCV present, he/ she should be screened for the virus (Rajan *et al.*, 2005; Stasi, 2009). Important risk factors that should prompt checking for HCV status include needle stick injury or mucosal exposure to HCV-positive blood, I/V drug abusers, multiple blood transfusions, haemodialysis, current sexual partners of HCV-infected persons or persons having multiple sexual partners, children born to HCV-infected mothers & unexplained abnormal aminotransferase levels. Multiple studies have demonstrated significant improvements in platelet counts following successful treatment of HCV infection suggesting the latter being a possible cause of thrombocytopenia (Iga *et al.*, 2005; Zhang *et al.*, 2003). In fact, several studies have suggested that thrombocytopenia is found in as much as 76% cases of cirrhosis of liver (Bashour *et al.*, 2000; Qamar *et al.*, 2009;). The severity of thrombocytopenia is generally directly proportional to the severity of the chronic liver disease (CLD) (Peck-Radosavljevic, 2000; Sallah & Bobzien, 1999). Although thrombocytopenia is generally less severe in HCV-infected patients compared to CITP patients, the former are more prone to major bleeding episodes due to liver disease associated coagulopathy & portal hypertension. Interestingly, a recent study (Giannini *et al.*, 2010) suggested that it is *thrombocytopenia rather than coagulopathy* that is the major determinant of bleeding risk in patients with CLD. The same study estimated the bleeding incidence to be 31% in patients with platelet count $< 75,000/mm^3$. WHO classifies bleeding into grade 1 (petechiae), grade 2 (mild blood loss), grade 3 (gross blood loss) & grade 4 (debilitating/life threatening blood loss) (Fogarty *et al.*, 2011).

Possible causes for HCV-related thrombocytopenia include:

1. *Decreased platelet production*: This in turn could be due to decreased hepatic production of thrombopoietin (a glycoprotein that promotes megakaryopoiesis) (Adinolfi *et al.*, 2001; Peck-Radosavljevic *et al.*, 1998) & direct suppressant effect of HCV on bone marrow (Ballard *et al.*, 1989; Bordin *et al.*, 1995).

2. *Increased peripheral destruction of platelets*: This in turn could be due to immune-mediated peripheral platelets destruction and hypersplenism leading to increased splenic platelet sequestration (McCormick & Murphy, 2000; Weksler, 2007). Since, HCV is known to cause thrombocytopenia even in well-compensated cases (in the absence of portal hypertension & hypersplenism) (Sakuraya *et al.*, 2002; Zhang *et al.*, 2003) and thrombocytopenia has been shown to persist after portal decompression in established cases of hypersplenism (decompensated cirrhotics) (Jabbour *et al.*, 1998), it appears logical to believe that probably *immune-mediated destruction of platelets* is more dominant a mechanism of thrombocytopenia than hypersplenism. HCV binding to platelet membrane with consequent binding of anti-HCV antibody and phagocytosis of platelets (called "innocent bystander" phagocytosis) (Hamaia *et al.*, 2001), and an HCV protein mimicking an epitope on platelet surface (called GPIIIa) triggering the production of anti-platelet antibodies[33] are the two most frequently postulated immune mechanisms explaining increased peripheral platelet destruction in HCV-infected cases (Bordin *et al.*, 1995; Hamaia *et al.*, 2001; Nagamine *et al.*, 1996; Pockros *et al.*, 2002).

3. *Iatrogenic*: Interferon (IFN) therapy is also known to suppress bone marrow with consequent 10 – 50% fall in the platelet count (Peck-Radosavljevic *et al.*, 1998). *Pegylated* interferon/ ribavirin (PEG-IFN/RBV) combination therapy has been shown to cause more severe thrombocytopenia than *non-pegylated* IFN/RBV combination therapy. Interestingly, thrombocytopenia is worst with PEG-IFN monotherapy (Fried *et al.*, 2002) suggesting that cocomitant ribavirin therapy probably has some protective effect (causes reactive thrombocytosis) (Peck-Radosavljevic *et al.*, 1998). In one study, PEG-IFN therapy-induced thromboctopenia lead to dose reductions in 19% cases and discontinuation in 2% cases (Sulkowski *et al.*, 2005). In cirrhotic patients, the incidence of treatment induced thrombocytopenia is generally higher than in non-cirrhotics (Bashour *et al.*, 2000).

Interestingly & paradoxically, advanced liver disease patients, such as cirrhotics, are not only predisposed to bleeding (secondary to thrombocytopenia & coagulopathy), but also to thromboembolic events (TEEs), especially portal/ splenic vein thrombosis. Reduced portal vein flow & possible presence of intra-abdominal cancer are two pertinent predisposing factors for the development of TEEs in such patients (Amitrano et al., 2007; Lisman et al., 2010; Tripodi et al., 2010). Performance of an invasive procedure in cirrhotics & hepatocellular carcinoma patients is also considered an independent risk factor for the development of portal vein thrombosis (incidence estimated to be up to 35%) (De Stefano et al., 2010; Kulik et al., 2008). It appears that patients who undergo an invasive procedure *involving splanchnic circulation* (e.g. variceal banding, radiofrequency ablation or transarterial chemoembolization) are particularly vulnerable to develop portal/ splenic vein thrombosis (Afdhal et al., 2012).

3   Pathophysiology of Thrombopoietin

Thrombopoietin (TPO), a glycoprotein primarily produced by hepatocytes, is the major regulator of both megakaryopoiesis and platelet production in human body. It is the key endogenous ligand for thrombopoietin receptor (TPO-R) found on the surface of megakaryocytes, and megakaryocytic precursors (Kuter & Begley, 2002; Kaushansky & Drachman; 2002). TPO binding to its receptor activates the Janus Kinase/Signal Transducer and Activator of Transcription (JAK-STAT) pathway ultimately leading to the release of platelets in the circulation (Ezumi et al., 1995; Rojnuckarin et al., 1999; Drachman et al., 1999). TPO also binds to circulating platelets enhancing their activation and function.

Platelets not only bind to TPO but also internalize and degrade it. Thus if platelet count increases, TPO degradation also increases and vice versa. This negative feed back system helps maintain normal platelet levels. In liver cirrhosis, the net production of TPO decreases thus predisposing to thrombocytopenia.[26,48] Studies have shown that the grade of liver fibrosis, the severity of TPO deficiency and the incidence of thrombocytopenia are all positively correlated (Adinolfi et al., 2001). Correction of TPO deficiency by 'liver transplantation' has been shown to improve megakaryopoiesis and thus circulating platelet levels (Goulis et al., 1999; Peck-Radosavljevic et al., 2000).

4   Different Therapeutic Strategies to Treat HCV-related Thrombocytopenia

Since successful treatment of HCV infection has clearly been shown to improve the platelet counts (Pockros et al., 2002; Rajan & Liebman, 2001), the therapeutic protocol for managing HCV-related thrombocytopenia ought to differ from that of primary (idiopathic) thrombocytopenic purpura. The therapeutic strategies employed in different studies to treat HCV-related thrombocytopenia include a reduction in the dose of IFN (Rajan & Liebman, 2001), addition of a new drug like oral steroids (Hernandez et al., 1998; Ramos-Casals et al, 2003; Sakuraya et al., 2002; Zhang et al., 2003), intravenous immunoglobulin (IVIG) (Garcia-Suarez et al., 2000), or anti-RhD Ig (Rajan et al., 2005), resorting to a invasive procedure like partial splenic embolization (Giannini & Savarino, 2008), splenectomy (Sakuraya et al., 2002; Zhang et al., 2003), or transjugular intrahepatic portosystemic stent shunt (TIPSS) placement. Although steroids are commonly used in CITP patients, their use in HCV-infected patients has shown to cause statistically-significant rises in transaminase levels & HCV viral loads, and worsening of liver damage (Rajan et al.,

2005). They have even shown to cause hyperbilirubinemia and development of overt jaundice (rarely). Because of these safety issues, steroid use in the treatment of HCV-related thrombocytopenia has never gained recognition despite conflicting reports of variable increases in platelet counts. Based on this it is recommended that all patients who are suspected to suffer from 'CITP' be investigated for Hep-C serology. This recommendation will hopefully prevent the potential adverse effect of prolonged corticosteroid usage on the underlying infection, if present. Splenic artery embolization & splenectomy are *often* effective in increasing the platelet levels in patients with portal hypertension regardless of Hep-C serology status (Sakuraya *et al.*, 2002; Zhang *et al.*, 2003). These however may be associated with such complications as splenic abscesses and portal vein thrombosis. Portal decompression with TIPSS placement may or may not improve platelet levels because of multifactorial pathogenesis of the latter (Jabbour *et al.*, 1998; Wong, 2006). The American Society of Clinical Oncology recommends platelet transfusions for cancer patients with platelet counts of 10,000/μL – 20,000/μL (Schiffer *et al.*, 2001). American Society of Hematology (ASH) suggests that in ITP patients without other risk factors, platelet levels of 30,000 – 50,000/μL are required to preclude most serious bleeding (intracerebral or major gastrointestinal) complications (George *et al.*, 1996). No consensus currently exists regarding the appropriate cut-off level of thrombocytopenia below which platelet transfusions may be indicated *prophylactically* in CLD patients. It appears that the appropriate cut-off value should be different in different patients. In *uncomplicated* thrombocytopenic patients, a cut-off value of < 10,000/μL may be considered appropriate; in *complicated* thrombocytopenic patients (e.g. those with fever, infection, splenomegaly etc), a higher cut-off value such as < 50,000/μL should be regarded as appropriate (Rebulla, 2000; Rinder *et al.*, 1999) (platelet levels of ≥ 50,000/μL are often considered 'safe' for 'most' invasive procedures) (George, 2004; Provan *et al.*, 2010).

The most practical strategy in treating HCV-related thrombocytopenia is based on the hypothesis that eradication of HCV infection should result in remission of thrombocytopenia. Pre-treatment platelet count of < 90,000/mm^3 is a *relative* contraindication to start PEG-IFN therapy (Calvaruso & Craxi, 2011). If pre-treatment platelet level is above this cut-off value, & thrombocytopenia develops following initiation of PEG-IFN therapy, one treatment option may be to continue PEG-IFN therapy but to reduce its dose (minimum effective dose is 1 μg/kg/week) if platelet count are < 30 × 10^9/L, or to discontinue it if < 20 × 10^9/L (Danish *et al.*, 2008; Sherman *et al.*, 2007). Reductions in the dosage schedule of PEG-IFN can compromise the success of the therapy. To help maintain optimal dosage schedule, adjunct eltrombopag (or romiplostim) may be considered to counteract thrombocytopenia in a sustained manner (Danish *et al.*, 2008, 2010). Eltrombopag is already recommended in CITP cases in two scenarios:

1. Post-splenectomy CITP patients who are refractory to other drug therapies (e.g. corticosteroids, immunoglobulins).

2. Patients in whom splenectomy is contraindicated and other medical agents have failed to correct thrombocytopenia.

Recently, eltrombopag has been used successfully in 2 cases of persistently thrombocytopenic, platelet transfusions-*dependent* patients following stem-cell transplantations (one allogeneic & one autologous) (Reid, 2012). In both cases, the patients became platelet transfusion *independent* with platelets counts ~30,000/uL & ~10,000/uL respectively *within ~2 weeks of starting eltrombopag treatment*. It is pertinent to mention here that the usefulness of repeated platelet transfusions is limited by their short duration of efficacy, risk of transfusion-related reactions & almost 50% incidence of alloimmunization (development of antiplatelet antibodies leading to refractory thrombocytopenia non-responsive to repeat platelet transfusions) (Poordad, 2007; Slichter, 2007; Trotter, 2006;). It thus appears that the therapeutic indications of eltrombopag may expand in the coming years (provided the drug proves relatively safe in human subjects, & the cost is not inhibiting).

5   Historical Note: Use of 1st-generation Thrombopoietic Growth Factors in Treating HCV-related Thrombocytopenia

Historically, multiple clinical trials (de Sauvage, 1994; Kaushansky, 1994a, 1994b; Wendling, 1994), showed improvements in platelet counts with 1st-generation thrombopoietic growth factors (recombinant human thrombopoietin [TPO] & pegylated recombinant human megakaryocyte growth and development factor [PEG-rHuMGDF]). However, their use was unexpectedly forsaken in 1998 when some patients paradoxically developed thrombocytopenia secondary to PEG-rHuMGDF use (Basser et al., 2002; Bartley et al., 1994; Harker et al., 2000; Li et al., 2001;). The possible explanation given was development of anti-PEG-rHuMGDF antibodies, which cross-reacted and thus neutralized the endogenous TPO. This led to efforts to develop nonimmunogenic 2nd-generation TPO-receptor agonists - Romiplostim [AMG-531, Nplate(R)] & Eltrombopag [SB-497115, Promacta(R), Revolade(R)] (Panzer, 2009).

Recently, the manufacturer of eltrombopag conducted an indirect comparison between eltrombopag and romiplostim in CITP. The aim was to evaluate the relative effectiveness of the two drugs in terms of platelet response and bleeding adverse event rates using placebo as the common comparator. The results showed no significant differences between the two drugs in terms of achieving either durable/sustained platelet responses, or overall platelet responses in all patients (splenectomised or non-splenectomised). Similarly, no significant differences in the incidence of bleeding adverse events (grade 2 or higher) were noted.

6   Role of Eltrombopag (2nd-generation Thrombopoietic Growth Factor) in Treating HCV-related Thrombocytopenia

6.1   Aim of Treatment

The ultimate aim of treating thrombocytopenia in HVC-positive cases is not to normalize the platelet counts (Vizcaíno et al., 2009) but to maintain them above the level of haemorrhagic risk (> 50,000/µl) thus conferring the advantage of possible avoidance of interferon dose reductions or interruptions.

6.2   Mechanism of Action

Eltrombopag is a thrombopoietin-receptor agonist (TPO-RA) (Erickson-Miller et al., 2005; Juan et al., 2004; Kalota et al., 2004). The ligand-receptor binding activates JAK2/STAT signalling pathways inducing increased proliferation and differentiation of human bone marrow progenitor cells into megakaryocytes. The net effect is an increase in the circulating platelets count (Erickson-Miller, 2004). It appears that eltrombopag binds the TPO receptor at a distance from the binding site for endogenous TPO and appears to initiate signal transduction by a different mechanism (Erickson-Miller, 2009). The two thus may have an *additive (& not competitive) effect* on platelet production. Endogenous TPO appears to be 7-9 times more potent than eltrombopag.

6.3   Pharmacokinetics

It appears that the pharmacokinetics of Eltrombopag (peak concentration 2 – 6 h after oral administration; average $T_{1/2}$ >12 hours) is linear and therefore it produces a dose-dependent increase in platelet proliferation and differentiation (higher doses are more effective & less safe!) (Bussel *et al.*, 2007; Erickson-Miller *et al.*, 2005; Jenkins *et al.*, 2007; Julian *et al.*, 2007; Luengo, 2004; Sellers *et al.*, 2004). Eltrombopag should be taken at least four hours before or after antacids, dairy products & multi-vitamin tablets/mineral supplements as these products chelate & thus significantly reduce the systemic absorption of eltrombopag (Williams *et al.*, 2009). Although the absolute oral bioavailability of eltrombopag in human subjects has not been well established, it is estimated to be at least 52%. 99.9% of absorbed eltrombopag circulates bound to plasma proteins, predominantly albumin. Circulating eltrombopag undergoes extensive hepatic metabolism through cleavage, oxidation & conjugation with glucuronic acid, glutathione or cysteine. Since individual UGT enzymes only show a limited contribution in the glucuronidation of eltrombopag, significant drug interactions involving glucuronidation are not anticipated with this drug. Also, eltrombopag doesn't appear to inhibit or induce CYP enzymes in both *in vitro* & *in vivo* studies. This implies that no clinically significant interactions should be expected when eltrombopag and CYP inducers or inhibitors are co-administered. Since eltrmbopag is primarily metabolized in the liver, *higher* plasma eltrombopag concentrations are reported in *HCV infected patients compared to CITP patients or healthy volunteers* (Bauman *et al.*, 2011). Inter-ethnic differences in the pharmacokinetics of eltrombopag have also been reported. It is suggested that low-dose 25 mg once daily eltrombopag therapy suffices in most patients of Asian origin (compared to Caucasians who usually require double this dose) (Gibiansky *et al.*, 2011). The underlying mechanism accounting for the observed inter-ethnic difference in the pharmacokinetics of eltrombopag is not clear; nonetheless, the most plausible explanation appears to be the difference in the body weight (less in East Asian population compared to the general Caucasian population) (Shida *et al.*, 2011). Since the clearance of eltrombopag increases with increase in body weight (Gibiansky *et al.*, 2011), *heavy* subjects need *higher* doses to produce an identical therapeutic effect. Another possible explanation is the known inter-ethnic differences (Mizutani, 2003; Zhang *et al.*, 2007) in the levels of activities of different drug metabolising enzymes involved in eltrombopag metabolism (e.g. cytochrome P450 (CYP) 1A2, CYP2C8, uridine diphosphate-glucuronosyltransferase (UGT) 1A1, and UGT1A3 etc) (Shida *et al.*, 2011). The predominant route of eltrombopag excretion is *via* faeces (59%) followed by urine (31%). Via the latter, only metabolites (& not the parent drug) are found to be excreted.

6.4   Evidence of Therapeutic Efficacy

The evidence of effectiveness of eltrombopag primarily comes from two phase-III, randomised, double-blind, placebo-controlled trials done on *CITP* patients.

In a recent phase-III, randomised, double-blind, placebo-controlled study (Cheng *et al.*, 2011), 197 *CITP* patients were randomised 2:1 (eltrombopag [n = 135] to placebo [n = 62]). Median platelet counts at baseline were 16,000/μL in both groups. The study showed that whereas only 17 (28%) patients in the placebo group responded to treatment, the treatment response (at least once during the study) was much higher (106 i.e. 79% patients) in the eltrombopag group. The odds of responding were demonstrated to be greater in the eltrombopag group compared with the placebo group throughout the 6-month treatment period (odds ratio 8.2, 99% CI 3.59 – 18.73; $p < 0.0001$). A platelet count between 50,000 – 400,000/μL in the absence of rescue medication (steroids, Ig) was achieved by significantly more patients in the eltrombopag treated group during the 6 month treatment period, $p < 0.001$. This rise in platelet count resulted in approximately 50% reduction in the incidence of clinically significant bleeding (WHO grades 2-4) from Day 15 to the end of treatment.

In another phase III, randomised, double-blind, placebo-controlled study (Bussel *et al.*, 2009), *CITP* patients having platelet counts of < 30,000/µL were given eltrombopag in a dose of 50mg once-daily (n = 76) or placebo (n = 38) for up to 6 weeks. The target was to achieve platelet counts of ≥ 50,000/µL at day 43. Whereas, only 16% placebo-treated patients achieved the target platelet count, the same was achieved in 59% of eltrombopag-treated patients (odds ratio [OR] 9·61 [95% CI 3.31 – 27.86]; p < 0.0001). Also eltrombopag-treated patients showed less instances of bleeding complications at any given time during the study compared to the placebo group (OR 0.49 [95% CI 0.26 – 0.89]; p = 0.021).

In a phase 2 study (McHutchison *et al.*, 2007), whereas only 6% of HCV-related cirrhotics in the placebo group completed the 12 weeks antiviral course, the same was completed by 36%, 53%, and 65% of patients receiving 30 mg, 50 mg, and 75 mg of eltrombopag respectively. Moreover, 75 to 95% of patients in the eltrombopag groups achieved the primary end point (a platelet count 100,000/mm^3 at week 4) in a dose-dependent manner. During this study, 7 patients reported serious adverse effects, namely:

- Ascites (in the group receiving 30 mg of eltrombopag). This led to withdrawal of eltrombopag in 3 patients. Ascites resolved subsequently.

- Retinal exudates (in the group receiving 75 mg of eltrombopag). This led to withdrawal of eltrombopag in 1 patient. Retinal exudates failed to resolve subsequently & investigators were of the view that these were unrelated to eltrombopag therapy.

In a recent double-blind, randomized, placebo-controlled, phase 3 clinical trial conducted in 13 countries (ELEVATE study), 292 patients with chronic liver disease (CLD) due to variable causes & with associated thrombocytopenia (platelet count < 50,000/mm^3) were randomly assigned to receive either eltrombopag (75 mg daily), or placebo for 14 days before a planned invasive procedure (last dose ~5 days before the procedure) (Afdhal *et al.*, 2012). Avoidance of platelet transfusion before, during & up to 7 days after the procedure was set as the primary end point. The results showed that primary end point was successfully achieved in 72 % (104 of 145) patients in eltrombopag group compared to only 19% (28 of 147) in the placebo group (*p* < 0.001). Bleeding episodes of WHO grade 2 or higher were reported in 17% & 23% of patients, respectively. Importantly, this study showed the development of *portal venous thrombosis in 6 patients receiving eltrombopag,* compared to only 1 in the placebo group. In total 10 thromboembolic events (TEEs) were recorded in 8 patients – 7 events in the eltrombopag group & 3 events in the placebo group (odds ratio with eltrombopag, 3.04; 95% CI, 0.62 to 14.82). All events occurred 1 – 38 days *after* cessating eltrombopag or placebo therapy. 9 out of 10 TEEs involved *symptomatic portal or splenic vein thrombosis – all occurring in the eltrombopag group*; the 1 TEE that occurred in the placebo group was MI. All affected patients in the eltrombopag group except 1, developed TEE at platelet levels of ≥ 200,000/mm^3. The post hoc analysis confirmed an association between platelet levels of ≥ 200,000/mm^3 & increased risk of portal venous thrombosis. The study concluded that till the time more data is being made available with further studies on the safety profile of eltrombopag, this drug is *NOT recommended as an alternative to platelet transfusion* in CLD patients (with thrombocytopenia) undergoing invasive procedures.

In another recent randomized, open-label, phase-II study (Kawaguchi), 12 CLD patients with platelet counts < 50,000/µL received 12.5 mg eltrombopag once daily for 2 weeks. After evaluating the safety of the drug, in the 2nd part of the study, 26 patients were randomly assigned to receive either 25 or 37.5 mg eltrombopag once daily for 2 weeks. At week 2, the mean increases in the platelet counts from the baseline were 24,800/μL (95 % CI 8,200 – 41,400), 54,000/μL (95 % CI 28,200 – 79,800), and 60,000/μL (95 % CI 29,300 – 90,700) in the 12.5, 25, & 37.5 mg groups, respectively. Most side effects were grade 1 or 2. Two patients in the 37.5 mg group developed serious side effects. It was therefore recommended that eltrombopag in a dose of 25 mg daily is effective in alleviating thrombocytopenia in CLD patients.

The safety and efficacy of *long-term use* of eltrombopag (299 CITP patients treated for *up to 3 years*) has been tested recently in the interim analysis (Mansoor *et al.*, 2012) of an ongoing, global, multi-center, open-label EXTEND study (Saleh *et al.*, 2010). The results showed that a platelet level of ≥ 50,000/μL was achieved at least once in both splenectomised and non-splenectomised patients (80% & 88% respectively for a median of 73 of 104 and 109 of 156 cumulative study weeks, respectively). ≥70% of patients who previously failed to respond or relapsed after either rituximab therapy or splenectomy achieved at least once the target platelet level of ≥ 50,000/μL. The same target was achieved for > 50% of study visits in almost 50% of patients who had been treated with ≥ 4 prior ITP treatments. Bleeding symptoms (WHO grades 1 – 4) decreased from a baseline of 56% to 20% at 2 years & 11% at 3 years reflecting the inverse relationship between platelets and bleeding severity in CITP patients (Provan *et al.*, 2010). 13% patients experienced ≥ 1 adverse events leading to study withdrawal. 6 of these patients withdrew due to hepatotoxicity. It was the conclusion of this interim analysis that long-term treatment with eltrombopag is effective in achieving & maintaining target platelet levels; also, this drug is well-tolerated and generally safe.

6.5   Starting criteria of eltrombopag therapy

1. Thrombocytopenia is the underlying reason in almost 6% cases of PEG-IFN dose reductions or withdrawals (Fried *et al.*, 2002). In an HCV-positive patient on antiviral therapy, consider initiating eltrombopag therapy if platelet count falls to < 50,000/μl AND Child-Pugh score is < 5 AND detailed history & examination suggests a realistic risk of bleeding. If Child-Pugh score is ≥ 5, it is better to avoid eltrombopag or used only when benefits clearly outweigh the risks with active monitoring (in the recent phase-II Japanese study (Kawaguchi), Child–Pugh score of 9 or less i.e. Child–Pugh classes A & B were part of the inclusion criteria).

2. *Pre-treatment* platelet count of < 90,000/mm^3 is a *relative* contraindication to start PEG-IFN therapy (Calvaruso *et al.*, 2012). If a pragmatic bleeding risk assessment suggests that a given patient is particularly at risk of developing bleeding in view of his/ her degree of thrombocytopenia & other comorbidities, eltrombopag therapy may be started to prime the platelet levels to help initiate PEG-IFN therapy (McHutchison *et al.*, 2007). More studies are needed to validate this indication.

3. CLD patients with thrombocytopenia who need to undergo an invasive procedure may be potential candidates for short 2 weeks courses of eltrombopag in the peri-procedural period. At least one phase 3, randomized-controlled trial (ELEVATE study) however concluded that because of the safety concerns (drug-induced thrombosis etc) eltrombopag should *NOT* be used as an *alternative to platelet transfusions* in CLD patients (with thrombocytopenia) undergoing invasive procedures.

6.6   Stopping Criteria of Eltrombopag Therapy

Each of the following should be considered an *independent* criterion to stop eltrombopag therapy:

1. If after a month of maximum-dose eltrombopag therapy (75 mg/day), the platelet count fails to rise to the target level of $\geq$ 50,000/μl.

2. The manufacturer recommends that eltrombopag therapy should be stopped if platelet count rises to > 250,000/μl. Nonetheless, platelet count should be monitored twice weekly (usual once weekly) and reinitiating eltrombopag therapy in a low dose of 25 mg once daily be considered if platelet count subsequently falls to $\leq$ 100,000/μl.

3. If serial peripheral blood films show signs of possible bone marrow fibrosis (e.g. teardrop cells, nucleated RBC's or immature WBC's). Eltrombopag is suggested to cause bone marrow fibrosis.

4. If significant hepatotoxicity develops with eltrombopag, which means a rise in ALT levels three times the upper normal limit AND one of the following:
    a) Progressively worsening transaminitis.
    b) Transaminitis that persists for $\geq$ 1 month.
    c) Transaminitis associated with hyperbilirubinemia.
    d) Development of liver-related clinical symptomatology (jaundice; signs of hepatic decompensation etc).

6.7   Dose of Eltrombopag

Although the exact indications and dosage of eltrombopag in HCV-related thrombocytopenia are not yet unanimously defined, a suggested protocol is given below:

*   The usual starting dose of eltrombopag in Caucasian population is 50 mg once daily. In patients of East Asian ancestry, a lower dose of 25 mg once daily appears to be equally effective (Kawaguchi) although eltrombopag shows linear pharmacokinetics, a recent randomized, open-label, phase-II study showed that rises in platelet counts apparently *saturate* at doses of 25 mg of eltrombopag in Japanese patients. Any higher doses (37.5 mg once daily in the given study) were associated with higher risk of potentially serious side effects (particularly portal vein thrombosis, ascites & pleural effusions).

*   In patients with Child–Pugh class B also, it is suggested to start eltrombopag at a lower dose of 12.5 – 25 mg once daily (the more the liver is diseased, the less is the hepatic eltrombopag metabolism & higher the plasma bioavailability).

*   It usually takes 1 – 2 weeks for measurable improvements in platelets counts to take place. Therefore, as a rule, wait for two weeks before increasing eltrombopag dose (and thereafter every time a dose adjustment is made).

*   If a platelet count of < 50,000/μl persists after two weeks of eltrombopag therapy, consider increasing the dose by 25 mg/day every two weeks to a maximum dose of 75 mg/day.

*   Aim to achieve and maintain a platelet count of $\geq$ 50,000/μl.

*   If after a month of high dose eltrombopag therapy at 75 mg/day, the platelet count fails to rise to the target level of $\geq$ 50,000/μl, probably it is best to stop this therapy.

*   If platelet count rises to > 150,000/μl, consider reducing the eltrombopag dose by 25 mg and wait for two weeks to see the effect of this or any subsequent dose reductions. Remember that a

platelet count of $\geq$ 50,000/µl should be maintained with the *minimum effective dose* of eltrombopag.

An alternative dosage regimen is '*intermittent*' eltrombopag therapy for 6 weeks followed by a 4 weeks drug holiday × 3 cycles. The starting dose remains 50 mg once daily with dose adjustments made to achieve & maintain a platelet count of $\geq$ 50,000/µl. One open label, repeat (TRA108057, REPEAT) dose study showed that this intermittent dosing schedule *does not* lead to loss of response to eltrmbopag therapy. More head-on studies are needed to compare the relative therapeutic efficacies, safety profiles and cost-effectiveness of the 'continuous' vs. 'intermittent' dosing schedules.

6.8 Monitoring Eltrombopag therapy

Full blood count (FBC), peripheral blood film and liver function tests (LFT's) should be requested at least once weekly till the target platelet count of $\geq$ 50,000/µl is maintained for at least one month continuously. Thereafter, the monitoring frequency can be reduced to once every two weeks and later once a month.

The rationale for doing FBC is obvious – to monitor platelet levels. Concomitantly requesting peripheral blood film is equally important because eltrombopag is suggested to cause bone marrow fibrosis in some cases. After having established the pre-eltrombopag treatment cellular morphology by a peripheral blood film, the subsequent films are done to monitor & compare the development of any new or worsening morphological abnormalities (e.g. teardrop cells, nucleated RBC's or immature WBC's). Any suggestion of bone marrow fibrosis and eltrombopag therapy should be stopped forthwith followed by a formal bone marrow biopsy. Besides the development of cellular morphological abnormalities, failure of platelet counts to '*maintain*' after an initial positive response despite increasing the eltrombopag dose to the maximum level is another clue to the possible development of bone marrow fibrosis.

Eltrombopag is potentially hepatotoxic (usually mild and reversible transaminitis can develop) and is known to predispose to portal vein thrombosis even at normal/ subnormal platelet counts. In patients with Child-Pugh score < 5, eltrombopag therapy can be initiated and dose adjustments made just like any other patient with no hepatic impairment. If Child-Pugh score is $\geq$ 5, eltrombopag should better be avoided. If benefits appear to clearly outweigh the risks, it may be started at a low dose of 25 mg once daily and dose adjustments made no earlier than after 3 weeks of active monitoring (normally dose adjustments are made on 2 weekly bases). Maximum-dose eltrombopag therapy (75 mg/day) has been found to particularly increase the risk of thromboembolism (portal vein thrombosis and even MI) *despite subnormal platelet counts* of $\leq$ 50,000/µl. Based on this, it is recommended that especially in patients with Caucasian ancestry, a dose of > 50 mg once daily should better be avoided/ used very cautiously in patients with Child-Pugh score of $\geq$ 5; probably, the same holds true for people with other ethnic backgrounds like Pakistanis & Indians.

Eltrombopag is highly bound to plasma proteins predominantly to albumin and thus lacks any significant renal excretion (main route of excretion is via faeces). Based on this it is recommended that *no* dose adjustments need to be made in patients with renal impairment. Nonetheless, patients who already have renal impairment, need to be actively monitored for any further derangement (eltrombopag is known to have caused renal tubular toxicity in animal studies).

In patient's $\leq$ 18 years of age, eltrombopag therapy is not recommended because of the lack of clinical data.

Older patient's ≥ 65 years of age should probably be treated similar to the younger subjects with no dose adjustments needed although more studies are needed in this age group to validate this recommendation.

6.9   Drug-drug Interactions

Antacids (containing aluminum & magnesium), high-calcium food (e.g. dairy products) & multi-vitamin tablets/ mineral supplements chelate and thus significantly reduce the systemic absorption of eltrombopag (Williams *et al.*, 2009). It is therefore recommended that eltrombopag should be administered at least four hours before or after these products. In the unusual scenario of eltrombopag overdosage (→ ↑ LFT's & ↑↑ platelet levels), oral administration of antacids and dairy products should be expected to limit eltrombopag absorption and cause increased faecal excretion. Since eltrombopag is not renally excreted, hemodialysis is unlikely to be effective in overdose cases.

Eltrombopag increases the therapeutic levels of statins particularly rosuvastatin. If needed it's best to switch to low-dose *atorvastatin or fluvastatin* and actively monitor the patients for the development of any statin-related side effects (e.g. myositis). Caution should also be exercised when coadministering eltrombopag & methotrexate. Lopinavir/ritonavir (LPV/RTV) coadministration with eltrmbopag seems to decrease oral absorption & thus bioavailability of the latter. If coadministration is necessary, platelet counts should be closely monitored to adjust the eltrombopag dose accordingly.

6.10   Safety Profile of Eltrombopag

Higher eltrombopag doses are associated with *higher* therapeutic efficacy & *higher* risk of side effects, & vice versa. Although almost 80% of the subjects on eltrombopag therapy develop one or the other side effects, the most commonly reported side effects in the published literature (headache [13% - the commonest side effect], cataract, dry eyes, dry mouth, pharyngitis, abdominal pain, nausea, vomiting, diarrhoea, constipation, insomnia, paresthesias, arthralgias, myalgias, peripheral edema) were of insufficient severity to require discontinuation of the drug.[103] Potentially serious side effects of eltrombopag therapy that may require discontinuation of the drug include:

1. Thromboembolism (portal vein thrombosis, MI, CVA; DVT; PE).

2. Rebound thrombocytopenia after discontinuation of eltrombopag therapy with secondary increased risk of bleeding.

3. Hepatotoxicity.

4. Bone marrow fibrosis.

Eltrombopag has been found to cause thromboembolism especially portal vein thrombosis *at normal or even subnormal platelet levels*. Therefore, eltrombopag should only be used when benefits clearly outweigh the risks in the following 'high-risk' patient groups:

• Patients who already have evidence of hepatic impairment (Child-Pugh score ≥ 5).

• Patients who have known risk factors for thromboembolism e.g. deficiencies of Factor V Leiden, AT-III, protein C, protein S or antiphospholipid syndrome etc. Likewise patients with poor mobility (due to advanced senility, post-surgery/ trauma, morbid obesity etc), cancer patients and patients on OCP's or HRT are also high-risk for thromboembolism.

In high-risk patients eltrombopag should be used in a dose that is *just sufficient* to achieve and maintain the target platelet count of $\geq 50,000/\mu l$. Ideally platelet count should not be allowed to rise above $100,000/\mu l$ in high-risk patients.

The reason why eltrombopag predisposes to thromboembolism despite normal or subnormal platelet counts is not yet clear. Eltrombopag therapy itself probably does not produce any ill-toward effect on platelet function as measured by platelet activation & aggregation, although more studies are needed to validate this observation (Erhardt *et al.*, 2004; Provan *et al.*, 2006). It has been postulated that both in HCV-related thrombocytopenia and CITP cases (regardless of whether treated with eltrombopag or not), the platelets become more *'sticky'* and thus may aggregate and form a thrombus despite low counts (Haselboeck *et al*, 2012; Severinsen *et al.*, 2011). A *rapid* increase in the platelet counts when eltrombopag is used in high doses of 75mg especially in patients with liver impairment probably also predisposes to thromboembolic events (TEEs). Additionally, an increased incidence of *endothelial damage* seen in liver disease may also be a contributory factor. These postulations may explain why *many patients with severe thrombocytopenia never develop any significant bleedin*g (Cuker & Cines, 2010). There are conflicting reports in the literature regarding whether or not eltrombopag further increases this 'physiological stickiness' of platelets. Whereas, several case reports incriminated eltrombopag to have cause increased 'reactivity' of platelets with consequent increased propensity to aggregation and thrombus formation (Cuker, 2010), small recent in-vitro and in-vivo studies have refuted any such link (Erhardt *et al.*, 2009; Psaila *et al.*, 2012). The first in vivo report on TPO-RAs on platelet reactivity *only studied 20 patients* (Lambert, 2012). Therefore, more studies on larger cohorts of patients are needed to clarify this controversy that may have important implications in the future acceptibility & use of this drug.

In great majority of the patients the platelet counts fall to the pre-treatment levels within 2 weeks of stopping eltrombopag therapy thus predisposing them to bleeding. To avoid this risk, adjunct eltrombopag therapy may need to be continued for several weeks in HCV-positive cases undergoing antiviral therapy (although the exact duration of eltrombopag therapy will vary from case-to-case; also data on continued use of eltrombopag for > 6 months is very limited) (Bussel *et al.*, 2010; Kuter *et al.*, 2010; Saleh *et al.*, 2009, 2010). Also, platelet counts should be monitored on weekly basis for at least 1 month following discontinuation of eltrombopag therapy. A recent study suggested that the observation of platelet counts returning to the baseline within 2 weeks post-treatment is based primarily on studies done in *CITP patients* (Afdhal, 2010; Cheng *et al.*, 2011). In *CLD patients* with thrombocytopenia, platelet counts have been shown to *continue to increase* 1 week post-treatment and thereafter fall rather *gradually* (Kawaguchi). The exact underlying reason accounting for this important difference is not yet clear; nonetheless, it is argued that since eltrombopag is primarily metabolized in the liver, in CLD patients the plasma eltrombopag concentrations during treatment & for a few days post-treatment are generally *higher* than CITP patients (Gibiansky *et al.*, 2011 Farrell *et al.*, 2010). More studies are needed to demonstrate the likely *reduced* risk of bleeding in the immediate post-treatment period in CLD patients compared to CITP patients.

Eltrombopag has been incriminated to have caused bone marrow fibrosis in different studies. Although the exact mechanism is not yet established, it is thought to be the release of TGF-β from eltrombopag-activated megakaryocytes, which in turn causes a reversible increase in reticulin deposition (Ulich *et al.*, 1996; Yanagida *et al.*, 1997). This finding is backed by similar observations made in animal studies in which use of 2nd-generation TPO-RA was shown to cause extensive bone marrow fibrosis with secondary extramedullary hematopoiesis (a picture comparable to human myelofibrosis) (Douglas *et al.*, 2002; Villeval *et al.*, 1997; Yan, 1995). Because of relative paucity of data in human subjects, more long-term exposure studies are needed to explore this potentially dangerous complication in humans (Arnold *et al.*, 2009) (a 2-year, longitudinal bone marrow study (NCT01098487), which includes baseline and repeated bone marrow examinations is currently ongoing) (Mansoor *et al.*, 2012). As mentioned before, if serial peripheral blood films suggest new or worsening cellular morphology indicating possible development of bone marrow fibrosis, it is one of the stopping criteria of eltrombopag therapy. Clinically, if platelet levels fail to improve or maintain despite optimal eltrombopag therapy in the recommended dosing range, we should suspect possible bone marrow fibrosis/ impairment.

An association between autoimmune diseases and risk of development of hematologic malignancies is well established in medical literature (Stern *et al.*, 2007). Autoimmune thrombocytopenia is known to be the first manifestation of a hematologic malignancy in many patients and actually may precede its onset by several years. Stimulation of hematopoietic stem cells by eltrombopag may thus increase the risk of development of hematologic malignancy, theretically speaking. Both pre-clinical studies (Erickson-Miller *et al.*, 2007; Will *et al.*, 2009) and EXTEND study (Mansoor *et al.*, 2012) showed that eltrombopag does not promote proliferation of *malignant cells* and thus *does not* increase the risk of hematologic malignancy.

Despite of some conflicting reviews in the literature, it is the opinion of this author that pregnancy be regarded as an *'absolute'* contraindication for interferon, ribavirin and eltrombopag therapies. Any HCV-infected woman of child-bearing age who wants to be treated for HCV infection must observe strict contraceptive measures for the entire duration of the therapy plus at least 6 months thereafter. This is because all three of these agents have repeatedly been shown to have teratogenic &/or embryocidal effects in animal studies and the potential risks in humans are unknown at this stage. Likewise, lactating mothers should not be offered any of these three agents because whereas the risk in human subjects is unknown, we know from animal studies that all three of these agents are likely secreted in the milk.

Eltrombopag doesn't appear to prolong QT interval in healthy subjects in doses between 50 – 150 mg in comparison to the placebo.

7   Cost-effectiveness of Eltrombopag Therapy

In UK one 50 mg tablet of eltrombopag costs £55, which makes one month course at 50 mg once daily dose cost £1650 (although due to negotiated procurement discounts the precise cost *on ground* may vary). Not much data is available on the cost-effectiveness of this novel agent in the treatment of *'HCV-related'* thrombocytopenia; nonetheless, a recent National Institute of Health & Clinical Excellence (NICE), UK technology appraisal on the use of eltrombopag in *'CITP'* patients concluded that eltrombopag is *not* a cost-effective use of NHS resources (Bowers *et al.*, 2009). Based on manufacturer's deterministic sensitivity analyses for the acquisition cost of eltrombopag (£50-£60 per 50 mg), it was reported that the incremental cost-effectiveness ratios (ICERs) ranged from £77,496 per QALY gained for splenectomised people to £90,471 per QALY gained for non-splenectomised people. The highest ICER reported was £99,441 per QALY gained for the non-splenectomised population (based on the acquisition cost of £60 per 50 mg tablet). The lowest ICER reported was £69,301 per QALY gained for the splenectomised population (based on the acquisition cost of £50 per 50 mg tablet). In a subsequent publication, Boyers et al reported that substantial reductions in the cost of eltrombopag are needed before the incremental cost per QALY drops to the recommended threshold of £30,000 per QALY gained (Boyers *et al.*, 2012).

8   Future considerations

1. Good quality RCTs need to be done regarding the role of eltrombopag in the treatment of '*HCV-related*' thrombocytopenia specifically.

2. More studies on larger cohorts of patients are needed to clarify whether or not eltrombopag causes increased *in-vivo* platelet reactivity (stickiness) and thus predisposes to thromboembolism.

3. Studies directly comparing eltrombopag with romiplostim (another TPO-RA) are needed to determine their relative therapeutic efficacies, safety profiles and cost-effectiveness. *Indirect* comparison of the data from RAISE trial suggested that eltrombopag is probably less efficacious than romiplostim (the latter has recently been approved by NICE, UK for use in CITP).

4. More head-on studies are needed to compare the relative therapeutic efficacies, safety profiles and cost-effectiveness of the 'continuous' vs. 'intermittent' dosing schedules of eltrombopag.

5. More long-term exposure studies & pharmacovigilance activities are needed to specifically explore the safety concerns of 2nd-generation thrombopoietic growth factors (eltrombopag; romiplostim) on bone marrow function in human subjects, hepatotoxicity, TEEs, recurrence of thrombocytopenia following cessating eltrombopag therapy, potential for increase in hematologic malignancies, cataracts/phototoxicity, renal tubular toxicity, & endosteal hyperostosis.

9   Conclusion

Although more studies are needed to validate true indications, dosage schedule, therapeutic efficacy and safety profile of eltrombopag adjunct therapy in HCV-related thrombocytopenia, from our knowledge of the use of this novel agent in CITP, it appears that it is an efficacious treatment modality for short-term amelioration of thrombocytopenia (Ikeda *et al.*, 2009). There are some relatively serious safety concerns related to the use of this drug in CLD patients, particularly treatment-related thrombosis. It doesn't appear to be a safe alternative to repeated platelet transfusions in CLD patients undergoing an invasive procedure. Nonetheless, if a last resort decision to use eltrombopag in the peri-procedural period is being made, this drug should normally be used for short-term periods of ~ 2 weeks and in the lowest possible effective doses (usually 12.5-50 mg once daily in CLD patients). At least at the time of writing this article, eltrombopag doesn't seem cost-effective (Tillmann *et al.*, 2009).

References

Adinolfi LE, Giordano MG, Andreana A, Tripodi MF, Utili R, Cesaro G et al. Hepatic fibrosis plays a central role in the pathogenesis of thrombocytopenia in patients with chronic viral hepatitis. Br J Haematol. 2001;113:590–595.

Afdhal N, Giannini E, Tayyab GN, Mohsin A, Lee JW, Andriulli A, et al. Eltrombopag in chronic liver disease patients with thrombocytopenia undergoing an elective procedure: results from ELEVATE, a randomized clinical trial. J Hepatol. 2010;52:S460 (Abstr 1185).

Afdhal N, McHutchison J, Brown R, Jacobson I, Manns M, Poordad F, et al. Thrombocytopenia associated with chronic liver disease. J Hepatol. 2008;48:1000–7.

Afdhal N., John McHutchison, Robert Brown, Ira Jacobson, Michael Manns, Fred Poordad, Babette Weksler, Rafael Esteban. Thrombocytopenia associated with chronic liver disease. Journal of Hepatology - June 2008 (Vol. 48, Issue 6, Pages 1000-1007, DOI: 10.1016/j.jhep.2008.03.009).

Afdhal, N, Giannini, E.G., Tayyab, G., et al. Eltrombopag before Procedures in patients with Cirrhosis and Thrombocytopenia. N Engl J Med 2012;367:716-24.DOI: 10.1056/NEJMoa1110709

Amitrano L, Guardascione MA, Ames PR. Coagulation abnormalities in cirrhotic patients with portal vein thrombosis. Clin Lab 2007;53:583-9.

Arnold DM, Nazi I, Kelton JG. New treatments for idiopathic thrombocytopenic purpura: rethinking old hypotheses. Expert Opin Investig Drugs. 2009;18(6):805-19.

Ballard HS. Hematological complications of alcoholism. Alcohol Clin Exp Res 1989;13:706-720.

Bartley TD, Bogenberger J, Hunt P, Li YS, Lu HS, Martin F, et al. Identification and cloning of a megakaryocyte growth and development factor that is a ligand for the cytokine receptor mpl. Cell 1994; 77:1117–1124.

Bashour FN, Teran JC, Mullen KD. Prevalence of peripheral blood cytopenias (hypersplenism) in patients with non-alcoholic chronic liver disease. Am J Gastroenterol 2000;95:2936-9.

Basser RL, O'Flaherty E, Green M, Edmonds M, Nichol J, Menchaca DM, et al. Development of pancytopenia with neutralizing antibodies to thrombopoietin after multicycle chemotherapy supported by megakaryocyte growth and development factor. Blood. 2002;99:2599–2602.

Bauman JW, Vincent CT, Peng B, Wire MB, Williams DD, Park JW. Effect of hepatic or renal impairment on eltrombopag pharmacokinetics. J Clin Pharmacol. 2011;51:739–50.

Bordin G, Ballaré M, Zigrossi P, Bertoncelli MC, Paccagnino L, Baroli A, et al. A laboratory and thrombokinetic study of HCV-associated thrombocytopenia: a direct role of HCV in bone marrow exhaustion? Clin Exp Rheumatol 1995;13:Suppl 13:S39-S43.

Bowers D, Jia X, Crowther M et al. Eltrombopag for the treatment of chronic idiopathic (immune) thrombocytopenic purpura (ITP): A Single Technology Appraisal (December 2009)

Boyers D, Jia X, Jenkinson D, Mowatt G. Eltrombopag for the treatment of chronic immune or idiopathic thrombocytopenic purpura: a NICE single technology appraisal. Pharmacoeconomics. 2012 Jun 1;30(6):483-95. doi: 10.2165/11591550-000000000-00000.

Bussel JB, Cheng G, Saleh MN, Psaila B, Kovaleva L, Meddeb B, et al. Eltrombopag for the treatment of chronic idiopathic thrombocytopenic purpura. N Engl J Med 2007;357:2237-2247.

Bussel JB, Kuter DJ, Pullarkat V, Lyons RM, Guo M, Nichol JL. Safety and efficacy of long-term treatment with romiplostim in thrombocytopenic patients with chronic ITP. Blood. 2009;113(10):2161-2171.

Bussel JB, Zhang J, Tang S, McIntosh J, Kuter DJ. Efficacy, safety and tolerability of E5501 (AKR501) in a 6-month extension study in subjects with chronic immune thrombocytopenia (ITP). Blood. 2010;116:Abstract 3695.

Bussel, J.B., Provan, D., Shamsi, T. et al. Effect of eltrombopag on platelet counts and bleeding during treatment of chronic idiopathic thrombocytopenic purpura: a randomised, double-blind, placebo-controlled trial. The Lancet 2009;373(9664):641-648.

Cacoub P, Renou C, Rosenthal E, Cohen P, Loury I, Loustaud-Ratti V et al. Extrahepatic manifestations associated with hepatitis C virus infection: A prospective multicenter study of 321 patients. Medicine. 2000;79:47–56.

Calvaruso, V. & Craxì, A. (2011). European Association of the Study of the Liver hepatitis C virus clinical practice guidelines. European Association of the Study of the Liver. Liver Int. 2012 Feb;32 Suppl 1:2-8. doi: 10.1111/j.1478-3231.2011.02703.x. Review. PMID: 22212565

Cheng G, Saleh MN, Marcher C, Vasey S, Mayer B, Aivado M, et al. Eltrombopag for management of chronic immune thrombocytopenia (RAISE): a 6-month, randomised, phase 3 study. Lancet. 2011 Jan 29;377(9763):393-402.

Chiao EY, Connie Erickson-Miller, Evelyn Delorme, Leslie Giampa, Christopher Hopson, Elizabeth Valoret, Shin-Shay Tian, et al. Biological activity and selectivity for Tpo receptor of the orally bioavailable, small molecule Tpo receptor agonist, SB-497115 [abstract]. Blood 2004; 104:796a Abstract 2912.

Cuker A, Cines DB. Immune thrombocytopenia. Hematology Am Soc Hematol Educ Program 2010;2010:377-384.

Cuker A. Toxicities of the thrombopoietic growth factors. Semin Hematol 2010;47(3):289-298.

Danish FA, Koul SS, Subhani FR, Rabbani AE, Yasmin S. Role of hematopoietic growth factors as adjuncts in the treatment of chronic hepatitis C patients. Saudi J Gastroenterol 2008;14:151-7.

Danish FA, Koul SS, Subhani FR, Rabbani AE, Yasmin S. Considerations in the management of hepatitis C virus-related thrombocytopenia with eltrombopag. Saudi J Gastroenterol 2010;16:51-6

de Sauvage FJ, Hass PE, Spencer SD, Malloy BE, Gurney AL, Spencer SA, et al. Stimulation of megakaryocytopoiesis and thrombopoiesis by the c-mpl ligand. Nature 1994; 369:533–538.

De Stefano V, Martinelli I. Splanchnic vein thrombosis: clinical presentation, risk factors and treatment. Intern Emerg Med 2010;5:487-94.

Douglas VK, Tallman MS, Cripe LD, Peterson LC. Thrombopoietin administered during induction chemotherapy to patients with acute myeloid leukemia induces transient morphologic changes that may resemble chronic myeloproliferative disorders. Am J Clin Pathol. 2002;117:844–850.

Drachman JG, Millet KM, Kaushansky K. Thrombopoietin signal transduction requires functional JAK2, not Tyk2. J Biol Chem 1999; 274:13480–13484.

Engels EA, Erhardt J, Erickson-Miller CL, Tapley P. SB 497115-GR, a low molecular weight TPOR agonist, does not induce platelet activation or enhance agonist-induced platelet aggregation in vitro. Blood 2004;104:3888-3888.

Erhardt JA, Erickson-Miller CL, Aivado M, Abboud M, Pillarisetti K, Toomey JR. Comparative analyses of the small molecule thrombopoietin receptor agonist eltrombopag and thrombopoietin on in vitro platelet function. Exp Hematol 2009;37(9):1030-1037.

Erickson-Miller , C.L., Delorme, E., Tian, S.-S. et al. Preclinical Activity of Eltrombopag (SB-497115), an Oral, Nonpeptide Thrombopoietin Receptor Agonist. Stem Cells 2009; 27(2):424 -430.

Erickson-Miller CL, DeLorme E, Tian SS, Hopson CB, Stark K, Giampa L, et al. Discovery and characterization of a selective, nonpeptidyl thrombopoietin receptor agonist. Exp Hematol. 2005;33:85–93.

Erickson-Miller CL, Payne PL, Moore S, Wert S, May RD. Eltrombopag decreases proliferation of human leukemia and lymphoma cell lines in vitro. Blood. 2007;110:Abstract 4089.

Erickson-Miller, C.L., Luengo, J.I., Nicholl, R. et al. In vitro and in vivo biology of a small molecular weight TPO receptor agonist, SB-497115. Poster presented at the 96th American Association for Cancer Research Annual Meeting, Anaheim, CA, April 16–20, 2005.

Ezumi Y, Takayama H, Okuma M. Thrombopoietin, c-mpl ligand, induces tyrosine phosphorylation of Tyk2, JAK2, and STAT3, and enhances agonist-induced aggregation in platelets in vitro. FEBS Letters 1995; 374:48–52.

Farrell C, Hayes S, Giannini EG, Afdhal NH, Tayyab GN, Mohsin A, et al. Gender, race, and severity of liver disease influence eltrombopag exposure in thrombocytopenic patients with chronic liver disease. Hepatology. 2010;52:920A.

Fazal A. Danish. Current Standards in the Pharmacotherapy of Chronic Hepatitis C and Local Practices. Infectious Diseases Journal 2008;17(3):93-7.

Fogarty PF, Tarantino MD, Brainsky A, Signorovitch J, Grotzinger KM. Selective validation of the WHO Bleeding Scale in patients with chronic immune thrombocytopenia. Curr Med Res Opin. 2012 Jan;28(1):79-87. Epub 2011 Dec 20.

Fried MW, Shiffman ML, Reddy KR, Smith C, Marinos G, Goncales FL Jr, et al. Peginterferon alfa-2a plus ribavirin for chronic hepatitis C virus infection. New England Journal of Medicine 2002; 347: 975–982.

Garcia-Suarez J, Burgaleta C, Hernanz N, Albarran F, Tobaruela P, Alvarez-Mon M. HCV-associated thrombocytopenia: clinical characteristics and platelet response after recombinant alpha2b-interferon therapy. Br J Haematol. 2000;110:98–103.

George JN, Woolf SH, Raskob GE, et al. Idiopathic thrombocytopenic purpura: a practice guideline developed by explicit methods for the American Society of Hematology. Blood. 1996;88(1):3-40.

George JN. For low platelets, how low is dangerous? Cleve Clin J Med. 2004;71(4):277-278.

Giannini E, Borro P, Botta F, et al. Serum thrombopoietin levels are linked to liver function in untreated patients with hepatitis C virus-related chronic hepatitis. J Hepatol. 2002; 572–577.

Giannini EG, Greco A, Marenco S, Andorno E, Valente U, Savarino V. Incidence of bleeding following invasive procedures in patients with thrombocytopenia and advanced liver disease. Clin Gastroenterol Hepatol 2010;8:899-902.

Giannini EG, Savarino V. Thrombocytopenia in liver disease. Curr Opin Hematol 2008;15(5):473-80.

Giannini EG. Review article: thrombocytopenia in chronic liver disease and pharmacologic treatment options. Aliment Pharmacol Ther. 2006;23:1055–1065.

Gibiansky E, Zhang J, Williams D, Wang Z, Ouellet D. Population pharmacokinetics of eltrombopag in healthy subjects and patients with chronic idiopathic thrombocytopenic purpura. J Clin Pharmacol. 2011;51:842–56.

Giordano TP, et al. Risk of immune thrombocytopenic purpura and autoimmune hemolytic anemia among 120 908 US veterans with hepatitis C virus infection. Archives of Internal Medicine [2009, 169(4):357-63].

Goulis J, Chau TN, Jordan S, et al. Thrombopoietin concentrations are low in patients with cirrhosis and thrombocytopenia and are restored after orthotopic liver transplantation. Gut. 1999; 754–758.

Hamaia S, Li C, Allain JP. The dynamics of hepatitis C virus binding to platelets and 2 mononuclear cell lines. Blood. 2001; 2293–2300.

Harker LA, Roskos LK, Marzec UM, Carter RA, Cherry JK, Sundell B, et al. Effects of megakaryocyte growth and development factor on platelet production, platelet life span, and platelet function in healthy human volunteers. Blood 2000; 95:2514–2522.

Haselboeck J, PabingerI, AyC, KoderS, PanzerS. Platelet activation and function during eltrombopag treatment in immune thrombocytopenia. Ann Hematol 2012;91(1):109-113.

Henderson L, Hernandez F, Blanquer A, Linares M, Lopez A, Tarin F, Cervero A. Autoimmune thrombocytopenia associated with hepatitis C virus infection. Acta Haematol. 1998;99:217–220.

Iga D, Tomimatsu M, Endo H, Ohkawa S, Yamada O. Improvement of thrombocytopenia with disappearance of HCV RNA in patients treated by interferon-alpha therapy: possible aetiology of HCV-associated immune thrombocytopenia. Eur J Haematol. 2005;75:417–423.

Ikeda Y, Miyakawa Y. Development of thrombopoietin receptor agonists for clinical use. J Thromb Haemost. 2009;7(Suppl 1):239-44.

Jabbour N, Zajko A, Orons P, Irish W, Fung JJ, Selby RR. Does transjugular intrahepatic portosystemic shunt (TIPS) resolve thrombocytopenia associated with cirrhosis? Dig Dis Sci. 1998;2459–2462.

Jenkins JM, Williams D, Deng Y, Uhl J, Kitchen V, Collins D, et al. Phase I clinical study of eltrombopag, an oral, nonpeptide thrombopoietin receptor agonist. Blood 2007;109:4739-4741.

Juan I. Luengo, Kevin J. Duffy, Anthony N. Shaw, Evelyne Delorme, Kenneth J. Wiggall, Leslie Giampa et al. Discovery of SB-497115, a small-molecule thrombopoietin (TPO) receptor agonist for the treatment of thrombocytopenia. Blood 2004;104:2910-2910.

Julian M. Jenkins, Daphne Williams, Yanli Deng, Joanne Uhl, Valerie Kitchen, David Collins et al. Phase 1 clinical study of eltrombopag, an oral, nonpeptide thrombopoietin receptor agonist. Blood 2007;109(11):4739-4741.

Kalota A, Brennan K, Erickson-Miller C, Danet G, Carroll M, Gewirtz A. Effects of SB559457, a novel small molecule thrombopoietin receptor agonist, on haematopoietic cell growth and differentiation. Blood. 2004;104 abstract 2913.

Kaushansky K, Drachman JG. The molecular and cellular biology of thrombopoietin: the primary regulator of platelet production. Oncogene 2002; 21:3359–3367.

Kaushansky K, Lok S, Holly RD, Broudy VC, Lin N, Bailey MC, et al. Cloning and expression of murine thrombopoietin cDNA and stimulation of platelet production. Nature 1994; 369(6481):565-68.

Kaushansky K, Lok S, Holly RD, Broudy VC, Lin N, Bailey MC, et al. Promotion of megakaryocyte progenitor expansion and differentiation by the c-mpl ligand thrombopoietin. Nature 1994; 369:568–571.

Kawaguchi, T., Komori, A., Seike, M., Fujiyama, S. et al. Efficacy and safety of eltrombopag in Japanese patients with chronic liver disease and thrombocytopenia: a randomized, open-label, phase II study. J Gastroenterol DOI 10.1007/s00535-012-0600-5

Kramer JR, Kulik LM, Carr BI, Mulcahy MF, et al. Safety and efficacy of 90Y radiotherapy for hepatocellular carcinoma with and without portal vein thrombosis. Hepatology 2008;47:71-81.

Kuter DJ, Begley CG. Recombinant human thrombopoietin: basic biology and evaluation of clinical studies. Blood 2002; 100:3457–3469.

Kuter DJ, Bussel JB, Newland A, et al. Long-term efficacy and safety of romiplostim treatment of adult patients with chronic immune thrombocytopenia (ITP): final report from an open-label extension study. Blood. 2010;116:Abstract 68.

Lambert MP. Platelets and eltrombopag: a not-so-sticky situation. Blood [2012, 119(17):3876-7].

Lavanchy D. Evolving epidemiology of hepatitis C virus. Clin Microbiol Infect 2011; 17:107–115.

Li J, Yang C, Xia Y, Bertino A, Glaspy J, Roberts M, et al. Thrombocytopenia caused by the development of antibodies to thrombopoietin. Blood. 2001;98:3241–3248.

Lisman T, Caldwell SH, Burroughs AK, et al. Hemostasis and thrombosis in patients with liver disease: the ups and downs. J Hepatol 2010;53:362-71.

Mansoor N. Saleh, James B. Bussel, Gregory Cheng, Oliver Meyer, Christine K. Bailey, Michael Arning, et al. Safety and efficacy of eltrombopag for treatment of chronic immune thrombocytopenia (ITP): results of the long-term, open-label EXTEND study. Prepublished online November 20, 2012; doi:10.1182/blood-2012-04-425512.

McCormick PA, Murphy KM. Splenomegaly, hypersplenism and coagulation abnormalities in liver disease. Baillieres Best Pract Res Clin Gastroenterol 2000;14:1009-1031.

McCullough J. Current issues with platelet transfusion in patients with cancer. Semin Hematol. 2000;37(2 Suppl. 4):3–10.

McHutchison JG, Dusheiko G, Shiffman ML, Rodriguez-Torres M, Sigal S, Bourliere M, et al. Eltrombopag for Thrombocytopenia in Patients with Cirrhosis Associated with Hepatitis C. N Engl J Med 2007;357:2227-36.

Mizutani T. PM frequencies of major CYPs in Asians and Caucasians. Drug Metab Rev. 2003;35:99–106.

Nagamine T, Ohtuka T, Takehara K, Arai T, Takagi H, Mori M. Thrombocytopenia associated with hepatitis C viral infection. J Hepatol. 1996;24:135–140.

Nurden AT, Viallard JF, Nurden P. New-generation drugs that stimulate platelet production in chronic immune thrombocytopenic purpura. Lancet. 2009 May 2;373(9674):1562-9. Epub 2009 Mar 25.

Panzer S. Eltrombopag in chronic idiopathic thrombocytopenic purpura and HCV-related thrombocytopenia. Drugs Today 2009;45(2):93-9.

Peck-Radosavljevic M, Wichlas M, Pidlich J, Sims P, Meng G, Zacherl J et al. Blunted thrombopoietin response to interferon alfa-induced thrombocytopenia during treatment for hepatitis C. Hepatology 1998; 28:1424–9.

Peck-Radosavljevic M, Wichlas M, Zacherl J, et al. Thrombopoietin induces rapid resolution of thrombocytopenia after orthotopic liver transplantation through increased platelet production. Blood. 2000; 795–801.

Peck-Radosavljevic M. Thrombocytopenia in liver disease. Can J Gastroenterol 2000;14:Suppl D:60D-66D.

Perrotta PL, Snyder EL. Non-infectious complications of transfusion therapy. Blood Rev. 2001;15:69–83.

Pietz K, Pockros PJ, Duchini A, McMillan R, Nyberg LM, McHutchison J, Viernes E. Immune thrombocytopenic purpura in patients with chronic hepatitis C virus infection. Am J Gastroenterol. 2002;97:2040–2045.

Poordad F. Thrombocytopenia in chronic liver disease. Aliment Pharmacol Ther 2007;26:Suppl 1:5-11.

Provan D, Stasi R, Newland AC, et al. International consensus report on the investigation and management of primary immune thrombocytopenia. Blood. 2010;115(2):168-186.

Provan, D., Saleh, M., Goodison, S., Rafi, R. et al. The safety profile of eltrombopag, a novel, oral platelet growth factor, in thrombocytopenic patients and healthy subjects. J Clin Oncol 2006;24:Suppl:18S-18S.

Psaila, B., Bussel J.B., Linden, M.D. et al. In vivo effects of eltrombopag on platelet function in immune thrombocytopenia: no evidence of platelet activation Blood 2012 119:4066-4072; published ahead of print January 31, 2012, doi:10.1182/blood-2011-11-393900

Pyrsopoulos NT, Reddy KR. Extrahepatic manifestations of chronic viral hepatitis. Curr Gastroenterol Rep. 2001;3:71–78.

Qamar AA, Grace ND, Groszmann RJ, et al. Incidence, prevalence, and clinical significance of abnormal hematologic indices in compensated cirrhosis. Clin Gastroenterol Hepatol 2009;7:689-95.

Rajan S, Liebman HA. Treatment of hepatitis C related thrombocytopenia with interferon alpha. Am J Hematol. 2001;68:202–209.

Rajan S, Espina BM, Liebman HA. Hepatitis C virus-related thrombocytopenia: clinical and laboratory characteristics compared with chronic immune thrombocytopenic purpura. Br J Haematol. 2005;129:818–824.

Ramos-Casals M, García-Carrasco M, López-Medrano F, Trejo O, Forns X, López-Guillermo A, et al. Severe autoimmune cytopenias in treatment-naive hepatitis C virus infection: clinical description of 35 cases. Medicine (Baltimore). 2003;82:87–96.

Rebulla P. Trigger for platelet transfusion. Vox Sang. 2000;78:179–182.

Reid, R., Bennett, J.M., Becker, M., Chen, Y. et al. Use of eltrombopag, a thrombopoietin receptor agonist, in post-transplantation thrombocytopenia. Published online 10 April 2012 in Wiley Online Library (wileyonlinelibrary.com). DOI: 10.1002/ajh.23225

Rinder HM, Arbini AA, Snyder EL. Optimal dosing and triggers for prophylactic use of platelet transfusions. Curr Opin Hematol. 1999;6:437–441.

Rojnuckarin P, Drachman JG, Kaushansky K. Thrompoietin-induced activation of the mitogen-activated protein kinase (MAPK) pathway in normal megakaryocytes: role in endomitosis. Blood 1999; 94:1273–1282.

Sakuraya M, Murakami H, Uchiumi H, Hatsumi N, Akiba T, Yokohama A et al. Steroid-refractory chronic idiopathic thrombocytopenic purpura associated with hepatitis C virus infection. Eur J Haematol. 2002;68:49–53.

Saleh MN, Cheng G, Bussel JB, et al. EXTEND study update: safety and efficacy of eltrombopag in adults with chronic immune thrombocytopenia (ITP) from June 2006 to February 2010. Blood. 2010;116:Abstract 67.

Sallah S, Bobzien W. Bleeding problems in patients with liver disease: ways to manage the many hepatic effects on coagulation. Postgrad Med 1999;106:187-90, 193-5.

Schiffer CA, Anderson KC, Bennett CL, Bernstein S, Elting LS, Goldsmith M, et al. Platelet transfusion for patients with cancer: clinical practice guidelines of the American Society of Clinical Oncology. J Clin Oncol. 2001;19:1519–1538.

Sellers T, Hart T, Semanik M, Murthyl K. Pharmacology and safety of SB-497115-GR, an orally active small molecular weight TPO receptor agonist, in chimpanzees, rats and dogs. Blood 2004;104:2063-2063.

Severinsen MT, EngebjergMC, FarkasDK, et al. Risk of venous thromboembolism in patients with primary chronic immune thrombocytopenia: a Danish population-based cohort study. Br J Haematol 2011;152(3):360-362.

Sherman M, Shafran S, Burak K, Doucette K, Wong W, Girgrah N, et al. Management of chronic hepatitis C: consensus guidelines. Can J Gastroenterol 2007; 21(Suppl C): 25C-34C.

Shida Y, Takahashi N, Nohda S, Hirama T. Pharmacokinetics and pharmacodynamics of eltrombopag in healthy Japanese males. Jpn J Clin Pharmacol Ther. 2011;42:11–20.

Slichter SJ. Evidence-based platelet transfusion guidelines. Hematology Am Soc Hematol Educ Program 2007:172-8.

Stasi R. Therapeutic strategies for hepatitis- and other infection-related immune thrombocytopenias. Semin Hematol. 2009;46(1 Suppl 2):S15-25.

Stern M, Buser AS, Lohri A, Tichelli A, Nissen-Druey C. Autoimmunity and malignancy in hematology--more than an association. Crit Rev Oncol Hematol. 2007;63(2):100-110.

Sulkowski MS. Management of the hematologic complications of hepatitis C therapy. Clin Liver Dis. 2005;:601–616.

Tillmann HL, Patel K, McHutchison JG. Role of growth factors and thrombopoietic agents in the treatment of chronic hepatitis C. Curr Gastroenterol Rep. 2009;11(1):5-14.

Tripodi A, Mannucci PM. Abnormalities of hemostasis in chronic liver disease: reappraisal of their clinical significance and need for clinical and laboratory research. J Hepatol. 2007;46:727–733.

Tripodi A, Primignani M, Mannucci PM. Abnormalities of hemostasis and bleeding in chronic liver disease: the paradigm is challenged. Intern Emerg Med 2010;5:7-12.

Trotter JF. Coagulation abnormalities in patients who have liver disease. Clin Liver Dis 2006;10:665-78.

Ulich TR, del Castillo J, Senaldi G, Kinstler O, Yin S, Kaufman S, et al. Systemic hematologic effects of PEG-rHuMGDF-induced megakaryocyte hyperplasia in mice. Blood. 1996;87:5006–5015.

Villeval JL, Cohen-Solal K, Tulliez M, Giraudier S, Guichard J, Burstein SA, et al. High thrombopoietin production by hematopoietic cells induces a fatal myeloproliferative syndrome in mice. Blood. 1997;90:4369–4383.

Vizcaíno G, Diez-Ewald M, Vizcaíno-Carruyo J. Treatment of chronic immune thrombocytopenic purpura. Looking for something better. Invest Clin. 2009;50(1):95-108.

Weksler BB. Review article: the pathophysiology of thrombocytopenia in hepatitis C virus infection and chronic liver disease. Aliment Pharmacol Ther. 2007;26 (suppl 1):13–19.

Wendling F, Maraskovsky E, Debili N, Florindo C, Teepe M, Titeux M, et al. C-mpl ligand is a humoral regulator of megakaryocytopoiesis. Nature 1994; 369:571–574.

Will B, Kawahara M, Luciano JP, et al. Effect of the non-peptide thrombopoietin receptor agonist eltrombopag on bone marrow cells from patients with acute myeloid leukemia and myelodysplastic syndrome. Blood. 2009;114(18):3899-3908.

Williams DD, Peng B, Bailey CK, Wire MB, Deng Y, Park JW et al. Effects of food and antacids on the pharmacokinetics of eltrombopag in healthy adult subjects: two single-dose, open-label, randomized-sequence, crossover studies. Clin Ther. 2009;31(4):764-76.

Wong F. The use of TIPS in chronic liver disease. Ann Hepatol. 2006;5:5–15.

Yan XQ, Lacey D, Fletcher F, Hartley C, McElroy P, Sun Y, et al. Chronic exposure to retroviral vector encoded MGDF (mpl-ligand) induces lineage-specific growth and differentiation of megakaryocytes in mice. Blood. 1995;86:4025–4033.

Yanagida M, Ide Y, Imai A, Toriyama M, Aoki T, Harada K, et al. The role of transforming growth factor-beta in PEG-rHuMGDF-induced reversible myelofibrosis in rats. Br J Haematol. 1997;99:739–745.

Zhang A, Xing Q, Qin S, Du J, Wang L, Yu L, et al. Intra-ethnic differences in genetic variants of the UGT-glucuronosyltransferase 1A1 gene in Chinese populations. Pharmacogenomics J. 2007;7:333–8.

Zhang L, Li H, Zhao H, Ji L, Yang R. Hepatitis C virus-related adult chronic idiopathic thrombocytopenic purpura: experience from a single Chinese centre. Eur J Haematol. 2003;70:196–197.

Zhang W, Nardi MA, Li Z, Borkowsky W, Karpatkin S. Role of molecular mimicry of hepatitis C-virus (HCV) protein with platelet GPIIIa in hepatitis C-related immunologic thrombocytopenia. Blood. 2008.

www.ingramcontent.com/pod-product-compliance
Lightning Source LLC
Chambersburg PA
CBHW050801220326
41598CB00006B/85